Handbook of Anticancer Drug Development

Handbook of Anticancer Drug Development

Edited by

Daniel R. Budman, M.D.
Don Monti Division of Oncology
North Shore University Hospital
New York University
Manhasset, New York

Alan Hilary Calvert, M.D.
Cancer Research Unit
Medical School
Newcastle-upon-Tyne, England

Eric Keith Rowinsky, M.D.
Institute for Drug Development
Cancer Therapy and Research Center
San Antonio, Texas

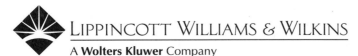

LIPPINCOTT WILLIAMS & WILKINS
A **Wolters Kluwer** Company
Philadelphia • Baltimore • New York • London
Buenos Aires • Hong Kong • Sydney • Tokyo

Editor: Jonathan Pine
Managing Editor: Stacey Baze
Marketing Manager: Julie Sikora
Production Editor: Jennifer Jett
Compositor: Maryland Composition Inc.
Printer: Edwards Brothers

351 West Camden Street
Baltimore, Maryland 21201-2436 USA

530 Walnut Street
Philadelphia, PA 19106

The publisher is not responsible (as a matter of product liability, negligence, or otherwise) for any injury resulting from any material contained herein. This publication contains information relating to general principles of medical care that should not be construed as specific instructions for individual patients. Manufacturers' product information and package inserts should be reviewed for current information; including contraindications, dosages, and precautions.

Printed in the United States of America

Library of Congress Cataloging-in-Publication Data

Handbook of anticancer drug development/edited by Daniel R. Budman,
Alan Hilary Calvert, Eric Keith Rowinsky.
     p. ; cm.
Includes bibliographical references and index.
  ISBN 0-7817-4010-X
1. Antineoplastic agents—Testing—Handbooks, manuals, etc.   2. Drug development—Handbooks, manuals, etc.
  [DNLM: 1. Antineoplastic Agents.   2. Drug Design.   3. Clinical Trials.   4. Drug Approval.   5. Drug Evaluation, Preclinical.   6. Models, Molecular.   QV 269 H2357 2004]   I. Budman, Daniel.   II. Calvert, A. Hilary.   III. Rowinsky, Eric K., 1956–

RS431.A64H357 2004
616.99′4061—dc22

                                                    2003056493

The publishers have made every effort to trace the copyright holders for borrowed material. If they have inadvertently overlooked any, they will be pleased to make the necessary arrangements at the first opportunity.

To purchase additional copies of this book, call our customer service department at **(800) 638-3030** or fac orders to **(301) 824-7390**. International customers should call **(301) 714-2324**.

Visit Lippincott Williams & Wilkins on the Internet: http://www.LWW.com. Lippincott Williams & Wilkins customer service representatives are available from 8:30 am to 6:00 pm, EST.

03 04 05 06 07
1 2 3 4 5 6 7 8 9 10

Contents

Part 8: Licensure Issues

Introduction

The field of anticancer drug development has undergone profound changes in the last two decades with the emergence of the critical roles of bioinformatics and computational power, the explosive growth of molecular biology and the success of the genome project, innovative methods of chemical synthesis and analysis, new delivery systems, new preclinical models with defined molecular targets, and the decline of empiric approaches leading to new entity discoveries with more focus on defined disease related targets. In addition, with the aging of the population in the industrialized countries and the emergence of diseases such as cancer being a major cause of morbidity and mortality, both governmental agencies and the pharmaceutical industry have delegated increased resources for drug development. As a consequence, the pharmaceutical industry in the United States has grown to 241,000 individuals, with an estimated value of pharmaceutical shipments from U.S. companies of US $121 billion (1). Similar statistics exist for the pharmaceutical industry in Europe, Japan, and part of Asia. The top ten largest pharmaceutical companies spent a total of US $27.9 billion on research in 2002 (2). The biotechnology industry, with more than 400 publicly traded companies, also continues to grow rapidly with better understanding of disease processes (3). Collectively, the biotechnology companies generated US $35.9 billion in 2001 (3).

A single laboratory or a small team of researchers can no longer successfully accomplish drug development. Rather, there is a complex interplay among the drug discovery staff, the preclinical formulation group, toxicology and metabolism, the analytic group, large scale purification or synthesis, the clinical group, and regulatory affairs (4). At each step in the drug discovery process, the lead candidate may fail despite enormous efforts. As a consequence, target validation, streamlined and focused drug development, and well-designed clinical trials become critical for the rapid introduction of new chemical entities. In the field of cancer, the successful development of new active compounds has come to be the result of a partnership among academia, government, and industry taking advantage of the expertise resident in these organizations. This partnership is reflected in the affiliations of the authors in this textbook.

Although only 400 targets for all of medicine have been identified for the currently commercially available drugs, up to 10,000 candidate targets for therapeutic intervention are postulated to exist on the basis of the recent discoveries in molecular biology. Target validation of the appropriate target thus becomes a critical role in drug development to minimize false leads. Algorithms used to identify candidate compounds whether developed *in silico* or by preclinical model systems thus become essential to filter potential leads into attractive drugs (5). As the new methodologies discussed in this textbook allow the generation of thousands of potential leads, methods to optimize each step in the drug discovery process are needed to contain resources and costs (6). The total preapproval costs of a drug reaching commercialization is estimated to be as high as US $802 million (7). Even design of drug discovery units is becoming limiting due to costs (8). Currently, most pharmaceutical companies are incorporating pharmacoeconomics early in clinical drug development in an attempt to curtail expenditures (9). No national economic system can support costs of drug development of this magnitude. Therefore, new approaches are needed to contain the cost at all stages of development.

Drug discovery remains a labor-intensive area of investigation with many leads not resulting in clinically useful drugs. Previous studies of phase I agents for cancer have indicated that approximately only 1 of 40 compounds that reaches clinical trials results in a commercially viable drug. Even with robotic screening and computer-aided design, candidate agents may fail to progress to clinical trial on the basis of inability to synthesize sufficient quantities, insolubility, poor biodistribution, toxic metabolites, or high prevalence of drug-drug interactions. In the *Handbook of Anticancer Drug Development*, the authors identify the potential pitfalls and the pathways useful in drug development.

At the present time, animal and human testing are still required to fully evaluate a new entity, and the regulatory agencies have established strict guidelines for safe and effective drug development. The steps needed for this pathway are major topics in this textbook. The emerging knowledge that different populations, such as children, the elderly, or patients with a polymorphic enzyme involved in the drug's activation or metabolism, may demonstrate differences of pharmacology or pharmacodynamics has also complicated drug development. These parameters are areas of active investigation to identify surrogate models that eventually will be able to identify lead compounds and to exclude compounds with potential adverse properties. In addition, drug development in these distinct populations requires a unique approach and is discussed by the authors. Pharmacogenomics, which remains a research tool, may be used in the near future to guide drug development and exclude application of a potentially toxic agent to selected patient populations. Quality-of-life evaluations and data auditing procedures are additional critical areas for successful new drug development.

Currently, the preclinical evaluation of a new agent for cancer may take more than 3 years and the clinical development more than 10 years (10), which is unacceptable to advance the treatment of these diseases. Hence, methodologies need to be developed to streamline drug development so that the time between initial drug discovery and advancement to New Drug Application is minimized without potentially harming patients. Clinical trials need to be focused and have adequate statistical power, yet not have the exposure of undue numbers of patients to a compound that might have unexpected side effects. Much of this book is devoted to discussions of methods to make these processes more efficient and safe, and the tasks accomplished in real time.

In the field of anticancer drug development, approximately 500 compounds are now in development with the potential of thousands of entities. To select appropriate compounds to advance requires well-integrated processes from the initial synthesis through clinical trials. The appropriate schedule of administration of a candidate substance and whether or not to combine the agent with other existing compounds lead to permutations that could overwhelm the current clinical trials structure. In the developed world, clinical trials mechanisms such as cancer centers and cooperative groups function to advance drug development as single agents, as combination therapies, and as combined modality therapies such as with radiation therapy. However, the number of patients entered into clinical trials in the United States remains low and many attractive leads cannot be pursued because of sample size or resource limitations. Trials that maximize the use of patients willing to participate in clinical trials must therefore be concise, able to ask a specific critical therapeutic question, and have the statistical power to answer the question.

Anticancer drug development parallels many of the approaches used for development of drugs for other disease categories. As such, this text is able to serve as a paradigm for rational approaches to much of drug development. Issues such as lead identification, formulation, preclinical models, initial human studies, pharmacology, quality-of-life measurements, and validation of records by the auditing process are generic issues for all areas of drug development. Obviously, because of the nature of malignancies, the use of toxic agents, and the potential unstable clinical nature of the patient with cancer, the differences in clinical development also diverge. These differences are discussed in this textbook. In some of the discussions, the authors differ in their interpretation of current approaches or conclusions. We have allowed these seemingly contradictory conclusions to be present so that the reader is aware of the limitations of current knowledge.

The authors would like to acknowledge Aventis for providing an unrestricted educational grant to support this book. Finally, the authors would like to thank the thousands of patients who participate in clinical trials for the betterment of humanity. Without their assistance, drug development would not occur.

Daniel R. Budman, M.D.
Alan Hilary Calvert, M.D.
Eric Keith Rowinsky, M.D.

REFERENCES

1. U.S. Census Bureau: Statistical Abstract of the United States. 2002.
2. Best Pipelines. *R and D Directions* 2003;9:32–58.
3. Lahteenmaki R, Fletcher L. Public biotechnology 2001–the numbers. *Nat Biotechnol* 2002;20: 551–555.
4. PeakmanT, Franks S, White C, et al. Delivering the power of discovery in large pharmaceutical organizations. *Drug Discov Today* 2003;5:203–211.
5. Terstappen G, Reggiani A. In silico research in drug discovery. *Trends Pharmacol Sci* 2001;22: 23–26.
6. Rooney K, Snoeck E, Watson P. Modelling and simulation in clinical drug development. *Drug Discov Today* 2001;6:802–806.
7. DiMasi J, Hansen, R. Grabowski, H. The price of innovation: new estimates of drug development costs. *J Health Econ* 2003;22:151–185.
8. Leon D. Innovation and the workplace. *Drug Discov Today* 1999;4:181–185.
9. DiMasi J, Caglarcan E, Wood-Armany M. Emerging role of pharmacoeconomics in the research and development decision-making process. *Pharmacoeconomics* 2001;19:753–766.
10. Dimasi JA. New drug development in the United States from 1963 to 1999. *Clin Pharmacol Ther* 2001;69:286–296.

Contributing Authors

Peter C. Adamson, M.D.
*Chief, Division of Clinical Pharmacology &
  Therapeutics
The Children's Hospital of Philadelphia
Philadelphia, Pennsylvania*

Jeffrey Augen, M.D.
*President, TurboWorx Inc.
New Haven, Connecticut*

Lasantha R. Bandara, M.D.
*Oxford GlycoSciences (UK) Ltd.
Abingdon, United Kingdom*

Martyn Banks, Ph.D.
*Lead Discovery
Bristol-Myers Squibb Pharmaceutical
  Research Institute
Wallingford, Connecticut*

Surendra K. Bansal, Ph.D.
*Hoffmann-La Roche, Inc.
Nutley, New Jersey*

Stefan D. Baral, M.D.
*National Cancer Institute of Canada Clinical
  Trials Group
Queen's University
Kingston, Ontario, Canada*

Donald A. Berry, Ph.D.
*Professor, Department of Biostatistics,
M.D. Anderson Cancer Center
Houston, Texas*

Martin Brandl, M.D.
*Department of Pharmaceutics and
  Biopharmaceutics
Institute of Pharmacy
University of Tromsø
Tromsø, Norway*

Daniel R. Budman, M.D., F.A.C.P.
*Experimental Therapeutics Section
Don Monti Division of Oncology
North Shore University Hospital
New York University
Manhasset, New York*

Adriana A. Byrnes, M.D.
*Clinical Research Specialist
Technical Resources International, Inc.
Bethesda, Maryland*

David Cella, Ph.D.
*Center on Outcomes, Research and Education
  (CORE)
Evanston, Illinois*

Alessandra Cesano, M.D.
*Senior Director of Clinical Research
Amgen, Inc.
Thousand Oaks, California*

A. Dimitrios Colevas, M.D.
*Senior Investigator
Investigational Drug Branch
NCI/CTEP
Rockville, Maryland*

Jerry M. Collins, Ph.D.
*Director, Laboratory of Clinical Pharmacology
Food and Drug Administration
Rockville, Maryland*

Kimberly Davis, Ph.D.
*Center on Outcomes, Research and Education
  (CORE)
Evanston, Illinois*

Robert B. Diasio, M.D.
*Department of Pharmacology and Medicine
Division of Clinical Pharmacology
Comprehensive Cancer Center
University of Alabama at Birmingham
Birmingham, Alabama*

Kelly Dineen, Ph.D.
*Center on Outcomes, Research and
  Education (CORE)
Evanston, Illinois*

Thomas M. Donnelly, D.V.M.
*The Warren Institute
Ossining, New York*

Ruth Duncan, M.D.
Centre for Polymer Therapeutics
Welsh School of Pharmacy
Cardiff University
Cardiff, United Kingdom

Merrill J. Egorin, M.D.
Professor of Medicine and Pharmacology
University of Pittsburgh Cancer Institute
Pittsburgh, Pennsylvania

Jane Endicott, M.D.
Laboratory of Molecular Biophysics
Department of Biochemistry
Oxford, United Kingdom

Hany Ezzeldin, Ph.D.
Department of Pharmacology and Medicine
Division of Clinical Pharmacology
Comprehensive Cancer Center
University of Alabama at Birmingham
Birmingham, Alabama

Ann T. Farrell, M.D.
United States Food and Drug Administration
Division of Oncology Drug Products
Center for Drug Evaluation and Research
Rockville, Maryland

Bruce Feistner, R.A.C.
OSI Pharmaceuticals, Inc.
Boulder, Colorado

Scott Z. Fields, M.D.
EISAI Medical Research, Inc.
Teaneck, New Jersey

Elizabeth Fox, M.D.
Pharmacology & Experimental
  Therapeutics Section
Pediatric Oncology Branch
National Cancer Institute
Bethesda, Maryland

Jay J. Greenblatt, M.D.
Head, Drug Regulatory Affairs Section
Regulatory Affairs Branch
Cancer Therapy Evaluation Program
Division of Cancer Treatment and Diagnosis
National Cancer Institute
Bethesda, Maryland

Roger J. Griffin, M.D.
Northern Institute for Cancer Research
School of Natural Sciences
University of Newcastle upon Tyne
Newcastle upon Tyne, United Kingdom

Ian R. Hardcastle, M.D.
Northern Institute for Cancer Research
School of Natural Sciences
University of Newcastle upon Tyne
Newcastle upon Tyne, United Kingdom

Jill I. Johnson
Office of the Associate Director
Developmental Therapeutics Program
Division of Cancer Treatment and Diagnosis
National Cancer Institute
Rockville, Maryland

Stanley B. Kaye, F.R.C.P., F.R.C.P.S., F.R.C.R., F.R.S.E.
Professor of Medical Oncology
Cancer Research United Kingdom
Department of Medicine
The Royal Marsden Hospital
Sutton, United Kingdom

Sandy Kennedy, M.D.
Oxford GlycoSciences (UK) Ltd.
Abingdon, United Kingdom

Jochen Kuhlmann, M.D., Ph.D.
Professor of Pharmacology and Toxicology
Bayer AG
Pharma-Research-Center
Wuppertal, Germany

John Leighton, Ph.D.
United States Food and Drug Administration
Division of Oncology Drug Products
Center for Drug Evaluation and Research
Rockville, Maryland

Zhenmin Liang, Ph.D.
Hoffmann-La Roche, Inc.
Nutley, New Jersey

Stuart M. Lichtman, M.D., F.A.C.P.
Associate Professor of Medicine
New York University School of Medicine
Section of Geriatric Oncology
Don Monti Division of Medical Oncology
North Shore University Hospital
Manhasset, New York

Iftekhar Mahmood, Ph.D.
Division of Clinical Trial Design and Analysis
Office of Therapeutic Research and Review
Clinical Pharmacology and Toxicology Branch
Center for Biologics Evaluation and Research
Food and Drug Administration
Rockville, Maryland

Elaine Meaker, M.S., R.A.C.
OSI Pharmaceuticals, Inc.
Boulder, Colorado

Martin Noble, M.D.
Laboratory of Molecular Biophysics
Department of Biochemistry
Oxford, United Kingdom

Bastiaan Nuijen, Pharm.D., Ph.D.
Department of Pharmacy and Pharmacology
Slotervaart Hospital, The Netherlands
Cancer Institute
Amsterdam, The Netherlands

Nicole Onetto, M.D., M.S.C.
OSI Pharmaceuticals, Inc.
Executive Vice President, Oncology Division Head
Boulder, Colorado

Ramesh Padmanabha, Ph.D.
Lead Discovery
Bristol-Myers Squibb Pharmaceutical Research
Institute
Wallingford, Connecticut

Richard Pazdur, M.D.
United States Food and Drug Administration
Division of Oncology Drug Products
Center for Drug Evaluation and Research
Rockville, Maryland

Jinee D. Rizzo, Ph.D.
Institute for Drug Development
Cancer Therapy and Research Center
San Antonio, Texas

Gary L. Rosner, Sc.D.
Department of Biostatistics
M.D. Anderson Cancer Center
Houston, Texas

Lawrence V. Rubinstein, Ph.D.
Biometric Research Branch
National Cancer Institute
Bethesda, Maryland

Christopher W. Ryan, M.D.
Assistant Professor
University of Chicago
Executive Officer
Cancer and Leukemia Group B (CALBG)
Chicago, Illinois

Edward A. Sausville, M.D., Ph.D.
Associate Director
Developmental Therapeutics Program
Division of Cancer Treatment and Diagnosis
National Cancer Institute
Rockville, Maryland

Richard L. Schilsky, M.D.
Professor and Associate Dean for
Clinical Research
Biological Sciences Division
University of Chicago
Chairman
Cancer and Leukemia Group B (CALBG)
Chicago, Illinois 60637

Lesley K. Seymour, M.D.
Professor of Oncology
Queen's University
Co-Director
Investigational New Drug Program
National Cancer Institute of Canada Clinical
Trials Group
Kingston, Ontario, Canada

Riyaz N.H. Shah, M.R.C.P., Ph.D.
Department of Medicine
The Royal Marsden Hospital
Sutton, United Kingdom

Richard M. Simon, D.Sc.
Biometric Research Branch
National Cancer Institute
Bethesda, Maryland

Howard Z. Streicher, M.D.
Senior Investigator
Investigational Drug Branch
Cancer Therapy Evaluation Program
Division of Cancer Treatment and Diagnosis
National Cancer Institute
Bethesda, Maryland

Chris H. Takimoto, M.D., Ph.D.
Associate Professor
University of Texas Health Science Center at San
Antonio
Cancer Therapy and Research Center
San Antonio, Texas

Robert H. tePoele, M.D.
The Cancer Research UK Centre for Cancer
Therapeutics
The Institute of Cancer Research
Sutton, United Kingdom

Theodora Voskoglou-Nomikos, M.D.
Study Coordinator
National Cancer Institute of Canada Clinical
*   Trials Group*
Queen's University
Kingston, Ontario, Canada

Christoph Wandel, M.D., Ph.D.
Bayer AG
Pharma-Research-Center
Wuppertal, Germany

Raymond B. Weiss, M.D., F.A.C.P.
Clinical Professor of Medicine
Lombardi Cancer Center
Georgetown University Medical Center
Washington, DC
Consultant in Oncology
Rockville, Maryland

Grant Williams, M.D.
United States Food and Drug Administration
Division of Oncology Drug Products
Center for Drug Evaluation and Research
Rockville, Maryland

Paul Workman, M.D.
The Cancer Research UK Centre for Cancer
*   Therapeutics*
The Institute of Cancer Research
Sutton, United Kingdom

PART 1

Introduction

1

How Oncology Drug Development Differs from Other Fields

Ann T. Farrell, John Leighton, Grant Williams, and Richard Pazdur

United States Food and Drug Administration, Division of Oncology Drug Products, Center for Drug Evaluation and Research, Rockville, Maryland 20852

DRUG DEVELOPMENT

Drug development is a stepwise process progressing from preclinical to clinical evaluation. Drug development programs differ because the "risk-benefit" ratio for a drug depends on the target disease and the patient population. Cancer is an aggressive and potentially fatal disease for which the patient receives therapy conventionally administered at or near maximally tolerated doses. The life-threatening nature of advanced cancer allows the acceptance of considerably more risk than would be acceptable in other conditions. Even within oncology drug development, differences exist for drugs being developed for chemoprevention compared with drugs being developed for the treatment of refractory disease because both the potential benefit of therapy and the acceptability of risk vary in different cancer settings. Oncology chemopreventive drug development more closely resembles that of drug development for non–life-threatening disease. Requirements for the preclinical and clinical data for oncology drugs also differ from those for other drugs.

General Considerations for Preclinical Drug Development

The goal of the preclinical safety evaluation is to ensure adequate characterization of toxic effects with respect to target organs, potential reversibility, dose dependence, and relationship to exposure (1). These preclinical studies should be conducted under Good

The views expressed are the result of independent work and do not represent the views or findings of the United States Food and Drug Administration or the United States Government.

Laboratory Practices. Preclinical studies determine the choice of an initial starting dose for clinical studies (2). The preclinical safety evaluation also identifies the potential organ toxicities to be monitored in the clinical studies. Serious adverse events observed during preclinical or clinical studies may warrant additional specific safety studies.

Toxicity Studies

Single-dose (acute) toxicity is usually assessed in two mammalian species (generally one rodent and one nonrodent species) (1,3). A dose-escalation study with an appropriate toxicity evaluation may substitute for an acute single-dose toxicity study (1). Toxicity studies that use doses high enough to cause toxicity assess clinical signs, body weight, food consumption, gross pathology, and histopathology. Repeat dose toxicity studies should use regimens similar to those planned for the clinical studies, including schedule, duration, and route of administration (3,4). If the drug will be administered subcutaneously, intramuscularly, dermally, or ophthalmologically, preclinical local tolerance studies should be performed, including single and repeat dose, if necessary (5).

National drug regulatory agencies differ somewhat concerning the preclinical data that are recommended prior to human use. The next two tables outline the duration of repeat-dose toxicity studies expected as support for clinical trials in the United States, the European Union, and Japan (1,3,6–9) (Tables 1.1 and 1.2).

Toxicokinetic Studies

Toxicokinetic studies generate pharmacokinetic data, which describe the systemic exposure achieved in

TABLE 1.1. *Duration of repeated-dose toxicity studies to support phase 1 and 2 trials in the European Union and phase 1, 2, and 3 trials in the United States and Japan*

Duration of clinical trials[a]	Minimum duration of repeated-dose toxicity studies	
	Rodents	Nonrodents
Single dose	2–4 wk	2 wk
Up to 2 wk	2–4 wk	2 wk
Up to 1 mo	1 mo	1 mo
Up to 3 mo	3 mo	3 mo
Up to 6 mo	6 mo	6 mo
> 6 mo	6 mo	Long-term

In Japan, if there are no phase 2 clinical trials of equivalent duration to the planned phase 3 trials, conduct of longer-duration toxicity studies should be considered as presented in Table 1.2. In the European Union and the United States, 2-week studies are the minimum duration. In Japan, 2-week nonrodent and 4-week rodent studies are needed. In the United States, as an alternative to 2-week studies, single-dose toxicity studies with extended examinations can support single-dose human trials.

[a] Data from 6 months of administration in nonrodents should be available before the initiation of clinical trials longer than 3 months. Alternatively, if applicable, data from a 9-month nonrodent study should be available before the treatment duration exceeds that which is supported by the available toxicity studies.

Revised from the International Conference on Harmonization Document M3. Guidance for industry: nonclinical safety studies for the conduct of human clinical trials for pharmaceuticals. Geneva: ICH, July 1997.

animals and its relationship to dose level, to any observed toxicity and the time course of the development of toxicity. This information may subsequently be used to adjust the choice of species for further study and for planning dosing schedule and study design in clinical trials. Pharmacokinetic data may be derived either from specially designed studies or from planned nonclinical toxicity studies, such as single-dose, repeat-dose, *in vivo* genotoxicity, carcinogenicity, or reproductive toxicity studies (10). Reproductive preclinical toxicokinetic data collection may involve exposure assessment in dams, embryos, fetuses, or the newborn. Tissue distribution studies provide information on the distribution and accumulation of the drug and its metabolites. Repeated-dose tissue distribution studies may be required under certain circumstances (11). Toxicokinetic study data should be available when clinical phase 1 studies are completed (1).

TABLE 1.2. *Duration of repeated-dose toxicity studies to support phase 3 trials in the European Union and marketing in Japan, the European Union, and the United States*

Duration of clinical trials	Minimum duration of repeated-dose toxicity studies	
	Rodents	Nonrodents
Up to 2 wk	1 mo	1 mo
Up to 1 mo	3 mo	3 mo
Up to 3 mo	6 mo	3 mo
> 3 mo	6 mo	Long-term

These data also reflect the marketing recommendations in Japan, the European Union, and the United States except that a long-term nonrodent study is recommended for clinical use exceeding 1 month.

Revised from the International Conference on Harmonization Document M3. Guidance for industry: nonclinical safety studies for the conduct of human clinical trials for pharmaceuticals. Geneva: ICH, July 1997.

Genotoxicity

Genotoxicity testing has been used to predict carcinogenicity. Pharmaceutical agents testing positive in genotoxicity tests have the potential to be human carcinogens and/or mutagens, which may induce cancer. In general, *in vitro* and *in vivo* genotoxicity testing detects direct or indirect genetic damage and should be performed prior to the initiation of phase 1 studies (6,12). However, in clinical studies of patients with end-stage disease, genetic testing may not be necessary at this stage of drug development. The standard battery of genotoxic tests includes the following: (a) a bacterial reverse mutation assay, (b) an *in vitro* test with cytogenetic evaluation of chromosomal damage with mammalian cells or *in vitro* mouse lymphoma thymidine kinase assay, and (c) an *in vivo* test for chromosomal damage using rodent hematopoietic cells. Negative results obtained with compounds to all three types of studies suggest the absence of genotoxicity. The standard battery may be modified when drugs are excessively toxic to bacteria, resulting in interference with the bacterial reverse mutation assay or with mammalian cell replication. In these situations, the performance of two mammalian cell *in vitro* tests using different cell types and different endpoints (e.g., chromosomal damage and gene mutation) should be considered.

Compared with *in vitro* testing, *in vivo* testing provides information on the absorption, distribution, metabolism, and excretion of the drug. The utility of *in vivo* testing is limited with agents that are not sufficiently absorbed, such as radioimaging agents. A single positive result in a genotoxicity assay does not necessarily imply that a genotoxic risk exists (12). Genotoxic test interpretation may be complicated by the concentration, culture conditions, and reproducibility of test results in drugs of the same or similar class. If *in vitro* genotoxicity results are equivocal or positive, additional *in vitro* or *in vivo* testing may be required.

Carcinogenicity Studies

Carcinogenicity studies identify tumorigenic potential in animals and evaluate possible human risk. These studies are performed primarily when the drug is expected to be administered regularly over a substantial part of a patient's life. Typically, these studies dose animals using the same administration route intended for humans. Several doses are tested. In the past, differences among international regulatory authorities existed concerning high dose selection. All regulatory authorities currently use a maximum feasible dose.

For most drugs used to treat advanced cancer, carcinogenicity studies may be completed later in drug development, including in the postapproval setting. In disease populations where the life expectancy is short, such as metastatic cancer, long-term carcinogenicity studies may not be required. However, in clinical situations where therapies are curative or have a pronounced effect on survival (e.g., patients receiving adjuvant chemotherapy or hormonal therapy to prevent cancer recurrence), carcinogenicity studies are usually necessary. Similarly, carcinogenicity studies are necessary for chemopreventive agents.

Carcinogenicity studies may be required if (a) the anticipated use of the drug is 3 to 6 months or longer, (b) concern exists about carcinogenic potential (e.g., carcinogenicity test results have been positive for other drugs in the product class, (c) the intended patient population has a life expectancy greater than 2 or 3 years, (d) the agent is an ophthalmologically or dermally applied product that may have extensive systemic exposure, and (e) the drug product is similar to an endogenous substance given as replacement therapy.

Completed carcinogenicity studies are usually not required when the pharmaceutical agent is unequivocally genotoxic (13). Regulatory authorities have usually required two long-term carcinogenicity rodent studies prior to marketing of a new drug (13). Regulatory authorities have recently considered the utility of one long-term and one short- or medium-term *in vivo* rodent test systems designed to clarify a particular carcinogenicity concern (e.g., initiation-promotion models in rodents) (14). Several regulatory guidances provide the study design, necessary monitoring, and required investigations (14–17). Mechanistic studies (e.g., specialized genotoxicity studies) may be useful in the interpretation of tumor findings in carcinogenicity studies (14).

Reproductive Toxicity Studies

Preclinical reproductive toxicity studies are used to investigate the drug's effect on mammalian reproduction (18). The necessity for these studies is based on the drug's anticipated use in relation to reproductive life cycle. Rats are the predominant species used. Embryotoxicity studies, however, require two species testing. Usually rabbits are the second mammalian species used for embryotoxicity studies because of the extensive prior background knowledge of this species. Reproductive toxicity testing is performed with study designs that focus on three periods: (a) fertility to early embryonic development (premating to conception to implantation), (b) prenatal to postnatal development, including maternal function (implantation to birth to sexual maturity), and (c) embryo/fetal development (implantation to end of pregnancy).

In the United States and European Union, men may be included in phase 1 and 2 clinical studies prior to a preclinical assessment of male fertility if an assessment of male reproductive organs was performed in repeat-dose toxicity studies (1,19). In Japan, prior to inclusion of men in studies, preclinical male fertility studies are usually performed. Ideally, preclinical male fertility testing should be performed prior to initiation of phase 3 trials.

Women who are not of childbearing potential can be included in clinical trials prior to completion of reproductive toxicity provided that an assessment of the female reproductive tract was performed in repeat-dose toxicity studies. In the United States, women of childbearing potential can be included in early studies without reproductive toxicity studies provided that highly effective birth control or pregnancy testing is used to minimize the risk (1). Highly effective birth control is defined as a method that results in a low failure rate (i.e., less than 1%) when appropriately used. Continued pregnancy testing and birth control compliance monitoring during the trial is performed to minimize risk. Informed consent forms should discuss potential risk, especially if no information is known.

In Japan, prior to the inclusion of women of childbearing potential using contraception in any trial, female fertility and embryo/fetal development testing should be performed. In the European Union, embryo/fetal assessment should be performed and completed prior to the inclusion of women of childbearing potential in phase 1 studies. In the United States, preclinical assessment of female fertility and embryo/fetal development should be performed prior to entering women of childbearing potential into phase 3 trials, even if the women are using adequate birth control. In the European Union, female fertility studies should be performed prior to phase 3. Preclinical prenatal and postnatal data should be available prior to marketing approval. For all three drug development regions, all female reproductive toxicity and standard battery of genotoxicity studies should be completed prior to the inclusion of women of childbearing potential who are not using highly effective birth control methods, or whose pregnancy status is uncertain.

Safety Pharmacology Studies

Safety pharmacology studies investigate the potential undesirable pharmacodynamic effects of a drug on physiologic function (20,21). These studies have three goals: (a) to identify undesirable pharmacodynamic effects of a drug on physiologic function, possibly relating to safety, (b) to evaluate adverse effects (e.g., pathophysiologic and/or pharmacodynamic) observed in toxicology and/or clinical studies, and (c) to investigate the mechanism of the observed or suspected adverse events. The most important adverse events to investigate are those that effect critical and essential functions (central nervous system, cardiovascular, and respiratory systems). Adverse events transiently effecting the hepatic, renal, or gastrointestinal system that do not cause irreversible effect may not warrant immediate study, except when there may be irreparable harm in a specific vulnerable patient population (e.g., gastrointestinal toxicity in an agent being developed for Crohn's disease). These studies may involve *ex vivo* and *in vitro* testing with isolated organs, tissues, cell cultures, cellular fragments, receptors, ion transporters, and enzymes (22).

Oncologic versus Nononcologic Preclinical Drug Development

Due to the life-threatening nature of an unresectable malignancy, conventional therapeutic strategies employ anticancer drugs, radiation therapy, and surgery with significant toxicity and complications, different risk/benefit considerations are used in regulatory decision making for cancer therapies (2,23). Preclinical studies for drugs to treat serious and life-threatening conditions may be abbreviated, deferred, or even omitted (1). Oncology preclinical drug development is tailored according to the intended use of the drug and the eventual patient population in the indication.

Starting Dose Determination for Traditional Cytotoxic Oncology Drugs

Like nononcology drugs, investigational cancer drugs should have two toxicology studies to support initial phase 1 clinical studies. One study is a required rodent study, which identifies the doses producing life-threatening and non–life-threatening toxicities. The rodent study identifies the dose (mg/m^2) that is severely toxic to 10% of the rodents (STD_{10}). If no life-threatening toxicity is observed in the rodent study, then the highest dose tested is taken to be the STD_{10}. The second study should confirm that this dose (STD_{10}) does not cause irreversible toxicity to nonrodents. The starting dose for a phase 1 study is one tenth of the STD_{10}. If life-threatening toxicity is observed in the nonrodent study at the proposed starting dose based on rodent studies, then the starting dose (mg/m^2) for clinical studies is one sixth of the highest dose tested in nonrodents that does not produce severe toxicity.

Dose Determination for Noncytotoxic Oncology Drugs

Many noncytotoxic oncology drugs use the approach for cytotoxic drugs to determine the starting dose. Preclinical pharmacodynamic information can facilitate dose determination in oncologic phase 1 drug development. The determination of the pharmacodynamically active dose may be more useful than maximum tolerated dose (MTD) determination for immunomodulators and noncytotoxic agents. For example, no additional benefit may occur from the administration of doses higher than that necessary to successfully block a receptor. Additional higher drug doses beyond the pharmacologically identified dose may incur toxicity without additional patient benefit.

Preclinical Data Required Prior to Investigational New Drug Application Filing

Preclinical studies necessary at the time of an Investigational New Drug (IND) and a New Drug Application (NDA) filings vary depending upon the drug product, proposed indication and patient population, the observed clinical outcome, characterization of toxicities observed in animals and humans, and the projected treatment duration. If a nononcologic drug is developed for a serious or life-threatening condition, the development may be similar to an oncologic drug. At the initial IND filing, the following preclinical studies are recommended: single-dose toxicity, repeat-dose toxicity, and genotoxicity. Genotoxicity studies may not be required at the IND filing for studies conducted in patients with advanced cancer. Additional preclinical studies may be required prior to IND filing for photosensitizing agents, antibody conjugate, liposomal delivery, and cytotoxics delivered via depot (2).

Preclinical Considerations for Cytotoxics

For cytotoxics prescribed in advanced disease, the necessary preclinical repeat-dose toxicity study may be only 28 days in duration. For cytotoxics used in the adjuvant setting, multiple-cycle toxicity studies may be required, especially if clinical data regarding repeat administration in a more advanced cancer/metastatic disease population do not exist. Preferentially, data from International Conference on Harmonization (ICH) stage C-D teratogenicity studies should be available prior to NDA submission but are not required prior to submission of a phase 1 protocol for treatment of advanced cancer. Carcinogenicity stud-

ies are usually not required for cytotoxics to treat advanced cancer, but may be required for these drugs used in adjuvant treatment, especially if the treatment duration would be longer than 6 months. Special safety pharmacology studies may be required to support an NDA filing (e.g., special cardiac studies for anthracyclinelike agents).

The initial evaluation of cytotoxic combination therapy has traditionally been performed in the clinical setting. This empirical approach has been relatively successful but may not be optimal. Preclinical testing of combinations provides the opportunity to explore various doses, dose ratios, schedules, and drug sequencing. Preclinical combination testing may not be necessary provided that each agent's toxicities have been fully characterized, and data do not indicate that the combination use would be unsafe. Concern may increase if one agent interferes with the metabolism or elimination of another, or if both cytotoxic agents target the same metabolic or cellular pathway, or cellular function. Additional safety testing may be required for the development of photosensitizers or for novel drug-delivery systems (e.g., copolymer implants, human albumin microspheres, monoclonal antibody–drug conjugates, and liposomal encapsulation).

Preclinical Considerations for Noncytotoxic, Chronically Administered Oncologic Drugs

Noncytotoxic, chronically administered oncologic agents (e.g., chemopreventives, hormones, and immunomodulators) should have repeat-dose toxicity studies. The duration will depend on the intended population because the development of these agents is similar to nononcologic drugs. In patients with advanced cancer, 28-day toxicology studies may be sufficient prior to phase 1 or 2 studies. Studies up to 6 months' duration in rodents and up to 12 months in nonrodents may be required prior to clinical studies involving high-risk or cancer-free patients, or those expected to have prolonged survival. The requirement for reproductive toxicity testing depends on the disease stage and intended patient population. ICH stage C-D (developmental) reproductive toxicity studies are important for NDA filing. In addition, ICH stage A-B (premating to implantation) reproductive toxicity studies are requisite for the development of hormonal agents and ICH A-B, C-F (implantation to offspring sexual maturity) reproductive toxicity studies are necessary for the development of chemopreventive agents. Carcinogenicity studies are usually not required for advanced disease, but would be required if the agent were administered to patients who are high-risk, cancer-free, or expected to have prolonged survival.

Preclinical Considerations for Chemotherapy Modulators

The development plan of chemotherapy modulators encompasses determining the modulator's starting dose and toxicities when given alone and the modulator's dose and toxicities when combined with other therapies (e.g., chemotherapy, radiation therapy). Prior to IND submission, single- and repeat-dose toxicity studies should be performed with the modulator alone and combined with intended agents. One study arm should replicate the intended treatment schedule. Genotoxicity testing prior to IND filing is needed in selected occasions when the modulator may be administered to healthy volunteers or patients believed to be cancer-free. If a chemoprotectant is being developed, the toxicology studies should include a histopathologic examination to evaluate the combination's toxicity and should evaluate the possibility of tumor protection. Toxicology studies of sufficient duration for the intended duration in the patient population should be conducted.

Phases of Clinical Drug Development

Phase 1

Phase 1 studies are the initial studies evaluating a new investigational agent in humans (24). For drugs developed for nonserious and non–life-threatening conditions, the phase 1 studies are conducted in normal, healthy volunteers. Phase 1 studies determine the drug's toxicity profile, pharmacodynamic/pharmacokinetic parameters, and the range of nontoxic doses for subsequent trials. In normal subjects, the highest allowed doses are limited by the highest nontoxic doses determined from preclinical animal data.

For drugs developed for serious and life-threatening conditions, the phase 1 studies are usually conducted in patients with the medical condition. The phase 1 studies identify acceptable doses, toxicities, and also provide initial signs of activity. The major goal of phase 1 oncology studies of cytotoxic drugs is to determine the MTD and the dose for subsequent phase 2 testing. A variety of dose-escalating designs exist (e.g., standard or modified Fibonacci, modified continual reassessment, accelerated titration, and pharmacokinetically guided dose strategies) (25,26). The highest doses used in clinical oncology studies are not restricted to those comparative doses used in the preclinical studies as long as the toxicities are easily monitored, reversible, and sufficiently precede lethality in animals. The maximum dose is usually defined by toxicities that are measured by accepted criteria, such as the National Cancer Institute Common Toxicity Criteria.

Prior to allowing a study to proceed, the US Food and Drug Administration (FDA) carefully evaluates the protocols, including starting dose and schedule, data (e.g., preclinical data, prior human use), dose-escalation plan, intended duration of administration, safety-monitoring plan, and the MTD definition. Deviations from common clinical study practices may be allowed provided safety is assured.

Phase 2

Phase 2 studies evaluate the drug's effectiveness for a specific disease and further describe its toxicities. In nononcologic fields, these studies may be dose-ranging, active, or placebo-comparator studies. Phase 2 studies serve as a template for the pivotal phase 3 studies. These nononcologic studies may be designed using the same inclusion and exclusion criteria, efficacy endpoints, and analysis plan as the phase 3 pivotal trials. In oncology, traditional phase 2 studies determine if cytotoxic drugs have activity against a particular tumor type and whether that activity justifies further drug development.

Phase 3

Phase 3 clinical trials are the confirmatory studies in a larger patient population and are intended to gather comparative effectiveness and safety information required to assess the drug's overall risk/benefit relationship. These trials are performed after preliminary evidence of effectiveness has been obtained from phase 2 studies. In most nononcology fields, these studies mimic the design and analysis of the phase 2 studies. In oncology, these phase 3 studies usually provide the first comparison of the drug to the standard treatment. Occasionally, oncology agents may be compared to best supportive care.

IND Exemptions for Nononcology and Oncology Studies

Lawfully marketed drugs or biological products may be exempt from filing an IND if the following criteria are met: (a) the trial is not intended to support FDA approval of a new indication or a significant change in the product labeling, (b) the trial is not intended to support a significant change in the advertising for the product, and (c) the clinical study does not involve a new administration route or dosage level or use in a patient population or other factor that significantly increases the risks (or decreases the acceptability of the risks) (27). The study must be conducted in accordance with institutional review board and informed consent regulations [21 Code of Federal Regulations (CFR) parts 50 and 56], and conducted in compliance with 21 CFR 312.7 regarding the promotion and charging for investigational drugs. The investigator may determine whether a study is exempt from submission. Although a study may be exempt from IND regulations, it still must be conducted with institutional review board oversight and must comply with the informed consent regulations (21 CFR parts 56 and 50).

Review and Approval Process

The NDA review and approval process ensures that safe and effective drugs are available for the American public. Approval occurs after the Agency has carefully considered the submitted preclinical and clinical study reports, manufacturing data, and a proposed product label. An NDA approval is for one or more specific indications. Once an NDA is approved, the pharmaceutical company may advertise and promote the drug's use consistent with the approved package insert.

A successful NDA must provide substantial evidence of effectiveness derived from adequate and well-controlled studies. The data must demonstrate that the drug is safe for its intended use. The application should define the appropriate patient population and provide adequate information to enable the product's safe and effective use.

Oncology Drug Approval

Recognizing the need for early access to promising medicines for the treatment of cancer and other serious and life-threatening diseases, the Agency has developed policies and procedures to facilitate drug development. These policies and procedures include: Accelerated Approval (28,29), Fast Track Program and Rolling NDA Submission (30), Priority Review (31), and Special Protocol Assessment (32).

Accelerated approval is granted for a new drug that provides benefit over available therapy for diseases that are serious or life threatening (29). Accelerated approval can be granted on a surrogate endpoint "reasonably likely to predict clinical benefit." Regulations mandate that sponsors subsequently demonstrate clinical benefit with due diligence after approval. Response rate is an example of a surrogate endpoint for clinical benefit in the treatment of solid tumors. Full approval could be granted when clinical benefit is demonstrated through an improvement in survival or symptom benefit in subsequent trials. Oncology applications receiving accelerated approval based on a surrogate endpoint in a refractory-disease population may subsequently demonstrate clinical benefit in an earlier stage of disease (e.g., accelerated approval in second-line metastatic breast cancer with full approval in first-line or in the adjuvant setting). Other regulatory authorities such as the European Agency for the Evaluation of Medicinal Products have published guidances on anticancer drug development and approval (33,34).

Drug development in oncology differs from other clinical disciplines because of a different risk/benefit relationship. Cancer is a potentially life-threatening disease that requires aggressive measures for treatment and justifies accepting increased toxicity in order to achieved increased efficacy. Drug development in oncology differs from other fields because of the breadth of agents being developed (e.g., cytotoxics, cytostatics, modulators, and chemopreventives). Because of the need to expedite oncology drug development, the quantity and types of preclinical and clinical data may differ from other therapeutic areas. Preclinical and clinical data requirements are tailored to the intended use of the drug and to the population who will eventually use this drug. Differences in preclinical and clinical study requirements may exist among the United States, Japan, and the European Union for the same pharmaceutical product being developed. Continuing consultation with regulatory authorities throughout the drug development process will expedite the approval process for oncology drugs.

REFERENCES

1. International Conference on Harmonization. Guidance for industry: nonclinical safety studies for the conduct of human clinical trials for pharmaceuticals. Geneva: ICH; July 1997; Document M3.
2. DeGeorge JJ, Ahn CH, Andrews P, et al. Regulatory considerations for preclinical development of anticancer drugs. *Cancer Chemother Pharmacol* 1998;41: 173–185.
3. US Department of Health and Human Services, Food and Drug Administration. Single dose acute toxicity testing for pharmaceuticals: revised guidance. *Federal Register* 1996 Aug 26;61:43934–43935.
4. The European Agency for the Evaluation of Medicinal Products Committee for Proprietary Medicinal Products. Note for guidance on repeated dose toxicity. London: EMEA; July 2000.
5. The European Agency for the Evaluation of Medicinal Products Committee for Proprietary Medicinal Products. Note for guidance on non-clinical local tolerance testing of medicinal products. London: EMEA; March 2001.

6. International Conference on Harmonization. Guideline for industry: specific aspects of regulatory genotoxicity tests for pharmaceuticals. Geneva: ICH; April 1996; Document S2A.

7. Choudary J, Contrera JF, DeFelice A, et al. Response to Monro and Mehta proposal for use of single-dose toxicology studies to support single-dose studies of new drugs in humans. *Clin Pharmacol Ther* 1996; 59:265–267.

8. International Conference on Harmonization. Guidance for industry: duration of chronic toxicity testing in animals (rodent and nonrodent). Geneva: ICH; July 1999; Document S4A.

9. US Department of Health and Human Services, Food and Drug Administration. International Conference on Harmonization: guidance on the duration of chronic toxicity testing in animals (rodent and nonrodent toxicity testing) availability. *Federal Register* 1999 Jun 25;64: 43934–43935.

10. International Conference on Harmonization. Guideline for industry toxicokinetics: the assessment of systemic exposure in toxicity studies. Geneva: ICH; March 1995; Document S3A.

11. International Conference on Harmonization. Guideline for industry pharmacokinetics: guidance for repeated tissue distribution. Geneva: ICH; March 1995; Document S3B.

12. International Conference on Harmonization. Guidance for industry: a standard battery for genotoxicity testing of pharmaceuticals. Geneva: ICH; July 1997; Document S2B.

13. International Conference on Harmonization Document S1A Document "Guideline for Industry: The Need for Long-term Rodent Carcinogenicity Studies of Pharmaceuticals." Geneva: ICH; March 1996.

14. International Conference on Harmonization. Guidance for industry: testing for carcinogenicity of pharmaceuticals. Geneva: ICH; July 1997; Document S1B.

15. International Conference on Harmonization. Guideline for industry: dose selection for carcinogenicity studies of pharmaceuticals. Geneva: ICH; March 1995; Document S1C.

16. International Conference on Harmonization. Guidance for industry: addendum to *Dose Selection for Carcinogenicity Studies of Pharmaceuticals:* addition of a limit dose and related notes. Geneva: ICH; March 1995; Document S1C (R).

17. The European Agency for the Evaluation of Medicinal Products Committee for Proprietary Medicinal Products. Note for guidance on carcinogenic potential. London: EMEA; July 2002.

18. International Conference on Harmonization. Guideline for industry: detection of toxicity to reproduction for medicinal products. Geneva: ICH; September 1994; Document S5A.

19. International Conference on Harmonization. Guideline for industry: detection of toxicity to reproduction for medicinal products: addendum on toxicity to male fertility. Geneva: ICH; April 1996; Document S5B.

20. International Conference on Harmonization. Guidance for industry: preclinical safety evaluation of biotechnology-derived pharmaceuticals. Geneva: ICH; July 1997; Document S6.

21. International Conference on Harmonization. Guidance for industry: safety pharmacology studies for human pharmaceuticals. Geneva: ICH; July 2001; Document S7A.

22. International Conference on Harmonization. Guideline: safety pharmacology studies for assessing the potential for delayed ventricular repolarization (QT interval prolongation) by human pharmaceuticals. Geneva: ICH; February 2002; Draft Consensus Document.

23. The European Agency for the Evaluation of Medicinal Products Committee for Proprietary Medicinal Products. Note for guidance on the pre-clinical evaluation of anticancer medicinal products. London: EMEA; July 1998.

24. 21 Code of Federal Regulations 312.21. 52 Federal Register 8831 (1981) codified at 210FR 312.21.

25. Nagamura F, Collins J, Kobayashi K, et al. Comparative review of oncology phase 1 dose escalation designs of new molecular entities. In: Proceedings of the American Society of Clinical Oncology; May 12–21, 2002; Orlando, FL. Abstract 352.

26. Simon R, Freidlin B, Rubinstein L, et al. Accelerated titration designs for phase 1 clinical trials in oncology. *J Natl Cancer Inst* 1997;89:1138–1147.

27. US Food and Drug Administration. Draft guidance for industry: IND exemptions for studies of lawfully marketed cancer drug or biological products. 67 Federal Register 17078 (2002).

28. 21 Code of Federal Regulations Part 314. 59 Federal Register 749 (1991) codified at 210FR 314.

29. 21 Code of Federal Regulations Subpart H Part 314.500. 57 Federal Register 58958 (1991) codified at 210FR 314.500.

30. US Department of Health and Human Services, Food and Drug Administration, Center for Drug Evaluation and Research, Center for Biologics Evaluation and Research. Guidance for industry: fast track drug development programs. Designation, development, and application review. September 1998.

31. Manual of Policies and Procedures 6020.3 Priority Review Policy April 22, 1996. Available at: http://www.fda.gov/cder/mapp/6020-3.

32. US Department of Health and Human Services, Food and Drug Administration, Center for Drug Evaluation and Research, Center for Biologics Evaluation and Research. Guidance for industry: special protocol assessment. May 2002.

33. The European Agency for the Evaluation of Medicinal Products Committee for Proprietary Medicinal Products. Note for guidance on evaluation of anticancer medicinal products in man. London: EMEA; November 2001.

34. The European Agency for the Evaluation of Medicinal Products Committee for Proprietary Medicinal Products. Accelerated evaluation of products indicated for serious disease (life-threatening or heavily disabling diseases). London: EMEA; September 2001.

PART 2

Drug Discovery

2

Natural Products

Riyaz N.H. Shah and Stanley B. Kaye

Department of Medicine, The Royal Marsden Hospital, Sutton SM2 5 PT, United Kingdom

The natural environment has provided a rich source of novel compounds that have had a great impact on clinical therapeutics. From digoxin for cardiac arrhythmias to penicillins for microbial infections, countless lives have been saved by these agents, and cancer therapeutics is no exception. At least two thirds of the anticancer agents in current everyday use either are directly isolated from other organisms or are semisynthetic derivatives of natural compounds (1).

Over the course of evolution, many living organisms have developed systems that confer an advantage over their competitors within the ecosystem. Such systems include chemicals that repel or destroy predators or alternatively increase their own predatory potential. These chemicals usually work at a subcellular level, affecting critical processes within the target cells resulting in cell cycle arrest, programmed cell death, or direct toxicity. Thus, living organisms provide a rich source of compounds with growth modulatory properties and have great potential as anticancer agents.

The ability to develop novel natural anticancer agents is dependent on a whole range of factors. Firstly, mechanisms need to be in place to acquire and store organisms isolated from a range of ecosystems. Novel chemicals isolated from such organic matter need screening methodologies to isolate compounds for further development. Given the huge amount of biological tissue that can be isolated, high-throughput screening systems are preferable.

The major factor determining whether a potential agent can be developed further is supply. Preclinical assessments usually involve *in vitro* work using cell line cultures as well as *in vivo* xenograft experiments, all of which require a large amount of the agent under investigation. Large-scale harvesting of living organisms has environmental implications and may not always be possible. Alternatives include large-scale production farming processes or the development of synthetic production systems. Structural elucidation of the novel agent is an integral part of its development, involving techniques such as nuclear magnetic resonance spectroscopy, mass spectroscopy, and infrared spectroscopy, and may allow the development of synthetic or semisynthetic alternatives more amenable to large-scale production. Synthesis can be a multistep and labor-intensive process, and the production of some of the newer marine investigational agents involves up to 100 stages.

Analytical testing of the novel agent involves assessing purity and minimization of batch-to-batch variation. The solubility of the product needs to be defined, especially for the development of a pharmaceutical-grade product. In many cases, solubilizing agents such as Cremophor EL have important implications as they add their own toxicity profile to that of the investigational agent (e.g., allergic reactions and thrombophlebitis). The development of a pharmaceutical-grade product often requires other factors such as bulking agents, stabilizers, and buffering agents, all of which may have toxicity implications.

As each new compound approaches potential clinical application as an investigational agent, factors such as its stability need to be assessed. Many agents have poor stability in solution and are prepared as lyophilized powders for reconstitution. In the case of intravenous agents, the stability in the administering solution needs to be documented (e.g., normal saline or 5% dextrose). In addition, issues regarding the administration kit need to be addressed, especially the use of filters and whether significant adsorption to the giving sets occurs.

All of these issues taken together suggest that pharmaceutical development is not always suitable for all novel agents that show activity against cancer cell lines in screens. These drug development factors need to be taken into account when making decisions about which agents to take forward for advanced clinical testing.

In this chapter, we will consider the three major sources for natural products: (a) the marine environment, (b) plants, and (c) microbes.

MARINE-DERIVED AGENTS

The marine environment provides a rich source of biodiversity from which potential anticancer agents may be found. Effective exploration of this ecosystem became possible with the advent of deep-sea diving technologies in the latter half of the last century. In addition, advances in aquaculture technology and semisynthetic chemistry have allowed the generation of adequate amounts of material for testing.

The first marine anticancer agents discovered, spongouridine and spongothymidine, were derived from the sea sponge *Cryptothethya crypta* (2,3). Cytosine arabinoside was synthesized from these agents, and this drug still plays a very important role in the treatment of acute leukemia. A survey conducted by the National Cancer Institute (NCI) in 1995 suggested that 4% of marine compounds probably have some type of anticancer activity. Today at least 10 different types of marine compound are actively being investigated with a view to formal clinical study (Table 2.1).

Ecteinascidins

Ecteinascidins were initially isolated from the Caribbean sea squirt, a marine tunicate that grows on the roots of mangroves. Their anticancer effects were shown as early as 1973 (4). ET-743 was taken forward for further clinical development because of its higher abundance. All have three fused tetrahydroisoquinolone rings and have been shown to exhibit sequence-specific DNA minor groove binding. Alkylation of the N2 position of guanine occurs in the minor groove, resulting in adduct formation and bending of the template towards the major groove (5,6). This re-

sults in the generation of topoisomerase I cleavage products. Two of the rings are involved in DNA interactions, and although there is no defined role for the third ring, it is postulated that it may interact with chromatin elements (7).

In vitro, ET-743 has shown slowing of the cell cycle in S phase and G2/M arrest with an associated hypersensitivity in G1 (8,9). Increased apoptosis is thought to be secondary to cell cycle effects. Although microtubule aggregation has been observed in cancer cells exposed to ET-743, no direct interaction is known between the cytoskeleton and this compound. ET-743 shows some sequence specificity in terms of DNA binding, preferred sites being 5′-PuGC-3′ and 5′PyrGG-3′ (5). These DNA adducts can inhibit the interaction of transcription factors with the template, thereby modulating the rates of transcription of nearby genes. This may result in increased or decreased expression of a particular encoded protein. ET-743 is known to inhibit the binding of transcription factors recognizing GC-rich elements (e.g., NF-Y, which recognizes the CCAAT box, Sp1, and the orphan nuclear receptor, SXR). ET-743 has been shown to downregulate *MDR1* gene expression at the mRNA level. This gene encodes P-glycoprotein (P-gp), a 170-kd membrane-bound transporter, which pumps some cytotoxic drugs (e.g., anthracyclines, paclitaxel, and vinca alkaloids) out of the cell, resulting in resistance to these agents in experimental models. P-gp belongs to the superfamily of ABC transporters, is overexpressed in many human cancers, and may be one factor involved in clinical drug resistance. Overexpression is often due to increased transcription of *MDR1*. *MDR1* promoter function requires recruitment of the transcription factors NF-Y and Sp1/Sp3 to a CCAAT box and Sp1 recognition site, respectively. These in turn recruit histone acetyl transferase–containing transcriptional activators such as P/CAF to form a viable transcription-initiation complex. ET-743 can inhibit the activation

TABLE 2.1. *A selection of promising new anticancer compounds derived from marine sources*

Marine compound	Source organism	Mechanism of action	Stage of clinical development
Ecteinascidin	*Ecteinascidia turbinata*	DNA minor groove binding (6)	Phase 2 and 3
Bryostatin	*Bugula neritina*	PKC interactions + other (48)	Phase 2
Dolastatin	*Dolabella auricularia*	Microtubule stabilization (50)	Phase 2
Didemnin B and aplidine	*Trididemnum sodium* and *Aplidium albicans*	Protein synthesis inhibition, antiangiogenis	Phase 1 completing Phase 2 soon
ES-285/Spisulosine	*Spisula polynyma*	Disrupts actin cytoskeleton	Preclinical

of endogenous *MDR1* transcription as well as reporter constructs in the presence of inducers (10) and does not affect basal *MDR1* transcription. The exact mechanism of this is not entirely clear, but it is postulated that it occurs via direct interference with NF-Y and/or Sp1 binding to the promoter or via epigenetic interactions with chromatin (11,12). SXR is an orphan nuclear receptor important in the activation of *CYP3A4* as well as *MDR1*. ET-743 inhibits *CYP3A4* activity and may potentiate the effects of drugs metabolized using this pathway. It is thought that this occurs via inhibition of SXR binding to the *CYP3A4* gene. In addition, the observation of ET-743–induced reduction in *MDR1* expression is thought to be mediated in part by the inhibition of SXR binding (13).

Dexamethasone induces *CYP3A4*, and evidence is emerging that it can potentiate the activity of ET-743 (14). This work has lead to the notion that ET-743 may be a useful drug in tumors that often overexpress P-gp or in combination with drugs that are pumped out by P-gp. However, the concentrations of ET-743 required to inhibit transcription factor binding to a DNA template are far higher than those required for tumor shrinkage in patients. The clinical relevance of these observations is therefore in doubt.

It now seems clear that the mechanism of ET-743 action is more complex. Cells with deficient transcription-coupled nucleotide excision repair mechanisms (TC-NER) tend to be hypersensitive to cisplatin and ultraviolet radiation but resistant to ET-743. ET-743 sensitivity requires an intact TC-NER mechanism. It is thought that ET-743 adducts prevent progression of the RNA polymerase II–containing complex during active gene transcription. Adducts recruit TC-NER systems that are unable to repair the defect, but enact programmed cell death pathways (9,15). Restoration of NER function results in acquired sensitivity to ET-743. In addition, cells defective in mismatch repair are relatively resistant to cisplatin but retain sensitivity to ET-743. ET-743 sensitivity is also associated with an intact DNA double-strand break repair pathway. This is enhanced in cells lacking DNA-dependent protein kinases (DNA-PK). Wortmannin inhibits DNA-PK and is known to increase sensitivity to ET-743 (16).

Synergism with cisplatin has already been reported in preclinical models (17). In addition, in similar *in vitro* models, it has been shown that ET-743 is particularly effective in P-gp–overexpressing cell lines, causes a reduction in P-gp expression levels, and potentiates the effect of doxorubicin and vincristine on these same cells (18).

ET-743 is in the advanced stages of clinical development. Phase 1 studies have been completed with successful documentation of a maximum tolerated dosage of 1.5 g/m^2 as a 24-hour infusion every 3 weeks (19). Common toxicities include a transaminitis, fatigue, myelosuppression, neutropenia, thrombocytopenia, nausea, and vomiting. During these preliminary studies, evidence was found of activity against anthracycline- and ifosfamide-resistant sarcomas (20). As a result, ET-743 is undergoing further clinical development, with advanced sarcoma as the first potential target for drug registration.

Recent data from a compassionate use program suggest a 12% response rate for ET-743; however, a quarter of patients in this study suffered from grade 3 or 4 neutropenia and a similar proportion demonstrated grade 3 or 4 thrombocytopenia (21). A rare observation has been the development of rhabdomyolysis, which is associated with a high mortality rate and is more frequent in patients with significant liver dysfunction. Different schedules of ET-743 are also being investigated. A 3-hour infusion of ET-743 (1.5 g/m^2) has shown higher response rates (24% clinical benefit rate) with similar dose intensity and rates of myelosuppression. However, this shorter infusion was associated with a higher rate of reversible transaminitis (22). Other schedules currently being examined include a weekly regimen with preliminary evidence of a better toxicity profile. Antitumor activity of ET-743 has also been observed in patients with breast and ovarian cancer, and combination studies with a range of other cytotoxics are ongoing. In addition, the potential for dexamethasone to ameliorate toxicity is being systematically explored.

Bryostatins

Bryostatins are a group of more than 20 macrocyclic lactones derived from the marine bryozoan *Bugula neritina*. Bryostatin 1 was initially isolated in 1982 and found to have antitumor activity against P388 murine leukemia models (23). Initially defined as a group of potential anticancer agents, subsequent work has suggested possible mechanisms of action. Most of the activity of this group of agents is thought to occur via interactions with protein kinase C (PKC), although other mechanisms may well apply as at least one active member of the family has little or no interaction with PKC. Apoptosis modulation occurs via alterations in the ratio of bax to bcl-2 (24) in addition to changes in the phosphorylation status of bcl-2 (25). Bryostatins have been shown to inhibit the activity of P-gp and in addition *MDR1* downregulation has also been documented (26). Bryostatins also have immune modulatory effects altering the cytokine profile and therefore the functionality of many immune effector cells, including T cells and neutrophils (27,28).

Bryostatins have anticancer effects in many cell line models both *in vitro* and *in vivo* (in xenograft models). In addition, promising synergistic activity has been described in a range of xenograft-plus-chemotherapy models, including chronic lymphatic leukemia and fludarabine, CHOP [cyclophosphamide, doxorubicin, vincristine (Oncovin), and prednisone] against lymphoma, Ara C against HL-60 leukemia cells, cisplatin in cervical carcinoma cells, and vincristine against the B cells in Waldenström's macroglobulinemia.

Bryostatin has undergone detailed phase 1 investigations (29–35). A range of different schedules has been assessed, and the least toxic dosage seems to be 25 $\mu g/m^2$ weekly for 3 out of 4 weeks as a 1-hour infusion. Other schedules examined include one 24-hour weekly infusion, two 72-hour weekly infusions, and two 1-hour weekly infusions. The main dose-limiting toxicity for all of these schedules seems to be myalgia. In addition, phlebitis is a common problem due to the ethanol- and polyethylene glycol–containing diluent used. These studies were also able to demonstrate that bryostatin administration increases lymphokine-activated killer cell activity in response to interleukin-2 (IL-2) and modulates PKC activity. There was some evidence in these studies of activity in malignant melanoma, lymphoma, and ovarian cancer, which resulted in progression to phase 2 evaluation.

The phase 2 data to date have been disappointing. Three studies have evaluated patients with metastatic melanoma (36–38) using a variety of schedules (25 $\mu g/m^2$ weekly for 3 out of 4 weeks and 40 $\mu g/m^2$ daily as a 72-hour infusion fortnightly). With the weekly schedule, 2 of 27 patients had stable disease for 9 and 4 months, respectively. Two additional patients demonstrated a reduction in the skin component of their disease. With the two weekly regimens, 1 partial response lasting 7 months was seen in 37 patients. Overall these levels of activity are low; however, there is evidence that IL-2 and bryostatin may have synergistic effects in terms of immune modulation (39,40). It will be interesting to see if clinical responses can be seen in these patients while receiving biotherapy.

Phase 2 studies in patients with relapsed non-Hodgkin's lymphoma have shown 1 complete response, 2 partial responses, and 1 sudden death in a total of 42 patients (41,42). No significant responses have been seen in patients with a range of other tumors including metastatic renal cancer, multiple myeloma, metastatic colorectal cancer, sarcoma, and head/neck cancers (43–47).

Further avenues are being explored, most notably the combination of bryostatin with other chemotherapeutic agents such as paclitaxel and platinum. These studies are ongoing, and only preliminary phase 1 reports have been published in abstract form (48). The results of current ongoing studies will determine whether this family of agents will ever have a role in the clinic.

Dolastatins

Dolastatins are a group of 15 related compounds isolated from the Indian Ocean sea hare *Dolabella auricularia*. They were initially found to strongly inhibit the growth of murine P388 leukemia cells (49). Dolastatin 10 and 15 were found to be most potent and were scheduled for further clinical development; however, research has been hampered by the lack of enough material and their highly lipophillic/water insoluble nature. More water-soluble analogues have been developed including LU103793 and auristatin PE, which are analogues of dolastatin 15 and 10, respectively.

Dolastatins have been shown to be potent inhibitors of tubulin polymerization causing accumulation of cells in metaphase (50,51). Their activity *in vitro* has been well documented in a range of cancer cell lines.

Phase 1 studies of dolastatins have been completed. For dolastatin 10, a maximum tolerated dose of 300 to 400 $\mu g/m^2$ has been defined with the main toxicity being cardiovascular (52,53). In addition, phase 1 studies of dolastatin analogues have shown better toxicity profiles (54–56).

In phase 2 studies, dolastatins have shown little or no activity in a range of tumor types including metastatic colorectal, renal, melanoma, prostate, and non–small cell lung cancers (57–61). Dolastatin analogues are currently in clinical trial, the most advanced in terms of development being LU103793. This agent has shown evidence of activity in malignant melanoma (62) and further studies are awaited.

Didemnin B and Aplidine

Didemnin B, a cyclic depsipeptide isolated from the tunicate *Trididemnum solidum* (63), has shown *in vitro* activity against immortal human tumor cell lines as well as fresh cultured tumor cells (64). Didemnin B was found to be the most potent antiproliferative isoform and was not cell cycle specific (65). It is a very potent inhibitor of protein synthesis (66). Didemnin B was developed further in a clinical setting. Phase 1 studies of didemnin B administered as a bolus infusion once every 4 weeks found significant toxicity with nausea, vomiting, and hepatic enzyme dysfunction. A maximum tolerated dose of 3.47 mg/m^2 was defined when combined with aggressive antiemetic scheduling.

Another phase 1 study of a weekly schedule found significant muscle weakness as the main toxicity (67). Nineteen phase 2 clinical trials of this agent have been published with very disappointing levels of activity in a wide range of solid tumors. Severe neuromuscular toxicity has also been found in a significant proportion of patients (68).

Aplidine is related to didemnin B and is isolated from the Mediterranean tunicate *Aplidium albicans.* Aplidine induces an oxidative stress that is thought to trigger an apoptotic program via activation of the JNK, p38, and ERK kinases (69).

Aplidine has potent anticancer properties *in vitro* (70) and in xenograft tumor models (71). Various schedules of aplidine have been tested in phase 1 studies and reported in abstract form (72–76). Myalgia and weakness are the main dose-limiting toxicities. This toxicity is often associated with a rise in noncardiac creatinine kinase levels as well as type 2 muscular atrophy on biopsy results. L-carnitine coadministration has been shown to counter this toxicity, allowing an up to 40% increase in the aplidine dose. Hepatic enzyme abnormalities and asthenia were also seen; however aplidine seems to have a better toxicity profile than didemnin B. Clinical benefit has been described within these studies in patients with a range of different tumors including non-Hodgkin's lymphoma, renal cancer, and medullary carcinoma of the thyroid. Phase 2 studies are ongoing.

Kahalalide F

This compound is a cyclic depsipeptide, initially isolated from the Hawaiian mollusc *Elysia rufescens,* and under development by PharmaMar. These herbivorous molluscs belong to the Sacoglossans family and feed on algae of the Bryopsis spp. Kahalalide F (KHF) is made by the feeding molluscs and has been shown to act as a chemical defence mechanism preventing algal predation by other marine species (77).

The structure of KHF has been elucidated (78); however, its mechanism of action is not entirely clear. There is evidence to suggest that it interferes with lysosomal membranes, encouraging intracellular acidification and apoptosis (79). In addition, there is evidence of inhibition of ErbB-2 tyrosine kinase activity and inhibition of TGFα gene expression (80). A lyophilized parenteral formulation has been developed to allow clinical administration (81).

Although negative in the NCI COMPARE analysis, KHF has shown *in vitro* activity in hormone-independent, HER-2–positive prostate cancer models (80). In addition, *ex vivo* responses can be seen in a wide range of human tumor types despite prior exposure to conventional chemotherapeutic agents. This suggests a novel mechanism of action and therefore a potentially wide range of oncologic clinical applications.

A phase 1 dose-escalation study in patients with androgen-resistant advanced prostate cancer has been reported in abstract form (82). KHF was given as a 1-hour infusion on days 1 to 5 of a 21-day cycle. The main toxicity was a rapidly reversible transaminitis and mild myalgia. A more than 50% reduction in prostate-specific antigen levels was seen in one patient and was associated with clinical palliative benefit. This study is ongoing as the maximum tolerated dose has not yet been reached. Another phase 1 study has been reported of a weekly 1-hour intravenous infusion. The dose-limiting toxicity of this regimen was asymptomatic grade 4 transaminitis. In addition, pruritus of the hands was commonly reported. Clinical benefit was seen in 3 out of 25 patients (83).

ES-285

ES-285, which is isolated from the North Atlantic mollusc *Spisula polynyma,* is another novel marine compound showing potential as an anticancer agent. Originally called Spisulosine, it is thought to work by interfering with the actin cytoskeleton (84). Work on this compound is still in the preclinical stages; however, wide-ranging anticancer effects have been seen *in vitro* (85). This agent is due to enter clinical trial very soon.

PLANT-DERIVED AGENTS

Plants have proved to be a very important source of pharmacologic substances. Many anticancer agents in daily use today have plant origins. In addition, other important drugs used in oncological practice have similar origins, such as morphine, which was isolated from *Papaver somniferum.* In many cases, plant extracts used in traditional remedies have provided a source from which pharmacologically active agents have been purified.

The vinca alkaloids vinblastine and vincristine were isolated from the Madagascar periwinkle *Cathranthus roseus.* This plant had been used in various cultures to treat diabetes, and attempts to isolate novel antidiabetic agents resulted in the isolation of this class of anticancer agent. Today the vinca alkaloids play an important role in the treatment of a wide range of tumors, particularly childhood tumors, leukemias, and lymphomas.

The bark of the Pacific yew tree *Taxus brevifolia* proved to be the source of the then-novel group of antimitotic agents called taxanes, exemplified by paclitaxel. Although originally isolated through a random collection and screening program between the US Department of Agriculture and NCI, Native Americans have used the tree bark for the treatment of a range of disorders. Additionally, in Asia, leaves of the Taxus species (including *T. baccata)* were being used in alternative treatments for cancer. Taxanes stabilize microtubules and disrupt the spindle. Today the taxanes (paclitaxel and docetaxel) play an important role in the treatment of a range of solid tumors including those of the breast, ovary, and lung. Their role in a range of tumors is currently being defined in large phase 3 studies.

Podophyllotoxin genus has long been used in American and Asian cultures for the treatment of warts and skin cancers. Podophyllotoxin was isolated from this genus and epipodophyllotoxin (an isomer of podophyllotoxin) was synthesized shortly afterwards. Semisynthetic derivatives of epipodophyllotoxin include etoposide and teniposide. These drugs block the cell cycle in G1 and S phase and play an important role in the treatment of a range of tumors. They work by inhibiting topoisomerase II, stabilizing cleavage complexes and resultant DNA breaks.

Camptothecin, isolated from the Chinese ornamental tree *Camptotheca acuminata*, was initially considered to be an exceptionally promising anticancer agent. However, early enthusiasm was tempered by the documentation of high and unacceptable toxicity including myelosuppression, severe diarrhea, and hemorrhagic cystitis. Semisynthetic derivatives of camptothecin have a much better toxicity profile and include topotecan and irinotecan, both of which inhibit DNA topoisomerase I, an enzyme involved in reducing the torsional stress of supercoiled DNA when undergoing processes such as replication, repair, transcription, and recombination. Activity has been shown in a range of tumor types. Topotecan is an acceptable second-line choice for the treatment of epithelial ovarian cancer (86). Irinotecan is used in combination with fluorouracil in the first-line treatment of colorectal cancer (87). Newer derivatives of camptothecin are in development (88,89), and the field has recently been reviewed (90).

A range of plant-derived products is currently under active development as potential anticancer agents. Homoharringtonine is a plant alkaloid isolated from the Chinese tree *Cephalotaxus harringtonia*. It has been shown to have activity in a range of hematologic malignancies including acute myeloid leukemia, acute promyelocytic leukemia, myelodysplastic syndromes, and chronic myeloid leukemia (91). Initially toxic in terms of hypotension and cardiac arrhythmias, this has been addressed by changing delivery schedules. Homoharringtonine has been shown to inhibit protein synthesis and block cell cycle progression (92). Although still an investigational agent, newer semisynthetic derivatives may have fewer side effects with increased efficacy.

Elliptinium is derived from the Fijian medicinal plant *Bleekeria vitensis*. It has also been found in a range of plants from the same genus (*Apocynaceae*). It has an anticancer effect through actions as a DNA intercalater and DNA topoisomerase II inhibitor. It has shown moderate activity in early studies in metastatic breast cancer (93–95). The main limitation to the clinical development of this agent has been its significant toxicity in terms of xerostomia and immune-mediated hemolysis due to immunoglobulin M antielliptinium antibodies.

Ipomeanol is a pneumotoxic furan derivative from the sweet potato *Ipomoeca batatas* when infected with the fungus *Fusarium solani*. It is converted into DNA-binding metabolites by the cytochrome P-450 group of enzymes predominantly within pulmonary Clara cells. Although *in vitro* this agent has activity against lung cancer cell lines, the results of clinical studies have been disappointing (96–98).

Combretastatins are a group of agents isolated from the African bush willow. Combretastatin A4-phosphaste (CA4P) is the most advanced in terms of clinical development. It has potent anticancer properties *in vitro*. The parent drug is rapidly metabolized from CA4-phosphate to CA4 and is thought to work via binding to the colchicine-binding site of tubulin, thereby inhibiting tubulin polymerization. In addition, it induces a rapid vascular shutdown via endothelial cell apoptosis within the tumor vasculature (99,100). One phase 1 study has been published (101). The main toxicity was tumor pain and the development of acute coronary syndromes in 2 of 25 patients; however, one patient with anaplastic thyroid cancer had a complete response. Several CA4P analogues have been developed and are entering clinical trials (102).

MICROBIAL-DERIVED AGENTS

Microbial organisms have been an important source of anticancer agents. Many chemotherapeutic agents in routine use have been derived from antibiotics. These include the anthracyclines (e.g., doxorubicin, danuorubicin, epirubicin, and idarubicin), bleomycin, actinomycin, and mitomycin. These agents play a critical role in the current treatment of a wide range of hematologic and solid tumors. A range of compounds derived from microbial sources is also currently under development and one of these will be discussed here.

Epothilone A (EpoA) and epothilone B (EpoB) are macrolides initially isolated from the myxobacterium *Sorangium cellulossum* in 1993 and recognized for their antifungal properties (103). Synthesis was described shortly afterwards (104), and it was soon recognized that these epothilones were potent inhibitors of the cell growth of a range of human cancer cell lines. Epothilones act by inducing microtubule stabilization and can competitively inhibit ^{3}H paclitaxel binding to microtubules, suggesting a common binding site (105,106). These compounds are interesting because in addition to being potent antiproliferative agents in taxane-sensitive models, high levels of anticancer activity have been documented in taxane-resistant models. This has been described in MDR phenotype cells overexpressing P-gp as well as cell lines with β-tubulin mutations (107).

Two closely related epothilone analogues have been clinically evaluated (EpoB and BMS-247550). Phase 1 studies of EpoB utilized both thrice-weekly and weekly schedules. In both cases, the drug is administered as a 5-minute intravenous bolus. The maximum tolerated doses are 6 mg/m^2 and 2.5 mg/m^2 for the thrice-weekly and weekly regimens, respectively. In both schedules, the main toxicity was diarrhea. In addition, nausea, fatigue, and sensory neuropathy were seen. Importantly, hair loss was not an issue unlike the case of taxanes (108,109). Phase 1 data on BMS-247550 were initially reported using a 1 hour infusion every 3 weeks in a series of abstracts presented at the 2001 and 2002 meetings of the American Society of Clinical Oncology. Significant problems were seen in terms of neurotoxicity, myelosuppression, and hyper-

sensitivity due to its Cremophor EL–containing formulation (110,111). These toxicity problems have been reduced by the use of a 1 hour infusion on days 1 to 5 every 3 weeks. A maximum tolerated dosage of 6 mg/m^2 daily without granulocyte colony stimulating factor (GCSF) support has been defined, the main toxicity being myelosuppression (112).

Phase 2 studies of BMS-247550 have recently been reported in abstract form. These studies all used the d1q21 schedule. Despite significant toxicity, evidence of activity was seen. Partial responses were seen in 53%, 10%, and 18% of patients with taxane-naïve metastatic breast cancer, metastatic gastric cancer, and non–small cell lung cancer, respectively (113–115). Although these studies are ongoing and numbers were small, they included a group of heavily pretreated patients. Phase 2 EpoB data are currently awaited.

CONCLUSION

Although this is the age of the molecularly targeted, rationally designed drug, there is no doubt that the natural environment continues to provide a rich source of novel anticancer agents. Organic material collected from the environment is likely to continue to be a source of new drugs. In addition, as we develop extensive libraries of these compounds, they will provide a useful reference for testing novel molecular targets. The structural analysis of these agents lends to the development of synthetic analogues, allowing minimization of the environmental impact. This important area of work should not be ignored in the new postgenomic age.

REFERENCES

1. Cragg GM, Newman DJ, Weiss RB. Coral reefs, forests, and thermal vents: the worldwide exploration of nature for novel antitumor agents. *Semin Oncol* 1997;24:156–163.
2. Bergmann W, Burke DC. Contributions to the study of marine products. XXXIX. The nucleosides of sponges. III. Spongothymidine and spongouridine. *J Org Chem* 1955;20:1501–1507.
3. Bergmann W, Feeney RJ. Contributions to the study of marine products. XXXII. The nucleosides of sponges. *J Org Chem* 1951;16:981–987.
4. Rinehart KL. Antitumor compounds from tunicates. *Med Res Rev* 2000;20:1–27.
5. Pommier Y, Kohlhagen G, Bailly C, et al. DNA sequence- and structure-selective alkylation of guanine N2 in the DNA minor groove by ecteinascidin 743, a potent antitumor compound from the Caribbean tunicate Ecteinascidia turbinata. *Biochemistry* 1996;35:13303–13309.
6. Zewail-Foote M, Hurley LH. Ecteinascidin 743: a minor groove alkylator that bends DNA toward the major groove. *J Med Chem* 1999;42:2493–2497.
7. Moore BM, Seaman FC, Hurley LH. NMR-Based Model of an Ecteinascidin 743-DNA adduct. *J Am Chem Soc* 1997;119:5476–5477.
8. Li WW, Takahashi N, Jhanwar S, et al. Sensitivity of soft tissue sarcoma cell lines to chemotherapeutic agents: identification of ecteinascidin-743 as a potent cytotoxic agent. *Clin Cancer Res* 2001;7:2908–2911.
9. Takebayashi Y, Pourquier P, Zimonjic DB, et al. Antiproliferative activity of ecteinascidin 743 is dependent upon transcription-coupled nucleotide-excision repair. *Nat Med* 2001;7:961–966.
10. Gorfajn BD, Jin S, Hu Z, et al. Et743, a novel transcription-targeted chemotherapeutic that inhibits activation of the Mdr1 promoter by multiple inducers. *Proceed Am Assoc Cancer Res 2000*. Abstract A5111.
11. Minuzzo M, Marchini S, Broggini M, et al. Interference of transcriptional activation by the antineoplastic drug ecteinascidin-743. *Proc Natl Acad Sci U S A* 2000;97:6780–6784.
12. Jin S, Gorfajn B, Faircloth G, et al. Ecteinascidin 743, a transcription-targeted chemotherapeutic that inhibits

MDR1 activation. *Proc Natl Acad Sci U S A* 2000;97: 6775–6779.

13. Synold TW, Dussault I, Forman BM. The orphan nuclear receptor SXR coordinately regulates drug metabolism and efflux. *Nat Med* 2001;7:584–590.

14. Faircloth GT, Grant W, Jimeno J, et al. Dexamethasone potentiates the activity of Ecteinascidin 743 in preclinical melanoma and osteosarcoma models. *Proc Am Assoc Cancer Res* 2002. Abstract 379.

15. Zewail-Foote M, Li VS, Kohn H, et al. The inefficiency of incisions of ecteinascidin 743-DNA adducts by the UvrABC nuclease and the unique structural feature of the DNA adducts can be used to explain the repair-dependent toxicities of this antitumor agent. *Chem Biol* 2001;8:1033–1049.

16. Damia G, Silvestri S, Carrassa L, et al. Unique pattern of ET-743 activity in different cellular systems with defined deficiencies in DNA-repair pathways. *Int J Cancer* 2001;92:583–588.

17. D'Incalci M, Erba E, Damia G, et al. The combination of ET-743 and cisplatin (DDP): from a molecular pharmacology study to a phase I clinical trial. *Proc Am Assoc Cancer Res 2002* Abstract 404.

18. Kanzaki A, Takebayashi Y, Ren X, et al. Overcoming multidrug resistance in P-Glycoprotein/MDR1-overexpressing cell lines by Ecteinascidin 743. *Proc Am Assoc Cancer Res 2002*. Abstract 4726.

19. Taamma A, Misset JL, Riofrio M, et al. Phase I and pharmacokinetic study of ecteinascidin-743, a new marine compound, administered as a 24-hour continuous infusion in patients with solid tumors. *J Clin Oncol* 2001;19:1256–1265.

20. Delaloge S, Yovine A, Taamma A, et al. Ecteinascidin-743: a marine-derived compound in advanced, pretreated sarcoma patients: preliminary evidence of activity. *J Clin Oncol* 2001;19:1248–1255.

21. Ruiz-Casado A, Lopez-Martin JA, Nieto A, et al. Ecteinascidin in heavily pretreated advanced sarcoma patients as a compassionate basis. *Proc Am Soc Clin Oncol 2002*. Abstract 1631.

22. George S, Maki RG, Harmon D, et al. Phase II study of ectinascidin-743 (ET-743) given by a 3-hour infusion in patients (pts) with soft tissue sarcomas (STS) failing prior chemotherapies. *Proc Am Soc Clin Oncol 2002*. Abstract A1630.

23. Pettit GR, Herald CL, Doubek DL, et al. Isolation and structure of bryostatin-1. *J Am Chem Soc* 1982;104: 6846–6848.

24. Mohammad RM, Beck FW, Katato K, et al. Potentiation of 2-chlorodeoxyadenosine activity by bryostatin 1 in the resistant chronic lymphocytic leukemia cell line (WSU-CLL): association with increased ratios of dCK/5′-NT and Bax/Bcl-2. *Biol Chem* 1998;379: 1253–1261.

25. May WS, Tyler PG, Ito T, et al. Interleukin-3 and bryostatin-1 mediate hyperphosphorylation of BCL2 alpha in association with suppression of apoptosis. *J Biol Chem* 1994;269:26865–26870.

26. Al-Katib AM, Smith MR, Kamanda WS, et al. Bryostatin 1 down-regulates mdr1 and potentiates vincristine cytotoxicity in diffuse large cell lymphoma xenografts. *Clin Cancer Res* 1998;4:1305–1314.

27. Berkow RL, Schlabach L, Dodson R, et al. In vivo administration of the anticancer agent bryostatin 1 activates platelets and neutrophils and modulates

protein kinase C activity. *Cancer Res* 1993;53: 2810–2815.

28. Trenn G, Pettit GR, Takayama H, et al. Immunomodulating properties of a novel series of protein kinase C activators. The bryostatins. *J Immunol* 1988;140: 433–439.

29. Prendiville J, Crowther D, Thatcher N, et al. A phase I study of intravenous bryostatin 1 in patients with advanced cancer. *Br J Cancer* 1993;68:418–424.

30. Philip PA, Rea D, Thavasu P, et al. Phase I study of bryostatin 1: assessment of interleukin 6 and tumor necrosis factor alpha induction in vivo. The Cancer Research Campaign Phase I Committee. *J Natl Cancer Inst* 1993;85:1812–1818.

31. Scheid C, Prendiville J, Jayson G, et al. Immunomodulation in patients receiving intravenous Bryostatin 1 in a phase I clinical study: comparison with effects of Bryostatin 1 on lymphocyte function in vitro. *Cancer Immunol Immunother* 1994;39:223–230.

32. Jayson GC, Crowther D, Prendiville J, et al. A phase I trial of bryostatin 1 in patients with advanced malignancy using a 24 hour intravenous infusion. *Br J Cancer* 1995;72:461–468.

33. Varterasian ML, Mohammad RM, Eilender DS, et al. Phase I study of bryostatin 1 in patients with relapsed non-Hodgkin's lymphoma and chronic lymphocytic leukemia. *J Clin Oncol* 1998;16:56–62.

34. Grant S, Roberts J, Poplin E, et al. Phase Ib trial of bryostatin 1 in patients with refractory malignancies. *Clin Cancer Res* 1998;4:611–618.

35. Weitman S, Langevin AM, Berkow RL, et al. A Phase I trial of bryostatin-1 in children with refractory solid tumors: a Pediatric Oncology Group study. *Clin Cancer Res* 1999;5:2344–2348.

36. Propper DJ, Macaulay V, O'Byrne KJ, et al. A phase II study of bryostatin 1 in metastatic malignant melanoma. *Br J Cancer* 1998;78:1337–1341.

37. Gonzalez R, Ebbinghaus S, Henthorn TK, et al. Treatment of patients with metastatic melanoma with bryostatin-1: a phase II study. *Melanoma Res* 1999;9: 599–606.

38. Bedikian AY, Plager C, Stewart JR, et al. Phase II evaluation of bryostatin-1 in metastatic melanoma. *Melanoma Res* 2001;11:183–188.

39. Curiel RE, Garcia CS, Farooq L, et al. Bryostatin-1 and IL-2 synergize to induce IFN-gamma expression in human peripheral blood T cells: implications for cancer immunotherapy. *J Immunol* 2001;167: 4828–4837.

40. Igor ED, Rottschafer S, Carmen G, et al. Bryostatin-1 and low-dose interleukin-2 (IL-2) is as efficient as high-dose IL-2 in reducing B16-BL6 melanoma growth in vivo without the acute toxicity (abstract). *Proc Am Soc Clin Oncol 1999*.

41. Varterasian ML, Mohammad RM, Shurafa MS, et al. Phase II trial of bryostatin 1 in patients with relapsed low-grade non-Hodgkin's lymphoma and chronic lymphocytic leukemia. *Clin Cancer Res* 2000;6:825–828.

42. Blackhall FH, Ranson M, Radford JA, et al. A phase II trial of bryostatin 1 in patients with non-Hodgkin's lymphoma. *Br J Cancer* 2001;84:465–469.

43. Pagliaro L, Daliani D, Amato R, et al. A phase II trial of bryostatin-1 for patients with metastatic renal cell carcinoma. *Cancer* 2000;89:615–618.

44. Zonder JA, Shields AF, Zalupski M, et al. A phase II trial of bryostatin 1 in the treatment of metastatic colorectal cancer. *Clin Cancer Res* 2001;7:38–42.

45. Varterasian ML, Pemberton PA, Hulburd K, et al. Phase II study of bryostatin 1 in patients with relapsed multiple myeloma. *Invest New Drugs* 2001; 19:245–247.

46. Brockstein B, Samuels B, Humerickhouse R, et al. Phase II studies of bryostatin-1 in patients with advanced sarcoma and advanced head and neck cancer. *Invest New Drugs* 2001;19:249–254.

47. Pfister DG, McCaffrey J, Zahalsky AJ, et al. A phase II trial of bryostatin-1 in patients with metastatic or recurrent squamous cell carcinoma of the head and neck. *Invest New Drugs* 2002;20:123–127.

48. Clamp A, Jayson G. The clinical development of the bryostatins. *Anticancer Drugs* 2002;13:673–683.

49. Miyazaki K, Kobayashi M, Natsume T, et al. Synthesis and antitumor activity of novel dolastatin 10 analogs. *Chem Pharm Bull (Tokyo)* 1995;43:1706–1718.

50. Bai R, Pettit GR, Hamel E. Dolastatin 10, a powerful cytostatic peptide derived from a marine animal. Inhibition of tubulin polymerization mediated through the vinca alkaloid binding domain. *Biochem Pharmacol* 1990;39:1941–1949.

51. Pathak S, Multani AS, Ozen M, et al. Dolastatin-10 induces polyploidy, telomeric associations and apoptosis in a murine melanoma cell line. *Oncol Rep* 1998; 5:373–376.

52. Pitot HC, McElroy EAJ, Reid JM, et al. Phase I trial of dolastatin-10 (NSC 376128) in patients with advanced solid tumors. *Clin Cancer Res* 1999;5:525–531.

53. Madden T, Tran HT, Beck D, et al. Novel marine-derived anticancer agents: a phase I clinical, pharmacological, and pharmacodynamic study of dolastatin 10 (NSC 376128) in patients with advanced solid tumors. *Clin Cancer Res* 2000;6:1293–1301.

54. Villalona-Calero MA, Baker SD, Hammond L, et al. Phase I and pharmacokinetic study of the water-soluble dolastatin 15 analog LU103793 in patients with advanced solid malignancies. *J Clin Oncol* 1998;16: 2770–2779.

55. Supko JG, Lynch TJ, Clark JW, et al. A phase I clinical and pharmacokinetic study of the dolastatin analogue cemadotin administered as a 5-day continuous intravenous infusion. *Cancer Chemother Pharmacol* 2000;46:319–328.

56. Michaelson MD, Ryan DP, Fram R, et al. A phase I clinical trial of ILX651, a Dolastatin analog, administered as a 30-minute intravenous infusion every other day × 3 doses every 21 days in patients with advanced solid tumours. *Proc Am Soc Clin Oncol 2002*. Abstract A414.

57. Aguayo A, Kraut E, Moore D, et al. Phase II study of Dolostatin 10 administered intravenously every 21 days to patients (pts) with metastatic colorectal cancer (CRC). *Proc Am Soc Clin Oncol 2000*. Abstract A1127.

58. Pitot HC, Frytak S, Croghan GA, et al. Phase II study of Dolostatin-10 (dola-10) in patients (pts) with advanced renal cell carcinoma. *Proc Am Soc Clin Oncol 2002*. Abstract A2409

59. Margolin K, Longmage J, Gandara D, et al. Dolastatin-10 (DOLA) in metastatic melanoma (MEL): A phase II trial of the California Cancer Consortium. *Proc Am Soc Clin Oncol 2000*. Abstract A2243.

60. Vaishampayan U, Glode M, Du W, et al. Phase II study of dolastatin-10 in patients with hormone-refractory metastatic prostate adenocarcinoma. *Clin Cancer Res* 2000;6:4205–4208.

61. Krug LM, Miller VA, Kalemkerian GP, et al. Phase II study of dolastatin-10 in patients with advanced non-small-cell lung cancer. *Ann Oncol* 2000;11:227–228.

62. Smyth J, Boneterre ME, Schellens J, et al. Activity of the dolastatin analogue, LU103793, in malignant melanoma. *Ann Oncol* 2001;12:509–511.

63. Rinehart KLJ, Gloer JB, Hughes RGJ, et al. Didemnins: antiviral and antitumor depsipeptides from a Caribbean tunicate. *Science* 1981;212:933–935.

64. Jiang TL, Liu RH, Salmon SE. Antitumor activity of didemnin B in the human tumor stem cell assay. *Cancer Chemother Pharmacol* 1983;11:1–4.

65. Crampton SL, Adams EG, Kuentzel SL, et al. Biochemical and cellular effects of didemnins A and B. *Cancer Res* 1984;44:1796–1801.

66. Urdiales JL, Morata P, Nunez DC, et al. Antiproliferative effect of dehydrodidemnin B (DDB), a depsipeptide isolated from Mediterranean tunicates. *Cancer Lett* 1996;102:31–37.

67. Maroun JA, Stewart D, Verma S, et al. Phase I clinical study of didemnin B. A National Cancer Institute of Canada Clinical Trials Group study. *Invest New Drugs* 1998;16:51–56.

68. Shin DM, Holoye PY, Murphy WK, et al. Phase I/II clinical trial of didemnin B in non-small-cell lung cancer: neuromuscular toxicity is dose-limiting. *Cancer Chemother Pharmacol* 1991;29:145–149.

69. Garcia-Fernandez LF, Losada A, Alcaide V, et al. Aplidin induces the mitochondrial apoptotic pathway via oxidative stress-mediated JNK and p38 activation and protein kinase C delta. *Oncogene* 2002;21:7533–7544.

70. Depenbrock H, Peter R, Faircloth GT, et al. In vitro activity of aplidine, a new marine-derived anti-cancer compound, on freshly explanted clonogenic human tumour cells and haematopoietic precursor cells. *Br J Cancer* 1998;78:739–744.

71. Faircloth G, Grant W, Nam S, et al. Schedule dependency on Aplidin, a marine depsipeptide with antitumor activity. *Proc Am Assoc Cancer Res 1999*. Abstract 40: 2612.

72. Maria E, Gil C, Twelves C, et al. Phase I clinical and pharmacokinetic study of the marine compound aplidine (APL) administered as a 3 hour infusion every 2 weeks. *Proc Am Soc Clin Oncol 2002*. Abstract A422.

73. Bowman A, Izquierdo M, Jodrell D, et al. Phase I clinical and pharmacokinetic (PK) study of the marine compound aplidine (APL), administered as a 1 hour weekly infusion. *Proc Am Soc Clinl Oncol 2001*. Abstract A476.

74. Armand JP, Ady-Vago N, Faivre S, et al. Phase I and Pharmacokinetic study of aplidine (APL) given as a 24-hour continuous infusion every other week (q2w) in patients (pts) with solid tumor (ST) and lymphoma (NHL). *Proc Am Soc Clin Oncol 2001*. Abstract A477.

75. Anthoney A, Paz-Ares L, Twelves C, et al. Phase I and pharmacokinetic (PK) study of aplidine (APL) using a 24-hour, weekly schedule. *Proc Am Soc Clin Oncol 2000*. Abstract A734.

76. Maroun JA, Goel R, Stewart DJ, et al. Phase I study of aplidine in a 5 day bolus Q 3 weeks in patients with

solid tumors and lymphomas. *Proc Am Soc Clin Oncol 2001*. Abstract A2082.

77. Becerro MA, Goetz G, Paul VJ, et al. Chemical defenses of the sacoglossan mollusk Elysia rufescens and its host Alga bryopsis sp. *J Chem Ecol* 2001;27: 2287–2299.

78. Lopez-Macia A, Jimenez JC, Royo M, et al. Synthesis and structure determination of kahalalide F (1,2). *J Am Chem Soc* 2001;123:11398–11401.

79. Garcia-Rocha M, Bonay P, Avila J. The antitumoral compound Kahalalide F acts on cell lysosomes. *Cancer Lett* 1996;99:43–50.

80. Faircloth G, Grant W, Smith B, et al. Preclinical development of Kahalalide F, a new marine compound selected for clinical studies. *Proc Am Assoc Cancer Res 2000*. Abstract A3823.

81. Nuijen B, Bouma M, Talsma H, et al. Development of a lyophilized parenteral pharmaceutical formulation of the investigational polypeptide marine anticancer agent kahalalide F. *Drug Dev Ind Pharm* 2001;27: 767–780.

82. Schellens JH, Rademaker-Lakhai J, Horenblas S, et al. Phase I and pharmacokinetic study of Kahalalide F in patients with advanced androgen resistant prostate cancer. *Proc Am Soc Clin Oncol 2002*. Abstract A451.

83. Ciruelos C, Trigo T, Pardo J, et al. A phase I and pharmocokinetic (PK) study with Kahalalide F (KF) in patients (pts) with advanced solid tumors (AST) with a continuous weekly (w) 1-hour iv infusion schedule (abstract). *Eur J Cancer* 2002;38:S33.

84. Cuadros R, Montejo dG, Wandosell F, et al. The marine compound spisulosine, an inhibitor of cell proliferation, promotes the disassembly of actin stress fibers. *Cancer Lett* 2000;152:23–29.

85. Jimeno JJ, Garcia-Gravalos D, Avila J, et al. ES-285, a marine natural product with activity against solid tumours. *Proc AACR-NCI-EORTC International Conference, 1999*.Washington. Abstract A314.

86. Gordon AN, Fleagle JT, Guthrie D, et al. Recurrent epithelial ovarian carcinoma: a randomized phase III study of pegylated liposomal doxorubicin versus topotecan. *J Clin Oncol* 2001;19:3312–3322.

87. Saltz LB, Cox JV, Blanke C, et al. Irinotecan plus fluorouracil and leucovorin for metastatic colorectal cancer. Irinotecan Study Group. *N Engl J Med* 2000; 343: 905–914.

88. Van Hattum AH, Schluper HM, Hausheer FH, et al. Novel camptothecin derivative BNP1350 in experimental human ovarian cancer: determination of efficacy and possible mechanisms of resistance. *Int J Cancer* 2002;100:22–29.

89. Prijovich ZM, Chen BM, Leu YL, et al. Anti-tumour activity and toxicity of the new prodrug 9-aminocamptothecin glucuronide (9ACG) in mice. *Br J Cancer* 2002;86:1634–1638.

90. Garcia-Carbonero R, Supko JG. Current perspectives on the clinical experience, pharmacology, and continued development of the camptothecins. *Clin Cancer Res* 2002;8:641–661.

91. Kantarjian HM, Talpaz M, Smith TL, et al. Homoharringtonine and low-dose cytarabine in the management of late chronic-phase chronic myelogenous leukemia. *J Clin Oncol* 2000;18:3513–3521.

92. Zhou DC, Zittoun R, Marie JP. Homoharringtonine: an effective new natural product in cancer chemotherapy. *Bull Cancer* 1995;82:987–995.

93. Rouesse J, Spielmann M, Turpin F, et al. Phase II study of elliptinium acetate salvage treatment of advanced breast cancer. *Eur J Cancer* 1993;29A:856–859.

94. Kayitalire L, Thomas F, Le Chevalier T, et al. Phase II study of a combination of elliptinium and vinblastine in metastatic breast cancer. *Invest New Drugs* 1992;10: 303–307.

95. Juret P, Couette JE, Delozier T, et al. [Hydroxy-9-methyl-2-ellipticinium (NSC 264-137) for osseous metastases from breast cancer. A 4 year experience (author's translation)]. *Bull Cancer* 1981;68:224–231.

96. Rowinsky EK, Noe DA, Ettinger DS, et al. Phase I and pharmacological study of the pulmonary cytotoxin 4-ipomeanol on a single dose schedule in lung cancer patients: hepatotoxicity is dose limiting in humans. *Cancer Res* 1993;53:1794–1801.

97. Kasturi VK, Dearing MP, Piscitelli SC, et al. Phase I study of a five-day dose schedule of 4-Ipomeanol in patients with non-small cell lung cancer. *Clin Cancer Res* 1998;4:2095–2102.

98. Lakhanpal S, Donehower RC, Rowinsky EK. Phase II study of 4-ipomeanol, a naturally occurring alkylating furan, in patients with advanced hepatocellular carcinoma. *Invest New Drugs* 2001;19:69–76.

99. Dark GG, Hill SA, Prise VE, et al. Combretastatin A-4, an agent that displays potent and selective toxicity toward tumor vasculature. *Cancer Res* 1997;57: 1829–1834.

100. Iyer S, Chaplin DJ, Rosenthal DS, et al. Induction of apoptosis in proliferating human endothelial cells by the tumor-specific antiangiogenesis agent combretastatin A-4. *Cancer Res* 1998;58:4510–4514.

101. Dowlati A, Robertson K, Cooney M, et al. A phase I pharmacokinetic and translational study of the novel vascular targeting agent combretastatin a-4 phosphate on a single-dose intravenous schedule in patients with advanced cancer. *Cancer Res* 2002;62:3408–3416.

102. Tozer GM, Kanthou C, Parkins CS, et al. The biology of the combretastatins as tumour vascular targeting agents. *Int J Exp Pathol* 2002;83:21–38.

103. Gerth K, Bedorf N, Hofle G, et al. Epothilons A and B: antifungal and cytotoxic compounds from Sorangium cellulosum (Myxobacteria). Production, physicochemical and biological properties. *J Antibiot (Tokyo)* 1996;49:560–563.

104. Nicolaou KC, Winssinger N, Pastor J, et al. Synthesis of epothilones A and B in solid and solution phase. *Nature* 1997;387:268–272.

105. Kowalski RJ, Giannakakou P, Hamel E. Activities of the microtubule-stabilizing agents epothilones A and B with purified tubulin and in cells resistant to paclitaxel (Taxol®). *J Biol Chem* 1997;272:2534–2541.

106. Giannakakou P, Gussio R, Nogales E, et al. A common pharmacophore for epothilone and taxanes: molecular basis for drug resistance conferred by tubulin mutations in human cancer cells. *Proc Natl Acad Sci U S A* 2000;97:2904–2909.

107. Giannakakou P, Sackett DL, Kang YK, et al. Paclitaxel-resistant human ovarian cancer cells have mutant beta-tubulins that exhibit impaired paclitaxel-driven polymerization. *J Biol Chem* 1997;272:17118–17125.

108. O'Neill V, Calvert P, Campbell S, et al. Phase I clinical and pharmacokinetic study of EPO906 (Epothilone B), given every three weeks, to patients with advanced solid tumors. *Proc Am Soc Clin Oncol 2000*. Abstract A829.

109. Oza A, Moore M, Siu L, et al. A phase I and pharma-
     cologic trial of weekly Epothilone B in patients with
     advanced malignancies. *Proc Am Soc Clin Oncol 2000*.
     Abstract A921.
110. Spriggs D, Soignet S, Bienvenu B, et al. Phase I first in
     man study of the Epothilone B analog BMS-247550 in
     patients with advanced cancer. *Proc Am Soc Clin On-
     col 2001*. Abstract A428.
111. LoRusso PM, Woznaik AJ, Flaherty LE, et al. Phase I
     clinical trial of BMS-247550 (aka Epothilone B ana-
     log;NSC710428) in adult patients with advanced solid
     tumors. *Proc Am Soc Clin Oncol 2001*. Abstract A2125.
112. Agrawal M, Kotz H, Abraham J, et al. A phase I clini-
     cal trial of BMS 247550 (NSC 71028), an epothilone B
     derivative, in patients with refractory neoplasms. *Proc
     Am Soc Clin Oncol* 2002. Abstract A410.
113. Roche H, Delord JP, Bunnel CA, et al. Phase II studies
     of the novel Epothilone BMS-247550 in patients (pts)
     with taxane-naive or taxane-refractory metastatic
     breast cancer. *Proc Am Soc Clin Oncol 2002*. Abstract
     A223.
114. Ajani JA, Shah MA, Bokemeyer C, et al. Phase II study
     of the novel epothilone BMS-247550 in patients (pts)
     with metastatic gastric adenocarcinoma previously
     treated with a taxane. *Proc Am Soc Clin Onco, 2002*.
     Abstract A619.
115. Delbaldo C, Lara PN, Vansteenkiste J, et al. Phase II
     study of the novel Epothilone BMS-247550 in patients
     (pts) with recurrent or metastatic non-small cell lung
     cancer (NSCLC) who have failed first line platinum
     based chemotherapy. *Proc Am Soc Clin Oncol 2002*.
     Abstract A1211.

3

History of the National Cancer Institute Drug Discovery Program

Edward A. Sausville and Jill I. Johnson

Developmental Therapeutics Program, Division of Cancer Treatment and Diagnosis, National Cancer Institute, Rockville, Maryland 20852

A shift is occurring in the methods used to discover anticancer drugs. Historically, "empirical" screens in which evidence of toxicity for tumor cells growing in tissue culture or in animals introduced enthusiasm that a compound might be useful as an antineoplastic agent. The drug's structure, dose, and administration schedule were then optimized in animal models responsive to the drug. Toxicology testing defined starting dose levels that could safely be used in a human clinical trial. This path did not necessarily consider the mechanism of action of the agent as an important feature in the discovery and development process. The relation of the pharmacologic features of the agent to molecular pharmacodynamic measures of drug action at the tumor site also was not considered as an important aspect in qualifying an agent for study.

Based on increased understanding and knowledge of the causative factors involved in malignancy, a shift to a more "rational" approach to drug development is occurring in the cancer drug discovery and development community. Primary assays for the selection of a lead drug structure are developed with a particular molecular target in mind. The strength of a target's importance is conveyed by an understanding of its role in the molecular "economy" of a tumor. The first screen for drug activity may occur at the level of a pure target, either as a biochemical reagent or using cells that have been engineered to overexpress the target or target-containing pathway. Drug optimization relies on understanding the pharmacology of the drug in relation to its effect on its respective target in animals, rather than simply on defining maximal tolerated dose activities in animals. Then, at a relatively late stage in the molecule's development, there can occur a focused *in vivo* efficacy evaluation in well-characterized animal models, again measuring the drug's effect on its cellular or biochemical target, as well as calibrating evidence of a potentially useful effect on tumor growth or progression.

The basis for these two potentially competing strategies in cancer drug development stems in part from the reality that prior to the modern elucidation of the basis for deregulated cancer cell growth, empirical tumor shrinkage was all that could be followed, and empirical activity *in vivo* was viewed as predictive of antitumor activity in humans. Even now, with use of "targeted" assays and engineered experimental tumor models, the most rationally conceived drug molecule may fail because of mutational changes "downstream" from its intended target, or metabolic features of tumors not allowing the drug to reach its target. Thus, one cannot yet view cancer drug discovery and development as totally "rational," as empiricism must at some level enter into the definition of new lead structures directed against biochemical targets, or in selecting leads that perform optimally in animals. On the other hand, the wealth of biochemical and genetic information defining cancer cell biology will lead to exciting new opportunities for clinical trials.

FORMER SCREENING PARADIGMS

The numbers of compounds tested at each phase of the development cycle decrease as the time, cost, and criteria for activity are continually refined. Various experimental animal and nonanimal models have been utilized in the past 50 years to select agents for evaluation as clinical candidates. The designs were based on the theory that empirically defined antitumor activity in a model, either cell or animal based, would translate into some likelihood of activity against human cancer. The first anticancer drug used in human clinical trials was nitrogen mustard, which was originally developed as an offensive weapon for use in World War I. Observations that nitrogen mustard impeded the growth of rapidly dividing cells and inhibited the development of induced tumors in animals led to the first anticancer chemotherapeutic human clinical trial in 1942 (1).

The National Cancer Institute (NCI) was created by President Franklin Roosevelt in 1937 with the signing of the National Cancer Institute Act. Support for cancer research at that time consisted of grants-in-aid and fellowships for cancer researchers. In 1946, the cancer control program appropriated money to the states in support of cancer control activities in six areas: biology, biochemistry, biophysics, chemotherapy, epidemiology, and pathology. The year 1953 witnessed the creation of the clinical research program at the Bethesda-based Clinical Center. In 1955, the Cancer Chemotherapy National Service Center (CCNSC) was established to coordinate the first national and voluntary cancer chemotherapy program, which was funded to acquire and screen potential anticancer therapeutic agents in appropriate models. The National Cancer Act of 1971 led to the establishment of four divisions within the NCI: Cancer Biology and Diagnosis, Cancer Cause and Prevention, Cancer Grants, and Cancer Treatment. The Division of Cancer Treatment has been restructured into the Division of Cancer Treatment and Diagnosis, of which the Developmental Therapeutics Program (DTP) is a part.

The stated mission of the DTP, derived from the functional role of the CCNSC, was to acquire chemical compounds and perform preclinical evaluations of these materials as potential cancer chemotherapy agents. From 1955 until 1998, the DTP maintained a drug discovery and development pipeline that began with the acquisition of 10,000 to 40,000 compounds per year for primary screening in murine tumor models, and had the goal of selecting at least five to eight candidates per year for phase 1 clinical trials (Fig. 3.1). Synthetic compounds, or purified "natural products" from plants, microorganisms, or native species, were submitted voluntarily by academic and industrial researchers from around the world. The program has acquired more than 500,000 samples of materials, both laboratory synthesized and pure natural products. Additionally, more than 50,000 plant and 10,000 marine samples have been collected and extracted.

The choice of specific mouse models was based primarily in response to agents already identified as clinically active (2,3). Initially, three transplanted mouse tumor models were used: Sarcoma 180, Carcinoma 755, and Leukemia L1210. The program was altered in 1960 to retain L1210, which was thought to be the most predictive of human clinical activity, plus a series of transplanted rodent tumor models. This scheme was replaced in 1975 by the murine P388 leukemia model, which was utilized as a prescreen and followed by a

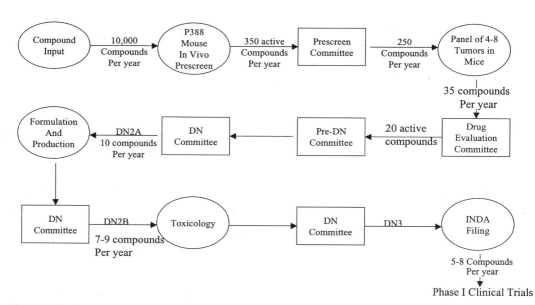

FIG. 3.1. The Developmental Therapeutics Program's drug discovery and development pipeline circa 1984. Up to 10,000 compounds were accepted annually supplied by academia and industries both domestic and foreign. Compounds were screened in a variety of animal models and results reviewed by National Cancer Institute committees. Five to eight compounds were selected each year for phase 1 clinical trials.

panel of tumors of various histologies. This panel first included only rodent tumors, but was later enhanced to include human tumor xenografts (4,5). Human tumor xenografts were employed with the intent of their serving as potentially better predictors of clinical activity against solid human tumors.

SHIFT TO *IN VITRO* SCREENING METHODOLOGY

After extensive consultation with external advisors, NCI decided to alter its screening strategy in 1985 in the hope of identifying agents with activity against solid tumors by conducting *in vitro* screening studies in a panel of human tumor cell lines derived primarily from solid tumors. In early 1990, after more than 5 years of development, the P388 prescreen was replaced by an *in vitro* human tumor cell line assay composed of 60 different cell types (6–8).

An unanticipated outcome of the screening endeavor was, in what could be considered one of the first incarnations of predictive bioinformatics, the ability of the *in vitro* drug screen to convey information about the mechanism of compound action. This information resulted from successful approaches to reduce the complexity of a 60-cell-line dose response produced by a given compound to a response pattern that can be utilized in computer-based pattern recognition algorithms (9). Using these algorithms, it is possible to postulate a known mechanism of action for a test compound, or to determine that the response pattern is unique and not similar to that of any of the prototype compounds included in the NCI database. The COMPARE pattern recognition algorithm quantitatively estimates the similarity of a test compound's pattern of activity in the screen to the pattern of known molecules. Use of COMPARE led to the recognition that compounds with the same or similar mechanisms of action, despite different chemical structure, often produced mean graph patterns that were closely correlated (10).

A further unanticipated dividend from the screening information emerged with the characterization of the cell line panel for expression of molecular targets potentially important for drug action. By defining patterns of molecular target expression compatible for use with the COMPARE algorithm, new compound structures that interacted with the molecular target could, in some instances, be determined. Examples where such molecular mechanisms have been confirmed by laboratory studies include multidrug resistance (MDR) (11) and epidermal growth factor receptor (12). These computationally based approaches ultimately resulted in identification of new

structures with tubulin-binding activity (13,14), topoisomerase I (15) and II activity (16), and novel antimetabolites (17,18). Additionally, compounds with unique profiles of growth inhibition, suggesting modes of action not shared with known clinically active classes of chemotherapeutic agents, have been identified (19).

The COMPARE algorithm, while valuable, is certainly not the only data-mining approach applied to the cell line data. Neural networks (20), cluster algorithms (21), microarray approaches (22), and self-organizing maps (23) offer differing methodologies to explore the mechanism of drug action with similar compound patterns or expressions of genes. Which is the best data-mining algorithm is a matter of current informatics-based investigation. The 60-cell-line screening data provide a richly diverse platform encouraging such endeavors. The 60-cell-line assay was originally designed to evaluate up to 10,000 compounds per year for potential anticancer activity. From 1990 to 1998, more than 70,000 compounds were evaluated in the 60-cell-line screen and yielded over 6,500 materials that were reviewed for possible *in vivo* testing. Agents selected on the basis of potency, selective activity against a particular disease category, and/or differential activity against a few specific cell lines were then evaluated against a small number of sensitive human tumors in the nude mouse xenograft model (24,25) as a basis for selecting compounds for further preclinical development. Owing to the large numbers of molecules emerging from the *in vitro* screen as candidates for xenograft testing, in 1995 this development path was further modified to include a hollow fiber (HF) assay (26), activity that was a prerequisite for study in classical xenograft models. The HF model, which is described in more detail below, involves the introduction of cell lines into semipermeable fibers in mouse intraperitoneal or subcutaneous space and intraperitoneal dosing of the test agent. The HF assay is a rapid and efficient means of selecting compounds with the potential for *in vivo* activity in conventional xenografts.

THE NEW PARADIGM

An analysis (27) was undertaken to determine the effectiveness of the drug discovery and development scheme instituted in 1995 including 60-cell-line results, HF testing, xenograft testing, and relating these data to the results of completed phase 2 clinical trial results. When xenograft activity was compared with clinical results from phase 2 trials (Fig. 3.2) for 39 clinical agents (Table 3.1), it became apparent that a histology-to-histology comparison of activity in

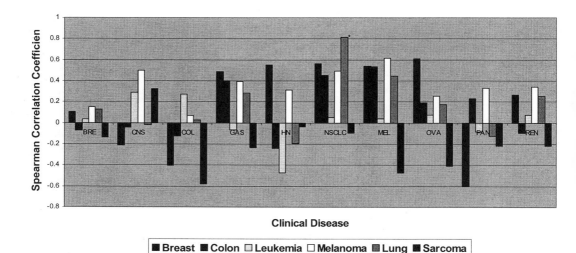

Clinical Disease

■ Breast　■ Colon　□ Leukemia　□ Melanoma　■ Lung　■ Sarcoma

FIG. 3.2. Correlation of *in vivo* activity with clinical activity by disease type. A comparison was made for compounds tested and shown to be active against various animal models (breast [BRE], brain [CNS], colon [COL], gastrointestinal [GAS], head and neck cancer [HN], non–small cell lung cancer [NSCLC], melanoma [MEL], ovarian [OVA], pancreatic [PAN], kidney [REN]) versus disease-category activity shown in phase 2 clinical trials. The Spearman correlation coefficients between animal model data and clinical data were calculated for each compound.

xenograft models to activity in the clinic could not be reliably discerned for compounds acting against non-molecularly characterized tumors selected for study, primarily because of successful growth in athymic mice. With the possible exception of lung tumors, histologic matches were not found between *in vivo* models and clinical response. However, activity in multiple xenograft models did appear to predict some degree of clinical activity (Fig. 3.3).

The results presented in Figures 3.2 and 3.3 may be taken to argue against the use of activity in an empirically selected xenograft model to predict activity in the same histologic type of cancer in the clinic, and indeed that result has influenced the current shift to characterizing drug action on its intended molecular target as a focus for development. For example, the clearly successful new agent STI-571 (Gleevec) was qualified for clinical development by observing schedule and pharmacology that resulted in suppression of the p210 brc-abl oncoprotein tyrosine phosphorylation (28). Other experience with farnesyl transferase inhibitors (29), proteasome inhibitors (30), and other kinase inhibitors clearly demonstrated the feasibility and value of filtering compounds for further development through a demonstration of activity affecting the intended molecular target in animal models.

Definition of an active agent in the appropriate xenografts allows optimization of schedule and phar-

macology, thus increasing the probability of clinical activity. It is therefore beneficial to have the ability to select agents with a likelihood of xenograft activity using a rapid and inexpensive test. The HF assay was developed to serve as a discriminator for compounds emerging from an empirical *in vitro* cell line screen. As with xenograft-to-clinical comparisons, activity against a single specific HF histology was generally not useful for predicting xenograft activity in the same histology, although there was a direct correlation between an increasing number of inhibited cell lines and ultimate xenograft activity (27). These results may be considered to define a "road-map" for charting the transition of a compound from an *in vitro* screening result to a clinical candidate.

In early 1995, an extensive review of the 60-cell-line data was undertaken. The purpose of the review was to determine if a subset of cell lines could be utilized to "prescreen" compounds that were likely to be active in the 60-cell-line screen. The initial observation was that many agents were completely inactive under the conditions of the 60-cell-line assay. Furthermore, if a prescreen could be developed that was faster and more economical to operate, this would create an opportunity for researchers to submit libraries of compounds on microtiter plates for evaluation. A protocol for a three-cell-line prescreen was developed. This prescreen would test for the presence of cytotoxicity at 10^{-4} molar drug concentration and could eliminate a

TABLE 3.1. *Cancer Chemotherapy National Service Center (NSC) numbers and common names for 39 phase 2 clinical agents*

NCS number	Common name
740	Methotrexate
3053	Actinomycin-D
3088	Chlorambucil
8806	Melphalan
19893	Fluorouracil
26271	Cyclophosphamine
26980	Mitomycin C
45388	Dacarbazine (USAN)
49842	Vinblastine
105014	2-CDA
119875	Cisplatin (USAN)
123127	Adriamycin hydrochloride
125066	Bleomycin
125973	Paclitaxel
141633	Homoharringtonine
172112	Spiromustine (USAN)
253272	Caracemide (USAN)
264880	Dihydro-5-Azacytidine
267469	Deoxydoxorubicin
269148	Menogaril
281272	Fazarabine
286193	Tiazofurin (USAN)
308847	Amonafide
312887	Fludarabine phosphate (USAN)
325319	Didemnin B
332598	Rhizoxin
336628	Merbarone
337766	Bisantrene
339004	Chloroquinoxaline sulfonamide
347512	Flavone acetic acid
349174	Piroxantrone hydrochloride
352122	Trimetrexate (USAN)
356894	Deoxyspergualin
361456	Pyrazine diazohydroxide
366140	Pyrazoloacridine
409962	BCNU
609699	Hycamptamine
616348	Irinotecan Camptothecin 11
628503	Taxotere (Docetaxel)

USAN, United States Adapted Names.

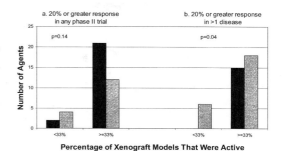

FIG. 3.3. Overall xenograft activity and clinical activity. **A**: Clinical activity was found in two of six agents (33%) with activity in fewer than one third or more of tested xenograft models, and in 21 of 33 agents (64%) with activity in one third or more of tested xenograft models ($p = 0.14$). **B**: Clinical activity in at least two diseases was found in zero of six agents (0%) that had activity in fewer than one third of tested preclinical xenograft models, whereas 15 of 33 agents (45%) with activity in one third or more of tested preclinical xenograft models had clinical activity ($p = 0.04$).

large proportion of the inactive agents, but preserve "active" agents for multidose 60-cell-line testing. Computer modeling indicated that approximately 50% of compounds could be eliminated from further consideration by this prescreen without a significant decrease in ability to identify active agents, and increase the throughput and efficiency of the main cancer screen with limited loss of information.

The three-cell-line assay has been in use since 1999, and currently utilizes the cell lines breast MCF7, CNS SF-268, and lung NCI-H460, against which potential chemotherapeutic agents are tested at a single dose for a 48-hour exposure period. Test agents that inhibit the growth of at least one of the cell lines to 32% or less of control cell growth are forwarded for testing in the 60-cell-line assay. The most current information concerning these assays is catalogued on the DTP Web site (http://dtp.nci.nih.gov).

This drug screening and development scheme remains an empirical one, as compounds are prioritized for development based on the definition of antiproliferative *in vitro* and *in vivo* responses. As our understanding of the molecular basis for human cancer gains force, researchers are placing a greater emphasis on transitioning from an empirical to a potentially more rational, molecular-target approach to the discovery and development of novel cancer therapeutics (31). Of particular interest is the design of models to detect the action of compounds on particular predefined targets. The antiproliferative activity of compounds that have been evaluated in empirical development schemes may be of value in serving as a baseline against which newer compounds and models may be compared. Likewise, performance in the screen may reveal important additional features about "targeted" agents.

CURRENT NATIONAL CANCER INSTITUTE PRACTICE

Stages of Drug Development

Compounds, which are submitted from both academic and corporate sources, that either have a defined molecular mechanism or are of a novel chemotype not previously explored are accepted for what is referred to as stage I screening evaluation in the three-cell-line prescreen. If the compound meets criteria for minimal growth inhibition as described previously, the compound is tested against the 60-cell-line panel at five concentrations (100–0.01 μmol/L). Compounds that are potent (average IC_{50} for growth less than 1 μmol/L), which display "differential" cytotoxicity across cell lines, or those that have selective activity for one or more cell types are considered for additional studies. Computer-based algorithms provide assurance that the compound's pattern of activity does not resemble known classes of approved agents. In that event, and with the compound supplier willing to provide more compound, the HF assay is conducted to provide preliminary evidence of *in vivo* activity.

The criteria selected for an *in vivo* efficacy prescreen included a high volume capacity, a short assay time, a limited need for compound, a low false-negative rate, and a minimal challenge for the test agent to overcome. The HF assay (26,32) allows screening of 50 or more compounds per week in a 10-day assay. The assay requires less than 500 mg of material and evaluates the activity of the test agent against a standard panel of 12 cell lines consisting of two lines each from the breast, colon, lung, melanoma, brain, and ovarian tumor subpanels. The cell lines used were selected by ranking the sensitivity of the *in vitro* cell lines to 3,500 compounds potentially suitable for *in vivo* testing, and selecting the two most sensitive cell lines from each histologic subpanel. The prostate and renal lines are not represented in the standard panel, as separate assays are conducted for compounds active against cells of these two histologic types. For the standard assay, compounds are evaluated at two dose levels based on the maximum tolerated dose (MTD) determined in mouse toxicity assays. A convenient extrapolation from the single-dose MTD to a multiple-day dosing scheme is afforded by setting the high test dose at [(1.5) (MTD)]/4, and the low dose at 67% of the high test dose. Hollow fiber cultures of each cell line are prepared *in vitro* and implanted into the subcutaneous and intraperitoneal compartments of mice. Since compound delivery is accomplished through intraperitoneal injection, the anticellular activity can be assessed in a same-site (ip/ip) and a distant-site (sc/ip) modality in the same mouse. The mice are treated with a vehicle or test agent for 4 days, and the fibers are retrieved for evaluation of viable cell mass using a formazan dye conversion assay. The percent net growth of each cell line is calculated by comparison to a set of control fibers assessed for viable cell mass on the day of implantation.

For a compound to be selected for additional testing, it must meet one of three referral criteria: (a) per-

cent net growth must be reduced by 50% or more in 10 of the 48 combinations tested; (b) the percent net growth of cells in the subcutaneous compartment must be reduced by 50% or more in 4 of the 24 combinations; and/or (c) a negative net cell growth (cell kill) must occur in one or more combinations. Each compound is evaluated in a total of 24 mice (four sets of cell lines × three mice/dose × two doses) with six data points generated in each mouse (three intraperitoneal and three subcutaneous fibers). This produces 144 data points for each compound tested in the HF assay. The basis for this scoring system is that its application to the selected cell lines would have resulted in detection of 95% of the currently available cytotoxic agents used in "standard" oncologic practice.

Compounds with evidence of activity in the HF system are candidates for detailed evaluation (stage IB). If a molecular target has been defined as a basis for compound activity, HF studies can be extended to clarify the modulation of the target in cells extruded from the fiber. In parallel, assessment of *in vitro* time and dose exposure for drug effect is correlated with activation pharmacology when the drug is administered by various routes. If a compound's molecular target is undefined, collaborative interactions with extramural scientists or the originating laboratory to address this issue are undertaken.

Following these initial studies, which strive to clarify a compound's capacity to achieve an effective concentration in a host organism, evidence of activity across pharmacologic barriers is sought. The model chosen is generally a classical subcutaneous xenograft in athymic mice, although intravenously administered tumors in severe compromised immunodeficient mice, orthotopic, or metastatic models may be employed.

Following demonstration of activity in at least one well-understood model encompassing the drug's intended target, the compound is advanced to stage IIA, defined as early preclinical development. Tasks at this stage include initial and range-finding toxicology, where evidence of a reversible toxic drug effect at concentrations above those conveying useful activity is sought. Development of a practical formulation occurs at this stage as well as refinement of *in vivo* activity in relation to the schedule intended for toxicologic and initial clinical development. Drugs that meet these criteria are proposed for advancement to late preclinical development, stage IIB. At this stage, two extramural experts review the compounds to assure that the candidate drug will address important scientific and clinical needs.

At the stage IIB phase of the development process, drugs undergo detailed Investigational New Drug (IND)-directed toxicology studies (Table 3.2).

TABLE 3.2. *NCI investigational drugs*

Chemical name	NSC number	Chemical name	NSC number
2-Cl-2′-deoxyadenosine	105014 (FDA approved)	Iododeoxyuridine	39661
3-Deazauridine	126849	Ipomeanol	349438
4-Nitroestrone	321803	L-Asparaginase	109229 (FDA approved)
6-Methylmercaptopurine riboside	40774 (FDA approved)	Leucovorin calcium	3590
9-Aminocamptothecin	603071	Levamisole	177023 (FDA approved)
Acivicin	63501	Lomustine (CCNU)	79037 (FDA approved)
Acodazole hydrochloride	305884	Melphalan	8806 (FDA approved)
Actinomycin D	3053 (FDA approved)	Menogaril	269148
ADR-529 (ICRF-187)	169780	Merbarone	336628
α-Interferon	377523 (FDA approved)	Methotrexate	740 (FDA approved)
Amascrine	249992	Methyl prednisone	63546 (FDA approved)
Aminothiadiazole	4728	Misonidazole	261037
Amonafide	308847	Mithramycin	24559 (FDA approved)
FR 901228 (Depsipeptide)	630176	Mitindomide	284356
Aphidicolin glycinate	303812	Mitoguazone	32946
Azacitidine	102816	Mitomycin C	26980 (FDA approved)
Bizelesin	615291	Mitoxantrone hydrochloride	301739 (FDA approved)
Bleomycin	125066 (FDA approved)	Mitozolomide	353451
Brefeldin A analog	656202	N-Methylformamide	3051
Bromodeoxyuridine	38297	O6-Benzylguanine	637037
Bryostatin	339555	o-p′-DDD	38721 (FDA approved)
CAI	609974	PALA	224131
Caracemide	253272	Pancratistatin	349156
Carboplatin	241240 (FDA approved)	PCNU	95466
Carmustine	409962 (FDA approved)	Penclomedine	338720
Chlorambucil	3088 (FDA approved)	Pentamethylmelamine hydrochloride	118742
Chlorosulfaquinoxaline sulfonamide	339004	Pentamidine isethionate	620107
Cisplatin	119875 (FDA approved)	Pentostatin	218321 (FDA approved)
Clomesone	338947	Perillyl alcohol	641066
Cyclocytidine hydrochloride	145668	Phyllanthoside	328426
Cyclodisone	348948	Pibenzimole hydrochloride	322921
Cyclopentenylcytosine	375575	Pipobroman	25154 (FDA approved)
Cyclophosphamide	26271 (FDA approved)	Piroxantrone	349174
Cytosine arabinoside (Ara-C)	63878 (FDA approved)	Porfimer sodium	602062 (FDA approved)
Dacarbazine	45388 (FDA approved)	Prednisone	63546 (FDA approved)
Daunomycin	82151 (FDA approved)	Pyrazine diazohydroxide	361456
Deoxyspergualin	356894	Pyrazoloacridine	366140
DHAC	264880	Quinocarmycin analog	607097
Diaziquone	182986	Rebeccamycin analog	655649
Didemnin B	325319	All trans-retinoic acid	122758 (FDA approved)
Dihydrotriazine benzenesulfonyl fluoride	127755	Rhizoxin	332598
Dolastatin 10	376128	Semustine (methyl CCNU)	95441 (FDA approved)
Doxorubicin	123127 (FDA approved)	Streptozotocin	85998 (FDA approved)
Ecteinascidin 743	648766	Suramin sodium	34936
Etanidazole	301467	Taxol	125973 (FDA approved)
Ethiofos (WR-2721)	296961	Taxotere	628503 (FDA approved)
Etoposide	141540 (FDA approved)	Temozolomide	362856 (FDA approved)

(continued)

TABLE 3.2. *Continued*

Chemical name	NSC number	Chemical name	NSC number
Fazarabine	281272	Terephthalamidine	57155
Flavone acetic acid	347512	Teroxirone	296934
Flavopiridol	649890	Thioguanine	752 (FDA approved)
Fludarabine phosphate	312887 (FDA approved)	Thiotepa	6396 (FDA approved)
Fostriecin	339638	Thymidine	21548
Fluorouracil	19893 (FDA approved)	Tiazofurin	286193
FUDR	27640 (FDA approved)	TMCA	36354
Gallium nitrate	15200	Topotecan	609699 (FDA approved)
Genistein	36586	Tributyrin	661583
GM-CSF	613795 (FDA approved)	Triciribine phosphate	280594
Hepsulfam	329680	Trimetrexate	249008
HMBA	95580	UCN-01	638850
Homoharringtonine	141633	Uridine	20256
Hydrazine sulfate	150014	Vincristine	67574 (FDA approved)
Hydroxyurea	32065 (FDA approved)	Zoladex	606864 (FDA approved)
Ifosfamide	109724 (FDA approved)		

FDA, US Food and Drug Administration.

Current US Food and Drug Administration (FDA) requirements for small molecules include studies in at least two species, including one nonrodent species, to define a dose at which there is little or no toxicity on a schedule that mimics the intended clinical use. The human starting dose is generally one sixth to one tenth the dose of no effect or low effect in the more sensitive of the two species. Stage IIB also includes the elaboration of a final good manufacturing practice (GMP) batch of drug, and manufacture of formulated and vialed material. The drug is then ready for advancement to clinical testing (stage III), where management of the clinical trials process passes to DTP's sister program, the Cancer Therapy Evaluation Program (CTEP). If the compound originates from a company that has already collected the information necessary to begin phase 1 clinical studies, review of the data by extramural advisors occurs prior to the CTEP's commitment to begin clinical studies.

Comparison with Past NCI Practice

The algorithm for drug development described previously, in place since 2000, differs substantially from the process that existed between 1975 and 2000 (Fig. 3.4). Compounds are no longer advanced to the clinic simply of the basis of empirical antitumor activity in animal models. Rather, pharmacologic suitability of the drug to modulate cancer-relevant targets creates enthusiasm for advancement to the clinic. The data package allows and indeed encourages the elaboration of early clinical trials that have biological endpoints in addition to the usual clinical and pharmacologic data collected in phase 1 and early phase 2

testing. In addition external reviewers provide guidance as to suitability for further development (at stage IIB for NCI screening-originated compounds; at stage III for company cross-filings.)

A Word About Biologics

New biologic therapies for cancer frequently utilize antibodies, recombinant proteins, genes in novel delivery strategies, or oligonucleotides. Commonly encountered problems are substances that arise in academic laboratories that have noteworthy activity but that can only be made available in small quantities. The many pitfalls of "scaling-up" production of these substances makes these projects high risk, leading to uncertainty or disinterest in the corporate sector in advancing the cause of these molecules. The

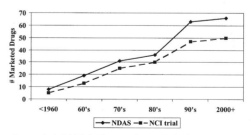

Note: Does not include biologics (e.g., vaccines, monoclonals, etc.)

FIG. 3.4. Cumulative New Drug Applications (NDAs) and National Cancer Institute (NCI)-sponsored trials. The number of anticancer agents for which NDAs where filed from the late 1950s to present are plotted (-x-) against those for which NCI sponsored a clinical trial (-o-).

Biopharmaceuticals Development Program (BDP) of the DTP collaborates actively with originating researchers to develop safe and reproducible formulations of these agents.

For example, intramural NCI research has proposed several versions of antibody-targeted toxins, using PE38, a modified toxin molecule derived from Pseudomonas exotoxin (33). Two of these immunotoxins were manufactured by the BDP, and are currently in clinical evaluation for lymphoma and leukemias, including hairy cell leukemia. BL-22 targets PE38 to the CD22 receptor on lymphocytes. A phase 1 trial of BL-22 involved 31 patients for a total of 115 cycles, resulting in 12 complete responses (CRs) in hairy cell leukemia (34). AlbaPharm Corporation has assumed support of BL-22 development, and is manufacturing material for a phase 2 trial. LMB-2 is another immunotoxin targeting PE-38 to the CD25 receptor on lymphocytes. BDP manufactured several lots of LMB-2 for phase 1 trials, in which 35 patients were treated with eight objective responses, including one CR (35).

DTP was instrumental in the development of these immunotoxins (ITs). Over the last 8 years, the DTP has evaluated the toxicity and kinetics in nonhuman primates (NHPs) of six different ITs, including BL22. While NHPs were much less sensitive to the toxic effects of these various ITs than humans, the NHPs completely predicted the dose-limiting toxicity in humans in almost all cases (gastrointestinal, liver, kidney, cardiac), whereas ITs simply produced hepatotoxicity in mice in every case. Other BDP efforts have involved collaboration with extramural grants, specifically the National Cooperative Drug Discovery Group (NCDDG) Program. One current effort utilizes a new construct of the interleukin-7 cytokine (36) that has been optimized through issues of fermentation, refolding, and purification process development to prepare for phase 1 and 2 clinical trials.

Natural Products

Despite intensive investigation of terrestrial flora, it is estimated that only 5% to 15% of the approximately 250,000 species of higher plants have been systematically investigated, chemically and pharmacologically (37). The potential of large areas of tropical rainforests remains virtually untapped and may be studied through collaborative programs with source country organizations, such as those established by the NCI. Of the plant-derived anticancer drugs currently in clinical use, those found to be most useful include vinca alkaloids, vinblastine and vincristine, isolated from the Madagascar periwinkle, *Catharanthus*

roseus. As *C. roseus* was used by various indigenous cultures for the treatment of symptoms attributed by some to diabetes, vinblastine and vincristine were first discovered during an investigation of the plant as a source of potential oral hypoglycemic agents.

More recent additions to the armamentarium of naturally derived chemotherapeutic agents are the taxanes and camptothecins. Paclitaxel initially was isolated from the bark of *Taxus brevifolia*, collected in Washington State as part of a random collection program by the US Department of Agriculture for the NCI (38). Likewise, the clinically active agents topotecan (hycamptamine), irinotecan (CPT-11), and 9-aminocamptothecin may be semisynthetically derived from camptothecin, isolated from the Chinese ornamental tree, *Camptotheca acuminata* (39). Camptothecin (as its sodium salt) was advanced to clinical trials by the NCI in the 1970s, but was dropped because of severe bladder toxicity. The flavone currently in phase 1 clinical trials, flavopiridol, is scheduled to be advanced to phase 2 trials against a broad range of tumors (40). While flavopiridol in its current form is totally synthetic, the basis for its novel structure is a natural product isolated from *Dysoxylum binectariferum*.

The marine environment is a rich source of bioactive compounds, many of which belong to totally novel chemical classes not found in terrestrial sources (41). As yet, no compound isolated from a marine source has advanced to commercial use as a chemotherapeutic agent, although several are in various phases of clinical development as potential anticancer agents. The most prominent of these is bryostatin 1, isolated from the bryozoan *Bugula neritina* (42). This agent exerts a range of biologic effects, thought to occur through modulation of protein kinase C. Phase 2 trials either are in progress or are planned against a variety of tumors, including ovarian carcinoma and non-Hodgkin's lymphoma (40).

The first marine-derived compound to enter clinical trials was didemnin B, isolated from the tunicate *Trididemnum solidum* (42). Unfortunately, it has failed to show reproducible activity against a range of tumors in phase 2 clinical trials, while demonstrating significant toxicity. Ecteinascidin 743, a metabolite produced by another tunicate *Ecteinascidia turbinata*, has significant *in vivo* activity against the murine B16 melanoma and human MX-1 breast carcinoma models, and is currently undergoing clinical evaluation in Europe and the United States (41). Sponges are traditionally a rich source of bioactive compounds in a variety of pharmacological screens (41). In the cancer area, halichondrin B, a macrocyclic polyether initially isolated from the sponge, *Halichondria okadai* in

1985, was accepted for preclinical development by the NCI in 1992. An analog (NSC 707389) derived from the total synthesis of halichondrin B has shown superior activity to the natural product (43), and is now advancing to clinical trials after preclinical development by the NCI in collaboration with Eisai Research Institute.

Antitumor antibiotics are among the most important of the cancer chemotherapeutic agents, which include members of the anthracycline, bleomycin, actinomycin, mitomycin, and aureolic acid families (44). Clinically useful agents from these families are the daunomycin-related agents, daunomycin itself, doxorubicin, idarubicin, and epirubicin; the glycopeptidic bleomycins A_2 and B_2 (blenoxane); the peptolides exemplified by dactinomycin; the mitosanes such as mitomycin C; and the glycosylated anthracenone, mithramycin. All were isolated from various *Streptomyces* species. Other clinically active agents isolated from *Streptomyces* include streptozocin and deoxycoformycin.

The future holds excitement in the untapped resources of the deep-sea vents occurring along ocean ridges, such as the East Pacific Rise and the Galapagos Rift. Several organizations are currently exploring these regions, and their rich biological resources of macroorganisms and microorganisms are being catalogued (45,46). Samples are being evaluated by the NCI in collaboration with chemists at Research Triangle Institute.

Agents in Development

The following section provides examples of agents that illustrate DTP's continuing contribution to various stages of development.

Histone Deacetylase Inhibitors

Acetylation of DNA-associated histones is linked to activation of gene transcription, whereas histone deacetylation is associated with transcriptional repression (47). Studies have shown that inhibitors of histone deacetylases (HDACs) can relieve transcriptional repression caused by the products of certain oncogenes. HDAC inhibitors developed with the assistance of DTP resources include Depsipeptide, Pyroxamide, and MS-275. Depsipeptide (NSC 630176) was first identified by DTP as a compound of interest for development because of its unique pattern of activity in the human tumor cell line assay, and was also structurally novel (48). Initial concerns that the compound would be unacceptably cardiotoxic were allayed by a DTP-designed schedule of administration that avoided cardiotoxicity. The originating company (Fujisawa) subsequently demonstrated potent HDAC inhibitory activity. DTP resources provided efficacy and toxicity evaluations in rodents on various dosing schedules, analytical methods for drug and dosage form stability, and formulation research. It was determined that an every fourth day for three doses schedule was least toxic; a unique lyophilized powder/PG:EtOH formulation was identified as clinically acceptable. An IND was filed and a clinical trial initiated in 1997. Clinical activity in cutaneous T cell lymphoma has emerged (49).

Pyroxamide (NSC 696085) (50) is an HDAC inhibitor that was presented along with seven analogs to DTP as a candidate for clinical development in March of 1997. DTP provided a bulk drug synthetic method, analytical methods for drug and dosage form, a liquid and a lyophilized formulation, all the necessary Chemical Manufacturing and Controls information for submission of the Drug Master File to the FDA, and completed pharmacology and toxicology studies for use by the sponsor (Memorial Sloan Kettering Cancer Center) in their IND filing.

MS-275 (NSC 706995) is an HDAC inhibitor with a novel synthetic benzamide structure (51). Tumor cell lines exposed to MS-275 demonstrated the accumulation of p21 in sensitive cell lines in a p53-independent manner. *In vivo* efficacy testing by the sponsor (Mitsui Pharmaceuticals) demonstrated activity of MS-275 against seven out of eight selected human tumor xenograft models using oral treatment on a 5-days-a-week schedule repeated for 4 weeks. NCI studies showed differential pattern of activity in NCI's 60-cell-line screen, *in vivo* activity in several tumor types including HL-60 TB with oral treatments on a 5-days-a-week schedule, myeloma RPMI-8226, and two small cell lung cancers (NCI-H209 and NCI-H510A). Toxicology studies in support of an IND filing were completed, and an NCI-held IND was filed and approved in January of 2001.

PS-341 (NSC 681239) is a boronic acid dipeptide brought to the DTP for potential codevelopment. It is a "first in class" inhibitor of the proteasome, which regulates degradation of numerous targets regulating transcription and cell cycle control (30). The boronic acid proteasome inhibitors represent a unique structural class of compounds in the DTP database of more than 500,000 agents, and are highly active in the *in vivo* HF assay. DTP data suggesting the selection of the clinical candidate, PS-341, were included in the initial public disclosure of the compound's antiproliferative properties. DTP tasks included *in vivo* assessment of several boronic acid analogs, development of a stable lyophilized formulation for clinical batches, and pharmacology and toxicology studies on the selected analog, PS-341. A suite of clinical trials across the country is being sponsored both by the originating commercial organization and by the NCI. Initial evidence of clinical activity has been observed in phase 1 trials in both prostate carcinoma (M. D. Anderson Cancer Center) and myeloma (University of North Carolina).

17-Allyaminogeldanamycin

NCI's interest in the preclinical development of geldanamycin was based in part on the initial evidence by extramural and intramural NCI researchers that geldanamycin (NSC 122750) can cause reversion of aspects of the transformed cell phenotype, is a potent growth inhibitor of several pediatric neural tumor cell lines, and was enhanced by the more recent demonstrations of high-affinity interactions between the geldanamycins and heat shock protein 90 (52). In order to support the investigations of geldanamycin and its analogs of interest, DTP produced kilogram quantities of geldanamycin from culture then synthesized 17-allyaminogeldanamycin (17-AAG) in large quantities. A stable, colloidal/liposomal formulation was also developed. 17-AAG is efficacious *in vivo* in two melanoma xenograft models and is less toxic than the parent compound (53). Clinical trials are underway in the United States and United Kingdom by the Cancer Research Campaign.

Pyrrolobenzodiazepine

SJG-136 is a pyrrolobenzodiazepine (PBD, NSC 694501) derivative developed in the United Kingdom and presented to the DTP for early development as a clinical candidate. The development of SJG-136 is part of a therapeutic strategy to produce low-molecular-weight antigene agents that operate by binding to long sequences of DNA. SJG-136 is one of several novel PBD derivatives whose syntheses are based on the chemical structure of the anthramycin family of naturally occurring antitumor antibiotics. The monomeric forms of PBD are somewhat limited in their sequence selectivity as they span only three DNA base pairs. The dimeric forms cross-link the guanine on one DNA strand to the guanine on the opposite strand. This novel class of compounds comprises the first sequence-selective agents that can cross-link guanine between opposite strands of DNA. SJG-136 was tested in NCI's *in vitro* 60-cell-line screen and was found to be very potent and to have a differential pattern of activity. Based on these data,

the compound was selected for *in vivo* evaluation in the HF assay. When tested against the standard panel of 12 human cell lines, the agent inhibited the growth of cell lines implanted both intraperitoneally and subcutaneously, with three cell lines killed (UACC-62 melanoma, OVCAR-3 ovarian cancer, and MDA-MB-435 breast cancer). SJG-136 was subsequently tested using various tumor xenograft models. The compound exhibited significant and selective activity against four of five subcutaneous human xenografts tested (UACC-62, OVCAR-3, MDA-MB-435, and SF-295 CNS tumor) following intravenous administration. Tumor-free animals were reported in the group of athymic nude mice bearing SF-295. Evidence of toxicity was observed with some tumor xenograft models; this toxicity might be reduced by optimizing the treatment schedule (54). NCI resources were utilized to scale-up synthesis of SJG-136, conduct detailed *in vivo* efficacy studies using sensitive tumor models to optimize the treatment schedule, initiate formulation development, and conduct preliminary pharmacology and dose-range-finding toxicology studies.

Rapamycin Analog CCI-779

Rapamycin (NSC 226080) was submitted to the NCI in 1974 by Wyeth Ayerst. This agent is a macrolide originally isolated from Streptomyces that was shown to exhibit activity in a variety of murine tumor systems, including weak activity against the P388 leukemia model (55). Rapamycin and other natural immunosuppressants, including cyclosporin A and FK-506, interact with signal transduction systems that operate in both normal T cells and tumor cells, albeit in a different manner (56). Rapamycin's poor solubility and instability compromised its preclinical development as an antitumor agent, although an oral formulation was successfully licensed for immunosuppression. NCI, in collaboration with Wyeth Ayerst, examined several derivatives of rapamycin in an effort to increase the solubility of the agent and facilitate parenteral administration into humans. The rapamycin analog CCI-779 (NSC 683864) was selected for further study (57,58). The most sensitive tumor cell lines *in vitro* were CNS, breast, and prostate cancer. In NCI *in vivo* efficacy studies, consistent antitumor activity of CCI-779 has been demonstrated in the PC3 and DU145 prostate cancer and AS283 non-Hodgkin's lymphoma xenograft models. Preclinical studies have shown that when given intermittently, the immunosuppressive effects of CCI-779 recover within 24 hours after the last dose is administered. These findings in part lead to the selection of CCI-779 as a candidate for clinical development. Preclinical toxicology studies as well as initial phase 1 clinical trials of CCI-779 were performed by Wyeth Ayerst. NCI and Wyeth Ayerst are now collaborating further, with NCI cross-filing on the existing IND for CCI-779 held by Wyeth Ayerst to allow more broad-based clinical trial opportunities.

Aminoflavone Prodrug

The aminoflavone NSC 686288 (Kyowa Hakko Kogyo) was originally selected as a development candidate on the basis of good differential activity in the NCI *in vitro* 60-cell-line screen plus marked drug effect in renal xenograft studies. Due to nonoptimal solubility, a lysine prodrug, NSC 710464, was prepared. NSC 710464 showed good in vitro correlation with the parent drug, and demonstrated activity *in vivo* against CAKI-1 renal and MCF-7 breast tumors. Aminoflavone requires metabolic activation by CYP1A1 to exert its antiproliferative effects, and the selectivity toward particular cell lines is related to the ability to induce CYP1A1 expression, which is mediated by the aryl-hydrocarbon receptor signal transduction pathway (59). Pharmacokinetic studies by NCI showed that the prodrug is rapidly converted to the parent 686288 in plasma. Additional studies performed by DTP included scale-up production, formulation, and IND-directed toxicology studies.

Benzothiazole Prodrug

The parent benzothiazole, NSC 674495, originally developed in the United Kingdom, was selected for development based on a unique pattern of *in vitro* growth inhibitory activity in the NCI 60-cell-line assay and *in vivo* efficacy against multiple human solid tumor models (60). Due to the poor aqueous solubility of this and other analogs, a prodrug was synthesized. The Lysyl prodrug, NSC 710305 (now known as Phortress), was subsequently selected as the lead compound after confirmation of activity and demonstration of its ability to achieve efficacious plasma concentrations. The mechanism of antiproliferative action is related to the enhanced expression of CYP1A1 and CYP1B1 as shown in a panel of sensitive breast cell lines. The benzothiazole prodrug has shown efficacy in the MCF-7 breast tumor model plus estrogen receptor-positive and receptor-negative breast tumor models. DTP studies were coordinated with those in the United Kingdom and included large-scale production, formulation, and IND-directed toxicology studies.

Benzoylphenylurea

The benzoylphenylurea class of compounds (Ishihara Sangyo Kaisha) were selected for development on the basis of differential cytotoxicity against breast and lymphoid cell lines in the NCI *in vitro* 60-cell-line screen. Mechanistic studies indicated that the benzoylphenylureas interact with the colchicine site but not the vincristine site on tubulin. *In vivo* activity was observed in the HF assay against breast cell lines and against AS-283 xenografts, an AIDS-related lymphoma (61). The lead compound NSC 639829 was selected from a list of five compounds on the basis of rapidity of cytocidal impact. NSC 639829, the N, N-dimethylaminophenylbenzoylurea compound, was also the only analog of the five that showed significant antitumor activity against breast and prostate tumor xenografts when administered orally. DTP studies included formulation, pharmacokinetics, toxicology, and continued mechanistic studies. Phase 1 clinical trials are in progress.

FACILITATING DRUG DISCOVERY AND DEVELOPMENT IN THE RESEARCH COMMUNITY

The preceding section focused on the role of DTP NCI as both a direct originator as well as a facilitator of compound development that in most (but not all) cases leads to an NCI-held IND. The following sections highlight new directions for the DTP mission from the operation of a drug pipeline as shown in Figure 3.1, to that of facilitator as shown in Figure 3.5. The following paragraphs detail the role of DTP NCI as a facilitator of drug discovery and development research at academic and business sites around the country, with particular emphasis on activities directed toward supporting the filing of investigator-held INDs.

Grant Mechanisms and Other Initiatives

The research grants program administered by the Grants and Contracts Operations Branch, (GCOB) that supports all aspects of preclinical anticancer drug discovery and treatment strategies, includes drug design, selective targeting of therapeutic agents, development of new preclinical models for drug discovery, and understanding, preventing, and overcoming drug resistance. GCOB resides in a unique situation in relation to the extramural grant community and the drug discovery/development activities of the DTP. Through management of a large grant and cooperative agreement portfolio, GCOB staff maintains extensive

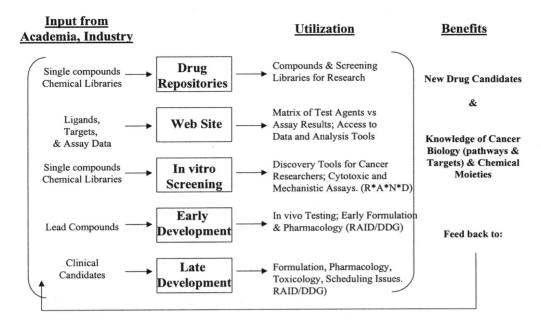

FIG. 3.5. The drug discovery and development interactions of the Developmental Therapeutics Program (DTP) in 2002. Various interactions between academia or industry and the DTP, and the means by which DTP facilitates anticancer drug discovery and development (e.g., drug repositories, the DTP Web site, *in vitro* screening, and early and late drug development assistance) are shown.

interactions with the external research community and can provide advice to foster the drug discovery mandate of the DTP. Such activities include assisting grantees to access the NCI drug and Natural Product repositories, arranging for scientists to participate in DTP seminar series, and for characterization of molecular targets in the 60-cell-line screen. Staff can advise grantees regarding availability of NCI resources for development of their agents to clinical trial, as well as answer questions regarding the subject material of their research. The DTP grant portfolio addresses agents involving DNA synthesis and repair, cell cycle, transcription, genomics, transgenics, knockouts, drug design, synthesis, combinatorial chemistry, structural biology, informatics, marine and plant natural products, animals, bioengineering, drug delivery, metabolic pathways, cell signaling, growth factors, apoptosis, mechanism of drug action, drug resistance, proteomics, high-throughput screening, pharmacology, toxicology, angiogenesis, metastases, pharmacogenetics, and gene therapy.

Recent grant initiatives include the FLAIR (Flexible System to Advance Innovative Research) for Cancer Drug Discovery for Small Business. This initiative provides a flexible system within the Small Business Innovative Research and Small Technology Transfer Research programs to accommodate the extensive needs of the complex drug and vaccine discovery and development process, at least partially, from basic discovery through proof of principle demonstration in clinical trial. The term *drug* is broadly defined to include any agent useful for the treatment or prevention of cancer. A second initiative is the Molecular Target Drug Discovery Grants. One of the priorities of the NCI 2001 Bypass Budget was to identify and use molecular targets for the discovery and clinical testing of new anticancer agents based on the molecular mechanisms that underlie neoplastic transformation, cancer growth and metastasis. DTP invited applications to exploit molecular targets for drug discovery. Rather than depending on *in vitro* and *in vivo* screens for antiproliferative activity, investigators were challenged to focus on new molecular targets and pathways essential for the development and maintenance of the cancer phenotype. The initiative also involves changes in the clinical evaluation of new agents that will include appropriate measurements to verify target modulation. Nonmammalian organisms share similar signaling and growth regulatory pathways with humans. Importantly, many sites in these pathways are altered in human tumors. These organisms could provide a valuable resource to understand more about human cancer and hopefully provide insight into new approaches for therapy. In 1999, NCI issued program announcements to support research activity in nonmammalian organisms as a means to develop new approaches for cancer treatment.

A final example of successful grant mechanisms is the National Cooperative Drug Discovery Groups. The NCDDG program, which was established in 1983, supports broad, innovative, multidisciplinary approaches to the discovery of new, synthetic or natural-source derived anticancer drugs. Although this program does not support clinical trials, a timely evaluation of products discovered by the groups is encouraged. Drugs licensed by the pharmaceutical industry from this program include Topotecan, an inhibitor of topoisomerase I (62). Topotecan is a semisynthetic, water-soluble analog of the natural product camptothecin and received approval from the FDA in 1996 for the treatment of ovarian cancer. Other NCDDG FDA-approved agents include Gliadel, a product consisting of BCNU impregnated in a wafer composed of a polyanhydride biodegradable polymer (63), approved in 1996 for the treatment of recurrent glioblastoma multiforme, and DAB389IL-2, a fusion protein composed of the catalytic and transmembrane domains of diphtheria toxin (64). This product was shown to be safe and well tolerated and to induce durable complete and partial remissions in hematologic malignancies characterized by expression of high-affinity interleukin-2 receptors. This product, known as ONTAK, interleukin-2 fusion protein, or Denileukin diftitox, was approved in 1998 for the treatment of adult patients with recurrent or persistent cutaneous T cell lymphomas (65).

Drug Development Support Available through DTP

There are two routes through which investigators can access DTP anticancer drug development resources resulting in the filing of an IND. The Drug Development Group (DDG) approves potential anticancer agents for access to DTP drug development contract resources. DDG-approved drugs are those for which NCI will be the IND-holding entity for eventual clinical trial, so coordination with the Cancer Therapy Evaluation Program (CTEP) of NCI to address compounds through DDG that fit into the CTEP portfolio of INDs is essential. DTP holds between 6 and 10 DDG meetings per year, depending on program need; the DDG is composed of NCI program staff. Applications for development services are accepted approximately 6 weeks prior to each meeting. Review criteria include strength of hypothesis,

scientific novelty, and the cost/benefit ratio. Each application is reviewed at some point in its development cycle by two nonvoting extramural experts, in addition to in house NCI staff. Successful DDG drug candidates lead to an NCI-held IND application and NCI sponsored clinical trials.

The Rapid Access to Intervention Development (RAID) program began in August of 1998 as a means of moving therapeutic agents from the laboratory to the clinic. It provides to academic researchers access to DTP's quality compound development (bulk synthesis, formulation, pharmacology, and toxicology) support contracts. Applications to RAID clearly outline the resources required to ready the proposed therapeutic agent for clinical trials. Applications are accepted twice yearly. The applications are reviewed by a panel of extramural experts within 2 months of receipt. Review criteria include strength of hypothesis, scientific novelty, and the cost/benefit ratio. The output (data, compound, formulations) are provided to the originating investigator, and may include GMP synthesized material, formulation research, pharmacologic methods, or IND-directed toxicology, for support of an investigator-held IND application and clinical trials.

The Inter-Institute Program for AIDS-Related Therapeutics (IIP) is a joint effort of the National Institute of Allergy and Infectious Diseases (NIAID) and the NCI designed to facilitate the preclinical development of novel anti-HIV therapies. In addition, the program supports development of novel approaches to AIDS-associated malignancies and opportunistic infections associated with AIDS. The program assists academic and nonprofit investigators as well as those from small biotechnology and pharmaceutical companies. IIP can help investigators advance their therapeutic or microbicide-based HIV-prevention strategy to the point where an IND application can be submitted to the FDA. Services include high-throughput screening, studies in animal models, formulation, pharmacology and toxicology studies, and bulk substances acquisition. Applications are accepted twice a year. All applications receive two levels of review. An ad hoc panel of experts from academia and industry evaluates the applications first for scientific and technical merit. Specific evaluation criteria include strength of the hypothesis, novelty, feasibility, and cost/benefit considerations. The IIP internal oversight committee then reviews the applications for importance of the project in addressing NIAID and NCI research agendas, portfolio diversity, and contract capacity. Approved projects receive assistance through NIAID or NCI drug contracts.

DTP initiated the Rapid Access to NCI Discovery Resources (R•A•N•D) program to assist academic and nonprofit investigators in the discovery stage of anti-cancer drug research. R•A•N•D can assist in the discovery of small molecules, biologics, or natural products through such initial efforts as the development of high-throughput screening assays, recombinant target protein production and characterization, and small-molecule library generation. Applications are accepted twice a year. Within 2 months after receipt of applications, an extramural review panel advised by NCI staff reviews applications for strength of the hypothesis, novelty, and cost/benefit ratio. Although the review panel considers the estimated costs in relation to possible payoffs, the applicant should not request specific funds or estimate costs. Approved projects are placed in DTP contract laboratories or in-house laboratories, and all output from the project is returned to the originator.

Submission of Compounds for Screening

Since 1998, the DTP has scaled back its empirical testing of new potential anticancer agents. Specifically, a targeted effort to screen at least 10,000 acquired new chemical entities per year has been replaced by an effort that emphasizes voluntary submissions from academic and small business suppliers who ideally have a hypothesis related to the compound's mechanism of action. Approximately 3,000 novel compounds are accepted yearly for initial anticancer evaluation. In order to submit compounds for evaluation, researchers access a Web-based, secure online form and enter structural and nonstructural information relating to the compounds they wish to have screened. The data are reviewed, and a decision regarding acceptance or rejection is relayed via electronic mail. This system has been used since August of 2000 and has proven an effective means of giving researchers access to the DTP screening program.

Plated Collections of Compounds

The NCI's Developmental Therapeutics Program has operated a repository of synthetic and pure natural products that in most cases have been evaluated as potential anticancer agents, and more recently as potential anti-HIV agents, for more than 40 years. These materials are from a variety of sources worldwide and were selected to represent unique structural diversity. The collection contains both synthetic compounds and fully characterized pure natural products. DTP has recently catalogued the structural

diversity of the nonproprietary portion of this collection with the goal of creating diverse sets of compounds to be utilized in cancer-relevant drug discovery research programs. Approximately 140,000 compounds comprise the "open" repository. For smaller-scale screening efforts, subsets of the open repository were created. The Structural Diversity set consists of 1,990 compounds representing, in terms of a ChemX software program, the chemical space of the full open repository. The mechanistic diversity set of 879 compounds are those that represent different patterns of cellular sensitivity and resistance in the 60-cell-line human tumor assay.

The DTP Web Site

The DTP Web site (http://dtp.nci.nih.gov) was launched in 1994 in an effort to increase awareness of the program and to allow for facile dissemination to the research community of screening data and other information.

The current web site includes 60-cell-line antiproliferative screening data for more than 31,000 compounds, downloadable structures for more than 250,000 compounds, yeast screening data for more than 50,000 compounds, anti-HIV screening data for more than 32,000 compounds, searchable data from the Botstein/Brown Microarray project (22), descriptions of all program functions and resources, generation of novel and publically accessible tools, and computational tools for biological and chemical analysis of screening data. The ability of researchers to access data and other information for compounds that they submitted using a secure login mode was recently added.

LOOKING TO THE FUTURE

Molecular Targets

An approach to cancer drug discovery that has gained tremendous momentum in recent years is one that targets molecules important in cancer pathogenesis. This approach may be of greater promise than the antiproliferative screens that discovered cytotoxic agents, and that have dominated cancer drug discovery for 60 years. The mapping of the human genome or even the identification of a specific mutation in the genome that leads the neoplastic state does not mean that the discovery of a new drug is imminent. Of the 40 plus small molecule, non-hormonally based drugs marketed today and utilized in cancer chemotherapy, most were discovered by empirical screens (31). Additionally, these newly discovered molecular targets exist in a cellular milieu consisting of additional influences on target function. Effective drug treatment will take into account drug uptake, metabolism, and elimination at the level of the cell as well as the organism. A key goal is to define for a new drug development paradigm a path that accounts for the cancer cell phenotype in its totality rather than as arising solely from single molecular targets.

The Possibility of ADMET

The DTP is committed to the support of genomics and proteomics research to identify new targets for therapy, and to the development of a comprehensive tox 'omics' program correlating clinical and microscopic pathology results with gene and protein changes. The aim is to develop patterns of gene and protein changes that can be correlated with specific types of toxicity and/or new biomarkers. Development of new *in vitro* ways of assessing drug absorption, distribution, metabolism, excretion, and toxicity (ADMET) potential can be used as high-throughput screens or to predict human sensitivity and phase 1 maximum tolerated doses. Continued expansion of an *in vitro* pharmacology program to predict better human kinetics, metabolism, and oral bioavailability of agents is also of importance. These two separate initiatives encourage the development, standardization, and validation of new and innovative assays that determine or predict specific organ toxicities (e.g., cardiotoxicity, gastrointestinal toxicity, hepatotoxicity, nephrotoxicity, ototoxicity, bladder toxicity, neurotoxicity, pulmonary toxicity, and endocrine toxicity, including pancreatic β-cell toxicity) of potential cancer therapeutic agents. These and other grant initiatives are described on the DTP Web site under "Grants and Contracts."

CONCLUSION

A key tenet of the assumed wisdom leading us down a new path for cancer drug discovery and development is that molecules with pathogenic significance in the *causation* of cancer will be key targets in the useful *treatment* of cancer. The anti–*bcr-abl*–directed protein kinase antagonist STI-571, a drug molecule crafted to be a specific kinase inhibitor, has emerged as a "poster child" for this new approach (66). STI-571 is a prototype that hopefully can be generalized to other drug molecules in addressing hematologic and pediatric neoplasms that utilize translocation-related fusion proteins as a basis for their existence. Yet, it is very unusual in adult oncology that a single target can be tied unequivocally to a cancer's pathogenesis. Common adult solid tumors actually contain dozens of interacting targets that deregulate cell cycle progression, convey cellular immortality (e.g., by activating telomerase), have disregulated cell death–promoting mechanisms, and in the majority of lethal tumors have become functionally enabled to induce new blood vessels, invade, and metastasize. Thus, a key feature of a hoped-for targeted therapeutic will be the ability to address multiple deranged targets in a way that is qualitatively different than current cytotoxics, whose value arises from the *cellular response* to the drug rather than from the nature of the drugs' targets. Furthermore, an additional factor leading to the success of this endeavor will be partnerships between chemists and biologists. Examples where such approaches have led to elucidation of lead structures by direct association with target (67) or by "smart" screening strategies (68) will become more frequent. DTP remains committed to providing an infrastructure that will support academic investigators and collaborators in commercial organizations to bring new agents forward that may be of value in the treatment of patients with cancer.

REFERENCES

1. Powis G. Toxicity of anticancer drugs to humans: a unique opportunity to study human toxicology. In: Powis G, Hacker MP, eds. *The toxicity of anticancer drugs.* New York, NY: Pergamon Press, 1991:1–9.
2. Gellhorn A, Hirschberg E. Investigation of diverse systems for cancer chemotherapy screening. *Cancer Res Suppl* 1955;3:1–125.
3. Zubrod CG, Schepartz S, Leiter J, et al. The chemotherapy program of the National Cancer Institute: history, analysis and plans. *Cancer Chemother Rep* 1966;50: 349–540.
4. Venditti JM. Preclinical drug development: rationale and methods. *Semin Oncol* 1981;8:349–361.
5. Venditti JM, Wesley RA, Plowman J. Current NCI preclinical antitumor screening in vivo: results of tumor panel screening, 1976–1982, and future directions. *Adv Pharmacol Chemother* 1984;20:1–19.
6. Alley MC, Scudiero DA, Monks A, et al. Feasibility of drug screening with panels of human tumor cell lines using a microculture tetrazolium assay. *Cancer Res* 1988;48:589–601.
7. Monks A, Scudiero D, Skehan P, et al. Feasibility of a high-flux anticancer drug screen using a diverse panel of cultured human tumor cell lines. *J Natl Cancer Inst* 1991;83:757–766.
8. Paull KD, Hamel E, Malspeis L. Prediction of biochemical mechanism of action from the in vitro antitumor screen of the National Cancer Institute. In: Foye WO, ed. *Cancer chemotherapeutic agents.* Washington, DC: American Chemical Society, 1995:9–45.

9. Paull KD, Shoemaker RH, Hodes L, et al. Display and analysis of patterns of differential activity of drugs against human tumor cell lines: development of mean graph and COMPARE algorithm. *J Natl Cancer Inst* 1989;81:1088–1092.

10. Paull KD, Hamel E, Malspeis L. Prediction of biochemical mechanisms of action from the *in vitro* antitumor screen of the National Cancer Institute. In: Foye W, ed. *Cancer chemotherapeutic agents*. Washington, DC: American Chemical Society, 1995.[1]

11. Alvarez M, Paull K, Monks A, et al. Generation of a drug resistance profile by quantitation of mdr-1/P-glycoprotein in the cell lines of the National Cancer Institute anticancer drug screen. *J Clin Invest* 1995;95: 2205–2214.

12. Wosikowski K, Schuurhuis D, Johnson K, et al. Identification of epidermal growth factor receptor and c-erbB2 pathway inhibitors by correlation with gene expression patterns. *J Natl Cancer Inst* 1997;89:1505–1515.

13. Bai R, Paull KD, Herald CL, et al. Halichondrin B and homohalichondrin B, marine natural products binding in the vinca domain of tubulin. Discovery of tubulin-based mechanism of action by analysis of differential cytotoxicity data. *J Biol Chem* 1991;266:15882–15889.

14. Paull KD, Lin CM, Malspeis L, et al. Identification of novel antimitotic agents acting at the tubulin level by computer-assisted evaluation of differential cytotoxicity data. *Cancer Res* 1992;52:3892–3900.

15. Kohlhagen G, Paull KD, Cushman M, et al. Protein-linked DNA strand breaks induced by NSC 314622, a novel noncamptothecin topoisomerase I poison. *Mol Pharmacol* 1998;54:50–58.

16. Leteurtre F, Kohlhagen G, Paull KD, et al. Topoisomerase II inhibition and cytotoxicity of the anthrapyrazoles DuP937 and DuP 941 (Losoxantrone) in the National Cancer Institute preclinical antitumor drug discovery screen. *J Natl Cancer Inst* 1994;86: 239–244.

17. Jayaram HN, Gharehbaghi K, Jayaram NH, et al. Cytotoxicity of a new IMP dehydrogenase inhibitor, benzamide riboside, to human myelogenous leukemia K562 cells. *Biochem Biophys Res Commun* 1992;186: 1600–1606.

18. Cleaveland ES, Monks A, Vaigro-Wolff A, et al. Site of action of two novel pyrimidine biosynthesis inhibitors accurately predicted by the compare program. *Biochem Pharmacol* 1995;49:947–954.

19. Bradshaw TD, Wrigley S, Shi DF, et al. 2-(4-aminophenyl) benzothiazoles: Novel agents with selective profiles of *in vitro* antitumor activity. *Br J Cancer* 1998;77:745–752.

20. Weinstein JN, Myers T, Buolamwini J, et al. Predictive statistics and artificial intelligence in the U.S. National Cancer Institute's Drug Discovery Program for Cancer and AIDS. *Stem Cells (Dayt)* 1994;12:13–22.

21. Weinstein JN, Myers TG, O'Connor PM, et al. An information-intensive approach to the molecular pharmacology of cancer. *Science* 1997; 275:343–349.

22. Ross DT, Scherf U, Eisen MB, et al. Systematic variation in gene expression patterns in human cancer cell lines. *Nat Genet* 2000;3:227–235.

23. Rabow AA, Shoemaker RH, Sausville EA, et al. Mining the National Cancer Institute's tumor-screening database: identification of compounds with similar cellular activities. *J Med Chem* 2002;45:818–840.

24. Dykes DJ, Abbott BJ, Mayo JG, et al. Development of human tumor xenograft models for in vivo evaluation of new antitumor drugs. *Contrib Oncol* 1992;42:1–22.

25. Plowman J, Dykes DJ, Hollingshead M, et al. Human tumor xenograft models. In: Teicher B, ed. *Anticancer drug development guide: preclinical screening, clinical trials, and approval*. Totowa, NJ: Humana Press, 1997: 101–125.

26. Hollingshead M, Plowman J, Alley M, et al. The hollow fiber assay. In: Fiebig H, Burger AM, eds. *Contributions to oncology volume 54: relevance of tumor models for anticancer drug development*. Freiburg: Karger,1999: 109–120.

27. Johnson JI, Decker S, Zaharevitz D, et al. Relationships between drug activity in NCI preclinical in vitro and in vivo models and early clinical trials. *Br J Cancer* 2001;84:1424–1431.

28. Sattler M, Verma S, Byrne CH, et al. BCR/ABL directly inhibits expression of SHIP, an SH2-containing olyinositol-5-phosphatase involved in the regulation of hematopoiesis. *Mol Cell Biol* 1999;19:7473–7480.

29. Sebti SM, Hamilton AD. Farnesyltransferase and geranylgeranyltransferase I inhibitors and cancer therapy: lessons from mechanism and bench-to-bedside translational studies. *Oncogene* 2000;19:6584–6593.

30. Adams J, Palombella VJ, Sausville EA, et al. Proteasome inhibitors: a novel class of potent and effective antitumor agents. *Cancer Res* 1999;59:2615–2622.

31. Sausville EA, Feigal E. Evolving approaches to cancer drug discovery and development at the National Cancer Institute, USA. *Ann Oncol* 1999;10:1287–1291.

32. Hollingshead MG, Alley MC, Camalier RF, et al. *In vivo* cultivation of tumor cells in hollow fibers. *Life Sci* 1995; 57:131–141.

33. Pastan I. Targeted therapy of cancer with recombinant immunotoxins. *Biochim Biophys Acta* 1997;1333: C1–C6.

34. Kreitman RJ, Wilson WH, Bergeron K, et al. Efficacy of the anti-CD22 recombinant immunotoxin BL22 in chemotherapy-resistant hairy-cell leukemia. *N Engl J Med* 2001;345:241–247.

35. Kreitman RJ, Wilson WH, White JD, et al. Phase I trial of recombinant immunotoxin anti-Tac(Fv)-PE38 (LMB-2) in patients with hematologic malignancies. *J Clin Oncol* 2000;18:1622–1636.

36. Sweeney EB, Foss FM, Murphy JR, et al. Interleukin 7 (IL-7) receptor-specific cell killing by DAB389 IL-7: a novel agent for the elimination of IL-7 receptor positive cells. *Bioconjug Chem* 1998;9:201–207.

37. Balandrin MF, Kinghorn AD, Farnsworth NR. Plant-derived natural products in drug discovery and development. An overview. In: AD Kinghorn, MF Balandrin, eds. *Human medicinal agents from plants*. Washington, DC: American Chemical Society, 1993;2–12.

38. Cragg GM, Schepartz SA, Suffness M, et al. The taxol supply crisis. New NCI policies for handling the large-scale production of novel natural product anticancer and anti-HIV agents. *J Nat Prod* 1993;56:1657–1668.

39. Wall ME, Wani MC. Camptothecin and taxol: discovery to clinic—thirteenth Bruce F. Cain Memorial Award Lecture. *Cancer Res* 1995;55:4753–4760.

40. Christian MC, Pluda JM, Ho TC, et al. Promising new agents under development by the Division of Cancer Treatment, Diagnosis and Centers of the National Cancer Institute. *Semin Oncol* 1997;24:219–240.

41. Carté BK. *BioScience* 1996;46:271–286.

42. McConnell O, Longley RE, Koehn FE. In: Gullo VP, ed. *The discovery of natural products with therapeutic potential*. Boston: Butterworth-Heinemann, 1994;109–174.

43. Towle MJ, et al. Highly potent in vitro and in vivo anticancer activities of synthetic macrocyclic ketone analogs of Halichondrin B. *Proc Am Assoc Can Res*, 2000;41:1370.

44. Foye WO, ed. *Cancer chemotherapeutic agents*. Washington, DC: American Chemical Society, 1995.

45. Lutz RA, Shank TM, Fornari DJ. *Nature* 1994;371:663–664.

46. Lutz RA, Kennish MJ. *Rev Geophys* 1993;31:211–242.

47. Zhou X, Richon VM, Rifkind RA, et al. Identification of a transcriptional repressor related to the noncatalytic domain of histone deacetylases 4 and 5. *Proc Natl Acad Sci U S A* 2000;97:1056–1061.

48. Sandor V, Robbins AR, Robey R, et al. FR901228 causes mitotic arrest but does not alter microtubule polymerization. *Anticancer Drugs* 2000;11:445–454.

49. Riekarz R, Robey R, Fojo T, et al. Analysis of molecular markers and targets in trials of depsipeptide, FR901228, a histone deacetylase inhibitor with clinical activity in T-cell lymphoma. *ASCO* 2002;21:23a.

50. Butler LM, Webb Y, Agus DB, et al. Inhibition of transformed cell growth and induction of cellular differentiation by pyroxamide, an inhibitor of histone deacetylase. *Clin Cancer Res* 2001;7:962–970.

51. Lee BI, Park SH, Kim JW, et al. MS-275, a histone deacetylase inhibitor, selectively induces transforming growth factor beta type II receptor expression in human breast cancer cells. *Cancer Res* 2001;61:931–934.

52. Buchner J. Hsp90 & Co.—a holding for folding. *Trends Biochem Sci* 1999;4:136–141.

53. Schulte TW, Neckers LM. The benzoquinone ansamycin 17-allylamino-17-demethoxy-geldanamycin binds to HSP90 and shares important biologic activities with geldanamycin. *Cancer Chemother Pharmacol* 1998;42:273–279.

54. Gregson SJ, Howard PW, Hartley JA, et al. Design, synthesis, and evaluation of a novel pyrrolobenzodiazepine DNA-interactive agent with highly efficient cross-linking ability and potent cytotoxicity. *J Med Chem* 2001;44:737–748.

55. Eng CP, Sehgal SN, Vezina C J. Activity of rapamycin (AY-22,989) against transplanted tumors. *J Antibiot (Tokyo)* 1984;37:1231–1237.

56. Bierer BE, Mattila PS, Standaert RF, et al. Two distinct signal transmission pathways in T lymphocytes are inhibited by complexes formed between an immunophilin and either FK506 or rapamycin. *Proc Natl Acad Sci U S A* 1990;87:9231–9235.

57. Hidalgo M, Rowinsky EK. The rapamycin-sensitive signal transduction pathway as a target for cancer therapy. *Oncogene* 2000;19:6680–6686.

58. Huang S, Houghton PJ. Inhibitors of mammalian target of rapamycin as novel antitumor agents: from bench to clinic. *Curr Opin Investig Drugs* 2002:295–304.

59. Kuffel MJ, Schroeder JC, Pobst LJ, et al. Activation of the antitumor agent aminoflavone (NSC 686288) is mediated by induction of tumor cell cytochrome P450 1A1/1A2. *Mol Pharmacol* 2002;62:143–153.

60. Bradshaw TD, Shi DF, Schultz RJ, et al. Influence of 2-(4-aminophenyl)benzothiazoles on growth of human ovarian carcinoma cells in vitro and in vivo. *Br J Cancer* 1998;78:421–429.

61. Hollingshead MG, Sackett DL, Alley MC, et al. The anticancer activity of six benzoylphenylurea compounds and their interaction with tubulin. *Proc Am Assoc Cancer Res* 1998;39:164.

62. Takimoto CH, Arbuck SG. Clinical status and optimal use of topotecan. *Oncology (Huntingt)* 1997;11:1635–1646.

63. Dang W, Daviau T, Brem H. Morphological characterization of polyanhydride biodegradable implant gliadel during in vitro and in vivo erosion using scanning electron microscopy. *Pharm Res* 1996;13:683–691.

64. Foss FM. DAB(389)IL-2 (ONTAK): a novel fusion toxin therapy for lymphoma. *Clin Lymphoma* 2000;110:110–116.

65. Kuzel TM. DAB(389)IL-2 (denileukin diftitox, ONTAK): review of clinical trials to date. *Clin Lymphoma* 2000;1:S33–S36.

66. Druker BJ, Talpaz M, Resta DJ, et al. Efficacy and safety of a specific inhibitor of the BCR-ABL tyrosine kinase in chronic myeloid leukemia. *N Engl J Med* 2001;344:1031–1037.

67. Liu S, Widom J, Kemp CW, et al. Structure of human methionine aminopeptidase-2 complexed with fumagillin. *Science* 1998;282:1324–1327.

68. Haggarty SJ, Mayer TU, Miyamoto DT, et al. Dissecting cellular processes using small molecules: identification of colchicine-like, taxol-like and other small molecules that perturb mitosis. *Chem Biol* 2000;4:275–286.

4

Combinatorial Chemistry in Anticancer Drug Development

Ian R. Hardcastle and Roger J. Griffin

Northern Institute for Cancer Research, School of Natural Sciences, University of Newcastle upon Tyne, Newcastle upon Tyne NE1 7RU, United Kingdom

Combinatorial chemistry has transformed the way medicinal chemists synthesize compounds for biological evaluation. In the traditional approach, compounds were made individually and sets of analogues built up serially. Each analogue prepared in this way may require an individualized reaction sequence and purification strategy. Consequently, this approach is labor intensive and costly. In contrast, combinatorial synthesis uses a defined pathway of bond-forming reactions to combine sets of simple molecules or building blocks to give complex products in a small number of steps. The process can be used repetitively, thus enabling libraries comprising large numbers of analogues to be created in an organized and efficient manner. The predefined and repetitive nature of combinatorial synthesis is amenable to automation, and libraries generated by this approach are typically arranged in a format suitable for high-throughput screening.

This chapter provides a very general introduction to the basic principles of combinatorial chemistry, followed by an overview of the application of this technology to one aspect of anticancer drug design and development. In common with other areas of drug discovery and development, combinatorial chemistry has found widespread application in anticancer drug design and development, both in the pharmaceutical sector and in academia. Consequently, the rapidly expanding literature relating to the subject could not possibly be discussed within a single chapter. We have instead attempted to illustrate some of the techniques employed in combinatorial synthesis, by drawing on selected examples from the literature relating to kinase enzymes of interest as therapeutic targets in cancer therapy. This discussion is by no means intended to be comprehensive, and the authors apologize in advance for any inadvertent omissions. For a detailed survey of combinatorial library synthesis, the reader is referred to excellent reviews covering the period 1992 to 2002 (1,2).

SOME BASIC PRINCIPLES OF COMBINATORIAL CHEMISTRY

Solid-phase Peptide Synthesis

R. B. Merrifield is credited with the first viable application of *solid-phase synthesis* (SPS), when, in 1963, he described the synthesis of a short peptide attached to a polystyrene resin (3). Reversible covalent attachment of the growing peptide onto a solid-support allowed multiple peptide coupling and deprotection (deblocking) steps to be conducted, without the need for lengthy purification of the intermediates at each synthetic step (Fig. 4.1). A final cleavage step was required to release the target peptide from the resin. This approach was subsequently applied to the preparation of oligonucleotides (4,5), but SPS failed to gain general acceptance in the chemistry community, owing to the limitations of conducting conventional organic synthesis on a solid support.

Some 30 years after Merrifield's seminal publication, the birth of combinatorial synthesis was heralded with publications from two independent groups, each detailing the synthesis of peptide libraries required for epitope-mapping experiments. In the Geysen method, the solid support comprised an array of "pins" arranged to fit into a standard 96-well microtiter plate, with each well containing an activated amino acid (6). Attachment of the amino acids to the individual pins of the solid support enabled the *multiple-parallel synthesis* (MPS) of peptides on the pins, with the washing and deblocking steps being performed in parallel. The 96 discrete peptides were finally cleaved from the pins directly into individual predetermined wells for subsequent analysis and biological evaluation.

Houghten's approach to the synthesis of peptide libraries involved the encapsulation of standard peptide synthesis resin within a porous, solvent-resistant packet or "tea bag" labeled with an indelible ink (7). Peptide synthesis was achieved on the resin by transferring the tea bags to reaction vessels containing the appropriate amino acids, and the bags were combined for the washing and deblocking steps prior to being sorted into the appropriate reaction vessels for the next amino acid coupling. This process of *directed sorting* of labeled or tagged portions of resin has become commonplace, with the tea bag often being replaced by a suitable porous container or "can." Each batch of resin is identified throughout the multistep procedure by a physical tag.

Nonpeptide or Small-Molecule Libraries

The independent publication of two solid-phase library syntheses of low-molecular-weight druglike molecules in the early 1990s demonstrated that combinatorial techniques were not confined to the synthesis of peptides (8,9). The past decade has seen enormous progress in the technologies associated with small-molecule combinatorial library synthesis, particularly with regard to novel solid supports and linkers, library quality control and product purification, and the generation of chemical diversity within a compound library. Many of the challenges associated with adapting synthetic organic reactions, normally conducted in solution, to the solid phase have been successfully addressed by the pharmaceutical industry and academia, and this rapidly expanding area of combinatorial chemistry has been very comprehensively reviewed (10–12).

The Split Synthesis Technique

The development of the *portion mixing* or *split synthesis* technique has revolutionized combinatorial chemistry by enabling the synthesis of very large compound libraries (13–15). For the preparation of peptide libraries, a bulk resin is divided into a number of equal portions, and a different amino acid is attached to each portion. The portions are recombined for the washing and deblocking steps, mixed, and divided again into portions for the next coupling step. This cycle is repeated until the desired length of peptide is achieved. The power of this approach resides in the large numbers of compounds that may be generated by the repetition of a few relatively simple operations. For example, a hexapeptide library with 10 amino acids at each position totaling 10^6 different peptide sequences can be prepared in 66 cycles of synthesis. Crucially, each resin bead bears only one peptide sequence and is, in essence, a micro–tea bag. This principle of *one-bead one-compound* offers the opportunity of directly screening resin bound peptides for biological activity, and selecting active beads for characterization, typically by Edman microsequenc-

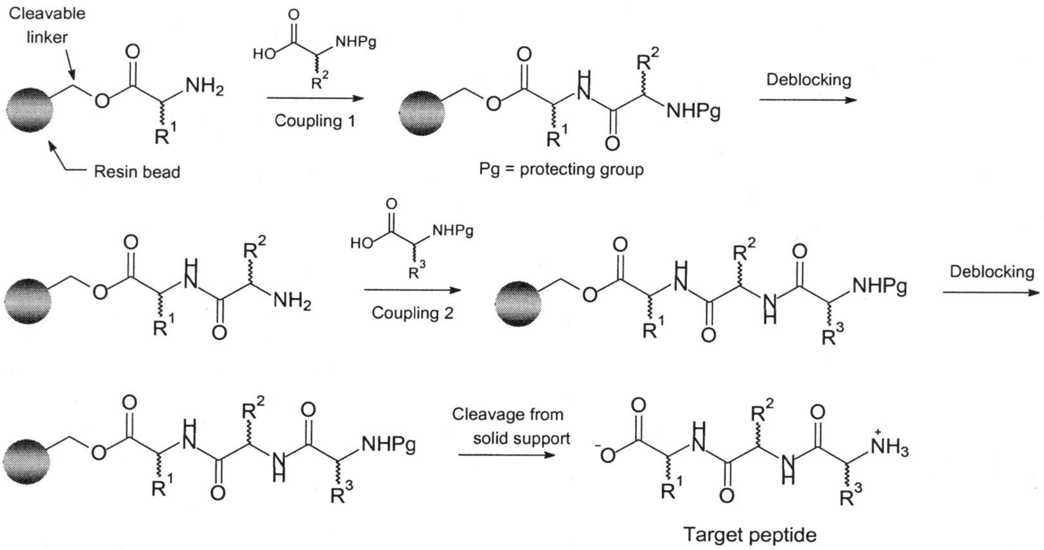

FIG. 4.1. Solid-phase synthesis of a tripeptide.

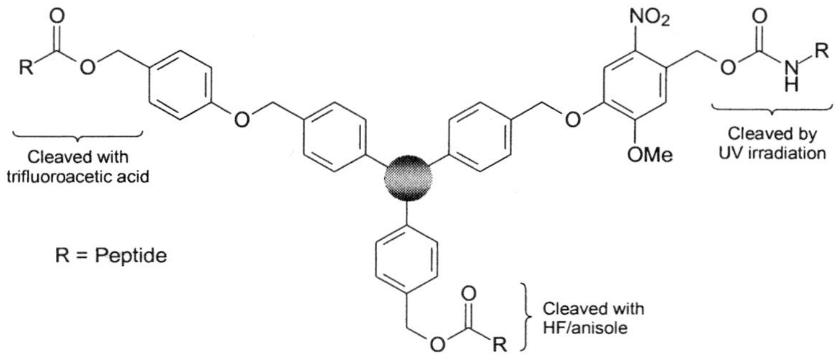

FIG. 4.2. A single polymer bead bearing three orthogonally cleavable linkers.

ing and mass spectrometry (16). The use of orthogonal multiple linkers (Fig. 4.2) on each individual bead has enabled active compounds to be identified from pools of beads, using an iterative cleavage-assay approach (17).

Application of the split synthesis method to the preparation of nonpeptide libraries requires a different approach for the identification of active compounds within the library. The *tagging* method entails the attachment of a unique identifier or tag to each bead or portion of beads, employing either a physical or chemical strategy (18). Physical tags include optically readable alphanumeric labels, barcodes, microdot code labels, and radiofrequency transponders, whereas chemical approaches using oligonucleotide or haloarene covalent tags have been reported. The physical tagging method is advantageous in allowing tracking of a particular resin throughout the library synthesis, and thus the application of a directed sorting approach, which enables resin portions to be allocated using a predetermined pathway such that every possible combination is prepared once. A prerequisite of the alternative *random distribution method* is that the total number of resin beads utilized to make the library must exceed the number of anticipated products by at least 10-fold, so as to ensure a representative statistical mixture of each combination. Directed sorting is not amenable to the preparation of solution phase libraries.

Multiple-parallel Synthesis

In contrast to libraries generated by split synthesis, those prepared by the MPS method comprise discrete spatially separated compounds (i.e., one compound per reaction vessel). Libraries are prepared in a matrix format, where the components of the matrix are defined by the building blocks used in the syntheses. For example, the preparation of a small library of amide derivatives could be achieved from a simple one-step reaction of anilines (**X**) with acid chlorides (**Y**). Thus an MPS involving five aniline (reagents A–E) and five acid chloride (reagents 1–5) building blocks would furnish a small library of 25 (5 × 5) products X–Y, with individual members of the library being readily identifiable from their relative positions within the matrix (Table 4.1).

Although libraries prepared by MPS are invariably smaller than those generated by split synthesis, the simplicity of the approach, coupled with the fact that single products of known chemical structure should, in principle, be obtained, renders this method attractive. Although suitable for both solid-phase and solution-phase reactions, MPS is frequently used in solution phase to avoid the additional complexities inherent to SPS. The technique is also very amenable to automation, by using modified liquid handling robots to dispense reagents to a reaction block incorporating an array of individual reaction vessels, typically in a 96-well format.

PEPTIDE-BASED COMBINATORIAL LIBRARIES IN ANTICANCER DRUG DEVELOPMENT

Synthetic Peptide Libraries

Synthetic peptide libraries have been used in cancer research both as chemical tools to probe site specificity for enzymes and protein–protein interactions, and as structural leads for inhibitor design. Peptide-based inhibitors are of value for validating potential therapeutic targets and establishing biological "proof-of-principle," and synthetic peptide libraries have proven useful for the rapid identification of tight-binding ligands. Although potent peptide inhibitors of a number of enzymes and protein–protein interactions have been reported, translation into clinically useful drugs has been hampered by the pharmacokinetic and chemical

TABLE 4.1. *Multiple-parallel synthesis (5 × 5 array) of a simple amide library*

stability problems inherent to peptides. The elaboration of peptide-based lead molecules into stable peptidomimetic or nonpeptide drugs continues to present a challenge to the medicinal chemistry community.

Targeting Kinases with Peptide Libraries

The substrate specificity of the tyrosine kinase p60[c-src] has been probed using peptide libraries (19). A random heptapeptide library comprising 19 natural amino acids was prepared on TentaGel beads by the split synthesis method, and a fraction of the library (~500,000 beads) was incubated with human recombinant p60[c-src] and [γ-^{32}P]-ATP. Substrate activity was detected by autoradiography, and active beads were collected individually and characterized by Edman microsequencing. Only two labeled beads were reportedly isolated by this technique, one of which proved to be the result of nonspecific binding of the peptide to ATP. The remaining active heptapeptide (YIYGSFK) was resynthesized and found to be an excellent substrate for phosphorylation by p60[c-src] compared with synthetic peptides derived from various cellular proteins, including the p60[c-src] autophosphorylation site.

Chan et al. (20) determined the substrate specificity of the HER2/Neu tyrosine kinase by two different methods, each utilizing peptide libraries generated by the split synthesis technique. In the first method, a solution library (AAXXXYAARRG) was prepared and incubated with HER-2/Neu and [γ-^{32}P]-ATP. Phosphorylated peptides were isolated by binding to a ferric iminodiacetate column, and purified by HPLC. The second approach entailed the synthesis of a solid-phase peptide library in the format (EDXXXYXXXG) on 100 μmol/L controlled pore glass beads. After incubation, the individual active beads were visualized by autoradiography and collected with microforceps. Of the four most active sequences identified from the two libraries by Edman microsequencing, AAEEIYAARRG (solution library) and EDKVDYRMHRRG (solidphase library) were found to give the best enzyme kinetic data.

The method of *positional scanning* has proven valuable for exploring the substrate specificity of kinases of potential interest as cancer therapeutic targets. For example, the type I and II receptors of transforming growth factor β (TGF-β) are transmembrane serine/threonine kinases, and the substrate specificity

TABLE 4.2. *The positional scanning approach for identifying active peptides (21)*

Library	-6	-5	-4	-3	-2	-1	0	+1	+2	+3	Polymer
X − 3			L	**X**	O	O	S	L	G	~	~ (wink)
X − 2 (R − 3)			L	R	**X**	O	S	L	G	~	~ (wink)
X − 2 (K − 3)			L	K	**X**	O	S/T	O	O	O	~ (wink)
X − 1			L	K	O	**X**	S/T	O	O	O	~ (wink)
X + 1			L	K	O	O	S/T	**X**	O	O	~ (wink)
X + 2			L	K	O	O	S/T	O	**X**	O	~ (wink)
X + 3			L	K	O	O	S/T	O	O	**X**	~ (wink)
X − 4	O	O	**X**	K	O	O	S/T	L	G	~	~ (wink)
X − 5	O	**X**	O	K	O	O	S/T	L	G	~	~ (wink)
X − 6	**X**	O	O	K	O	O	S/T	L	G	~	~ (wink)

O, random peptide position; X, defined peptide position; ~, linker to polymer wink.

of these kinases was probed with peptide libraries prepared using a positional scanning approach (21). Libraries were synthesized on porous polyethylene discs or "winks," with the amino acid at positions denoted **X** fixed, and a mixture of 17 amino acids incorporated at positions labeled **O** (Table 4.2). Determination of the degree of phosphorylation of the 19 winks with differing amino acids at position **X** revealed the preferred amino acid at each position, and additional libraries were prepared and screened with **X** located at other positions in a seven to nine amino acid peptide, thereby allowing the optimum sequence to be generated. The synthesis of a total of 186 analogous libraries spanning a 10 amino acid peptide enabled elucidation of the optimum amino acid sequence for both TGF-β type I and II receptors as KKKKKK(S/T)XXX. Importantly, the peptide libraries were found to have general application as probes for serine/threonine kinases. For example, the optimal substrate sequence for protein kinase A was determined as RRXS(I/L/V), which is in agreement with the sequence obtained by other methods.

A positional scanning strategy was also used to identify the optimal peptide substrates for death-associated protein kinase (DAPK), a calmodulin-regulated serine/threonine protein kinase implicated in apoptosis, tumor suppression, and ischemia-induced neuronal cell death (22). Using the available crystal structure of DAPK in conjunction with molecular modeling, positional scanning studies were conducted with peptide libraries based on the motif KKRPQRATSNVF. Two structurally similar peptides (KKRPQRRY(L)SNVF) were identified as excellent substrates for DAPK.

A library affinity approach was exploited to study the Src homology domain of phosphatidylinositol 3-kinase (PI 3-kinase) (23). Using the split synthesis approach, a solid-phase combinatorial library of $361 (19^2)$ peptides was synthesized with the format G(F_2Pmp)X_1-PX_3S-amide (X = standard 19 L-amino acids except cysteine), where F_2Pmp is the nonhydrolyzable phosphotyrosine surrogate (phosphonodifluoromethyl)phenylalanine (**1**). After cleavage from the resin, active peptides were isolated by affinity chromatography and characterized by electrospray tandem mass spectrometry (ES-MS/MS), thereby avoiding the need for library encoding or on-bead assays. The ES-MS/MS technique gave sequence information but was unable to distinguish between amino acids with identical molecular masses (e.g., Ile and Leu). Nevertheless, a clear preference for a hydrophobic residue at the +1 site and a methionine residue at the +3 site, relative to the phosphotyrosine, was demonstrated. In principle, and subject to the detection limits of the mass spectrometer (10–50 pmol), this approach can be used for the analysis of large peptide libraries.

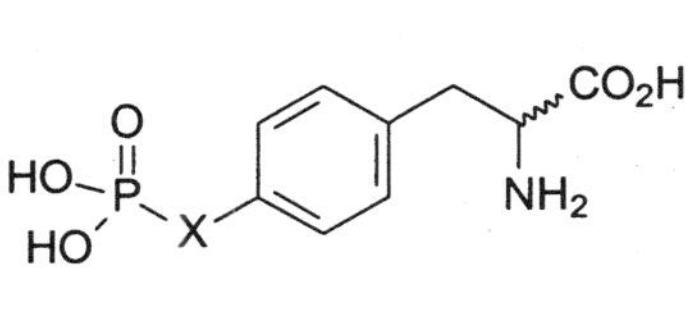

(**1**); X = CF₂
(**2**); X = CHF
(**3**); X = CHOH

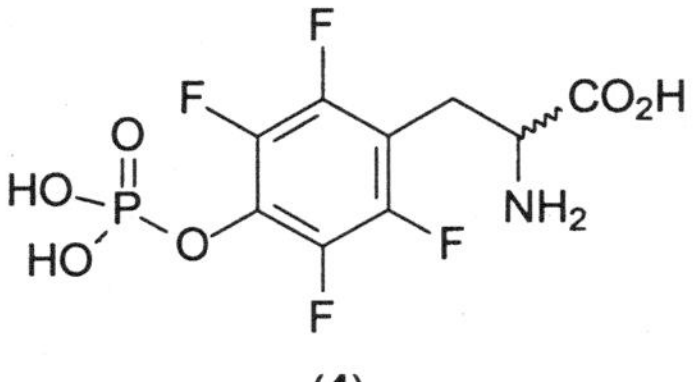

(**4**)

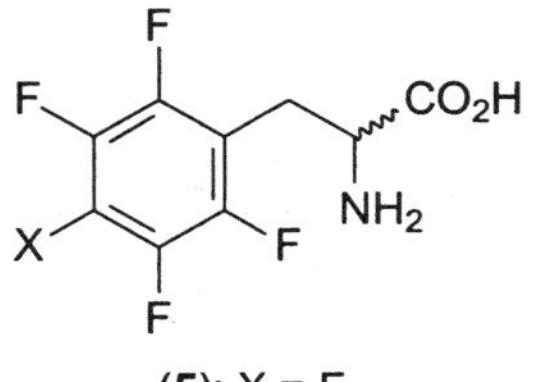

(**5**); X = F
(**6**); X = OH

Peptide libraries encompassing nonhydrolyzable phosphotyrosine surrogates have also been prepared as probes for the p56^{lck} SH2 domain of the lympho-cyte-specific tyrosine kinase, with a view to identi-fying phosphatase-stable high-affinity ligands as lead compounds for inhibitor design (24). Using the high-affinity ligand (EPQpYEEIPIYL) as the tem-plate, a solid-phase library comprising the sequence EPQXEEIPIYL was synthesized, where X denotes tyrosine (Y), phosphotyrosine (pY) or a phosphoty-rosine surrogate (2–6). Libraries were evaluated by incubation of beads with a GST-SH2 fusion protein, peptide binding being determined by a bead-binding ELISA assay. The results of this study enabled refinement of the initial template to QpYEEIP and GpYVPML, and focused libraries were prepared based on these shorter sequences. From these studies, 4-(μ-fluoro)phosphonomethyl-DL-phenylala-nine (2) and 4-(μ-hydroxy)phosphonomethyl-DL-phenylalanine (3) were identified as potentially in-teresting surrogates for O-phosphotyrosine in the QpYEEIP motif.

COMBINATORIAL APPROACHES TO IDENTIFYING SMALL-MOLECULE PROTEIN KINASE INHIBITORS

Cyclin-dependent Kinase Inhibitors

The cyclin-dependent kinase (CDK) family of en-zymes plays a pivotal role in the control of cell cycle progression, particularly at cell cycle checkpoints,

and aberrant cell cycle control, resulting from tumor suppressor gene malfunction or oncogene activation, is associated with increased CDK/cyclin activity in human tumors. CDKs are thus currently attracting considerable attention as therapeutic targets in cancer as well as nonneoplastic proliferative diseases (25–27).

The majority of small-molecule CDK inhibitors are competitive at the ATP-binding domain, and the purine pharmacophore has been widely ex-ploited for inhibitor design, as exemplified by the benchmark CDK inhibitors olomoucine (7) and (R)-roscovitine (8). The 2,6,9-trisubstitution pattern common to 7 and related compounds is very amenable to systematic variation by a combinatorial approach, and the development of synthetic methodology for the preparation of libraries has been extensively investigated.

Schultz et al. (28) employed a "binary library" ap-proach for the solid-phase synthesis of spatially sep-arated combinatorial libraries of 2,6,9-trisubstituted purines derived from 7, where one position on the purine ring was held invariant to allow attachment to the solid support. Iterative combinatorial variation of the other two positions on the purine enabled a de-termination of the optimal substitution pattern for CDK inhibition, resulting in the identification of the selective CDK1/CDK2 inhibitors purvalanol A (9) and purvalanol B (10), which were some 1,000-fold more potent than olomoucine (7) (Table 4.3). The structural basis for CDK selectivity was confirmed by determination of the crystal structure of 10 in

TABLE 4.3. *Inhibition of cyclin-dependent kinases (CDKs) by selected 2,6,9-trisubstituted purines*

(A)   (B)

Number	Structure	R	R′	IC$_{50}$(μ mol/L) CDK1/cyclin B	IC$_{50}$(μ mol/L) CDK2/cyclin A	Reference
7	A	H	Me	7.0	7.0	27
8	A	Et	CH(CH$_3$)$_2$	0.45	0.70	27
9	B	H	H	0.035	0.070	28
10	B	H	CO$_2$H	0.006	0.006	27
11	B	NH$_2$	H	0.033	0.033	29

IC$_{50}$, 50% inhibition/inhibitory concentration.

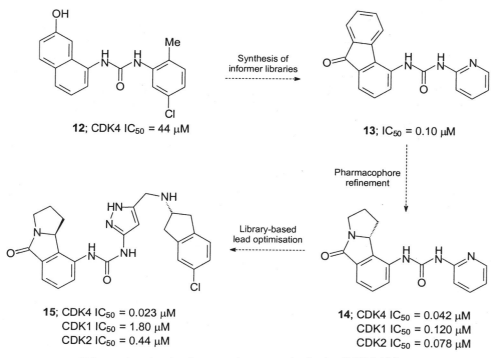

12; CDK4 IC$_{50}$ = 44 μM

13; IC$_{50}$ = 0.10 μM

Synthesis of
informer libraries

Pharmacophore
refinement

Library-based
lead optimisation

15; CDK4 IC$_{50}$ = 0.023 μM
CDK1 IC$_{50}$ = 1.80 μM
CDK2 IC$_{50}$ = 0.44 μM

14; CDK4 IC$_{50}$ = 0.042 μM
CDK1 IC$_{50}$ = 0.120 μM
CDK2 IC$_{50}$ = 0.078 μM

FIG. 4.3. Iterative development of potent and selective CDK4 inhibitors.

complex with human CDK2, and growth inhibition was demonstrated for **9** against a panel of human tumor cell lines, albeit at micromolar inhibitor concentrations.

The authors utilized SAR correlations obtained from these initial studies, together with information obtained from selected CDK2-ligand complexes, to further refine subsequent inhibitor design (29). The limitations of the original binary library approach were overcome through the development of new solid- and solution-phase syntheses, which enabled the combinatorial variation of groups at the 2, 6, and 9 positions in several libraries. The effect of substituents at these positions on the purine on CDK2 inhibitory activity was found to be approximately additive, and a number of specific and potent CDK inhibitors were identified that elicited interesting effects on the cell cycle. In addition to exhibiting potent CDK1/CDK2 inhibitory activity, several purines including **11** [50% inhibition/inhibitory concentration (IC$_{50}$) = 0.02 μmol/L] were also potent inhibitors of CDK5/p35.

A very elegant example of the use of library synthesis to complement rational drug design was recently reported for the development of highly selective CDK4-cyclin D inhibitors (30,31). A CDK4 homology model was constructed from the activated form of CDK2, and used for computational lead generation by employing a *de novo* design strategy in conjunction with database searching. Biological evaluation of candidate inhibitors identified by this approach resulted in the selection of a diarylurea template (**12**), from which informer libraries were prepared by MPS, leading to the identification of the lead inhibitor **13**. Structure-activity studies, guided by the docking of **13** with the CDK4 homology model, enabled further refinement of the pharmacophore, and the predicted binding mode in the ATP pocket of CDK4 was validated through a crystal structure determination of **14** in complex with CDK2. Selectivity for CDK4 overrelated CDKs was achieved by subsequent modification of **14**, guided by the CDK4 homology model and the CDK2-**14** complex. The preparation of defined compound libraries derived from **14** enabled optimization of the substitution pattern, resulting in the identification of **15** as a potent and highly selective CDK4 inhibitor (Fig. 4.3). G$_1$ arrest, consistent with CDK4 inhibition, was observed with submicromolar concentrations of **15** in the Rb(+) Molt-4 tumor cell line.

Protein Kinase C Activators and Inhibitors

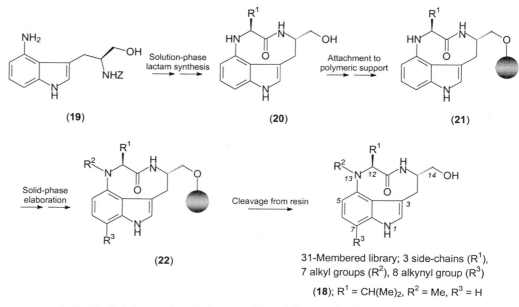

(16)   (17)

Protein kinase C (PKC) comprises a family of at least 12 closely related serine-threonine kinase isoforms, the distribution of which is partially tissue specific. Although a potentially interesting target in cancer chemotherapy, the development of clinically useful PKC inhibitors has proven challenging, in part because of the highly complex nature of the PKC signal transduction pathway and the lack of isoform-specific modulators of PKC activity. Certain classical PKC family members are activated and recruited transiently to the plasma membrane by the second messenger diacylglycerol (DAG). In order to probe the DAG C1 binding domain of PKC, Marquez et al. (32) prepared a 16-member focused combinatorial library (16) derived from the active DAG enantiomer. All possible combinations of four acyl side-chain groups,

varied with respect to size and degree of unsaturation, were introduced at two positions (R), from which compound 17 was identified as the most potent DAG ligand reported to date. Molecular modeling studies provided evidence of a preferred binding orientation for 17 in the DAG C1 domain, arising through favorable protein–ligand interactions.

A number of exogenous agents, notably the phorbol esters and bryostatin, are able to mimic the role of DAG in PKC activation and membrane translocation. (−)-Indolactam V (18), a member of the teleocidin class of tumor promoters, is also a PKC activator, and a combinatorial approach has been utilized to delineate SARs for this interesting heterocycle (33). From a consideration of established structural requirements for biological activity, the authors chose to introduce

(19)   Solution-phase lactam synthesis   (20)   Attachment to polymeric support   (21)

Solid-phase elaboration   (22)   Cleavage from resin

31-Membered library; 3 side-chains (R^1),
7 alkyl groups (R^2), 8 alkynyl group (R^3)

(18); R^1 = CH(Me)$_2$, R^2 = Me, R^3 = H

FIG. 4.4. Solution- and solid-phase combinatorial synthesis of an indolactam library.

structural diversity at the C12, N13, and C7 positions of **18**, while retaining the essential C14 hydroxyl substituent. For this purpose, a combination of solution- and solid-phase synthesis was employed (Fig. 4.4). Thus, the core indole scaffold **19** was synthesized and reacted in solution with three α-hydroxy acid ester triflates to introduce diversity at C12 (R^1). The resulting lactams (**20**) were then attached to a polymeric resin through the C14 hydroxyl group (**21**), via a suitable linker, and the combinatorial incorporation of groups at N13 (R^2) and C7 (R^3) was achieved by appropriate reactions with seven aldehydes and eight alkynes, respectively, in parallel syntheses (**22**). Cleavage from the resin afforded a library of 31 indolactam derivatives, and selected library members were evaluated as PKC activators in Swiss 3T3 fibroblasts, using a cell-based assay involving phosphorylation of MARCKS (myristoylated alanine-rich C kinase substrate). All derivatives evaluated exhibited PKC activating activity to a variable degree, but were less potent than the parent (-)-indolactam V or the standard phorbol ester PDB. The authors suggest that the varying activity observed may enable structure-function relationships to be determined, as a prelude to identifying isoform-specific PKC activators based on the indolactam pharmacophore.

The development of inhibitors of PKC has inevitably centered on agents that are competitive at the ATP-binding site, with the indolylcarbazole staurosporine A (**25**) representing the prototypic PKC inhibitor. However, although a very potent PKC inhibitor (IC$_{50}$ = 2.5 nmol/L), staurosporine A is a "pan kinase" inhibitor exhibiting potent inhibitory activity against a wide range of other kinases (34). Efforts to achieve improved PKC selectivity have been made by modifying the staurosporine core scaffold, and also through investigations with other inhibitor classes, including the fungal metabolite balanol (**23**), a potent but nonspecific PKC inhibitor. In attempting to optimize the activity of **23**, Nielson and Lyngsø (35) devised a combinatorial solid-phase synthesis for the preparation of balanol analogues, although no screening data were reported. A simple three-component linear synthesis utilizing two monoprotected diacids, four protected amino-alcohols, and four benzoic acids enabled the generation of a 32-membered library (**24**) using standard split synthesis methodology. This approach serves to illustrate how combinatorial synthesis may be used for the construction of libraries of relatively complex natural products, starting from simple building blocks.

Smith et al. (36) recently reported an interesting example of the advantages offered by combinatorial

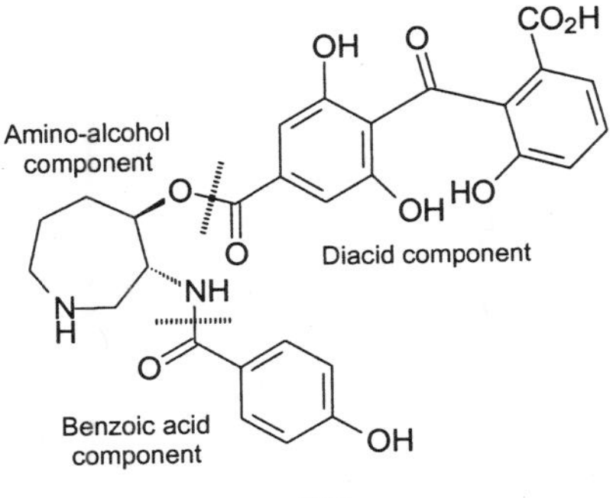

(23)

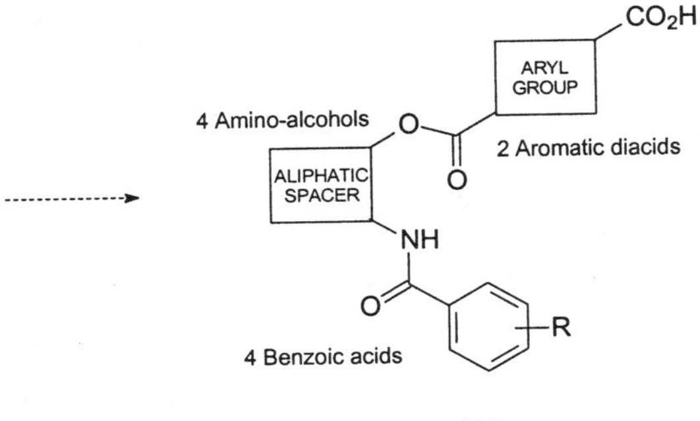

(24)

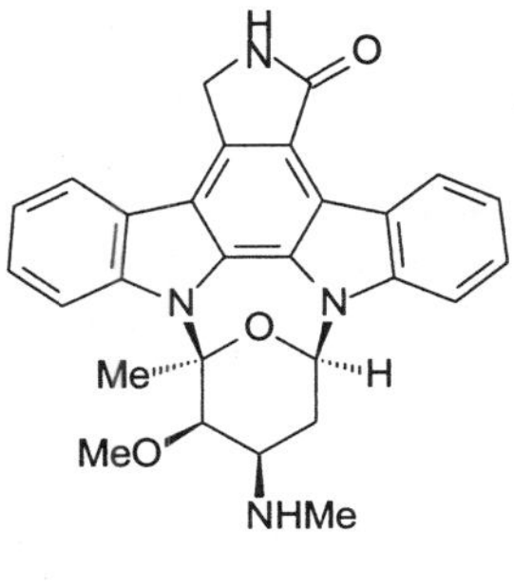

(25)

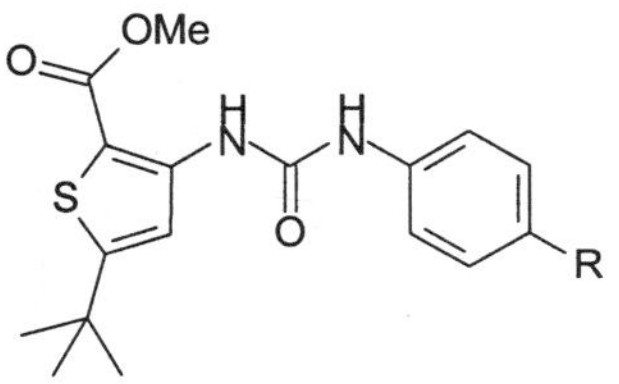

(26); R = H
(27); R = Me
(28); R =

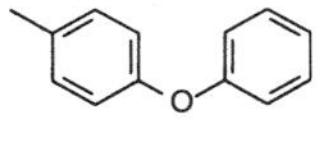

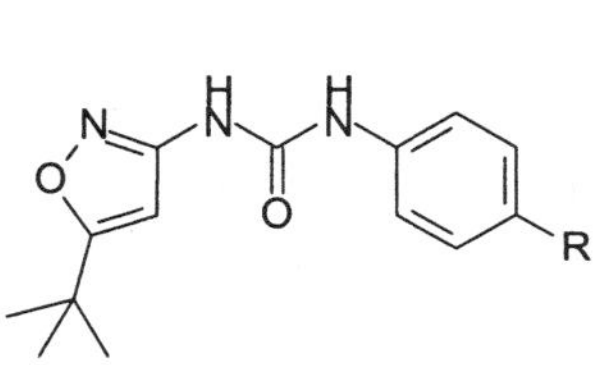

(29); R = Me
(30); R =

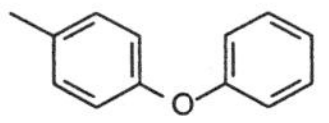

chemistry over the more conventional sequential analogue synthesis approach to lead elaboration in the development of raf kinase inhibitors at Bayer. Raf kinase, a serine-threonine kinase that functions as a downstream effector in the ras signal transduction pathway, is an attractive therapeutic target in cancer chemotherapy. The 3-thienylurea (26) was identified from high-throughput screening of the Bayer compound collection, and although only a modest inhibitor of raf kinase (IC$_{50}$ = 17 μmol/L) with higher activity against p38 MAP kinase (IC$_{50}$ = 0.29 μmol/L), the heterocyclic urea offered potential as a privileged kinase inhibitor pharmacophore. Exploration of the SAR of 26 was undertaken jointly by a conventional sequential analogue synthesis approach, where modifications to the heterocyclic and anilino substituents were made independently, and also through the synthesis of a combinatorial library varied with respect to both the heterocycle and the aniline. A library of approximately 1,000 analogues was prepared by reacting amines with isocyanates in solution phase, using a modular parallel

candidate was eventually developed. It is of interest to note that compounds encompassing either the 4-phenoxyphenyl (28) or the 5-*tert*-butyl-3-isoxazoyl substituents (29) common to 30 were both weak raf kinase inhibitors (IC$_{50}$ > 25 μmol/L). Consequently, a conventional SAR analysis based on these results would have resulted in the rejection of these fragments, and 30 would not have been synthesized.

Inhibitors of DNA-dependent Protein Kinase

The serine/threonine protein kinase DNA-dependent protein kinase (DNA-PK), a member of the phosphatidylinositol (PI) 3-kinase–like kinase (PIKK) family, plays a key role in the detection and repair of DNA double-strand breaks (37). Specific inhibitors of DNA-PK thus have potential application as radiosensitizers and chemosensitizers in cancer therapy. Our own studies, conducted in collaboration with KuDOS Pharmaceuticals, have resulted in the identification of DNA-PK inhibitors that are more potent and selective

(32)   (33)

(31)   (34)

synthesis workstation in conjunction with robotic liquid handling, and an orbital shaker heating block. The result of the traditional sequential analoging approach, involving "single-point modifications" to the structural lead, was disappointing, in that only a 10-fold improvement in potency was achieved for analogue 27. In contrast, the "multiple-point modification" of 26 achieved through a combinatorial approach, resulted in the identification of an interesting second-generation lead (30; IC$_{50}$ = 0.54 μmol/L), from which a clinical

than the benchmark PIKK family inhibitor LY294002 (31) (38). Structure-activity relationships for one such inhibitor class, the thiopyranones, were investigated using a solution-phase MPS approach. Suzuki coupling reactions conducted with the bromothiopyranone (32), afforded a library of derivatives (33) bearing a diverse range of substituents on the thiopyranone template, from which (34) was identified as one of the most potent DNA-PK inhibitor reported to date (IC$_{50}$ = 0.19 μmol/L).

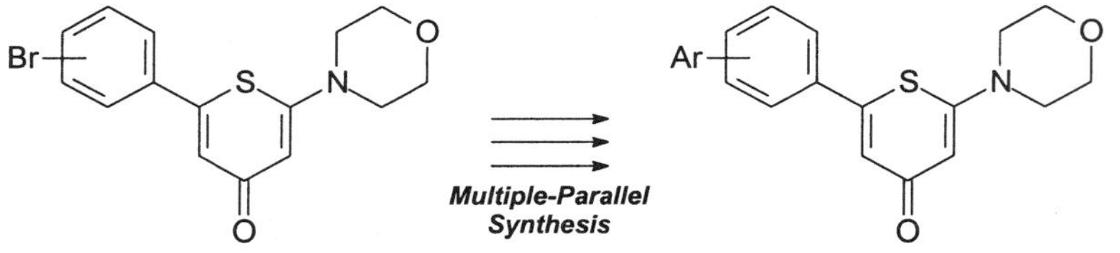

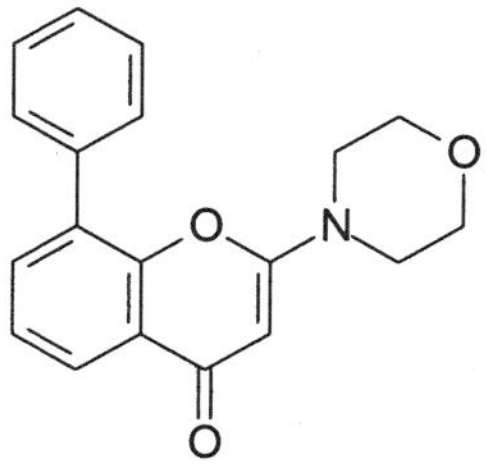

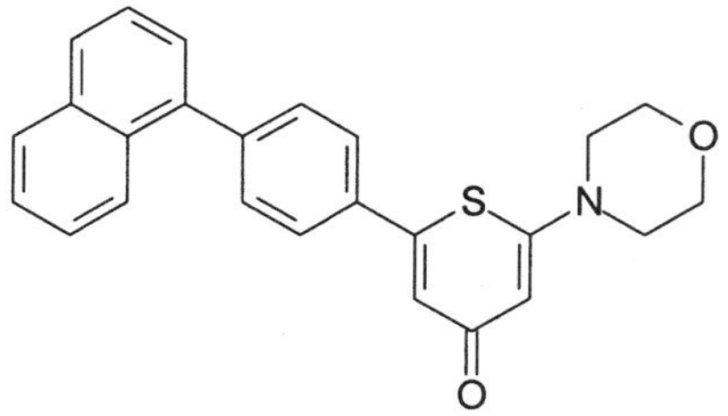

Tyrosine Kinase Inhibitors

Receptor and nonreceptor protein tyrosine kinases (PTKs) are established targets for cancer chemotherapy, and a large number of small-molecule inhibitors have been developed as prospective antitumor agents (34,39). The majority of these compounds target the ATP-binding site, and selectivity within a particular kinase family has proven challenging. In one of the earliest documented examples of combinatorial chemistry based on a natural product, Green (40) used a solid-phase synthesis strategy to prepare a library of 60 analogues of the PTK inhibitor lavendustin A (35), varied with respect to the three aryl substituents (X–Z). Unfortunately, no biological data were reported for these analogues. In a pioneering study, Czarnik et al. (41) developed a solid-phase directed sorting method, which employed reusable radiofrequency identification tags to track each stage of a multistep library synthesis. Using the tyrphostin PTK inhibitor AG490 (36)

synthesis of combinatorial libraries based on the benzodiazepine scaffold, a pharmacophore known to have peptidomimetic properties. By employing a three-component solid-phase synthesis comprising 2-aminobenzophenones, amino acids, and alkylating agents, a library of 1,680 benzodiazepines was synthesized. Compounds were cleaved from the solid support, prior to evaluation in a high-throughput kinase screen for activity against a range of PTKs, including Src, Yes, Csk, FGFr, Abl, and Lck. Several benzodiazepines were identified exhibiting 50% or greater Src inhibitory activity at 100 μmol/L, with structure-activity correlations indicating a preference for a biphenylmethyl and L-tyrosine ring substitution pattern. Compound 37 was selected as the most potent selective Src inhibitor (IC$_{50}$ = 73 μmol/L), and detailed kinetic studies revealed noncompetitive inhibition kinetics against ATP and mixed binding kinetics against the peptide substrate. Low toxicity was observed against human fibroblasts, and 37 inhibited

(35)   (36)   (37)

as a template, a 432-member library (18 × 8 × 3) was synthesized in a set of 432 tube-shaped reactors, each comprising a functionalized polystyrene matrix with a chemical linker group attached, and containing one radiofrequency identification tag. Stepwise assembly of the tyrphostin library on the reactor matrix was achieved in 29 (18 + 8 + 3) parallel reactions, and reading the radiofrequency identification tag after each reaction step enabled the products to be obtained as discrete compounds rather than as mixtures, after final cleavage from the resin. Although PTK inhibition data were not reported for the library, the authors demonstrated that the compounds obtained were sufficiently pure for direct biological evaluation without the need for further purification.

Ellman et al. (42) sought to identify selective non–ATP-competitive inhibitors of the membrane associated nonreceptor PTK pp60$^{c\text{-}Src}$ (Src) through the

colony formation in the HT29 colon adenocarcinoma, a tumor cell line known to have a high dependency for Src activity.

Another example of the use of a natural product as a biologically validated lead compound for combinatorial library synthesis relates to the nakijiquinone (38) class of inhibitors of the HER-2/Neu receptor PTK (43). The authors considered 38 as a modular structure comprising a hydrophobic terpene group, a quinone core, and a pendant amino acid substituent. By employing a solution-phase convergent synthesis approach, a 56-member library of nakijiquinone derivatives was prepared in which the quinone function was retained, the terpene was replaced with simple hydrophobic groups, and the nature of the amino acid substituent was varied. The compounds were screened against a range of receptor PTKs, and although activity was not observed against HER-2/Neu, the bis-threonine derivative (**39**) was inhibitory against Tie-2 (IC_{50} = 5 μmol/L), VEGFR-3 (IC_{50} = 3 μmol/L), and insulin-like growth factor 1 receptor (IGF1R) (IC_{50} = 6 μmol/L). Selective inhibitory activity against Tie-2 was also observed for compounds **40** and **41**, with IC_{50} values of 18 and 14 μmol/L, respectively. A kinetic analysis of **39** confirmed ATP-competitive inhibition, and molecular modeling of selected inhibitors within the ATP-binding domains of Tie-2, vascular endothelial growth factor receptor (VEGFR)-2, and VEGFR-3 revealed molecular interactions consistent with the subclass selectivity observed.

The utility of conventional combinatorial chemistry approaches for the generation of biologically active small compounds is invariably constrained by the availability of a structural lead molecule and/or knowledge of the biological target. The Ellman group has developed an innovative combinatorial strategy to enable the identification of small-molecule ligands in the absence of such information (44). This method requires the initial synthesis of a set of binding elements incorporating a common chemical linkage group, and these are evaluated at high concentrations (~1 mmol/L) to allow identification of all binding elements that interact with the biological target, however weakly. A combinatorial library is then constructed that incorporates the most active binding elements, connected through the common chemical linkage group via a set of flexible linkers, and the library of linked binding elements is screened to identify the tightest binding ligands. Preselection of the most potent binding elements in this manner, reduces the total number of compounds to be prepared, while the use of flexible linkers of varying length increases the probability of both binding elements interacting with proximal binding sites on the biological target.

The viability of this approach was exemplified through the development of potent subtype specific inhibitors of the nonreceptor PTK c-Src (44). An initial library of potential binding elements was prepared by the reaction of 305 diverse aldehydes with *O*-methylhydroxylamine, affording the corresponding *O*-methyloximes (Fig. 4.5A). These were screened for inhibitory activity against c-Src at a concentration of 1 mmol/L, and compounds exhibiting greater than 60% inhibition were reevaluated at 500 μmol/L, from which 37 potential binding elements were selected for further evaluation. To ensure that any contribution to biological activity made by the common chemical linkage group was retained, the linked binding elements were synthesized by condensing all possible combinations of the aldehyde precursors of the selected potential binding elements with an equimolar mixture of 5 *O,O'*-diaminoalkanediols ($H_2NO(CH_2)_n ONH_2$) of varying chain length (n = 2–6) in microtiter plates (666 wells) to afford a library of dioximes (Fig. 4.5B). Screening of this library of linked binding elements for c-Src activity, using a microtiter-based enzyme-linked immunosorbent assay format, enabled the selection of four wells showing greater than 50% inhibition at 1 μmol/L, and each of the component linked binding elements from these wells was resynthesized on a larger scale to allow accurate IC_{50} values to be determined. This resulted in the identification of a single linked binding element (**42**) that exhibited potent c-Src inhibitory activity (IC_{50} = 64 ± 38 nmol/L), and excellent selectivity over closely related PTKs. The relative contributions of the individual binding elements were also determined, and defined SARs were observed for **42**, with the chain length of the linker group and the catechol group both proving critical determinants of potency and kinase specificity.

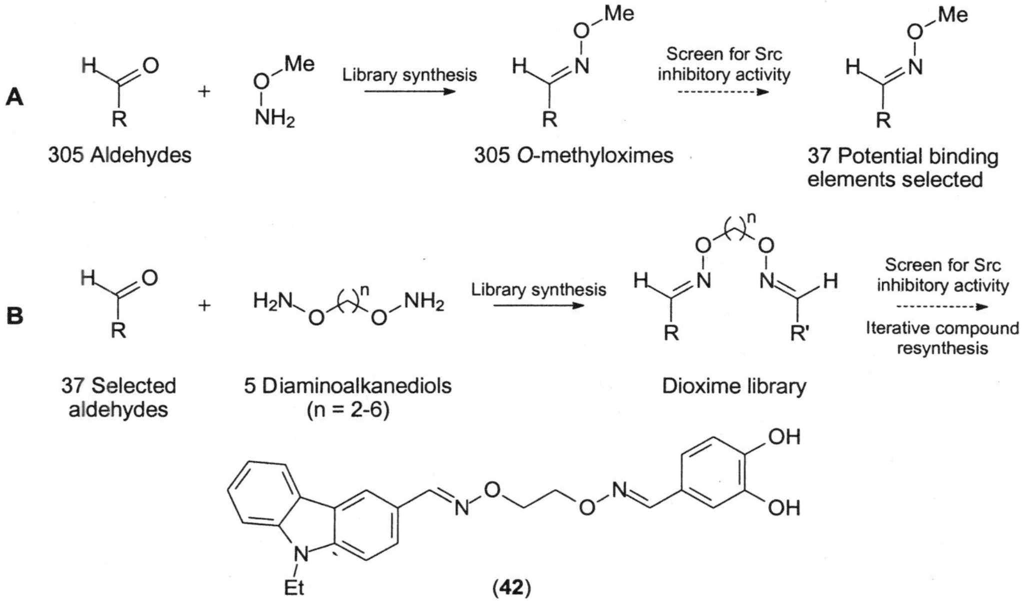

FIG. 4.5. Identification of c-Src inhibitors by combinatorial target-guided assembly.

CONCLUSIONS

Combinatorial chemistry is now a firmly established component of the drug discovery and development process, and a wide range of technologies have become available to enable the generation of chemical libraries for biological evaluation. Initial enthusiasm for the generation of large compound mixtures has been tempered by problems encountered with library deconvolution and biological screening, not least of which is the identification of "false positives," resulting in a change of emphasis towards the preparation of single-compound libraries. The quality of a chemical library is now also recognized as being of equal importance to size and diversity, and the development of validated synthetic methodology is a major factor in the design of combinatorial libraries.

Although we decided to select protein kinases to illustrate some aspects of the application of combinatorial chemistry to anticancer drug design and development, a number of other therapeutic targets, including matrix metalloproteinases, protein phosphatases, and farnesyl protein-transferases, would have been equally as appropriate. Anticancer drug development is an interdisciplinary science, and interactions at the biology–chemistry interface will be crucial to the successful exploitation of potential therapeutic targets arising from an understanding of the molecular pathology of cancer. Combinatorial chemistry is set to play an important role in this process.

The authors thank Professor B. T. Golding, School of Natural Sciences, University of Newcastle upon Tyne, for comments regarding the manuscript, and Cancer Research UK for financial support.

REFERENCES

1. Dolle RE. Comprehensive survey of combinatorial library synthesis: 2001. *J Comb Chem* 2002;4:1–50.
2. Hall DG, Manku S, Wang F. Solution- and solid-phase strategies for the design, synthesis and screening of libraries based on natural product templates: a comprehensive survey. *J Comb Chem* 2001;3:125–150.
3. Merrifield RB. Solid phase peptide synthesis I. The synthesis of a tetrapeptide. *J Am Chem Soc* 1963;85:2149–2154.
4. Letsinger RL, Mahadevan V. Stepwise synthesis of oligodeoxyribonucleotides on an insoluble polymer support. *J Am Chem Soc* 1966;88:5319–5324.
5. Cramer F, Koster H. Synthesis of oligonucleotides on a polymeric carrier. *Angew Chem Int Ed Engl* 1968;7:473–474.
6. Geysen HM, Meloen RH, Barteling SJ. Use of peptide synthesis to probe viral antigens for epitopes to a resolution of a single amino acid. *Proc Natl Acad Sci USA* 1984;81:3998–4002.
7. Houghten RA. General method for the rapid solid-phase synthesis of large numbers of peptides: specificity of antigen-antibody interaction at the level of individual amino acids. *Proc Natl Acad Sci USA* 1985;82:5131–5135.

8. Hobbs DeWitt S, Kiely JS, Stankovic CJ, et al. 'Diversomers': an approach to non-peptide, non-oligomeric chemical diversity. *Proc Natl Acad Sci USA* 1993;90: 6909–6913.

9. Bunin BA, Ellman JA. A general and expedient method for the solid phase synthesis of 1,4-benzodiazepine derivatives. *J Am Chem Soc* 1992;114:10997–10998.

10. Balkenhohl F, Bussche-Hünnefeld C, Lansky A, et al. Combinatorial synthesis of small organic molecules. *Angew Chem Int Ed Engl* 1996;35:2288–2337.

11. Nefzi A, Ostrech JM, Houghten RA. The current status of heterocyclic combinatorial libraries. *Chem Rev* 1997;97:449–472.

12. Obrecht D, Villalgordo JM. *Solid-supported combinatorial and parallel synthesis of small-molecular-weight compound libraries.* Elsevier: Oxford University Press, 1998.

13. Furka A, Sebestyén F, Asgedom M, et al. General method for rapid synthesis of multicomponent peptide mixtures. *Int J Pept Protein Res* 1991;37:487–493.

14. Lam KS, Salmon SE, Hersh EM, et al. A new type of synthetic peptide library for identifying ligand-binding activity. *Nature* 1991;354:82–84.

15. Houghten RA, Pinilla C, Blondelle SE, et al. Generation and use of synthetic peptide combinatorial libraries for basic research and drug discovery. *Nature* 1991;354: 84–86.

16. Lam KS, Wade S, Abdul-Latif F, et al. Application of a dual color detection scheme in the screening of a random combinatorial peptide library. *J. Immunol Methods* 1995;180:219–223.

17. Salmon SE, Lam KS, Lebl M, et al. Discovery of biologically active peptides in random libraries: Solution-phase testing after staged orthogonal release from resin beads. *Proc Natl Acad Sci USA* 1993;90: 11708–11712.

18. Ohlmeyer MHJ, Swanson, RN, Dillard LW, et al. Complex synthetic chemical libraries indexed with molecular tags. *Proc Natl Acad Sci USA* 1993;90: 10922–10926.

19. Lam KS, Wu JZ, Lou Q. Identification and characterization of a novel synthetic peptide substrate-specific for Src-family protein-tyrosine kinases. *Int J Pept Protein Res* 1995;45:587–592.

20. Chan PM, Nestler HP, Miller WT. Investigating the substrate specificity of the HER2/Neu tyrosine kinase using peptide libraries. *Cancer Lett* 2000;160:159–169.

21. Luo KX, Zhou P, Lodish HF. The specificity of the transforming growth-factor-beta receptor kinases determined by a spatially addressable peptide library. *Proc Natl Acad Sci USA* 1995;92:11761–11765.

22. Velentza AV, Schumacher AM, Weiss C, et al. A protein kinase associated with apoptosis and tumor suppression: structure, activity, and discovery of peptide substrates. *J Biol Chem* 2001;276:38956–38965.

23. Kelly MA, Liang HB, Sytwu II, et al. Characterization of SH2 ligand interactions via library affinity selection with mass spectrometric detection. *Biochemistry* 1996;35:11747–11755.

24. Broadbridge RJ, Sharma RP. p56(lck) SH2 domain binding motifs from bead binding screening of peptide libraries containing phosphotyrosine surrogates. *Lett Pept Sci* 1999;6:335–341.

25. Sielecki TM, Boylan JF, Benfield PA, et al. Cyclin-dependent kinase inhibitors: Useful targets in cell cycle regulation. *J Med Chem* 2000;43:1–18.

26. Sausville E. Complexities in the development of cyclin-dependent kinase inhibitor drugs. *Trends Mol Med* 2002;8:32–37.

27. Knockaert M, Greengard P, Meijer L. Pharmacological inhibitors of cyclin-dependent kinases. *Trends Pharm Sci* 2002;9:417–425.

28. Gray NS, Wodicka L, Thunnissen AWH, et al. Exploiting chemical libraries, structure, and genomics in the search for kinase inhibitors. *Science* 1998;281:533–537.

29. Chang Y-T, Gray NS, Rosania GR, et al. Synthesis and application of functionally diverse 2,6,9-trisubstituted purine libraries as CDK inhibitors. *Chem Biol* 1999;6:361–375.

30. Honma T, Hayashi K, Aoyama T, et al. Structure-based generation of a new class of potent Cdk4 inhibitors: new *de novo* design strategy and library design. *J Med Chem* 2001;44:4615–4627.

31. Homma T, Yoshizumi T, Hashimoto N, et al. A novel approach for the development of selective Cdk4 inhibitors: library design based on locations of Cdk4 specific amino acid residues. *J Med Chem* 2001;44:4628–4640.

32. Nacro K, Sigano DM, Yan S, et al. An optimized protein kinase C activating diacylglycerol combining high binding affinity (K_i) with reduced lipophilicity (log P). *J Med Chem* 2001;44:1892–1904.

33. Meseguer B, Alonso-Diaz D, Griebenow N, et al. Natural product synthesis on polymeric supports: synthesis and biological evaluation of an indolactam library. *Angew Chem Int Ed Engl* 1999;38:2902–2906.

34. Cohen P. Protein kinases: the major drug targets of the twenty-first century. *Nat Rev Drug Discov* 2002;1: 309–315.

35. Nielson J, Lyngsø LO. Combinatorial solid-phase synthesis of balanol analogues. *Tetrahedron Lett* 1996;46: 8439–8442.

36. Smith RA, Barbosa J, Blum CL, et al. Discovery of heterocyclic ureas as a new class of raf kinase inhibitors: identification of a second generation lead by a combinatorial chemistry approach. *Bioorg Med Chem Lett* 2001;11:2775–2778.

37. Smith GCM, Jackson SP. The DNA-dependent kinase. *Genes Dev* 1999;13:916–934.

38. Griffin RJ, Calvert AH, Curtin NJ, et al. Structure-activity relationships and cellular activity of chromenone and pyrimidoisoquinoline inhibitors of DNA-dependent protein kinase (DNA-PK). *Proc Am Assoc Cancer Res* 2002;43:4210.

39. Bridges AJ. Chemical inhibitors of protein kinases. *Chem Rev* 2001;101:2541–2571.

40. Green J. Solid phase synthesis of lavendustin A and analogues. *J Org Chem* 1995;60:4287–4290.

41. Shi S, Xiao X, Czarnik AW. A combinatorial synthesis of tyrphostins via the "directed sorting" method. *Biotechnol Bioeng* 1998;61:7–12.

42. Ramdas L, Bunnin BA, Plunkett MJ, et al. Benzodiazepine compounds as inhibitors of the Src protein tyrosine kinase: screening of a combinatorial library of 1,4-benzodiazepines. *Arch Biochim Biophys* 1999;368: 394–400.

43. Stahl P, Kissau L, Mazitschek R, et al. Natural product derived receptor tyrosine kinase inhibitors: identification of IGF1R, Tie-2, and VEGFR-3 inhibitors. *Angew Chem Int Ed Engl* 2002;41:1174–1178.

44. Maly DJ, Choong IC, Ellman JA. Combinatorial target-guided ligand assembly: identification of potent subtype-selective c-SRC inhibitors. *Proc Natl Acad Sci USA* 2000;97:2419–2424.

5

Protein Crystallography in Drug Discovery

Martin Noble and Jane Endicott

Laboratory of Molecular Biophysics, Department of Biochemistry,
Oxford OX1 3QU, United Kingdom

Crystallography is a technique that provides a direct image of a molecular structure at an effectively atomic resolution. This image can be interpreted as an atomic model that is accurate to within a few tenths of an angstrom of the time-averaged positions of the atoms in the crystallized target. Our understanding of the physical principles that govern molecular action and interactions can allow us, in principle, to exploit this knowledge to select or tailor molecular properties of an inhibitor to achieve the goals of accessing and binding to a potential drug target so as to treat a disease. The potential contribution of structural information to the understanding of the molecular pathology, and ultimately to the treatment of disease conditions, was immediately recognized by the founding father of the discipline of protein crystallography, Max Perutz. After determining the first structure of an oligomeric protein, hemoglobin, in 1959, he began to look for ways in which the structure might be exploited to address genetic hemoglobin diseases such as sickle cell anemia, and went on to study agents that addressed hypoxic diseases such as angina (1).

In this chapter, we will describe the principles and practice of protein crystallography, with some reference to recent developments that impact the role of crystallography in drug discovery. We will then describe the ways in which crystallography is contributing to the development of novel anticancer therapies. Blundell and Johnson (2) provide a more detailed description of the theory of x-ray crystallography.

DETERMINING TARGET STRUCTURES

Protein crystallography yields high-resolution information about the atomic structure of a drug target or target/lead complex that can make a unique and substantial contribution to an interdisciplinary drug design program. However, the method remains expensive and time consuming and has a high failure rate.

For these reasons, a great deal of effort is properly spent in selecting and validating a target. In addition to the target validation criteria discussed elsewhere, drug discovery programs that rely on crystallographic input have additional constraints in that the target must be available in a biologically relevant form and in large amounts. Typically, tens to hundreds of milligrams of pure protein will be used in the structural experiments surrounding a structure-based drug design program. A final consideration is that to make a significant impact on the drug discovery process, the structure of a target protein has to be determined at an early time point. If not, drug discovery is likely to proceed efficiently through such techniques as multiple-parallel synthesis and high-throughput screening.

The four main steps in macromolecular crystallography are crystallization, diffracted-intensity data collection, phase determination, and model building/refinement (Fig. 5.1). Improvements in technology have addressed the challenges of each of these steps, but the current rate-limiting step is protein crystallization.

Crystallization

High-throughput cloning and expression strategies are currently being developed to allow the production of a validated target in sufficiently large quantities for structural studies (3). The challenge of crystallizing these targets is effectively a search in the multidimensional space that defines solution conditions, and has been reviewed elsewhere (4). This process can be described in terms of physical chemistry, whereby crystalline states are considered as one of the potential phases accessible to a target, and conditions are sought that favor those states over the dissolved or randomly aggregated states that the protein can alternatively adopt.

The testing of each condition generally involves the mixing of a small sample (typically 0.1–10 μL)

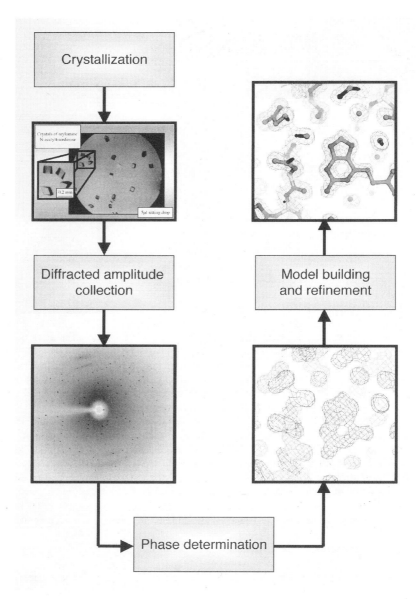

FIG. 5.1. Steps in protein structure determination by x-ray crystallography.

of a solution of the target protein at relatively high concentration (typically 0.1–10 mmol/L), with an approximately equal volume of a solution that contains reagents that encourage the target to leave the solution phase (the "precipitant solution"). Nucleation of crystal growth occurs when small ordered clusters of molecules form. These nuclei are stabilized by only a few intermolecular interactions, and therefore require a high protein concentration to form and to be maintained. Nucleation is the key step in crystallization, and the conditions that favor the formation of well-ordered crystals tend to be rather narrow. In order to slowly approach those conditions from the initial solution environment of a protein, the crystallization droplet is generally prepared with initial conditions that do not cause protein precipitation. Subsequent concentration of the protein and precipitant solution is achieved by setting the droplet close to a reservoir containing the precipitant. Volatile components of the reservoir and the droplet equilibrate slowly through the process of vapor diffusion, and under ideal conditions a small number of nuclei are formed.

Crystal growth can be supported at lower protein and precipitant concentrations than are required for nucleation. Subsequent growth occurs as additional molecules encounter the crystal nucleus in an appropriate orientation and typically macromolecular crystals seldom grow to a size greater than a few hundred micrometers in length. Successful structure determinations have been reported from crystals less than 5 μm (5). In searching for appropriate crystallization conditions, the parameters that are routinely varied include pH, temperature, ionic strength, and precipitant concentration. When using a heterologous expression system, the choice of start and end residues of a fragment of a larger multidomain protein can also be a critical determinant of a successful crystallization trial.

Diffracted Intensity Data Collection

Crystallization perfectly aligns many copies of the target molecule with respect to each other. In this arrangement they interact with x-rays to produce a scattered pattern that depends on their structure. By contrast, a single copy of a biological macromolecule would be destroyed by the dose of x-rays that would be needed to image it from current x-ray sources. The x-rays scattered from a crystal form a diffraction pattern of discrete spots. The directions in which diffracted spots occur depend on the shape of the repeating unit within the crystal, whereas the intensities and phases of the diffracted spots depend on the structure of the crystallized molecule.

X-rays for crystallography are produced in one of two ways. Laboratory-scale ("in-house") x-ray generators produce x-rays by colliding electrons with a metallic (usually copper) target. The wavelengths of peaks in the resulting x-ray emission spectrum are characteristic of the metal used in the target, and typically only a single wavelength is used for data collection. Synchrotrons exploit a different phenomenon to produce x-rays. These x-rays are substantially more intense, and have the characteristics of being intrinsically more parallel and of a selectable or tuneable wavelength.

Crystalline samples are generally exposed to x-rays under cryogenic conditions in order to mitigate the effects of radiation damage. A stream of cooled nitrogen maintains a temperature of approximately 100 K, and the crystal is protected from forming potentially damaging ice crystals by pretreatment with a cryoprotecting agent such as glycerol. The diffraction pattern is collected upon either a storage phosphor or a charged couple detector. A three-dimensional image of the target can only be achieved if the diffraction pattern of the crystal is collected in a sufficient range of orientations. Individual images are collected over a short rotation range (0.1°–2.0°), with many such images required for a complete "dataset."

Phase Determination

Available technology for recording the diffraction pattern measures the intensity of the individual diffraction spots, but is not able to record their relative phases. This removes an important part of the information required to calculate an image of the electron density distribution of the target molecule and is referred to as the "phase problem," historically a rate-limiting step in a structure determination.

The diffracted phases can be determined by implementation of methods that utilize one of four principles. Most simply, recording of a set of diffraction intensities to a sufficient resolution can allow phases to be determined essentially directly. This process requires that the crystal be sufficiently well ordered so that individual atomic positions (generally separated by approximately 1.5 Å) are resolved. The second principle is that of isomorphous replacement. Methods for phase determination that employ this principle infer the diffracted phases from a comparison of diffraction patterns collected in the absence (native crystals) and presence (derivative crystals) of a specifically binding, intensely scattering atom (heavy atom). The third principle is anomalous scattering. Methods based on this principle rely on a breakdown in some of the symmetry normally observed in a diffraction pattern that occurs if incident x-rays are used that match an absorption energy of a heavy atom that is intrinsic to the target (e.g., copper atoms in metalloproteins) or introduced in a soaking experiment. The final principle, one that is particularly important in drug design programs, is molecular replacement. Molecular replacement protocols take advantage of the fact that a reasonable estimate of diffracted phases can be calculated from an approximate atomic model of the molecule within a crystal. The model can come either from a previous structure determination of the target molecule or from a previously determined structure of a homologue. However, to be optimistic of a successful solution, this homologue should represent more than 50% of the contents of the target crystal and be more than 30% identical in sequence.

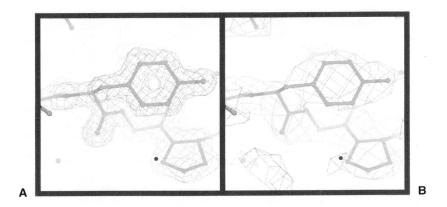

FIG. 5.2. Electron density maps. Representative electron density for a tyrosine residue calculated using observations to respectively relatively **(A)** high (1.5 Å) or **(B)** low (3.0 Å) resolution. At the higher resolution, the shape of the tyrosine side-chain is clearly discernible. The protein is drawn in ball-and-stick mode.

Model Building and Structure Refinement

Combining estimates of the diffraction phases with the measured diffraction amplitudes allows the computer-aided generation of an image of the target molecule(s). Because x-ray scattering is a property of the electrons of the atoms that constitute a molecule, the image is actually one of the electron density of the molecule, and thus is strongest for more electron-dense atoms (e.g., Cu, Fe), moderately strong for the main constituents of biological macromolecules (C, N, O, S, P), and extremely weak for hydrogen atoms. The final challenge in crystallography is to interpret an electron density image in terms of an atomic model. Where the data allow the resolution of features separated by less than 1.5 Å, individual peaks in the electron density can be correlated with individual atoms of the target molecule. Otherwise, computers (or crystallographers) have to be able to recognize the characteristic electron density shapes of the monomers (amino acids or nucleic acid bases) that constitute the target molecule. Figure 5.2 shows the difference in electron density for a part of a molecule that results from using observations to relatively high (1.5 Å, Fig 5.2A) and low (3.0 Å, Fig. 5.2B) resolution. In practice, map interpretation is generally achieved in a semiautomatic way, provided that the diffraction extends beyond 2.5-Å resolution.

Refinement is the procedure whereby parameters of the atomic model (i.e., the coordinates and displacement factors of the constituent atoms) are modified to maximize the agreement with observed diffraction data and known stereochemical preferences of the groups involved.

Determining Structures of Complexes

The structure of a target in complex with a lead compound can be determined either by soaking experiments or by cocrystallization. Each technique has its strengths and weaknesses. In a soaking experiment, preformed "apo"-crystals of the target are incubated with the ligand in a step subsequent to crystal growth. In a cocrystallization trial, the compound is present in the droplet in which the protein crystal grows. This experimental design allows the target protein to undergo the full range of ligand-induced structural changes that reflect inhibitor binding in solution. It may enable a more accurate picture of ligand binding to be gained, which can inform further inhibitor development and it may also be a required procedure where ligand-induced conformational changes in the target would damage a preformed crystal. The strength of cocrystallization can, however, also be a weakness: ligand binding prior to crystallization may change the structure or flexibility of the target in such a way as to preclude crystal growth under previously identified apoenzyme crystallization conditions. Hence, cocrystallization may require repeated broad screening of crystallization conditions for each ligand studied. In practice, this need not be a substantial hurdle where different ligands do not have a dramatically different effect on target structure or flexibility. Nevertheless, crystal-soaking experiments remain the technique of choice for high-throughput determination of protein/ligand complex structures.

THE ROLES OF PROTEIN CRYSTALLOGRAPHY IN DRUG DISCOVERY

Figure 5.3 presents a flow diagram of the stages in a drug discovery program. We will use this chart to illustrate how crystallography can and does contribute to many aspects of drug discovery.

Target Identification

Although historically crystallography has not contributed to target identification, it is hoped that this will change in a postgenomic world (6). High-throughput structural genomics initiatives will provide structures for a number of proteins for which potential function cannot be predicted by bioinformatics. For these proteins, structure determination may reveal a previously observed fold that suggests function, while for others a novel fold will be the starting point for a functional study. For any protein, validation as a target for potential therapeutic intervention should precede an initiative to identify potent and selective inhibitors.

Target Validation

To be a validated therapeutic target, the cellular function of a protein has to be fully characterized. Genetic methods are usually employed to disrupt protein function in such a way that its roles in the cell can be identified. Traditionally, such techniques include gene disruption and generation of conditional mutant alleles and/or of overexpression strains. However, these approaches have unwanted "side effects" that can make interpretation of the results difficult. This is particularly the case in the study of molecules involved in signal transduction where the inherent redundancy and overlapping nature of signaling pathways means that identifying the unique contribution of any one component of the signaling network is difficult.

To complement these approaches, once a protein has been suggested as a target for therapeutic intervention, a crystallographic structure can contribute to its validation in two main ways. Firstly, a high-resolution molecular structure can direct the selection and/or design of small-molecule inhibitors that can confirm the efficacy of specific inhibition of the target in disease treatment. Reverse chemical genetics is a very powerful extension of this approach. Secondly, structures may help to establish the existence and "druggability" of potential ligand-binding sites that might offer an opportunity for inhibition.

Selective knockout of protein activity by specific inhibition, when used as a probe of the cellular role of that protein, is part of the field of chemical genetics. Whereas "forward" chemical genetics studies the phenotype induced by treatment of a system with a given chemical and does not require any structural insight into the molecular targets of the chemical being used, "reverse" chemical genetics requires a structure of the target protein at atomic resolution. With this knowledge, the protein can be specifically mutated to accommodate the novel ligand. The foundation of the technique was laid by Hwang and Miller (7) in their work on elongation factor Tu, where they discovered that by selectively mutating residue Asp 138 to an asparagine, they changed the enzyme's base specificity from guanosine to xanthosine. Since this early work,

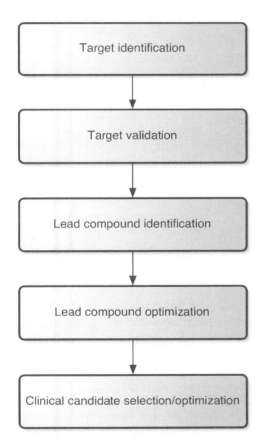

FIG. 5.3. Flow diagram illustrating the steps in a drug discovery program.

reverse chemical genetics has been used successfully to study the roles of GTPases, kinesin, and myosin motors and protein kinases (8).

Protein kinases are key components of signal transduction pathways, the deregulation of which can contribute to the development of a cancer phenotype. As such, they offer a good example of the ways in which structural knowledge combined with reverse chemical genetics can be used for target validation. In order to assess the roles of specific kinases in both normal and diseased cells, Shokat et al. (9) used structural information to design and produce versions of several kinases that can be specifically and selectively addressed in a cellular environment. Addressing in this context means either enabling the kinase activity, by providing the modified kinase with an adenosine triphosphate (ATP) analogue that can be utilized by that kinase but no other kinase within the cell, or alternatively inhibiting activity by specifically challenging the enzyme with an inhibitor that binds uniquely to it.

The design of suitable ligands and the corresponding active site mutations has relied heavily on the availability of structures of both protein kinases and protein-kinase/ligand complexes. Selective protein kinase activation or inhibition is achieved by using site-directed mutagenesis to reveal a "hole" in the kinase active site. At the back of the protein kinase ATP binding site is a so-called "gatekeeper" residue [equivalent to Phe 80 in cyclin-dependent kinase 2 (CDK2)] that in all human protein kinase sequences has a large side-chain that blocks entry into a back pocket. This hole is able to accommodate a bulky group such as a benzyl moiety on a ligand that binds into the adenine binding pocket (i.e., an inhibitor or ATP analogue). Mutation of the gatekeeper residue to one with a small side-chain such as glycine or alanine allows the resulting enzyme (a so-called "bump" mutant) to bind to the modified ligand while all other protein kinases present in the cell cannot.

When the ligand is modified N6-benzyl ATP, radioactively labeled at its γ-phosphate group, then it can be used to directly identify the bump mutant protein's substrates as part of the target validation process. When the benzyl group is appropriately synthesized into a potent and selective ATP-competitive inhibitor of the protein, then the approach effectively parallels the experimental technique of protein ablation through gene-knockout, antisense RNA, or Tet-on/Tet-off methods. However, it has three advantages over these techniques. Firstly, it is inducible: the inhibitor can be selectively added to or depleted from the growth medium of cells under study. Secondly, it acts rapidly: the inhibitor knocks out function at the protein level and the only limiting factor is the rate of inhibitor diffusion from the media to its site of action within the cell. Finally, it is domain specific: in a multidomain protein, only the function of the domain that binds the inhibitor is inactivated.

Confirming the existence of interaction sites that can be targeted by subsequent structure-based drug design as part of target validation can also be achieved by reference to a suitable crystallographically determined protein structure. Using another twist on the chemical genetics approach, Schultz et al. (10) mutated human growth hormone and the extracellular domain of the human growth hormone receptor so that the binding affinity between the two proteins is significantly (by a factor of 10^6) reduced. A small molecule was then identified that, by binding into the cavity created by the two mutations, restored the interaction.

Signal transduction pathways rely on protein-protein interactions, and proteins that are commonly mutated in various cancers are known to act through forming stable complexes with regulators and effectors. Targeting the extensive surface areas that are generally involved in such interactions is a challenge for any form of rational drug design. These interfaces are, in general, unsuitable for competitive inhibition through the type of relatively small molecule that is likely to have acceptable pharmacokinetic properties. However, a number of complex structures have provided the starting point for anticancer drug design programs. These include the CDK2/cyclin A/p27 (11), MDM2/p53 peptide (12) (Fig. 5.4), Bcl-2/Bak BH3 domain peptide (13) and SH2/peptide complexes (14). These complex structures have excited interest because the key protein–protein interfaces are localized to recessed patches or grooves on the surface of the molecules and have a marked core region that is predominantly hydrophobic. These characteristics are typical of known drug-binding sites and suggest that these sites are "druggable" (15–18).

Lead Compound Identification

In structure-based drug design, a lead compound is often related to a substrate or cofactor. Information about how one might modify this backbone is frequently provided by structural analysis of complexes of the target protein bound to chemically diverse ligands including both the substrate itself, and inhibitors that have been identified by high-throughput screening (HTS). Structure/activity relationships in the different series identified by HTS ultimately provide a pharmacophore model of the inhibitor binding site that includes detailed information about available

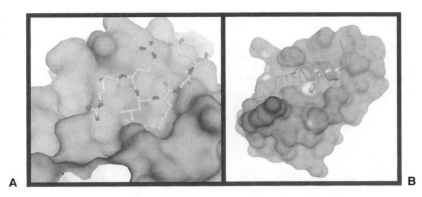

FIG. 5.4. Protein–protein interactions amenable to small molecule inhibition. **A:** Cyclin A-p27. **B:** MDM2-p53. The Connelly molecular surfaces of (A) cyclin A and (B) MDM2 are colored according to hydrophobic potential from dark gray (low affinity) to light gray (high affinity) using the program Aesop (M. Noble, 2003, unpublished results). The cyclin A recruitment site binds to a short peptide consensus sequence RXLF present in a number of cyclin-dependent kinase 2 (CDK2) substrates and inhibitors including p27. This interaction is illustrated by the peptide RRLFGE derived from the retinoblastoma-related protein p107 (32). The p107 peptide is drawn in ball-and-stick mode. **B:** MDM2 recognizes the hydrophobic face of a p53 α-helix. The p53 peptide backbone is shown together with the side chains of residues Phe 19, Trp 23, and Leu 26 that bind into the deep hydrophobic cleft on the MDM2 surface.

protein/inhibitor interactions. Figure 5.5 illustrates the diverse chemical series that have been used to define the pharmacophore of CDK2.

Two main technologies exploit crystallography to accelerate the process of lead identification, both of which require knowledge of the target protein structure. In the "fragment library" approach, small chemical fragments (molecular weight typically 100–200 d) that represent the synthons from which inhibitors may be constructed (Fig. 5.6) are cocrystallized with the target protein or soaked at high concentrations into apoprotein crystals (19,20). The fragments themselves are likely to be only poor inhibitors of protein activity (kd > 100 μmol/L), but their binding can nevertheless be detected in a crystallographic experiment in which they are present at concentrations in the millimolar range. Such binding studies can be pursued efficiently by use of synthon cocktails, where each constituent can be readily distinguished on the basis of shape in an electron density map. As well as serving as a binding assay for these fragments, the crystallographic experiment provides knowledge of their binding mode that can subsequently guide construction *in silico* of potential high-affinity ligands amenable to chemical synthesis.

This method lends itself to protein targets that are readily crystallized and that diffract to high resolution. Although such targets have often been the subject of more conventional inhibitor-binding studies, this may not continue to be the case as high-throughput methods provide structures for proteins that have had little biochemical or biological characterization. The method has an interesting counterpart in the area of drug design assisted by nuclear magnetic resonance, where "SAR by NMR" techniques can be used to quickly assemble fragments into high-affinity inhibitors (21).

The holy grail of computational drug design is the ability to predict the molecular structure of a potent and selective inhibitor of a validated drug target, with excellent pharmacokinetic properties, solely by reference to the three-dimensional structure of that target. While this goal has not yet been realized, two main approaches have been developed to identify high-affinity ligands from a crystallographically determined structure of the apotarget. The first of these is to map the inhibitor-binding site of the drug target in terms of chemical character, and then to infer the structure of a chemical moiety that presents complementary functional groups in the appropriate geometric constellation. The second related method is to use computational techniques to search for potential binding sites for large, hypothetical collections of chemicals within the known structure of a drug target. This process of "virtual screening" is a direct computational equivalent to the process of experimental HTS, but has been found to offer some advantages when used in combination with the more experimental approach. Specifically, the number of false positive (i.e., compounds that do not prove to have the indi-

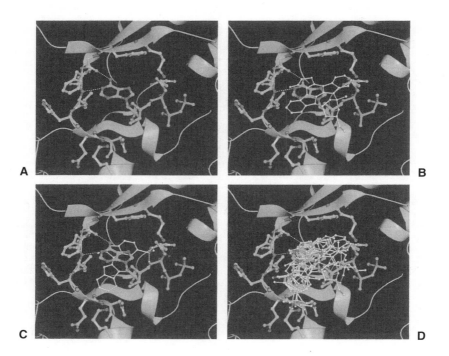

FIG. 5.5. Defining a pharmacophore model for cyclin-dependent kinase 2 (CDK2). The elucidation of the binding modes of multiple adenosine triphosphate (ATP)-competitive inhibitors to CDK2 have helped define a pharmacophore model for the enzyme. The CDK2 fold is rendered in ribbon mode and the side-chains of selected residues within the CDK2 ATP binding site that make contacts to the ligand are drawn in ball-and-stick mode. Dotted lines represent hydrogen bonds. For comparison, ATP bound to CDK2 is included in each panel. The inhibitor backbones are overlaid on ATP as ball-and-stick models in a light color. **A:** CDK2-ATP (PDB code 1HCK). **B:** CDK2-staurosporine (PDB code 1AQ1). **C:** CDK2–indirubin-5-sulphonate (33). **D:** Overlay of multiple CDK2–small-molecule inhibitor complexes.

cated effect upon further characterization), nonspecific, and nondruglike compounds that are identified in HTS has made the method less effective than initially expected (22).

Programs that carry out virtual screening are differentiated in two main ways: the way in which putative target/ligand complexes are scored (i.e., in which their relative affinity is estimated), and the search algorithm that is used to generate atomic models of those complexes. Scoring schemes can be characterized either as empirical [e.g., LUDI (23)] or as derived by "inverse Boltzmann" approaches [e.g., PMF (24)]. In an empirical scoring scheme, simplified mathematical descriptions of the underlying physics of nonbonded interactions and internal strain in ligand and receptor are used to produce an estimate of the energy of a receptor/ligand complex. "Inverse Boltzmann" approaches are related, but derive the parameters for evaluating the strengths of nonbonded interactions

from surveying the available known structures of small molecules and protein/ligand complexes. Favorable interactions are identified as those that occur most frequently in such complexes, and a pseudoforce constant can be derived from the distribution of observed interatomic distances for each different type of atom pair. In practice it is often found that different scoring schemes perform best for certain receptors, presumably as a consequence of their different handling of polar and nonpolar interactions. Overall, combined scoring schemes are found to offer the best enrichment of useful hits (25).

Search algorithms seek either to transfer the molecule from solution to the optimal binding site in an energetically steered random walk [e.g., DOCK (26)], or to use constraints of shape and chemical character to elaborate the range of binding "poses" that place inhibitor atoms close to complementary regions of the receptor surface [e.g., FlexX (27)].

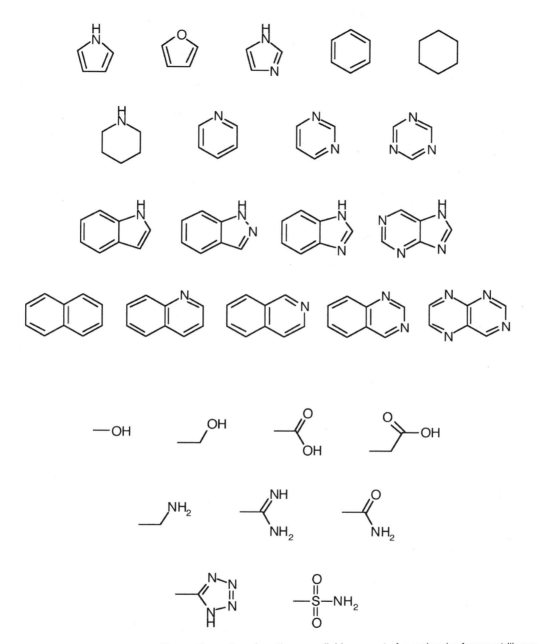

FIG. 5.6. A molecular fragment library. Examples of synthons available as part of a molecular fragment library that can be used to enumerate, by x-ray crystallographic analysis, potential interactions of a ligand to a protein target as part of a lead-compound identification program.

Lead Compound Optimization

Macromolecular crystallography contributes to lead-compound optimization as part of an iterated cycle that includes compound synthesis, biological evaluation, lead-target complex structure determination, and further design (Fig. 5.7). A perfect predictive understanding of the forces that bind small molecules to macromolecular receptors would allow this process to be completed in a single pass. Unfortunately, efforts to identify the optimum modification to apply to a lead compound are confounded by the complex energy terms that underlie nonbonded interactions, as well as the problems of flexibility in the macromolecular target and the lead compound itself. Although these phenomena can be relatively accurately modelled, to do so requires a great deal of computing power—a requirement that limits the range of chemical modifications that can be tested *in silico* in a reasonable time. Iteration of a structure-based drug design cycle, in which the efficacy of comparatively small suggested modifications is confirmed biologically and the anticipated binding mode is confirmed experimentally, allows a broad chemical space to be explored in a stepwise process, with each step based on firm observation.

Early successes of this approach (28) have benefited from visualization of the ligand/receptor complex and the chemical intuition of a team involved in inhibitor design. At the simplest level, the structure of the complex identifies key interactions that drive inhibitor binding, and that should be preserved in sub-sequent generations. Optimization of the interaction is then achieved by increasing the complementarity of the inhibitor to the extended interaction site in terms of both shape and atomic property. Experience has shown that free energy of interaction can effectively be won by: (a) minimizing the introduction of uncompensated polar binding functions that occur when a complex is formed, and (b) maximizing the apolar:apolar contact surface area of the complex. Beyond this observation, the crystallographic structure can identify points of strain or unusual conformation in the inhibitor or the target. Such locations indicate chemical modifications to maintain the desired interactions, while either (a) providing a more optimal geometry in the combining site, or (b) preforming the bound inhibitor conformation by locking it chemically or sterically through, for example, cyclization.

From an experimentally determined structure of the complex of a target with a lead compound, a number of computational approaches have been used to identify modifications that are likely to improve potential druglike properties. These all use the principles outlined in this chapter to predict the binding energy of a slightly modified lead compound, but can be characterized as growing or assembling the next generation compound. Growing strategies involve the addition of atoms or fragments to the scaffold offered by the lead compound in order to produce a new compound, whereas assembling strategies explore the region surrounding a lead compound to discover potential binding sites for chemical fragments, using techniques analogous to docking. The next-generation compound is subsequently designed by identifying how to link the scaffold to the neighboring fragments.

The ability to identify a chemical species that would form optimal interactions with a drug target would not of itself allow the instant design of a drug; even before considerations such as pharmacokinetics, a computationally designed molecule would need to be amenable to chemical synthesis. Historically this problem has been addressed in less automated iterations of a drug design cycle by using the chemical intuition of inhibitor designers (i.e., by asking the chemists). Automation of this process requires that two areas of computational science be brought together: docking/modeling approaches to identify molecules that are anticipated to have improved druglike properties, and expert systems of organic synthesis to identify synthetic routes to those compounds. As well as applying the requirement that a molecule should be amenable to synthesis as a screening step after the process of design, efforts are being made to integrate the principles of retrosynthesis into packages that propose candidate molecules.

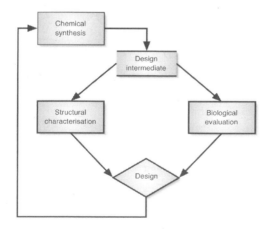

FIG. 5.7. Lead-compound optimization. Optimization of a lead compound results from iteration of a cycle that includes the steps of compound synthesis, biological evaluation, lead-target complex structure determination, and design.

Clinical Candidate Selection

Conventionally, the contribution of crystallography to drug discovery has finished with the emergence of a tight binding inhibitor. Unfortunately, this is far from the ultimate target of a therapeutic. Today, crystallography can also contribute to the refinement of pharmacokinetic properties that distinguish a useful drug from a potent inhibitor. Since the emergence of empirical rules that relate inhibitor structure to pharmacokinetics (29), it has been possible to identify ways in which to improve properties of drug uptake and stability. Structural information about inhibitor binding allows targeted modification of inhibitors so that they conform with such rules without losing chemical potency. The future holds still more promise. Available structures for major drug metabolizing enzymes such as cytochrome P450 will further allow prediction of the metabolic stability of compounds in advance of costly experiments. Structural studies have already been used to rationalize the emergence of drug resistance in chronic myeloid leukemia patients treated with the c-Abl protein drug imatinib (Gleevec, formerly known as STI571 and Glivec) (30,31) (Fig. 5.8). It is to be hoped that this understanding will allow the design of subsequent generations of compound that can overcome this problem.

The authors thank E. Lowe, J. Sinclair and S. Holton for their assistance with the figures. Work in the authors' laboratories is supported by the Medical Research Council (MRC, UK), Biological Sciences Research Council (BBSRC, UK), The Wellcome Trust, the Human Frontier Science Program (HFSP), and Oxford University.

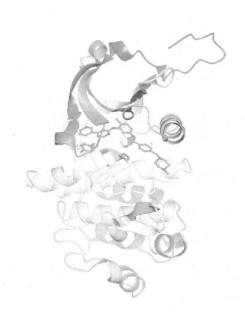

FIG. 5.8. Structure of the imatinib–c-Abl kinase complex. The c-Abl kinase domain is drawn in ribbon representation. Imatinib (Gleevec) is drawn in ball and stick mode bound within the c-abl ATP binding site cleft [PDB code 1IEP, (30)]. The tyrosine side-chain located close to imatinib is one site where point mutations have conferred drug resistance.

REFERENCES

1. Perutz MF, Fermi G, Abraham DJ, et al. Hemoglobin as a receptor of drugs and peptides: X-ray studies of the stereochemistry of binding. *J Am Chem Soc* 1986;108: 1064–1078.
2. Blundell TL, Johnson LN, eds. *Protein crystallography.* New York, Academic Press, 1976.
3. Yokoyama S. Protein expression systems for structural genomics and proteomics. *Curr Opin Chem Biol* 2003; 7:39–43.
4. McPherson A, ed. *Crystallization of biological macromolecules.* New York: Cold Spring Harbor Laboratory Press, 1999.
5. Brown NR, Noble ME, Endicott JA, et al. The crystal structure of cyclin A. *Structure* 1995;3:1235–1247.
6. Russell R.B, Eggleston DS. New roles for structure in biology and drug discovery. *Nat Struct Biol* 2000; 7[Suppl]:928–930.
7. Hwang YW, Miller DL. A mutation that alters the nucleotide specificity of elongation factor Tu, a GTP regulatory protein. *J Biol Chem* 1987;262:13081–13085.
8. Bishop A, Buzko O, Heyeck-Dumas S, et al. Unnatural ligands for engineered proteins: new tools for chemical genetics. *Annu Rev Biophys Biomol Struct* 2000;29: 577–606.
9. Bishop AC, Ubersax JA, Petsch DT, et al. A chemical switch for inhibitor-sensitive alleles of any protein kinase. *Nature* 2000;407:395–401.
10. Guo Z, Zhou D, Schultz PG. Designing small-molecule switches for protein-protein interactions. *Science* 2000;288:2042–2045.
11. Russo AA, Jeffrey PD, Patten AK, et al. Crystal structure of the p27Kip1 cyclin-dependent-kinase inhibitor bound to the cyclin A-Cdk2 complex. *Nature* 1996; 382:325–331.
12. Kussie PH, Gorina S, Marechal V, et al. Structure of the MDM2 oncoprotein bound to the p53 tumor suppressor transactivation domain. *Science* 1996;274:948–953.
13. Sattler M, Liang H, Nettesheim D, et al. Structure of Bcl-xL-Bak peptide complex: recognition between regulators of apoptosis. *Science* 1997;275:983–986.

14. Waksman G, Shoelson SE, Pant N, et al. Binding of a high affinity phosphotyrosyl peptide to the Src SH2 domain: crystal structures of the complexed and peptide-free forms. *Cell* 1993;72:779–790.
15. Chen YN, Sharma SK, Ramsey TM, et al. Selective killing of transformed cells by cyclin/cyclin-dependent kinase 2 antagonists. *Proc Natl Acad Sci U S A* 1999; 96:4325–4329.
16. Stoll R, Renner C, Hansen S, et al. Chalcone derivatives antagonize interactions between the human oncoprotein MDM2 and p53. *Biochemistry* 2001;40:336–344.
17. Degterev A, Lugovskoy A, Cardone M, et al. Identification of small-molecule inhibitors of interaction between the BH3 domain and Bcl-xL. *Nat Cell Biol* 2001; 3:173–182.
18. Garcia-Echeverria C. Antagonists of the Src homology 2 (SH2) domains of Grb2, Src, Lck and ZAP-70. *Curr Med Chem* 2001;8:1589–1604.
19. Blundell TL, Jhoti H, Abell C. High-throughput crystallography for lead discovery in drug design. *Nat Rev Drug Discov* 2002;1:45–54.
20. Nienaber VL, Richardson PL, Klighofer V, et al. Discovering novel ligands for macromolecules using X-ray crystallographic screening. *Nat Biotechnol* 2000;18: 1105–1108.
21. Shuker SB, Hajduk PJ, Meadows RP, et al. Discovering high-affinity ligands for proteins: SAR by NMR. *Science* 1996;274:1531–1534.
22. Rishton G. Reactive compounds and *in vitro* false positives in HTS. *Drug Discov Today* 1997;2:382–384.
23. Bohm HJ. The development of a simple empirical scoring function to estimate the binding constant for a protein-ligand complex of known three-dimensional structure. *J Comput Aided Mol Des* 1994;8:243–256.
24. Muegge I, Martin YC. A general and fast scoring function for protein-ligand interactions: a simplified potential approach. *J Med Chem* 1999;42:791–804.
25. Bissantz C, Folkers G, Rognan D. Protein-based virtual screening of chemical databases. 1. Evaluation of different docking/scoring combinations. *J Med Chem* 2000; 43:4759–4767.
26. Ewing TJ, Makino S, Skillman AG, et al. DOCK 4.0: search strategies for automated molecular docking of flexible molecule databases. *J Comput Aided Mol Des* 2001;15:411–428.
27. Rarey M, Kramer B, Lengauer T, et al. A fast flexible docking method using an incremental construction algorithm. *J Mol Biol* 1996;261:470–489.
28. Wlodawer A, Vondrasek J. Inhibitors of HIV-1 protease: a major success of structure-assisted drug design. *Annu Rev Biophys Biomol Struct* 1998;27:249–284.
29. Lipinski CA, Lombardo F, Dominy BW, et al. Experimental and computational approaches to estimate solubility and permeability in drug discovery and development settings. *Adv Drug Deliv Rev* 2001;46:3–26.
30. Schindler T, Bornmann W, Pellicena P, et al. Structural mechanism for STI-571 inhibition of abelson tyrosine kinase. *Science* 2000;289:1938–1942.
31. Capdeville R, Buchdunger E, Zimmermann J, et al. Glivec (STI571, Imatinib), a rationally developed targeted anticancer drug. *Nat Rev Drug Discov* 2002;1: 493–502.
32. Brown NR, Noble ME, Endicott JA, et al. The structural basis for specificity of substrate and recruitment peptides for cyclin-dependent kinases. *Nat Cell Biol* 1999; 1:438–443.
33. Hoessel R, Leclerc S, Endicott JA, et al. Indirubin, the active constituent of a Chinese antileukaemia medicine, inhibits cyclin-dependent kinases. *Nat Cell Biol* 1999;1:60–67.

6

High-Throughput Screening

Ramesh Padmanabha and Martyn Banks

Lead Discovery, Bristol-Myers Squibb Pharmaceutical Research Institute, Wallingford, Connecticut 06492

Full many a gem of purest ray serene, the dark unfathomed caves of ocean bear.

—Thomas Gray

Drug discovery is a critical component within a pharmaceutical company's research and development process. Early drug discovery is challenged to rapidly add new compounds to the drug development pipeline. This has lead to a continuous drive to increase the efficiency of this process so new medicines with improved efficacy and fewer side effects can be delivered to patients (1).

Screening for new chemical entities has been around for many decades; for example, scientists like Paul Ehrlich screened hundreds of compounds trying to find an antisyphilitic "magic bullet." Through the middle of the twentieth century there was a concerted effort to screen compounds *in vivo* to detect biological activity. This approach was essentially serendipitous and low capacity, and often the mechanism of action of the compounds was not clear. Today, after a series of scientific and technological advances in our ability to clone, express, and isolate human proteins, opportunities have been created for different drug discovery paradigms. Critically, through functional genomics and bioinformatics there is a growing understanding of the complexities of the disease state at a molecular level, which in turn has lead to a growing number of potential therapeutic targets (2–6). From a chemistry perspective there are numerous robust synthetic platforms capable of generating thousands of compounds in relatively short timeframes (7). To complement this growth in the number of available compounds, there has been significant investment in the infrastructure to store and distribute compounds for testing. The essential challenge has been to integrate the opportunity presented by more compounds and more targets.

High-throughput screening (HTS) is one technological solution to this problem. Simply put, HTS is the ability to perform a large number of assays in a short period of time.

High-throughput screening itself has undergone a tremendous change over the last decade (8,9). These changes have been both evolutionary and revolutionary (10,11). The evolutionary changes have involved the gradual movement towards miniaturization, the concomitant improvements in assay automation technology, and the improvements in the information technology (IT) infrastructure to enable the handling of increasing volumes of data (12–14). The revolutionary changes have been a paradigm shift in the way HTS is performed. Previously, HTS was treated as a "mere" scale up of regular laboratory assays and practices (15). This was adequate in the days of small compound decks (less than 100,000) and low-throughput assays (which took months to complete). However, once throughput and output increased, it became obvious that a truly industrialized approach was needed to ensure that HTS was successful in generating starting points for medicinal chemistry programs (16). This industrialization of drug discovery has resulted in a major shift in the way HTS is conducted and includes changes in assay design, quality control, automation, and informatics support for data capture and analysis (12,17).

This chapter will focus on the process of HTS rather than a catalog of screening methods or technologies (18). For more detailed information about assay methods, suppliers, automation solutions, and some of the theoretical and statistical underpinnings of HTS, the reader is directed to the hts.net (www.htsscreening.net) and SBS (www.sbsonline.org) Web sites, two of the many HTS-related resources available on the Internet.

A generalized HTS process is illustrated in Figure 6.1. A screen can be considered the intersection of

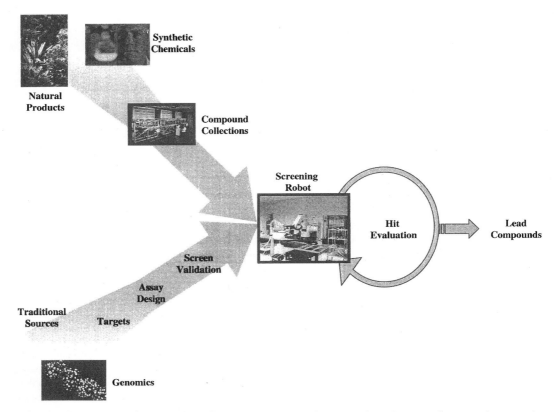

FIG. 6.1. High-throughput screening (HTS) is the intersection of compounds and assays. Compound sources include natural products and synthetic compounds and are stored and managed usually by automated compound inventory systems. Assays from traditional sources and from genomics are designed and validated into HTS formats. After screening compounds, hits are evaluated in an iterative fashion before being deemed leads of interest for further investigation and application of biological and chemistry resources.

chemical space (as represented by the compounds to be tested) and biology space (as represented by the specific target) (19).

COMPOUNDS

The traditional sources of compounds for screening have been natural product extracts and compounds from medicinal chemistry projects collected over many years. Recently, combinatorial chemistry-derived compounds have also been added to compound collections.

Natural Products

One third of the current top-selling drugs are natural products or their derivatives (20–22). The proportion increases to almost two thirds for antitumor and anti-infective agents. Despite this rich heritage, there has

been a trend to move away from using natural products as sources for new leads in the drug discovery programs of many large pharmaceutical research organizations. There are many reasons for this, some scientific and others cultural. The rapid advances in the technology of screening has resulted in changes in process that have made the traditional methods of natural product screening and bioassay-guided isolation of active molecules incompatible with the demands of early drug discovery. One result of this technology gap has been that natural products are often "behind the progress curve" and thus the compounds generated have little impact on already progressing chemistry programs. However, there is still an appreciation of the untapped diversity present in natural products, and methods and techniques currently being developed may result in a resurgence of this important resource (23–25). For example, prefractionation of extracts has been used to reduce the time taken after screening to identify the active components in a crude mixture (26).

Medicinal Chemistry Collections

Large pharmaceutical houses have the products of years of medicinal chemistry efforts stored in compound banks or libraries. These continue to be a rich source of leads for novel targets. One disadvantage of relying too heavily on in-house programs to populate a deck of compounds is that inevitable biases result in the collection (27). These collections are now being augmented by the purchase of compounds.

Combinatorial Chemistry Libraries

With the advent of parallel synthesis methods, the number of compounds being synthesized has grown exponentially over the years (28,29). Many of these "libraries" are now part of the compound collections of companies and are available for screening. While this certainly increases the number of compounds available to be screened, most libraries are made around common cores, which could result in an overall loss of diversity (30–33).

One outcome of this increase in the sizes of compound libraries has been the expansion and automation of compound inventory and management systems (34). There is also a growing awareness of the need to monitor and maintain the quality of the collection over time. These efforts include quality control of the incoming compounds to experiments to determine the best long-term storage conditions. Adding to this complexity is that different parts of the organization have very different needs vis-à-vis compound access and delivery. For example, animal study groups typically require a few compounds in high milligram quantities in dry form, whereas HTS groups require thousands of compounds in a microtiter plate format. The challenge facing compound management groups is to effectively serve all user communities while still maintaining and growing the compound collection.

This explosion in the number of compounds available for screening has raised questions of how many compounds need to be screened to obtain a lead (33,35). The usual approach has been to attempt to screen the entire compound collection. This approach, while completely valid if doable, is often the default since the alternatives are more difficult to implement and often require a reorganization of compound collections and relevant automation and IT infrastructures to be in place. Alternatives to full-deck screening include selecting a subset of compounds to sample the chemotypes present in the full collection ("diversity decks"), focused libraries, sequential screening, and reorganizing the full deck such that related compounds are in blocks of plates (36,37). Each of these approaches has its advantages and disadvantages. Unfortunately, some of these approaches require opposing methods of deck organization. In the end, the decision as to what to screen has to be made on an individual basis and has to take into account the ease and costs of the assay, the diversity and organization of a particular compound collection, and the infrastructure available in the compound management organization.

TARGET SOURCES

The targets for pharmaceuticals have traditionally come from basic discovery research involving metabolic pathways, explorations of disease etiologies, and genetic studies for both human diseases and antiinfective therapy. The advent of genome sequencing has radically changed the target identification opportunities, with the biggest potential impact being the sequencing of the human genome.

The number of potential drug targets has risen exponentially, and the challenge facing the biomedical community is to identify the most relevant and tractable targets (4,5). A combination of high-throughput biology, high-throughput compound management, and lead identification is now needed. One approach that is being tried is to bin the potential targets by class (e.g., kinases, G-protein-coupled receptors, proteases, ion channels). In this scenario, a panel of proteins in a target class is screened against a library of compounds and the intersections of biology space with chemistry space are mapped out. The idea here is that chemotypes then emerge that are active against one subclass of targets versus another. Taking this idea to its logical end would entail the screening if every potential target versus as large a chemistry space as possible. The work would then shift to target validation using the chemical tools identified. This is essentially a disease-independent process, and as a model of drug discovery is radically different from current practice and would require a major paradigm shift in both academia and industry.

Oncology has traditionally relied on cytotoxic compounds for therapy, even when the exact mechanism of action of the compound is unclear. While still very valuable, there is now a shift to more defined molecular targets, such as tyrosine kinases, matrix metalloproteinases, and DNA repair enzymes

(38–40). This shift is based on knowledge of the mechanism of action of a particular protein or pathway in growth control and regulation.

ASSAY DESIGN

Assay design for HTS and assay design for "normal" assays used to be seen as separate entities. This dichotomy is largely artificial and was often driven by the technology differences that existed between high-throughput methods and more traditional assay methods (Fig. 6.2). With a dovetailing of methods ("traditional" methods being converted to higher-throughput formats and HTS techniques being adopted widely), this difference is starting to disappear and the focus in HTS assay design is in optimizing the screen to the specific goals of hit identification, rather than simply making an assay robust enough to be automated.

Assay design consists of two main parts: screen construction and screen validation. Screen construction consists of determining the optimum conditions for the assay within the constraints of the particular HTS environment. It is at this stage that critical decisions regarding the ultimate goal of the screen, assay format, and kinetic parameters under which the screen will be run are made and the best conditions established. For example, running a tyrosine kinase assay at the Km for ATP will allow the identification of both competitive and noncompetitive compounds with respect to ATP, but running well below the Km will bias to screen towards ATP-competitive compounds. As can be appreciated, this exercise requires a compromise between the best possible assay and the exigencies of an efficient high-throughput screen. The determination of the final conditions of the assay is still, to a large degree, a linear process and can be quite time consuming. However, the application of industrial Design of Experiments (DOE) principles coupled to automation has started to streamline this aspect of assay design (41). Put simply, DOE allows multiple variables to be assessed simultaneously through the application of statistics (42). This approach allows the researcher to quickly

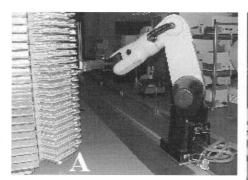
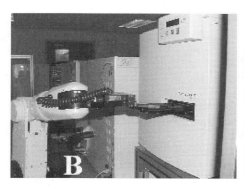
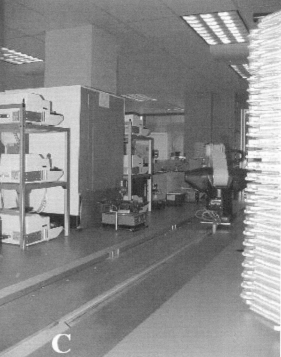

FIG. 6.2. Throughput and quality is achieved by the application of technology. **A:** A robotic arm is used to retrieve a plate from a plate store. **B:** The arm places a plate into a plate reader. **C:** A view of the integrated system showing liquid handlers, incubators, and plate hotels.

identify those variables that have the greatest effect on the assay. This greatly reduces the number of experiments that need to be performed, conserving both resources and time. For example, Taylor et al. (43) described the use of experimental design statistics with automated liquid handling to derive optimal assay conditions.

REAGENT DESIGN

Reagent design is an integral part of good assay design and will enable an efficient screening process. For example, the use of particular tags on fusion proteins may preclude the use of particular assay formats due to cost or interference with other assay components. Another criterion is the ease of scale up of reagents from bench quantities to HTS quantities. This aspect of scale up is often overlooked in the early design phase and can greatly delay a project or make it prohibitively expensive. A commonly used rule of thumb for estimating reagents is $1.5\times$ the number of wells to be screened. This takes into account factors such as the dead volumes encountered on the liquid handlers and the amounts used in the testing phase. The scale up of cells for screening presents particular problems (e.g., ensuring consistency of signaling from an engineered cell line throughout a screen). The demands of this labor-intensive process have been somewhat alleviated by automation. An example of an automated cell growth system is shown in Figure 6.3.

SCREEN VALIDATION

Assay and screen validation as it applies to HTS has a very specific meaning and context. An assay that works in low throughput (tubes or a small number of plates) may behave very differently when expanded to thousands of plates and automated liquid handling. The process of screen validation establishes that the assay performs within the biological parameters determined in the assay design in a predictable and reproducible manner on the screening equipment throughout the length of the screening run. It is important to note that validation is a *process* and involves the testing and monitoring of a diverse set of parameters and includes both biology (e.g., reagent stability, assay sensitivity, day-to-day variability) and instrumentation (e.g., liquid handling, plate reader sensitivity). The goal of assay design and validation is to determine the conditions that allow the activity due to compounds to be distinguished from the variability and noise of the assay.

Screening

HTS laboratories now have the capacity to routinely screen 10^5 to 10^6 compounds in relatively short timeframes, usually 2 to 4 weeks. To achieve this level of efficiency there is a strong reliance on automation. Current HTS screening platforms exist at differing degrees of sophistication, ranging from semiautomated workstations to fully automated turnkey systems (44). All of the systems however share the same basic components: (a) a method for physically moving microtiter plates (stackers to robotic arms), (b) a series of liquid-dispensing devices (individually controlled tips to bulk dispensing systems), (c) incubators (open shelves to fully environmentally controlled), and (d) appropriate detectors for measuring the output of the assay.

The key difference between workstations and fully automated systems is the way plates are handled through the screen process. In workstation mode, plates are moved in batches, with the batch size depending on the particulars of the assay and the equipment. This is an efficient method for robust assays where timing of each step is not a critical factor. These include, for example, reactions with long incubation times where slight differences in the timing of each step have a minimal effect, or reactions that reach equilibrium. A fully automated mode on the other hand allows for far greater flexibility in assay design and can ensure that each plate is treated in exactly the same way. This mode is preferred for those assays that require precise incubation times or have unstable readouts. The control of plate flow through the system is managed by scheduling software that also controls all of the liquid handling and readers. The more advanced schedulers have rule-based artificial intelligence to optimally manage the screening process.

Quality Control

It is important to keep in mind that HTS is a stochastic process. The activity (e.g., percent inhibition of an enzyme, binding of a ligand) measured in the assay is a representation of the intersection of several parallel processes and as such reflects the accumulated errors in each of those processes. For example, the activity is directly related to the test compound concentration in the assay. The method by which the compound is dissolved and delivered to the assay obviously has a direct bearing on the final concentration; however, the history and properties of the compound (purity, solubility, stability, age, storage conditions) all have an influence to varying degrees on the final concentration

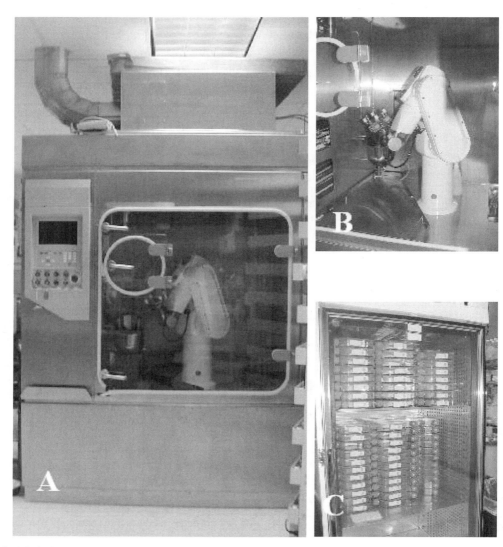

FIG. 6.3. Labor-intensive tasks such as cell culture are facilitated by automation. **A:** The front view from the **Cellmate (The Automation Partnership, Wilmington, DE)**. The device is a fully automated cell culture hood that replicates all of the standard steps for adding and removing media (e.g., scrapping cells from flasks) in a sterile environment. **B:** A close-up view of the robotic arm. **C:** A view of the flask store illustrating the capacity of the system.

of that compound. On the biology side, the purity of the reagents, kinetic properties, and stability all affect the measured activity. In addition, the very method used to detect the activity has its own influence. The goal of good assay design and validation is to minimize the variability of as many of these components as possible, thus increasing ones confidence in the measured activity. Quality control throughout the process helps quantify and monitor these inherent variations. An example of quality control in HTS is the running of control compounds with known activity under the conditions of the screen. Ideally, several compounds with varying degrees of activity should be run every day at the beginning and end of each HTS run. Plotting the observed activity of the compounds and comparing with the known activity allows the screener to quickly assess the quality of the previous days run before starting the next.

Data Analysis

One of the biggest challenges facing most HTS groups is handling the volume of data that a fully automated screening system can produce. For example, a screen can easily run 100,000 samples in a 24-hour period. An example of the types of automation used in HTS is illustrated in Figure 6.4. This will include controls, quality control plates, and compound plates. At this rate, a week of screening produces 500,000 data points. Normally, these plates are all uniquely identified by barcodes and the data collected from each plate can be saved directly onto servers. Many of the routine operations of data handling, such as matching barcodes to plates and alignment of activity with compound identifications, and basic calculations of activity such as percent inhibition are all relatively simple and are automated to the point of transparency to the end-user of the data. The real challenge is in the analysis of the data because the fundamental goal of this exercise is to be able to select a list of potential hits with some degree of confidence. The analysis of the quality of the screen is essential to this task, and there are statistical methods available for this purpose. For example, a common measure of screen performance is the Z-factor (or Z'-factor) (45). This a measure of the separation between the high and low signals for the screen and takes into account the variability (measured as the standard deviation) of the activity as well as the average value. The following formula is used to calculate the Z'-factor, which normally lies between 0 and 1:

$$ 1 - \frac{3*s_3 + 3*s_1}{\bar{x}_3 - \bar{x}_1}. $$

The greater the value of Z', the more confidence one has in the ability of the screen to identify active compounds outside the noise of the assay.

Data-visualization methods are also increasingly being used to both assess the quality of the data and to aid in hit selection (46). Figure 6.4 shows examples of the types of data visualization commonly used in analyzing HTS data. Other visualization methods at the plate and well level allow one to identify any systematic patterns both within and between plates. These patterns usually arise due to pipetting errors, but other sources include plate-reader biases and temperature gradients across plates. Regardless of the source, these patterns can bias the data and need to be accounted for.

The standard method of hit identification is to use a threshold activity value as a cut-off point for selection. This method has the advantage of ease of list generation and generally identifies the most potent compounds; however, it suffers from some drawbacks. If the screen has a high proportion of false positives (e.g., quenchers), these will be selected and will thus reduce the number of true actives selected. Another disadvantage to using a cut-off value as the only criterion for selection is the problem of false negatives (i.e., compounds that are true actives but had an activity just below the selected cut-off value). One way around this is to use the primary list of actives to search the mass of inactive compounds with a view to identify similar chemotypes for testing. This is usually done in a linear fashion with a small number of chemotypes for which accurate IC_{50} (50% inhibition/inhibitory concentration) values are available. This linear iterative approach is time consuming and is often a drain on resources. An alternate approach is to perform the clustering analysis immediately after the primary screen and to then select families of compounds with a range of activities for retest, rather than just the most active ones. A stumbling block for this approach has been the perception of the general unreliability of primary screening data for reasons discussed previously in the chapter (see "Quality Control"). However, with improvements in the technology and IT infrastructures supporting HTS, and with decreased timelines and increasing costs as additional drivers, a lot more attention has been paid to improving the quality and predictability of primary screening data. This has included miniaturization with the possibility of screening in duplicates, a better understanding of compound delivery issues, and a general trend towards a robust industrialized approach to improving HTS.

Hits to Leads

The purpose of HTS is to identify chemotypes that have a desired activity. It is the first step in the very long process of converting an initial activity into a drug. The goals of a particular HTS campaign may vary, but usually it is to try and identify as many different chemotypes as possible such that a range of chemical (and other biological) properties is present. These early molecules are usually termed "hits." These hits progress to "leads" after they have passed a battery of tests. A lead (or leads) is a chemotype that is now subjected to actual chemistry to try and achieve very specific goals. The process of converting hits to leads is an extensive triage where the liabilities of each of the molecules is weighed and measured against the desired properties of the drug, and decisions are made on the probability of achieving those

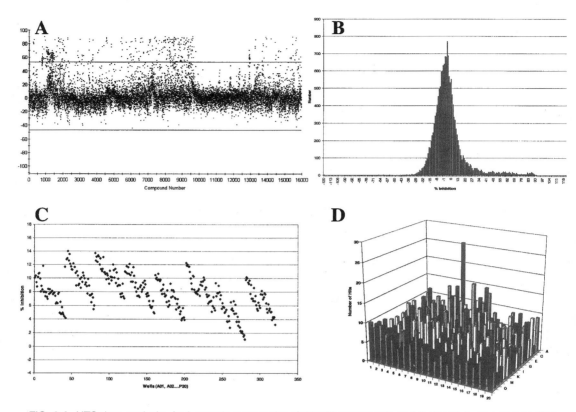

FIG. 6.4. HTS data analysis. **A:** A sample scatter plot of 32,000 compounds and their activity in a screen. The data show that most compounds are inactive with activities centered around zero and that there are no obvious patterns. **B:** A different view of the same data where the activities of the compounds are plotted as a distribution. This shows that this screen had a tight distribution, implying that the variability of the assay was low. A noisy assay would have broadened the distribution. **C:** Trends in an assay can bias the data. Each point on the plot is the average activity of each well of a set of plates and shows a systematic bias from well A01 to P22. **D:** The location of hits on the plate can reveal hidden errors. Well B8 in this case had an unusual number of hits. One can also see that more hits appeared to come from the top of the plate rather than being randomly distributed across the plate.

goals for each of the molecules (or series) (47). A common paradigm that is used at this stage is "fail early" or "fail fast" (48). Since the costs of the latter stages of drug development far outweigh the early stages, it makes sense to determine as quickly as possible all of the potential liabilities a candidate molecule possesses, so that go/no-go decisions can be made. The usual liability assays include cytochrome P-450 activity, cytotoxicity, cell permeability, Human-ether-a-go-go related gene (hERG) K$^+$-channel activity, rate of metabolism, and pharmacodynamic and pharmacokinetic properties (49–54).

With the advent of parallel synthesis and combinatorial chemistry, the elucidation of early structure/activity relationships (SAR) often generates thousands of compounds to be tested (30). This is often performed in a high-throughput mode and represents an extension of the role of HTS, and is enabled due to technological improvements in compound and plate handling. With the advent of HTS methods for liability assays as well, there is now the concept of a "chemical dossier" for each lead chemotype. This dossier contains all of the relevant selectivity assays, liability, and other relevant chemical properties of the molecules (or series), in addition to any early SAR information. This wealth of information being provided in a short time frame will allow medicinal chemistry groups to quickly judge each molecule for development feasibility and will allow efficient use of resources.

THE FUTURE OF HIGH-THROUGHPUT SCREENING

What impact HTS has had on the drug discovery process over the last decade and whether technology is the answer are two legitimate questions (55). A recent worldwide study involving HTS directors and suppliers reported on the trends, successes, and challenges facing HTS (56). One theme that emerged was that given the long lead times from discovery to market, it may still be too early to determine the real impact of HTS on the drug discovery process. There was also an emphasis on improving the overall quality of the process to increase impact.

In the last decade, there have been tremendous technological and process improvements in the field to the point where in many organizations, good HTS practice is almost routine. The current challenge is to disseminate this knowledge into the rest of drug discovery to avoid a widening of the technology gap and to reap the benefits of high-throughput methods in all areas of drug discovery. This process is inevitable, and the next decade will see the spread of HTS technology to "standard" biological research laboratories. This process of technology spread has taken place in the past (e.g., molecular biology in the early days was a specialty field), but now the methods and techniques are standard practice.

REFERENCES

1. Hughes D. Dizzying but scary: looking towards R&D in 2005. *Drug Discov Today* 1999;4:393–395.
2. Ommen G, Bakker E, Dunnen J. The human genome project and the future of diagnostics, treatment, and prevention. *Mol Med* 1999;354:SI5–SI10.
3. Roses A. How will pharmacogenetics impact the future of research and development. *Drug Discov Today* 2001;6:59–60.
4. Searls D. Using bioinformatics in gene and drug discovery. *Drug Discov Today* 2000;5:135–143.
5. Lenz G, Nash H, Jindal S. Chemical ligands, genomics and drug discovery. *Drug Discov Today* 2000;5:145–156.
6. Wells T, Feger G. Discovery research in the co-genomic era: biology goes industrial. *Drug Disc World* 2000:16–21.
7. Appleton T. Combinatorial chemistry and HTS: feeding a voracious process. *Drug Discov Today* 1999;4:398–400.
8. Mander T. Beyond uHTS: ridiculously HTS? *Drug Discov Today* 2000;5:223–225.
9. Beggs M. HTS: where next. *Drug Disc World* 2000:25–30.
10. Fernandes P. Technological advances in high-throughput screening. *Curr Opin Chem Biol* 1998;2:597–603.
11. Fox S, Farr-Jones S, Yund M. High throughput screening for drug discovery: continually transitioning into new technology. *J Biomol Screen* 1999;4:183–186.
12. Beggs M, Blok H, Diels A. The high throughput screening infrastructure: the right tools for the task. *J Biomol Screen* 1999;4:143–149.
13. Burbaum J. The evolution of miniaturized well plates. *J Biomol Screen* 2000;5:1–8.
14. Eglen R. High throughput screening: myths and future realities. *J Biomol Screen* 1999;4:179–181.
15. Cox B, Denver JC, Binnie A, et al. Application of high-throughput screening techniques to drug discovery. *Prog Med Chem* 2000;37:83–133.
16. Norrington I. Laboratory automation for high throughput screening. *Pharm Manuf Int* 2000:37–40.
17. Archer R. Faculty or factory? Why industrializing drug discovery is inevitable. *J Biomol Screen* 1999;4:235–237.
18. Hertzberg R, Pope A. High-throughput screening: new technology for the 21st century. *Curr Opin Chem Biol* 2000;4:445–451.
19. Houston J, Banks M. The chemical-biological interface: developments in automated and miniaturized screening technology. *Curr Opin Biotechnol* 1997;8:734–740.
20. Shu Y. Recent natural products based drug development: a pharmaceutical industry perspective. *J Nat Prod* 1998;61:1053–1071.
21. Buss A, Waigh R. Natural products as leads for new pharmaceuticals. *Med Chem Drug Discov* 1995;1:983–1033.
22. Sampson J, Phillipson, J, Bowery N, et al. Ethnomedicinally selected plants as sources of potential analgesic compounds: indication of in vitro biological activity in receptor binding assays. *Phytother Res* 2000;14:24–29.
23. Harvey A. Strategies for discovering drugs from previously unexplored natural products. *Drug Discov Today* 2000;5:294–300.
24. Quinn R, Moni R, Feckner G, et al. Browsing biodiversity: HTS and natural product libraries. *Chem Int Aust* 1998;9:8–11.
25. Cordell G. Biodiversity and drug discovery: a symbiotic relationship. *Phytochemistry* 2000;55:463–480.
26. Schmid I, Sattler II, Grablev S, et al. Natural products in high throughput screening: automated high-quality sample preparation. *J Biomol Screen* 1999;4:15–25.
27. Spencer R. High-throughput screening of historic collections: observations on file size, biological targets, and file diversity. *Biotechnol Bioeng* 1998;61:61–67.
28. Parrill A, Reddy M. Adapting structure-based drug design in the paradigm of combinatorial chemistry and high-throughput screening. *J Am Chem Soc* 1999;121:226–238.
29. Myers P. Re-engineering of the drug discovery process, utilising a unique combination of library design and parallel synthesis. *High Throughput Screen* 2000;37–42.
30. Teague S, Davis A, Leeson P, et al. The design of lead-like combinatorial libraries. *Angew Chem Int Ed Engl* 1999;38:3743–3748.
31. Li J, Murray C, Baxter C, et al. Structure-based filtering and design of chemical libraries. 2000:87–96.
32. Mcmillan K, Auld D, Lin T, et al. Successful application of combinatorial chemistry to lead identification. 2000:83–86.

33. Teig S. Informative libraries are more useful than diverse ones. *J Biomol Screen* 1998;3:85–88.
34. Harrison W. Automation in compound library management. *Pharm Manuf Int* 2000:99–102.
35. Bailey D, Brown D. High-throughput chemistry and structure-based design; survival of the smartest. *Drug Discov Today* 2001;6:57–59.
36. Hodgkin E, Andrews-Cramer K. Compound collections get focused: smaller, well-designed compound collections make better use of HTS resources. *J Am Chem Soc* 2000;122:55–60.
37. Valler M, Green D. Diversity screening versus focused screening in drug discovery. *Drug Discov Today* 2000;5:286–293.
38. Sedlacek HH. Kinase inhibitors in cancer therapy. *Drugs* 2000;59:435–476.
39. Curran S, Murray G. Matrix metalloproteinases in tumour invasion and metastasis. *J Pathol* 1999;189: 300–308.
40. Gunatilaka AA, Kingston D. DNA-damaging natural products with potential anticancer activity. *Stud Nat Prod Chem* 1998;20:457–505.
41. Lutz M, Menius A, Choi T, et al. Experimental design for high-throughput screening. *Drug Discov Today* 1996;1:277–286.
42. Haaland P, ed. *Experimental design in biotechnology.* New York: Marcel Dekker Inc, 1989.
43. Taylor P, Stewart FP, Dunnington DJ, et al. Automated assay optimization with integrated statistics and smart robotics. *J Biomol Screen* 2000;5:213–225.
44. Harding D, Banks M, Fogarty S, et al. Development of an automated high-throughput screening system: a case history. *Drug Discov Today* 1997;2:385–390.
45. Zhang J, Chung T, Oldenburg K. A simple statistical parameter for use in evaluation and validation of high throughput screening assays. *J Biomol Screen* 1999;4: 67–73.
46. Wedin R. Visual data mining speeds drug discovery: computers promised fountains of wisdom but delivered only floods of data. *J Am Chem Soc* 1999;121:39–47.
47. Oprea T, Davis A, Teague S, et al. Is there a difference between leads and drugs? A historical perspective. *J Chem Inf Comput Sci* 2001;41:1308–1315.
48. Brennan M. Drug discovery: filtering out failures early in the game. *Chem Engineer News* 2000;63–74.
49. Eddershaw P, Beresford A, Bayliss M. ADME/PK as part of a rational approach to drug discovery. *Drug Discov Today* 2000;5:409–414.
50. Tarbit M, Berman J. High-throughput approaches for evaluating absorption, distribution, metabolism and excretion properties of lead compounds. *Curr Opin Chem Biol* 1998;2:411–416.
51. Smith D. High throughput drug metabolism. In: Gooderman N, ed. *Drug metabolism: towards the next millennium.* Amsterdam: 10S Press, 1998:137–143.
52. Spalding D, Harker A, Bayliss M. Combining high-throughput pharmacokinetic screens at the hits-to-leads stage of drug discovery. *Drug Discov Today* 2000;5: S70–S76.
53. Watt A, Morrison D, Evans D. Approaches to higher-throughput pharmacokinetics (HTPK) in drug discovery. *Drug Discov Today* 2000;5:17–24.
54. Rodrigues A. Preclinical drug metabolism in the age of high-throughput screening: an industrial perspective. *Pharm Res* 1997;14:1504–1510.
55. Archer J. Does technology deliver the goods? *High Throughput Screen* 2000;9.
56. Fox S, Wang H, Sopehak L, et al. High throughput screening 2002: moving toward increased success rates. *J Biomol Screen* 2002;7:313–316.

7

Bioinformatics and Data Mining in Support of Drug Discovery

Jeffrey Augen

TurboWorx, Inc., New Haven, Connecticut 06150

During the past few years, advanced computing technologies have evolved into core components of both the drug discovery process and biotechnology in general. Bioinformatics is the discipline that focuses these technologies on the drug discovery process by allowing *in silico* experiments. During the past decade, bioinformatics tools have evolved from simple adjuncts for wet chemistry, in most cases designed to accelerate target identification, lead optimization, or combinatorial chemistry, to sophisticated and indispensable parts of the discovery process. High-performance computing infrastructure and data management software are now making possible the rapid industrialization of many of the processes that comprise the drug discovery pipeline. The transformation is evident across all processes and includes, but is not limited to, gene discovery, structure and function determination of target proteins, combinatorial chemistry and molecular dynamics of lead compound/target protein interaction, and selection of subjects for clinical trials. Subject selection is often based on computerized analysis of messenger RNA (mRNA) expression profiles and medical histories of the candidate patients.

The basic drug discovery pipeline, a well-known entity within the pharmaceutical industry, consists of seven basic steps: disease selection, target hypothesis, lead-compound identification, lead optimization, preclinical trial testing, clinical trial testing, and pharmacogenomic optimization (1). In actuality, each step of the pipeline involves a complex set of interactions, and each interaction has an information technology component that facilitates its execution. Although the simple pipeline model is both complete and correct with regard to logistics, the interactions between critical components of the system must be described in detail to be useful to someone designing computer infrastructure to support a specific development environment. Various relationships among the pipeline's information components are outlined in Figure 7.1.

The flow of the diagram in the figure begins at the upper right with information about the basic biology of various disease states. Initial information is combined from a variety of sources, including physiological databases, medical records, and sources containing data obtained from animal models of human diseases. The next section of the diagram depicts various activities related to target selection and validation. Information from protein structure/sequence and genomic sequence databases is combined to help drive this process. Lead-target binding is the subject of the next section of the diagram. These interactions are often predicted as a result of combinatorial chemistry experiments and high-throughput screening as well as *in silico* modeling. Once lead compounds are selected and clinical trials are launched, the information technology focus shifts to medical informatics, the goal being to relate clinical results to the specific genetic makeup of the patient. These studies often rely on the results of microarray experiments that reveal the up-regulation and down-regulation of individual genes and gene clusters as a result of the treatment. Finally, results from clinical trials are fed back to enhance the next round of target selection and lead identification/optimization.

Each step in the process involves several different informatics tools that are often related and may even overlap. For example, much of today's animal model work involves comparative genomics, including tools for multiple-sequence homology and pattern recognition. Many of the same tools are also used to find genes that code for specific target proteins. Likewise, both target validation and lead optimization are enhanced by the use of computer programs that facilitate the prediction of three-dimensional structures of targets, lead compounds, and target–lead complexes.

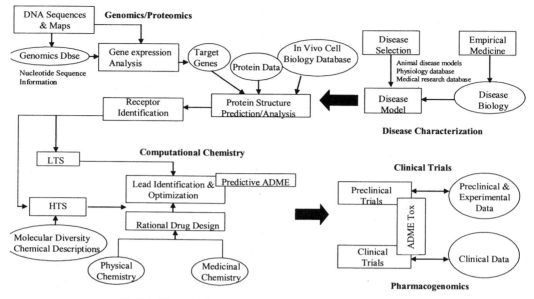

FIG. 7.1. Flow of information through the drug discovery pipeline.

In general, bioinformatics problems span two broad technical categories: floating point and integer. Floating-point problems are computationally intensive because they involve complex algorithms borrowed from physical chemistry and quantum mechanics. Molecular dynamics, protein folding, and metabolic systems modeling are representative floating-point problems. Integer problems, although often as computationally intensive, are typically built on algorithms that compare characters in sequences or search for matching phrases and terms. Most of contemporary molecular biology, including genome sequencing, is built on the solution to such problems. Gene sequence alignment and pattern discovery are relevant examples of high-speed integer-style problems. One of the most significant applications in this class is the assembly algorithm that was used to construct the human genome from millions of fragments obtained through a process known as "shotgun sequencing." The execution of this algorithm required enormous computer horsepower and represents one of the most complex logic problems ever solved.

The floating-point—intensive applications listed above—molecular dynamics, tertiary protein structure prediction, and kinetic modeling—are focused on optimizing the high-throughput screening process by replacing much of the wet chemistry required for lead compound optimization. As these tools mature, much of the drug discovery process will migrate from the lab bench to the computer with *in silico* modeling re-

placing more traditional methods. The ultimate goal is to be able to model a disease process at the molecular level, predict which specific chemical compounds are best suited to treating the disease for a genetically defined patient population, perform docking experiments *in silico*, and accurately predict absorption, distribution, metabolism, and excretion of the compound. Achieving these goals *in silico* will dramatically improve the drug discovery process and pave the way for personalized medicine based on a molecular-level understanding of both the patient and the illness.

Finally, systems that combine the power of statistical analysis with insights gained through pattern discovery are emerging as a new force in bioinformatics and medicine. These systems rely on "data mining" to discover complex and subtle relationships among apparently unrelated items, such as the clinical record, demographic history, gene-expression profiles, and treatment outcomes. Such systems are currently being developed as tools to increase the accuracy of patient selection for clinical trials and will ultimately be used for presymptomatic testing of disease. One prominent example involves the analysis of mRNA-expression profiles to select patients that exhibit particular genetic up-regulation and down-regulation patterns known to be diagnostic for the onset of a particular illness. The profiles are stored in large databases along with details regarding each patient's treatment and medical history. Pattern discovery is used to correlate treatment outcomes with specific gene-expression profiles and medical histories. Likewise, data-mining techniques have the power to advance pharmacogenomics so that drug discovery becomes intertwined with systems biology—the study of complex interrelated metabolic pathways.

Today's advanced pharmaceuticals often result from a molecular-level understanding of gene expression at the single-gene level. A well-known example is the development and testing of trastuzumab (Herceptin, Genentech Inc., South San Francisco, CA) for the treatment of patients with breast cancer. Overexpression of the *HER2/neu* oncogene (also known as c-*erb*B2) is a frequent molecular event in many human cancers (2). The humanized anti-HER2/neu antibody, Herceptin, has proven to be effective in patients with metastatic breast cancer who overexpress the *HER2/neu* oncogene. However, the efficacy of drugs like Herceptin also depend on the up-regulation and down-regulation of many related genes, some that control the expression of enzymes that metabolize the drug in question. Further calibration of dosing and the prescription of combination chemotherapies could potentially be enhanced through the use of data-mining technologies that reveal the relationships among hundreds of genes, the disease state, and proposed treatments (3). Additionally, it is impossible to use these techniques without robust data infrastructure and, in most cases, query tools that allow access to heterogeneous data sources. Some of these data sources are proprietary (e.g., clinical records) and many exist in the public domain. Ultimately, the combination of wet chemistry, *in silico* modeling, pattern discovery, and data-mining technologies will lead to realization of the ultimate goal, personalized medicine based on a molecular-level understanding of disease and the results of various drug therapies.

GENE IDENTIFICATION

Widespread availability of the complete sequence of the human genome has created a backdrop for discovery that begins with the basic process of gene identification (4,5). While this process might appear to be straightforward, it is actually one of the most difficult challenges in contemporary bioinformatics. Initial estimates of the number of genes in the human genome varied from 30,000 to over 100,000. After much analysis, it is now believed that there are approximately 40,000 coding sequences present in the genome. The number is shocking for a variety of reasons. Based solely on the count, the human genome is only 10 times more complex than that of the lowly *Escherichia coli* bacterium; 40,000 coding sequences account for less than 3% of the three billion bases in

the genome, and the long-accepted dogma—"one gene one protein"—was shattered when it was established that individual mRNA molecules often have hundreds of splice variants.

The fact that 40,000 genes ultimately code for as many as 2 million different proteins hints at the enormous complexity of human gene expression. Gene identification is a complex process that requires transforming the basic biology of gene expression into a mathematical problem. Before we can discuss that problem, it makes sense to review the basics of gene structure and expression with a view towards the underlying themes that will become the foundation of modern bioinformatics.

Much of the increased complexity arises from the basic structure of eukaryotic genes. While bacterial genes are built from an uninterrupted stretch of nucleotides, gene-coding sequences of higher organisms contain coding regions (exons) interrupted by long noncoding sequences (introns) that are spliced out in the final mRNA transcript. The process involves creation of a primary mRNA transcript, which is then spliced by a complex of RNA-processing enzymes before the final transcript, the one that will be translated into a protein, is transported across the nuclear membrane and into the cytoplasm. Alternative splicing of primary transcripts is the primary driver of complexity in the human genome because it makes the protein synthesis process much more versatile by allowing different proteins to be produced from the same gene. The splicing process has also become a driver of evolution and biodiversity because it facilitates genetic recombination of introns, allowing the evolution of new proteins from portions of preexisting amino acid sequences. These sequences, which have become the basic building blocks for proteins in all organisms, have been catalogued and extensively studied in recent years (6–8). The ends of all introns contain well-characterized "consensus" sequences at their 5′ (donor) and 3′ (acceptor) ends. The enzymatic splicing mechanism that removes introns is often unable to distinguish between alternative pairings, which leads to the production of splice variants. A more directed mechanism for RNA splicing involves regulatory molecules that control the splicing machinery's access to portions of the transcript. It is important to note that the fidelity of the process must be very high because shifting the reading frame by a single base completely destroys the protein.

Another important transcriptional feature is the addition of a poly-A tail to the end of the messages. The addition is mediated by a special-purpose RNA polymerase enzyme, poly-A polymerase, and occurs at a specific site identified by the sequence AAUAAA approximately 20 nucleotides upstream of the cut site at the 3' end of the message. The addition of 100 to 200 adenine nucleotides at the 3' cut site completes the message. Finally, during the transcription process, at about the 30-nucleotide stage, a "cap" composed of a methylated G nucleotide is added to the 5' end (the end where transcription begins). This 5' cap serves as the binding site for the ribosome during translation of the message into protein. After binding to the site, the ribosome begins "scanning" the message until it encounters the first AUG sequence: the codon for methionine. All eukaryotic proteins begin with an N-terminal methionine, which is often enzymatically removed after translation. The translation mechanism is another source of sequence diversity because the ribosome sometimes fails to recognize the first AUG start codon and skips to the second one, producing a completely different protein. This process is called "leaky scanning." Both the proximity to the cap and nucleotide composition of sequences that surround the start codon determine the efficiency of the recognition process (9).

Upstream of the complex of introns and exons are promoters and other regulatory elements that control transcription. Transcription in higher eukaryotes involves the assembly of a protein complex composed of "general transcription factors" that functions to induce the binding of RNA polymerase II at the promoter site. The promoter site almost always contains the sequence TATA, which is recognized by one of the general transcription factors. The TATA sequence, often referred to as a TATA box, usually resides 25 nucleotides upstream of the point where transcription will begin. Another conserved sequence, CCAAT, is associated with transcription start sites in higher organisms and appears in approximately 50% of vertebrate promoters. The CCAAT sequence is normally found upstream from the TATA box. Once the general transcription factors and RNA polymerase II are bound at the promoter, transcription of the gene begins. The transcription rate is tightly regulated by control proteins that bind to sites scattered across a very large area associated with each gene—often as wide as 50,000 nucleotides, upstream and downstream of the promoter and even the gene itself. This effect, often referred to as "control at a distance," is a common theme in the human genome. Thousands of different proteins bind to these regulatory sites; some "up-regulate" and some "down-regulate" the transcription process. The regulation mechanism seems to be based on loop structures in the DNA that bring control regions into contact with the promoter. Finally, each cell type has a different population of regulatory proteins to match its gene-expression pattern. The

present discussion refers to one of three RN- synthesizing enzymes, RNA polymerase II. The other major RNA polymerases (I and III) are primarily responsible for synthesizing RNA molecules that have structural or catalytic roles within the cell, mostly related to the protein-synthesizing machinery used for translation: RNA polymerase I synthesizes large ribosomal RNAs, whereas RNA polymerase III synthesizes the transfer RNAs, amino acid carriers for translation, and the small structural 5S ribosomal RNA. Conversely, RNA polymerase II synthesizes the thousands of genes coding for proteins and the small catalytic RNAs often referred to as snRNPs (small nuclear ribonucleoproteins). The present discussion is focused on genes that code for proteins and, therefore, RNA polymerase II (10).

An accurate view of transcription reveals a relatively small coding sequence (the actual gene) surrounded by a much larger region of nucleotides that contains a promoter, binding sites for regulatory proteins, structural sequences that cause the DNA to fold into loops, consensus sequences that facilitate RNA splicing, sequences that signal the 3' cut site where the poly-A tail is added, and a ribosomal-binding site near the 5' end of the molecule (the site where the methylated guanine cap is added). Each of these elements provides a piece of information that can be used algorithmically in gene-finding experiments.

SEARCHING THE GENOME

Unfortunately, the protein synthesis process, which begins with a DNA sequence and ends with a folded protein, cannot be completely described, most notably with regard to the specific signal sequences required for recognition and processing of the components. For example, because 30% of promoters do not contain the signature TATA box, this signal is not a completely reliable mechanism for locating transcription start sites. Furthermore, there is no specific set of rules for unambiguous identification of introns. Even if such rules were defined, there is no precise way to predict for a given gene which introns will be spliced into a final message.

Despite these complexities, bioinformaticians have succeeded in developing a combination of approaches to gene identification that have proven to be reliable. These approaches can be grouped into three categories (11):

1. *Content Based.* Content-based analyses are based on statistical parameters of a sequence, such as the frequency of occurrence of particular codons and periodicity of repeated sequences. DNA sequences

can also be translated into amino acids and scored against weighting functions that use a statistical basis to predict the formation of basic protein features: α helix, β sheet, and reverse-turn structures.

2. *Feature Analysis.* Feature-analysis methods are based on the identification of donor and acceptor splice sites at the ends of introns, long polyadenine sequences that signal the 3′ end of a transcript, binding sites for transcriptional factors, and start/stop codons that signal the beginning and end of an open reading frame. Open reading frame analysis based on identification of a 3′ end start codon (ATG, the code for methionine) and a 5′ end stop codon (TAA, TAG, or TGA) is perhaps the most straightforward method of gene identification. However, the complexities of the splicing process can obscure start and stop codons with interruptions in the prespliced mRNA or add invalid stop codons by shifting the reading frame after the start.

3. *Database Comparison.* These methods rely on sequence homology studies that search databases containing thousands of known protein sequences. In many cases, the protein sequences are subdivided into small motifs used to populate dictionaries of known structures. Amino acid sequences in the dictionary are back translated into their corresponding nucleotide sequences and scanned against the complete DNA data. Many of these sequences are conserved throughout evolution and have served as the basis for annotation of the human genome. Sequence homology algorithms use various measures of complementarity to compare the data, which almost always contain inexact matches, frame shifts, spaces, and "wildcard" characters representing "wobble" bases in the sequence.[1] (12,13).

Regardless of the algorithm used, it is important to remember that every gene-coding region contains six possible reading frames: three that commence at positions 1, 2, and 3 on one DNA strand, and a corresponding set of three frames beginning at the 5′ end of the complimentary strand. Modern bioinformatic programs are designed to examine all six possible reading frames. The realization that a single gene-coding region can contain multiple reading frames superimposed on a large number of splice variants with open reading frames on both strands of the DNA helix has added tremendous complexity to the gene finding process. Not surprisingly, modern gene-identification

programs are designed to scan both strands in each of the three reading frames in the 5′ to 3′ direction. Furthermore, algorithms that scan DNA sequences must take into account the fact that splice sites within the coding region almost always shift the reading frame while separating nucleotides that are destined to be joined in the final transcript. These issues are especially critical for researchers using sequence homology algorithms because the sequences that are being compared may be sparse and differ with regard to the specific lengths of intervening segments. Problems of this nature have driven the development of unbounded pattern-discovery programs that can identify sparse and complex patterns.

Fifty years of statistical analysis have contributed to an understanding of the relative frequency of codon usage in various genomes, most recently the human genome (14,15). The distribution of codons in the human genome is depicted in Table 7.1.

Two content-based statistical approaches have been used for open reading frame identification in genomes. The first is based on an unusual property of coding sequences: namely, every third base tends to be duplicated more often than would be expected by random chance alone (16). This observation holds true for all coding sequences in all organisms and is a result of the nonrandom nature of protein structure. The second approach involves comparing the distribution of codons in the test region to the known distribution for coding sequences in the rest of the organism (17–20).

Feature identification as a tool for genomic analysis is at least 25 years old and has advanced as rapidly as molecular biology itself. Today there are many popular algorithms, most in the public domain, designed to identify the various features associated with coding sequences (e.g., introns, exons, and promoter sites). Most use tables and weighting functions along with some type of sequence-specific statistical analysis to predict the presence and frequency of key features (21,22). Feature-analysis techniques are much more powerful when combined with known information about protein and genetic structure. Such information is housed in public databases, such as the National Center for Biotechnology Information's GenBank DNA sequence database (23,24). One such algorithm, PROCRUSTES, forces a fit between a test DNA sequence and potential transcription products that have already been sequenced. A spliced-alignment algorithm is used to sequentially explore all possible exon assemblies in an attempt to model the best fit of gene and target protein. PROCRUSTES is designed to handle situations where the query DNA sequence contains either partial or multiple genes

---

[1] The genetic code is degenerate in the sense that most amino acids are specified by more than one nucleotide triplet. The code contains some variability in the third base, which is known as the "wobble" base.

TABLE 7.1. *Frequency of each codon per 100,000 codons in the human genome*

UUU	16.6	UCU	14.5	UAU	12.1	UGU	9.7
UUC	20.7	UCC	17.7	UAC	16.3	UGC	12.4
UUA	7.0	UCA	11.4	UAA	0.7	UGA	1.3
UUG	12.0	UCG	4.5	UAG	0.5	UGG	13.0
CUU	12.4	CCU	17.2	CAU	10.1	CGU	4.7
CUC	19.3	CCC	20.3	CAC	14.9	CGC	11.0
CUA	6.8	CCA	16.5	CAA	11.8	CGA	6.2
CUG	40.0	CCG	7.1	CAG	34.4	CGG	11.6
AUU	15.7	ACU	12.7	AAU	16.8	AGU	11.7
AUC	22.3	ACC	19.9	AAC	20.2	AGC	19.3
AUA	7.0	ACA	14.7	AAA	23.6	AGA	11.2
AUG	22.2	ACG	6.4	AAG	33.2	AGG	11.1
GUU	10.7	GCU	18.4	GAU	22.2	GGU	10.9
CUC	14.8	GCC	28.6	GAC	26.5	GGC	23.1
GUA	6.8	GCA	15.6	GAA	28.6	GGA	16.4
GUG	29.3	GCG	7.7	GAG	40.6	GGG	16.5

Source: GenBank Release 128.0 [database online]. Available at: http://www.kazusa.or.jp/codon. Updated February 15, 2002.

(25). Another approach involves using neural networks that have been trained to recognize characteristic sequences of known exons, intron/exon boundaries, and transcription start sites in a particular organism. Such networks, once trained, are often capable of discerning complex and subtle relationships between sequence elements that are not otherwise detectable (26,27).

Despite the steady and rapid improvement in computer-based sequence analysis, one simple charting technique, dot-matrix two-dimensional comparison, lives on as a core component of the modern bioinformatics toolkit. This straightforward method facilitates the comparison of two sequences written across the axes of a two-dimensional grid. Dots are placed within the grid to mark positions where the two sequences match, and the emerging pattern of diagonal lines is used to visually identify homologous regions. The two-dimensional nature of the grid facilitates identification of regions that are locally similar, even when the complete sequences do not align well. Additional simplification is often accomplished by filtering regions that contain a threshold number of exact matches. Figure 7.2 contains a dot-matrix plot for two sequences containing several homologous regions.

Understanding and predicting the genetic level structure of specific coding regions is critical to the drug discovery process because specific differences at the DNA-sequence level are responsible for aberrations in protein structure that become the basis for new therapeutics and diagnostics. Such differences are especially significant when the elucidation of a metabolic pathway reveals a key role for a specific protein and the coding region for that protein is dis-

covered to contain mutations that are linked to a specific phenotype. These mutations often take the form of a single-nucleotide polymorphism (SNP) that maintains the reading frame but causes replacement of a single amino acid. Other anomalies, such as frame-shift mutations, are more complex and usually lead to a nonfunctioning protein or no protein at all. Because most coding regions contain many splice variants, a given mutation is likely to show up in many different proteins, some of which may be completely unrelated to the original target under investigation. As bioinformatic sophistication has grown, the volume of literature relating tumor biology and

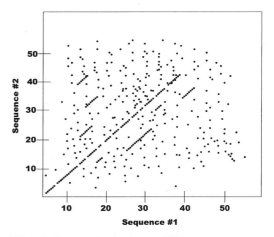

FIG. 7.2. Dot-matrix plot for two DNA sequences containing several short homologous regions.

cancer to specific genetic changes has increased exponentially during the past several years. The elucidation of various molecular mechanisms of oncogenesis has led to an understanding of the role that tumor suppressors, oncogenes, and DNA-repair genes play in the development of various cancers. Many of these alterations can occur sporadically, whereas others are inherited. Finally, the presence of specific genetic alterations is often used to diagnose a cancer that otherwise would be difficult to verify. Genetic mutations also can be prognostic indicators and guide the treatment plan of the physician (28).

One of the best-characterized genetic regulatory pathways, p53, is a perfect model for the linkage between DNA sequence information and drug therapy. Mutations in the *p53* gene occur in half of all human cancers, and aberrant regulation of the protein is present in many others. Many known oncogenes become active in the absence of p53, and animals lacking p53 are extraordinarily prone to tumor development (29). New strategies that target p53 for cancer therapy include gene therapy, customized viruses designed to replicate only in p53-inactive cells, and small-molecule drugs designed to reactivate p53. Finally, a downstream gene, *mdm-2*, regulates p53 through a complex negative-feedback loop. Wild-type p53 is an upstream transcriptional activator of *mdm-2*, which in turn interacts with p53 and functions as a ubiquitin E3 ligase that promotes the conjugation of p53 to ubiquitin. This conjugation serves as a tag that causes the degradation of p53 by the proteasome, serving to keep the level of p53 low in nonstressed cells. *Mdm-2* is also rapidly degraded by the ubiquitin system and consequently has a very short half-life in wild-type cells (30). Gene-level strategies for treating p53-associated tumors often include inhibition of *mdm-2* transcription (e.g., in human sarcomas where overexpression of *mdm-2* is common).

Another excellent example that links a phenotype to a genetic aberration involves a variety of known mutations in the gene for the cystic fibrosis transmembrane conductance regulator (CFTR), a mediator of chloride transport in epithelial cells lining the respiratory tract. The first aberration identified, often referred to as the AF508 mutation, is caused by the deletion of three nucleotides that code for phenylalanine in position 508 (31–33). However, since the discovery of the first *CFTR* mutation, over 500 additional alterations have been identified. Some prevent translation of the CFTR message, whereas others interfere with the chloride transport function of the protein and a few affect the primary structure or posttranslational processing of CFTR so that the final protein cannot be inserted into the epithelial membrane (34). Many of these mutations are associated with other diseases such as pancreatic cancer and non–cystic fibrosis pulmonary disease (an illness that mirrors some of the classic symptoms of cystic fibrosis but fails the standard sweat chloride diagnostic test). The latter has been well characterized and involves a C-to-T point mutation in intron 19 of the *CFTR* gene. The aberration creates a partially active splice site in intron 19 and causes the insertion of a new 84-base-pair exon, containing an in-frame stop codon, between exons 19 and 20 (35,36).

Genetic polymorphisms are also significant modulators of drug response and toxicity, and it is well established that aberrations in genes encoding drug-metabolizing enzymes, drug transporters, and/or drug targets significantly affect an individual's response to therapy. For example, a polymorphism in the gene for thiopurine S-methyltransferase has a dramatic effect on the pharmacokinetics and ADME (absorption distribution metabolism and excretion) of thiopurine-based drugs, and individuals with this enzyme deficiency must be treated with less than 10% of the normal dose (37). Such pharmacokinetic effects are almost always determined by the interplay of several gene products and SNPs. Unraveling the polygenic determinants that drive these effects is a complex information technology problem that includes kinetic modeling of metabolic pathways, algorithms for gene identification and gene-structure prediction, and SNP databases. Another notable example involves metabolism of the anticonvulsant drug mephenytoin, which is dramatically affected by a genetic polymorphism. Furthermore, frequency of the low-metabolizer phenotype is fivefold higher in Asian populations than in white populations. Impaired metabolism of mephenytoin and several other commonly prescribed drugs results from a defect in the cytochrome P-450 enzyme CYP2C19. The principal defect is a single base-pair mutation (G to A) in exon 5 of the enzyme, which creates an aberrant splice site (38).

TRANSCRIPTIONAL ANALYSIS

The development of a complete molecular-level picture of health and disease involves understanding processes at four distinct levels: DNA sequence, mRNA profile, protein structure, and metabolic pathway. Bioinformatics is part of an evolving toolkit that includes a variety of technologies that together are allowing researchers to build this molecular-level understanding:

• DNA-sequence information is directly relevant to the development of genetic tests for illnesses that exhibit a pattern of inheritance. DNA-sequence information also provides a context for understanding polygenic diseases and complex phenotypes. Complexities associated with the splicing process make it important to interpret DNA sequence information in the context of phenotype, because a single mutation can affect many proteins and create a complex phenotypic change.

- Messenger-RNA profiles are important diagnostics that can delineate a pattern of up-regulation and down-regulation of a large number of related genes. This information can be used experimentally to help drive the target discovery process or as a clinical diagnostic to predict the onset or progression of disease. It is important to note that many messages serve a regulatory function and are not translated into protein.
- Proteomics is a discipline focused on understanding the structures and interactions of the millions of proteins encoded in the genome. Final protein structures are normally achieved only after posttranslational modifications (e.g., acetylation, glycosylation, methylation, removal of n-terminal amino acids) have been made; however, it is not currently possible to predict these modifications from DNA-sequence or mRNA-sequence information. However, computational modeling of protein structure can be a useful tool for predicting potential sites for posttranslational modification, as well as the extent of change to protein folding that is likely to result from those modifications.
- Systems biology is an attempt to study the complex and subtle relationships among the millions of proteins that make up an organism. Systems experiments often involve perturbing a system at the mRNA level and measuring the complex downstream results. Modeling of biological systems is a complex bioinformatic challenge that has recently become feasible because of rapid advances in information technology (39).

Messenger-RNA profiling technologies are emerging as standard tools in all of the areas mentioned above, both for research and clinical use. On the research side, transcription profiling has five major applications:

- Clarification of details surrounding the splicing process for sequenced coding regions
- Identification of key messages for previously unidentified proteins (many of these protein are minor messages present in small copy numbers and previously unidentified)
- Delineation of metabolic pathways through "perturbation" experiments

- Identification of regulatory sequences that are not translated into protein
- Analysis of molecular-level responses to various stimuli, such as stress, drugs, hormone signals, and genetic mutations

On the clinical side, transcription profiling is beginning to play a role in identifying patients for clinical trial, predicting the onset of disease, and customizing treatment regimens for individual patients. Central to these advances are pattern-matching technologies that facilitate rapid large-scale database similarity searches. The task is similar to that of scanning a database containing millions of fingerprint records for patterns that are similar to a reference fingerprint. In the majority of situations where thousands of genes are involved, it is necessary to correlate up-regulation and down-regulation patterns for a given set of expressed genes with the treatment outcomes as measured by phenotypic changes. Over the next several years, such techniques are likely to become core components of clinical medicine.

Over the past several years, it has become apparent that the "one gene at a time" approach to understanding complex metabolic events is simply not adequate. Some estimates indicate that as many as 10% of the 10,000 to 20,000 mRNA species in a typical mammalian cell are differentially expressed between cancer and normal tissues. As a result, several technologies have been developed to quantify the expression of many genes in parallel. One of the many technologies, the DNA hybridization array (which is also referred to as a microarray, expression array, and gene chip) has become dominant because of its low cost and flexibility.

Because microarray analysis is highly parallel in nature, typical experiments produce thousands, sometimes millions, of data points. Microarrays are often referred to as "gene chips" because they are built on technologies adapted from the semiconductor industry—photolithography and solid-phase chemistry. Each array contains densely packed oligonucleotide probes whose sequences are chosen to maximize sensitivity and specificity allowing consistent discrimination between closely related target sequences. A typical pharmaceutical-microarray experiment involves the following steps (40,41):

1. A microarray containing thousands of single-stranded gene fragments, including known or predicted splice variants and potential polymorphisms, is constructed or purchased. The sequences are selected to support a large number of cross comparisons to confirm complex results.
2. Messenger RNA is harvested from selected cells in treated and untreated individuals (untreated sam-

ples will be used as an internal control in the array).

3. Messenger RNA is reverse transcribed into more stable complimentary DNA (cDNA) with the addition of fluorescent labels (green for cDNA derived from treated cells, red for cDNA derived from untreated cells), which are composed of 5-aminopropargyl-2′-deoxyuridine 5′-triphosphate coupled to Cy3 or Cy5 fluorescent dyes (Cy3-dUTP or Cy5-dUTP, respectively).

4. Samples of fluorescently labeled cDNA are applied to the array and exposed to every spot. A sequence match results in binding between the test cDNA test sequence and a complimentary DNA sequence on the array. Each match contains a double-stranded fluorescently labeled spot that results from the combination of the two fluorescent dies and the amount of die containing cDNA in each of the samples.

5. A laser fluorescent scanner is used to detect the hybridization signals from both fluorophores, and the resulting pattern of colored spots is stored in a database—red for strongly expressed genes in the treated sample, green for weakly expressed genes in the treated sample, yellow for genes that are equally expressed in both samples, and black for sequences that are not expressed in either sample. Since the sequence of every spot in the chip is known, the identity of each expressed cDNA can

be determined, and the amount and source (treated or untreated sample) inferred from the color and intensity of the spot.

6. Differences in intensity correspond both to expression levels of the genes in the sample and to the exactness of the match. Similar sequences containing various combinations of single-base and multiple-base changes are used as internal controls to provide more precise sequence information about genes expressed in the test sample. For example, the identity of a single base can be deduced by measuring the binding affinity of a test sequence to four slightly different probes that vary only at the position of the base in question (each contains one of the four possible bases).

The steps involved in a typical two-color microarray experiment are outlined in Figure 7.3.

One drawback of microarray analysis is related to its ability to distinguish low-abundance transcripts, those present in single-digit copy counts. Increasing the absolute amount of the hybridized target is not usually helpful because it is the relative abundance of each transcript within the RNA pool, coupled with probe characteristics, that determines the sensitivity of the array for each sequence (42). Unfortunately, it is often difficult to identify transcripts that are upregulated by less than 50%, a significant problem for researchers in areas such as oncology and neuroscience

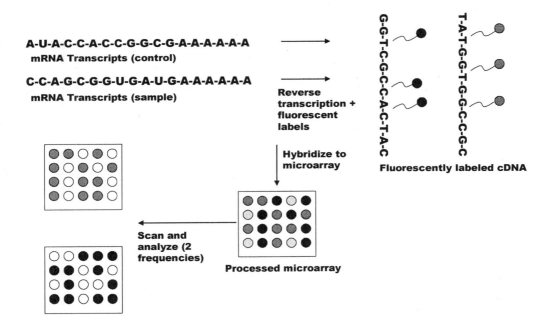

FIG. 7.3. A diagrammatic representation of a typical microarray experiment.

where subtle changes in gene expression are critical to understanding the differences between disease and health. However, the downstream effects of subtle changes in gene regulation are often more dramatic and straightforward to measure. Many of the minor messages that are difficult to detect are likely to be regulatory genes and microarray analysis can still reveal the more pronounced levels of up-regulation and down-regulation associated with more downstream members of these gene pathways—the messages most likely to code for druggable targets. In addition, several new techniques are being developed to solve the minor message problem with the goal of detecting and precisely counting the number of molecules of every transcript in the cell, even those with copy counts in the single-digit range.

The major goal of microarray data analysis is to identify statistically significant differences between genes expressed in the control and test samples. One of the most straightforward and commonly used analysis techniques involves construction of a simple scatterplot where each point represents the expression level of a specific gene in two samples: one assigned to the x-axis and one to the y-axis. For each point, position relative to the main diagonal (the identity line) directly relates the ratio of expression levels for the test and control sequences. Messages with identical expression levels in both samples appear on the identity line, whereas differentially expressed sequences appear at some point above or below the diagonal as determined by the level of expression on each axis points that appear above the diagonal are overexpressed in the sample represented by the y-axis, whereas points that appear below the diagonal are overexpressed in the sample represented on the x-axis. The absolute expression level for any gene can be determined by measuring the overall distance from the origin. A microarray scatterplot is depicted in Figure 7.4.

Scatterplots are excellent visual representations because they allow rapid and simple comparisons of two datasets. However, it is frequently necessary to identify groups of genes with similar expression profiles across a large number of experiments. The most commonly used technique for finding such relationships is cluster analysis, which produces functional groupings of genes and is helpful for identifying biochemical pathways.

Hierarchical Clustering

Hierarchical clustering, the most frequently used technique, attempts to group genes into small clusters

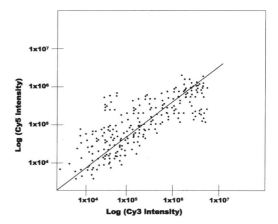

FIG. 7.4. Microarray scatterplot for two samples.

and to group clusters into higher-level systems. The resulting hierarchical tree is easily viewed as a dendrogram (43,44). Most studies involve comparing a series of experiments to identify genes that are consistently coregulated under some defined set of circumstances (e.g., disease state, increasing time, increasing drug dose). A two-dimensional grid is constructed with each row corresponding to a different gene sequence and each column to a different set of experimental conditions. Each set of gene expression levels (each row in the matrix) is compared to every other set of expression levels in a pairwise fashion, and similarity scores are produced in the form of statistical correlation coefficients. These correlation coefficients can be thought of as representing the Euclidean distances between the rows in the matrix. The correlations are ordered and a node is created between the highest-scoring (geometrically closest) pair of rows—the two gene sequences that were most nearly coregulated across each of the experiments. The matrix is then modified to represent the joined elements as a single node and all distances between the newly formed node and other gene sequences (rows) in the matrix are calculated. It is not necessary to recalculate all correlations because only those involving the two rows joined in the new node have changed. Typically, the node is represented by a link in the dendrogram, the height of the link being directly proportional to the strength of the correlation. The process of creating proportional links and joining genes into clusters continues until all genes in the experiment have been joined into a single hierarchical cluster through links of appropriate length. If more than two nodes are related by the same correlation coefficient (same geometric distance), the conflict is resolved according to a predetermined set of rules.

It is sometimes meaningful to cluster data at the experiment level rather than at the individual-gene level. Such experiments are most often used to identify similarities in overall gene-expression patterns in the context of different treatment regimens, the goal being to stratify patients based on their molecular-level responses to the treatments. The hierarchical techniques outlined in this section are appropriate for such clustering, which is based on the pairwise statistical comparison of complete scatterplots rather than on individual gene sequences. The data are represented as a matrix of scatterplots, which is ultimately reduced to a matrix of correlation coefficients. The correlation coefficients are then used to construct a two-dimensional dendrogram in the exact same way as in the gene-cluster experiments previously described.

The overall process of constructing a two-dimensional dendrogram using hierarchical clustering data is depicted in Figure 7.5.

Messenger-RNA profiling techniques have become a cornerstone of modern disease classification. These advances are especially significant in oncology where complex phenotypes have recently been found to correlate with specific changes in gene expression, the result being more precise patient stratification both for clinical trials and treatment. A significant example that illustrates the utility of hierarchical clustering is the method by which distinct tumor subclasses were identified in diffuse large B-cell lymphoma (DLBCL). Two distinct forms of DLBCL have been identified using hierarchical clustering techniques, each related to a different stage of B-cell differentiation. The fact that the cluster correlates are significant is demonstrated by direct relationships to patient survival rates (45).

Despite its proven utility, hierarchical clustering has many flaws. Interpretation of the hierarchy is complex and often confusing because (a) the deterministic nature of the technique prevents reevaluation once points are grouped into a node; (b) all determinations are strictly based on local decisions and a single pass of analysis; (c) it has been demonstrated that the tree structure can lock in accidental features reflecting idiosyncrasies of the clustering

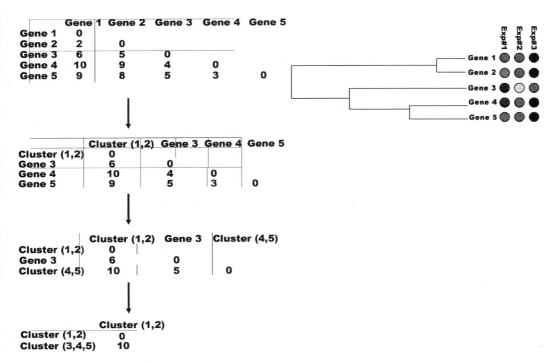

FIG. 7.5. Construction of a two-dimensional dendrogram representing a hierarchical cluster of related genes. Each column represents a different experiment, and each row a different spot (oligonucleotide sequence) on the microarray. The height of each link is proportional to the strength of the correlation.

rules; (d) expression patterns of individual gene sequences become less relevant as the clustering process progresses, and (e) an incorrect assignment
made early in the process cannot be corrected (46).
These deficiencies have driven the development of
additional clustering techniques that are based on
multiple passes of analysis and utilize advanced algorithms borrowed from the artificial intelligence
community. Two of these techniques, k-means clustering and self-organizing maps (SOM), have
achieved widespread acceptance in research oncology, where they have been enormously successful in
identifying meaningful genetic differences among
patient populations.

When discussing clustering algorithms, it is essential to recognize the limitations of two-dimensional
and three-dimensional representations of individual
gene-expression values across a collection of experiments. Figure 7.6 depicts a simple analysis composed
of two experiments. Each experiment is represented
by a dimension in the grid, and clusters of the genes
are readily apparent. Likewise, a three-dimensional
image containing three sets of expression data
from three experiments is also readily represented in
Figure 7.7.

Each of the 10 genes in these experiments is represented on one of the axes of the grid and clusters of the
genes are readily apparent. Higher-dimensional representations—those containing more than three sets of
experimental results—are much more complex to
imagine because absolute distances between individual genes and gene clusters do not lend themselves to

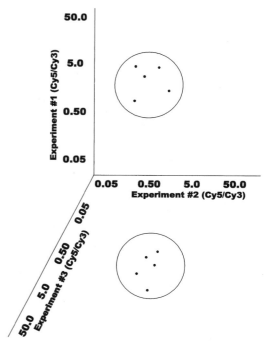

FIG. 7.7. A three-dimensional (three-experiment)
gene-clustering analysis containing 10 different sequences. Each axis in the drawing represents a different experiment, and a single vector defined in three
dimensions represents each set of expression levels.
As in the two-dimensional case, grouping of the sequences is accomplished by determining the geometric
distance between each vector. Higher-dimensional
models representing more than three experiments cannot be visualized as single vectors, and different graph-
ical techniques must be used.

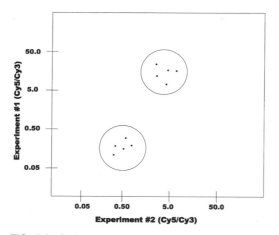

FIG. 7.6. A simple clustering case composed of two
experiments and 10 gene sequences. Each experiment is represented on one of the axes of the grid and
clusters of the genes are readily apparent.

visual representation. Despite the complexities associated with visual representation of microarray data, it
is always possible to calculate a single vector to
represent all the expression values for any gene
sequence, regardless of the number of dimensions/ex-
periments. It is the distance between these vectors that
determines the degree to which a pair of genes is
coregulated. Clustering is the process of defining
boundaries that partition vectors into meaningful
groups. Datasets with many dimensions are often visualized in a simple two-dimensional plot, with time
or experiment number on the x-axis and expression
ratio on the y-axis (expression ratios are normally represented logarithmically). When many different gene
sequences are shown on the same grid, it is often possible to visually identify groups. A two-dimensional
grid containing expression-level information for several different genes measured across 10 different time

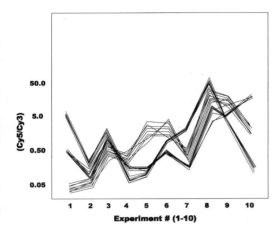

FIG. 7.8. A two-dimensional grid containing expression level information for several different genes measured across 10 different time points. The expression data represented in these 10 experiments reveal three distinct clusters of coregulated genes.

points is displayed in Figure 7.8. Although many of the expression curves overlap and individual sequences are difficult to dissect out from the mix, it is clear that the data fall into three distinct clusters of coregulated genes. Representations of this type are often used to set starting conditions for more complex algorithmic clustering procedures, such as those described in the next few sections.

K-means Clustering

K-means clustering is most useful when the number of clusters that should be represented is known. An example might include microarray classification of a group of patients that have morphologically similar diseases that fall into three clinically distinct categories (k = 3). The clustering process would proceed as follows (47):

- Each expression vector is randomly assigned to one of three groups or clusters (k = 3).
- An average expression vector (called the center) is calculated for each group, and these vectors are used to compute the distances between groups.
- Each gene-expression vector is reassigned to the group whose center is closest. Expression vectors are allowed to remain in a cluster only when they are closer to the center of that cluster than to a neighboring one.
- Intercluster and intracluster distances are recomputed, and new expression vectors for the center of each cluster are calculated.

- The process is repeated until all expression vectors are optimally placed. At this point any additional changes would increase intracluster distances while decreasing intercluster dissimilarity.

K-means clustering has proven to be a valuable tool for identifying coregulated genes in systems where biochemical or clinical knowledge can be used to predict an appropriate number of clusters. The tool is also useful when the number of appropriate clusters is unknown if the researcher experiments with different values of k. However, the unstructured nature of the technique tends to proceed in a local fashion and this effect intensifies as additional clustering centers are added to the analysis. Excessive locality eventually leads to incorrect groupings and important gene associations can be lost. It follows that as the number of clustering centers is increased, initial placement of the centers becomes increasingly critical; for analyses that involve large numbers of clustering centers, it makes sense to use more structured techniques. Algorithms based on SOMs solve many of these problems and have demonstrated tremendous utility in anticancer drug discovery and research oncology.

Self-Organizing Maps

The SOM analysis technique bears much resemblance to k-means clustering because both techniques involve an iterative approach to locating the center of each cluster. However, SOM analysis is much more structured, and the user must initialize the system with a specific geometric construct representing the initial location of each cluster center. More than a simple list of locations, the construct is a complete topology where SOM cluster centers, which are referred to as centroids, are part of a symmetrical structure. Many successful experiments have been conducted utilizing a simple two-dimensional 3 × 2 grid as the starting point. Alternative structures based on hexagonal rings, grids, and lines have also been used, and each has a pronounced effect on the outcome of the analysis. More structured than k-means clustering and far less rigid than hierarchical techniques, SOM is emerging as the technique of choice for analyzing complex datasets with high-dimensional character and many gene sequences (48). An eight-node SOM based on two experiments is depicted in Figure 7.9.

Each iteration involves the random selection of a gene-expression vector. Reference vectors for nearby centroids are adjusted to make them more similar to the selected gene; the nearest centroid is adjusted by the largest amount, and smaller adjustments are made with other local centroids to move them towards the

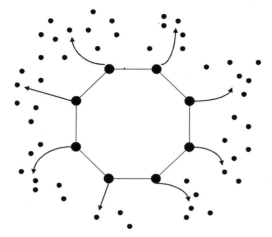

FIG. 7.9. Depicts a simple self-organizing map analysis composed of eight centroids, 51 genes, and two dimensions (two sets of experimental conditions or time points). Large circles denote centroids and small dots represent gene-expression vectors. Successive iterations of the system generate the trajectories, shown as centroids, which migrate to fit the data. Additional experiments require additional dimensions and are difficult to visualize in a drawing. Many other topologies (e.g., hexagonal rings, lines, and complex grids) are also possible, and have a pronounced effect on the outcome.

selected gene, the degree depending on their proximity to the selected point. The process typically continues for 20,000 to 50,000 iterations.

In a seminal article on this topic, Golub and Slonim (49) compared expression profiles from tissue samples recovered from patients with acute myeloid leukemia and acute lymphoblastic leukemia using the Affymetrix HU6800 GeneChip. The goal was to identify a gene or small number of genes that are consistently upregulated in one disease class and down-regulated in the other. Once such a grouping is located cluster analysis can be used to locate "nearby" genes that behave in similar fashion. The array contained probes for 6,817 different human genes, and final results revealed 1,100 that were coregulated in one of the disease classes. Each of these can be thought of as providing a "weighted vote" based on its statistical significance in the analysis. The system is tested on a well-characterized sample (known disease class) that is not included in the training set for the SOM. Of the 1,100 genes identified, the 50 genes that had the highest correlation with class distinction were selected as predictors and tested against samples from 38 patients with carefully diagnosed conditions. Of the 38 samples, 36 were correctly assigned as belonging to the

acute myeloid leukemia or acute lymphoblastic leukemia group strictly on the basis of up-regulation or down-regulation of these 50 genes. Two of the 38 predictions were statistically uncertain. Finally, the selection of 50 genes was arbitrary in the sense that more than 50 genes displayed expression patterns well correlated with one of the disease states. Further refinement of the technique might include additional genes, and in practice it often makes sense to adjust the predictor set once the function of each of the genes is known. Such an approach links microarray analysis to further biochemical experimentation and may require extensive experimentation to determine function for previously unknown genes. Conversely, if a gene is found to be a strong correlate with a specific disease state, and if the function of that gene is not currently known, it makes excellent scientific sense to select that particular sequence for further analysis. Approaches of this sort are driving the use of microarray analysis as a core component of research oncology.

Two additional procedural points are important to note. First, all expression data should be passed through a variation filter to remove genes that do not show significant up-regulation or down-regulation. This additional step prevents centroids from being attracted to groups of inactive genes. Second, expression levels must be normalized across all experiments to focus attention on the shape of the expression curves rather than absolute expression levels.

Additional Microarray Analysis Techniques

Neural networks are algorithmic approaches to machine learning that are designed to simulate the input/output structure biological neurons. Like their biological counterparts, neural networks learn by adjusting weighting functions and combining outputs to create trigger situations when inputs exceed certain thresholds. SOM-clustering algorithms can be thought of as "unsupervised" neural networks. The system proceeds through thousands of iterations of learning until a solution is discovered that optimally places the centroids in the centers of gene clusters. Conversely, supervised neural networks are similar in their iterative approach to learning but proceed until a predefined endpoint determined by the user is reached. The simplest case of a supervised neural network is a single two-dimensional matrix referred to as a perceptron (50). Values contained in the matrix are used as the basis of a scoring system whose ultimate goal is to distinguish between two sets of data. An iterative process is used to score individual members of each dataset and make modifications to the matrix until a satisfactory endpoint is reached. More complex systems use multiple layers of perceptrons; scores in the first layer are combined and used as triggers for the second layer, and so on through as many layers as are built into the system. Modern neural networks often use three layers of perceptrons—an input layer, a hidden layer that combines data from the input layer, and a final output layer. Each iteration involves comparison to the predetermined endpoint, and a decision is made regarding modification of one of the layers. One of the most important features of multilayer perceptron-based supervised neural networks is that they can be designed to perform multiset classifications of complex datasets. Recent experiments have demonstrated the utility of this approach for studying gene-expression signatures from multiclass microarray data representing gene clusters for major metabolic pathways. One of the most intriguing outcomes of the research involved the detailed examination of "false positives"—results that seemed to artificially cluster genes not thought to be directly related. However, deeper analysis revealed that these false positives were found to represent related metabolic pathways with overlapping enzymatic reactions (51).

PROTEIN STRUCTURE PREDICTION AND DATA MINING OF CHEMICAL STRUCTURE DATABASES: NEW TOOLS FOR PREDICTING TARGETS AND IDENTIFYING LEAD COMPOUNDS

An important part of target validation involves purifying and studying a specific receptor to identify the parameters most likely to affect lead-compound binding. Pharmaceutical companies often rely on combinatorial chemistry and high-throughput screening to predict these interactions. Additionally, during the past several years, *in silico* techniques for predicting these molecular events have advanced to the point where biotech companies are beginning to skip much of the laboratory benchwork involved in combinatorial chemistry and synthesize only the most promising compounds based on a structural understanding of the receptor and associated ligands. Both target validation and lead optimization are enhanced by the use of programs that facilitate the prediction of three-dimensional structures of proteins and protein–ligand complexes.

Computational structure prediction techniques are critical because they can provide three-dimensional information about the vast majority of proteins whose structures cannot be determined experimentally— membrane-bound proteins, large complexes, certain glycoproteins, and other molecules that cannot readily be crystallized (52). IBM Research recently announced its intent to build a supercomputer, called Blue Gene/L, which will be optimized for protein structure prediction and other similar problems that lend themselves to parallelization. It was determined that the smallest machine that can be reasonably used to simulate the folding process will be capable of operating in the range of 1 petaflop—1×10^{15} floating point operations per second. Furthermore, such a machine will require on the order of 1 month to model the folding of even the smallest proteins. Table 7.2 below depicts the complexity of the folding process in terms of time steps (53).

The calculation assumes that the protein being folded is very small (less than 100 residues), requiring an environment of only about 6,000 water molecules, and that it folds quickly (in less than 0.1 msec). With a time step of 5×10^{-15}, a petaflop size machine would still require 20 days to fold this small protein. By comparison, the largest supercomputer in use today is approximately 12 teraflops. Such a machine, despite its size and complexity, is two orders of magnitude too small to be useful for protein folding simulations. Therefore, it is necessary to restrict the size of the problem.

Fortunately, many alternatives to using structure prediction as part of the target identification process are available. For example, in many cases the molecule being modeled is membrane bound and the calculation is focused on the portion known, through chemical analysis, to be exposed outside the cell membrane. This approach has been helpful to researchers working to identify antibody targets on the surface of infected T-helper cells in human immunodeficiency virus (HIV)-seropositive patients. A recently created monoclonal antibody is believed to bind to a region of the gp41 transmembrane glycoprotein close to a transmembrane domain. This region is accessible to neutralizing antibodies, and could form a useful target for vaccine design (54).

TABLE 7.2. *Computational complexity of protein folding*

No. of atoms	2×10^4
No. of instr./atom/time step	5×10^6
No. of instr./time step	1×10^{11}
Physical time for folding (second)	1×10^{-4}
Physical time step (second)	5×10^{-15}
No. of time steps needed	2×10^{10}
No. of instr.	2×10^{21}
No. of seconds in 20 days	1.7×10^6
No. of instr./second	1×10^{15}

Another example involves using bioinformatic tools to predict which portion of a protein sequence is likely to be a biologically active binding site, and to model the specific structure of that site. An interesting example is the Gp120 glycoprotein, a cell surface protein that, like Gp41, mediates HIV entry into target cells initiating the replication cycle of the virus. The crystal structure of the core of gp120 has been recently solved (55,56). It reveals the structure of the conserved HIV-1 receptor binding sites and some of the mechanisms evolved by HIV-1 to escape Ab response. The protein consists of three faces. One is largely inaccessible on the native trimer, and two faces are exposed but apparently have low immunogenicity, particularly on primary viruses. The investigators modeled HIV-1 neutralization by a CD4 binding site monoclonal antibody, and propose that neutralization takes place by inhibition of the interaction between gp120 and the target receptors as a result of steric hindrance. Such structural knowledge is central to the discovery of new drugs across a variety of disease categories and is especially relevant to oncology where cell—cell signaling plays a crucial role in disease progression (57).

Target modeling represents half the computational problem because a complete solution must also include correct identification of appropriate lead compounds. Furthermore, because compounds that bind to a target may still be toxic, ADME predictions are also a critical part of lead-compound optimization. It is not possible to synthesize or even generate all the possible lead compounds; some estimates set the number of chemical structures in the molecular weight range of a typical pharmaceutical (less than 500 d) at more that 10^{20} different molecules. As a result of this explosive diversity, pharmaceutical companies have build tremendous compound libraries containing tens of thousands of promising compounds. Likewise, many data sources are now available that contain libraries of two-dimensional and three-dimensional structures, the National Cancer Institute's Drug Information System (NCI DIS) three-dimensional database being one of the most significant examples (58).

The NCI DIS three-dimensional database contains over 400,000 compounds and is maintained by the National Cancer Institute's Developmental Therapeutics Program Division of Cancer Treatment (Rockville, MD). The structural information stored in the DIS represents the connection table for each drug—a list that details the connections between atoms in the compound. This information can be searched to find drugs that share similar bond patterns, which are often a predictor of biological activity. As mentioned previously, it is often possible to model the points of interaction between a drug and its target with only a small number of atoms. This geometric arrangement of atoms, typically referred to as a pharmacophore, can be used to search three-dimensional structural databases to find compounds with similar biological activity (despite the fact that these compounds may have very different patterns of chemical bonds). A diverse set of lead compounds increases the chance of finding an appropriate drug with acceptable properties for clinical development (59). Alternatively, if a lead compound is known, then similarity searches are often used to identify other compounds with similar structures and chemical properties.

One problem with this approach is that three or four point pharmacophore are often too restrictive, whereas slightly more open-ended searches will usually return an unwieldy number of hits from a large structure database. Furthermore, it is often impossible to score or rank the hits. As a result, pharmacophore searches have a tendency to return "already known" solutions. A more sophisticated and unbiased approach involves exhaustive receptor-ligand docking experiments. Such experiments, which require that every compound in the library be tested for binding against the target structure, have been made possible by recent improvements in computer performance (target structures are determined experimentally using x-ray crystallography or nuclear magnetic resonance, or through *in silico* modeling). Each docking event receives a score based on a calculation of the free energy of binding—typically based on the geometry of hydrogen bond contacts, lipophilic contacts, metal binding contacts, and other factors related to entropic penalties that describe the freezing of ligand conformational flexibility on binding (60).

Finally, *in silico* ADME modeling is often used prior to clinical trials to predict metabolic behavior of the drug. Such modeling will require a detailed understanding all related metabolic pathways and the effects the drug has on the up-regulation and down-regulation of key genes whose protein products modulate those pathways (61).

SYSTEMS BIOLOGY: THE NEW VISTA

Emerging technologies that measure the simultaneous expression levels of thousands of genes, and those that discover the relationships that link those genes to regulated networks, represent one of the most exciting areas of contemporary molecular biology. The ultimate application of these technologies is the detailed modeling of interacting pathways to make phenotypic predictions, also known as systems biology (62).

One specific project conducted at the Institute for Systems Biology involved construction of a global model based on 20 systematic perturbations of a system containing 997 mRNAs from the yeast galactose-utilization pathway (63). The experiments provided direct evidence that 15 of 289 detected proteins were posttranscriptionally regulated, and the model that emerged identified explicit physical interactions governing the cellular response to each perturbation. Such experiments, which demonstrate that it is possible to develop and test complete systems models that have the potential to rapidly advance the cause of predictive medicine, represent an important milestone in the history of drug discovery. They form the basis of a new emergent science sometimes referred to as "information-based medicine." It is also important to note that such efforts merge two distinct but related fields: molecular biology and information technology.

Over the past several years, bioinformatics has evolved from a new science focused on sequence matching and pattern discovery to a branch of mathematics focused on the modeling of complex and dynamic biological systems. As a result, bioinformatics has emerged as a core component of the drug discovery process.

REFERENCES

1. Clulow M, Phillippe J, Bar-Nahum G. Life science informatics. UBS Warburg LLC report; April 12, 2001.
2. Slamon DJ, Godolphin W, Jones LA, et al. Studies of the HER-2/neuproto-oncogene in human breast and ovarian cancer. *Science* 1989;244:707–712.
3. Sakamoto M, Kondo A, Kawasaki K, et al. Analysis of gene expression profiles associated with cisplatin resistance in human ovarian cancer cell lines and tissues using cDNA microarray. *Hum Cell* 2001;14:305–315.
4. International Human Genome Sequencing Consortium. Initial sequencing and analysis of the human genome. *Nature* 2001;409:860–921.
5. Venter JC, Adams MD, Myers EW, et al. The sequence of the human genome. *Science* 2001;291:1304–1351.
6. Rigoutsos I, Floratos A, Ouzounis C, et al. Dictionary building via unsupervised hierarchical motif discovery in the sequence space of natural proteins. *Proteins* 1999;37:264–277.
7. Martí-Renom MA, Stuart A, Fiser A, et al. Comparative protein structure modeling of genes and genomes. *Annu Rev Biophys Biomol Struct* 2000;29:291–325
8. Pieper U, Eswar N, Stuart AC, et al. MODBASE, a database of annotated comparative protein structure models. *Nucleic Acids Res* 2002;30:255–259.
9. Kozak M. Initiation and translation in procaryotes and eukaryotes. *Gene* 1999;234:187–208.
10. Alberts BD, Bray J, Lewis M, et al. *Molecular biology of the cell,* 3rd ed. New York: Garland Publishing, 1994:365–430
11. Baxevanis A, Ouellette F. *Bioinformatics a practical guide to the analysis of genes and proteins.* New York: John Wiley and Sons, 2001:235–242.
12. Claverie JM. Computational methods for the identification of genes in vertebrate genomic sequences. *Hum Mol Genet* 1998;6:1735–1744.
13. Claverie JM. Exon detection by similarity searches. *Methods Mol Biol* 1997;68:283–313.
14. Mount D. *Bioinformatics: sequence and genome analysis.* New York: Cold Spring Harbor Laboratory Press, 2001:337–373.
15. Sharp PM, Li WH. The codon adaptation index: a measure of directional synonymous codon usage bias, and its potential applications. *Nucleic Acids Res* 1987;15:1281–1295.
16. Fickett JW. Recognition of protein coding regions in DNA sequences. *Nucleic Acids Res* 1982;10:5303–5318.
17. Uberbacher EC, Mural RJ. Locating protein-coding regions in human DNA sequences by a multiple sensor-neural network approach. *Proc Natl Acad Sci U S A* 1991;88:11261–11265.
18. Uberbacher EC, Xu Y, Mural RJ. Discovering and understanding genes in human DNA sequence using GRAIL. *Methods Enzymol* 1996;266,:259–281.
19. Burge CB, Karlin S. Finding genes in genomic DNA. *Curr Opin Struct Biol* 1998;8:346–354.
20. Burste M, Guigo R. Evaluation of gene structure prediction programs. *Genomics* 1996;34:353–367.
21. Chen QK, Hertz GZ, Stormo GD. MATRIX SEARCH 1.0: a computer program that scans DNA sequences for transcriptional elements using a database of weight matrices. *Comput Appl Biosci* 1995;11:563–566.
22. Prestridge DS. SIGNAL SCAN: a computer program that scans DNA sequences for eukaryotic transcriptional elements. *Comput Appl Biosci* 1991;7:203–206.
23. Gish W, States DJ. Identification of protein coding regions by database similarity search. *Nat Genet* 1993; 3:266–272.
24. Kolchanov NA, Ponomorenko MP, Frolov AS, et al. Integrated databases and computer systems for studying eukaryotic gene expression. *Bioinformatics* 1999;15:669–686.
25. Gelfand MS, Mironov AA, Pevzner PA. Gene recognition via spliced sequence alignment, *Proc Natl Acad Sci U S A* 1996;93:9061–9066.
26. Farber R, Lapedes A, Sirotkin K. Determination of eukaryotic protein coding regions using neural networks and information theory. *J Mol Biol* 1992;226:471–479.
27. Reese MG, Harris N, Eeckman F. Large scale sequencing specific neural networks for promoter and splice site recognition. In: Hunter L, Klein TE, eds. *Biocomputing: proceedings of the 1996 Pacific Symposium.* Singapore: World Scientific, 1996.
28. Ganjavi H, Malkin D. Genetics of childhood cancer. *Clin Orthop* 2002;401:75–87.
29. Donewower LA. The p53 deficient mouse: a model for basic and applied cancer studies. *Semin Cancer Biol* 1996;7:269–278.
30. Lane D, Lain S. Therapeutic exploitation of the p53 pathway. *Trends Mol Med* 2002;8(Suppl):S38–S42.
31. Collins F. Cystic fibrosis: molecular biology and therapeutic implications. *Science* 1992;256:774–779.

32. Riordan J. The cystic fibrosis transmembrane conductance regulator. *Annu Rev Physiol* 1993;55:609–630.

33. Welsh MJ, Anderson MP, Rich DP, et al. Cystic fibrosis transmembrane conductance regulator: a chloride channel with novel regulation. *Neuron* 1992;8:821–829.

34. Zielenski J, Tsui L. Cystic fibrosis and phenotypic variations. *Annu Rev Genet* 1995;29:777–807.

35. Highsmith WE, Burch LH, Zhou Z, et al. A novel mutation in the cystic fibrosis gene in patients with pulmonary disease but normal sweat chloride concentrations. *N Engl J Med* 1994;331:974–980.

36. Malatsa N, Casalsc T, Portaa M, et al. Cystic fibrosis transmembrane regulator (CFTR) AF508 mutation and 5T allele in patients with chronic pancreatitis and exocrine pancreatic cancer. *Gut* 2001;48:70–74.

37. William Evans W, Johnson J. Pharmacogenomics: the inherited basis for interindividual differences in drug response. *Annu Rev Genomics Hum Genet* 2001; 2:9–39.

38. de Morais SM, Wilkinson GR, Blaisdell J, et al. The major genetic defect responsible for the polymorphism of S- mephenytoin metabolism in humans. *J Biol Chem* 1994;269:15419–15422.

39. Ideker T, Thorsson V, Ranish J, et al. Integrated genomic and proteomic analysis of a systematically perturbed metabolic network. *Science* 2001;292:929–934.

40. Friend S, Roland S. The magic of microarrays. *Sci Am* 2002;286:44–49.

41. Shalon D, Smith SJ, Brown PO. A DNA microarray system for analyzing complex DNA samples using two-color fluorescent probe hybridization. *Genome Res* 1996;6:639–645.

42. Mimics K, Middleton F, Lewis A, et al. Analysis of complex brain disorders with gene expression microarrays: schizophrenia as a disease of the synapse. *Trends Neurosci* 2001;24:479–486.

43. Kuklin A, Shah S, Hoff B, et al. Data management in microarray fabrication, image processing, and data mining. In: Grigorenko E, ed. *DNA arrays: technologies and experimental strategies.* Boca Raton, CRC Press, 2002:115–128.

44. Eisen MB, Soellman PT, Brown PO, et al. Cluster analysis and display of genome-wide expression patterns. *Proc Natl Acad Sci U S A* 1998;95:14863–14868.

45. Alizadeh AA, Eisen MB, Davis RE, et al. Distinct types of diffuse large B-cell lymphoma identified by gene expression profiling. *Nature* 200;403:503–511.

46. Tamayo P, Slonim D, Mesirov J, et al. Interpreting patterns of gene expression with self-organizing maps: methods and application to hematopoietic differentiation. *Proc Natl Acad Sci U S A* 1999;96:2907–2912.

47. Quackenbush J. Computational analysis of microarray data. *Nat Rev Genet* 2001;2:418–427.

48. Kohonen T, Huang T, Schroeder M, eds. *Self organizing maps,* 3rd ed. New York: Springer-Verlag, 2001.

49. Golub TR, Slonim DK, Tamayo P, et al. Molecular classification of cancer: class discovery and class prediction by gene expression monitoring. *Science* 1999;286: 531–537.

50. Rosenblatt F. The perceptron: a probabilistic model for information storage in the brain. *Psych Rev* 1958;65: 386–407.

51. Mateos A, Dopazo J, Jansen R, et al. Systematic learning of gene functional classes from DNA array expression data by using multi-layer perceptrons. Bioinformatics unit, Centro Nacional de Investigaciones Oncologicas, Madrid, Spain; Department of Molecular Biophysics and Biochemistry, Yale University, New Haven, CT; IBM Computational Biology Center, York Town Heights, NY. Manuscript in preparation.

52. Baker D, Sali A. Protein structure prediction and structural genomics. *Science* 2001;294:93–96.

53. IBM Blue Gene Team. Blue gene: a vision for protein science using a petaflop supercomputer. *IBM Syst J* 2001;40:310.

54. Zwick MB, Labrijn AF, Wang M, et al. Broadly neutralizing antibodies targeted to the membrane-proximal external region of human immunodeficiency virus type 1 glycoprotein gp41. *J Virol* 2001;75:10892–10905.

55. Malenbaum SE, Yang D, Cavacini L, et al. The n-terminal v3 loop glycan modulates the interaction of clade A and B human immunodeficiency virus type 1 envelopes with CD4 and chemokine receptors. *J Virol* 2000;74: 11008–11016.

56. Ye YJ, Si ZH, Moore JP, et al. Association of structural changes in the v2 and v3 loops of the gp120 envelope glycoprotein with acquisition of neutralization resistance in a simian-human immunodeficiency virus passaged in vivo. *J Virol* 2000;74:11955–11962.

57. Poignard P, Ollmann Saphire E, Parren P, et al. Gp120: Biologic aspects of structural features. *Annu Rev Immunol* 2001;19:253–274.

58. Milne GWA, Nicklaus MC, Driscoll JS, et al. The NCI drug information system 3D database. *J Chem Inf Comput Sci* 1994;34:1219–1224.

59. Ooms F. Molecular modeling and computer aided drug design. Examples of their applications in medicinal chemistry. *Curr Med Chem* 2000;7:141–158.

60. Waszkowycz B, Perkins TDJ, Li J. Large-scale virtual screening for discovering leads in the postgenomic era. *IBM Syst J* 2001;40:360–376.

61. Augen J. The evolving role of information technology in the drug discovery process. *Drug Discov Today* 2002;7: 315–323.

62. Kitano H. Systems biology: a brief overview. *Science* 2002;295:1662–1664.

63. Ideker T, Thorsson V, Ranish J, et al. Integrated genomic and proteomic analysis of a systematically perturbed metabolic network. *Science* 2001;292:929–934.

8

Genomics and Drug Development

Robert H. tePoele and Paul Workman

The Cancer Research UK Centre for Cancer Therapeutics, The Institute of Cancer Research, Sutton SM2 5NG, United Kingdom

In the last few years, our understanding of what goes wrong at the molecular level in a normal cell to form a malignant cell has increased dramatically. Although numerous unanswered questions remain, our knowledge is such that a significant number of novel and interesting molecular targets for therapeutic intervention have already been identified. The growing feeling is that drugs targeting the specific abnormalities that are responsible for the malignant phenotype will be more effective and less toxic than the current anti-cancer agents (1). The challenge is to develop agents targeting those causative changes as effectively and expediently as possible (1,2).

With the publication of the draft human genome sequence (3), and the consequent development of techniques such as high-throughput DNA sequencing (4) and genome-wide expression profiling (5), the drug discovery and development process can be accelerated and made more efficient. Furthermore, expression profiling and high-throughput sequencing of cancer genomes will identify additional molecular targets for drug development, and will also facilitate the targeting of drug treatment according to the genomics of the individual patient. In this chapter, we will illustrate how genomics is having a major impact on the contemporary discovery and development of new anticancer agents.

During the development of new molecular therapeutics, it is essential to define factors that confer sensitivity or resistance. This will be of even greater importance with the emergence of agents targeted at the molecular pathology of cancer, as compared to cytotoxic drugs targeting all proliferating cells, especially because in many cases only a genetically defined subgroup of a particular cancer may be responsive. Examples of such agents that have already received regulatory approval include imatinib mesylate (Gleevec), trastuzumab (Herceptin), and ZD1839 (Iressa).

Of equal importance is to identify molecular pharmacodynamic markers to assess whether the drug is actually modulating the intended molecular target and the biochemical pathways and biological processes in which it operates. Such proof of concept is important in the preclinical discovery phase and in early clinical trials. Sensitivity and resistance to anticancer drugs is determined by the biology of the particular cell, which in turn is largely controlled by the expression of genes in that cell. With modern screening technologies such as genome-wide expression profiling and proteomics, we now have very powerful means to interrogate the biology and molecular pharmacology of cancer.

The science of genomics can be distinguished from molecular biology and molecular genetics by analysis on a genome-wide scale. We will therefore pay particular attention in this chapter to genome-wide sequencing and global gene-expression profiling. It is also important to mention that while the emphasis is on novel molecular therapeutics that exploit modern cancer genome targets, the genomic methodologies discussed are equally applicable to new agents acting on more traditional targets.

MULTISTEP ONCOGENESIS

Until recently, one of the major bottlenecks in drug development has been target identification. Compounds were commonly screened in cell-based assays, and were selected on the basis of antiproliferative or cytotoxic properties rather than specific anticancer characteristics. Often these compounds were developed into drugs without knowing the cellular target of the agent, which proved subsequently to involve interference with fundamental cellular processes that are equally essential in both the cancer cell and the normal cell.

In the last two decades, the molecular basis for carcinogenesis has come into view. It is now understood that cancer results from the progressive acquisition of genetic and epigenetic abnormalities in susceptible cells (6). These typically involve somatic mutations, but can also be inherited. Tumorigenesis is a multistep process. Multiple mutations ("hits") are required before a fully malignant cancer develops. The genetic alterations in the development of colorectal cancers are the best understood (7), but the mutations involved also apply to numerous other cancers.

Tumors arise from the activation of oncogenes and the inactivation of tumor-suppressor genes. Oncogenes can be defined as gene-encoding products, the increased activity of which leads to increased proliferation and survival, whereas tumor-suppressor genes are negative regulators that when inactivated lead to loss of growth control. To date about 30 tumor suppressors and 100 oncogenes have been identified. The deregulation of cancer genes results in a wide range of changes in cellular structure and function, all contributing in various ways to the malignant phenotype (Table 8.1) (8).

Because human colorectal cancer develops through well-defined morphological stages, it has been possible to define the sequence of mutations in particular detail (7). Development of colorectal tumors appears to be initiated by mutations in the *APC* (adenomatous polyposis coli) tumor-suppressor gene, usually resulting in the truncation of the protein. Mutations in the *APC* gene can occur somatically, causing a single tumor, or in the germline, leading to a genetic predisposition to colorectal cancer known as familial adenomatous polyposis. Inactivation of the *APC* gene leads to cellular atypia and disordered growth. Interestingly, restoring APC function leads to apoptosis in these cells (9).

Hereditary nonpolyposis colorectal cancer (HNPCC) is associated with inherited mutations in mismatch repair (MMR). The MMR machinery recognizes base mismatches and extrahelical loops of nucleotides. Repair of such damage is important in preventing microsatellite instability. Mutations in HNPCC families have been found in the *hMSH2*, *hMLH1*, and *hPMS2* genes (10). These result in a mutator phenotype, with mutation rates in cells of HNPCC patients being two to three orders of magnitude higher than those in normal cells (11). The increased mutation rate in HNPCC patients provides an explanation for tumor progression; however, MMR defects do not seem to be initiating events in colorectal carcinogenesis.

Mutations in the *ras* genes are often the second step in colorectal tumorigenesis. Introduction of activated *ras* into susceptible cells confers neoplastic properties to these cells (12). However, mutations of the *ras* loci have little effect on the proliferative capacity of epithelial cells in the absence of other mutations, indicating that *ras* mutations do not initiate tumorigenesis but rather occur as a later event promoting the malignant process. This is consistent with the Vogelstein/Kinzler model in which K-*ras* mutations tend to occur during the progression from a benign to a malignant tumor (7). Loss of *p53* function is observed in the majority of colorectal tumors. The *p53* tumor suppressor gene, located on chromosome 17p, is lost through chromosomal recombination in about 80% of colorectal tumors, whereas this loss is only sporadic in adenomas. Loss of p53 function is associated with transition from late adenoma to carcinoma.

Most emphasis has been focused on identifying genes that are mutated, amplified, or deleted in human cancers. However, it has recently become clear that epigenetic alterations, especially DNA methylation, are frequently involved in the deregulation of both tumor suppressors and oncogenes, and are an important driving force in tumorigenesis (13–15). DNA methylation is a covalent modification of cytosine residues in CpG dinucleotides and is inherited in somatic cell division. Methylation of CpG-rich sequences, CpG islands, in the promoter regions of genes often results in the transcriptional silencing of these genes. Whereas CpG islands in normal cells are usually unmethylated, they are frequently methylated in tumors. Epigenetic inactivation of genes involved in growth control, such as tumor-suppressor genes, cell cycle genes, DNA-repair genes, and genes involved in invasion and metastasis, has been reported in numerous cancers. The retinoblastoma, *p14ARF*, *APC*, and *BRCA1* genes are examples of genes that are frequently epigenetically inactivated in human cancer (16).

Our understanding of the multistep progress of human colorectal cancer has established a paradigm that is now being applied to other cancers. Ultimately, our aim must be to understand in comprehensive molecular detail the complete repertoire of genomic pathology that drives each and every cancer. This will

TABLE 8.1. *Malignant phenotype*

Self-sufficiency in proliferative growth signals
Insensitivity to growth-inhibitory signals
Evasion of apoptosis
Acquisition of limitless replicative potential
Induction of angiogenesis
Induction of invasion of mestastasis

Modified with permission from Morin PJ, Weinberg RA. The hallmarks of cancer. *Cell* 2000;100:57–70 (8).

in turn provide the basis for the development and use of cocktails of individualized molecular therapeutics. In the meantime, we already have sufficient information to develop specific new agents that act on particular genomically defined molecular targets in cancer cells.

CURRENT AGENTS TARGETING GENETIC ABNORMALITIES

The first generation of therapeutic agents targeting a specific genetic abnormality in cancer cells are now being tested in clinical trials (Table 8.2) (23–30). ZD1839 (Iressa) is a selective small-molecule inhibitor of the epidermal growth factor (EGF) receptor tyrosine kinase, which plays a key role in tumorigenesis in epithelial cancers and is frequently overexpressed therein (17). Iressa has shown significant activity as a single agent in non–small cell lung (NSCL), head and neck, and hormone-refractory prostate cancer (18). However, phase 3 clinical trials of Iressa in combination with chemotherapy did not show any improvement over chemotherapy alone in the treatment of NSCL cancer (19,20). Trastuzumab (Herceptin), the first anticancer drug targeted at a tyrosine kinase to receive marketing approval, is a humanized monoclonal antibody to the extracellular domain of the ErbB2 (HER-2) receptor. Herceptin is used to treat breast cancer patients who show overexpression of the ErbB2 receptor. In this subpopulation, responses of up to 60% to 70% have been obtained in combination with doxorubicin, paclitaxel, or docetaxel, and median survival is increased compared to chemotherapy alone (21,22). Herceptin can, however, also increase the cardiotoxicity of anthracycline-based chemotherapy.

The most encouraging results obtained to date with the new molecular therapeutics have been the very high response rates achieved with the c-ABL kinase inhibitor imatinib mesylate (Gleevec, formerly known as STI571) in the treatment of chronic myelogenous leukemia (CML) (31). CML is characterized by deregulated c-ABL kinase activity arising from a chromosomal translocation involving the BCR and c-ABL genes, resulting in continuous activation of the ABL kinase function. Some encouraging results with imatinib mesylate have also been obtained in the treatment of metastatic gastrointestinal stromal tumors (GIST) (32,33). GIST are characterized by the expression of the tyrosine kinase Kit, commonly present in a mutated and activated form. The Kit tyrosine kinase is effectively inhibited by imatinib mesylate. Interestingly, patients with particular KIT gene mutations have a much higher response rate.

It can be argued that CML and GIST are homogeneous diseases driven by a single genetic abnormality. Hence the results obtained with imatinib mesylate in CML may not be readily repeated in other types of cancer where multiple genetic defects are involved. However, with the implementation of modern technologies and the increasing speed of elucidation of the pathways involved in multistep carcinogenesis, additional targets will be defined and new small molecule inhibitors, antisense constructs and antibody-based molecular therapies will become available. If multiple pathways combine to drive the particular cancer, a cocktail of inhibitors may be required to block the malignant phenotype (Table 8.1). It will be critical to be able to predict which drugs will be effective in subgroups of individual patients, depending on which genetic abnormalities and hijacked pathways are driving the particular cancers.

In an interesting and important paper (34), a transgenic model system was used to address the fundamental question of whether an oncogene that was required for the initial development of a specific tumor is still required to maintain the malignant phenotype of that tumor at a later stage, when additional genetic abnormalities have been acquired. The authors engi-

TABLE 8.2. *Examples of genomic targets in clinical and preclinical development*

Target	Agent
EGF tyrosine kinase	ZD1839 (Iressa) (17)
ErbB2	Trastuzumab (Herceptin) (23)
Bcr/Abl kinase	Imatinib mesylate (Gleevec) (24)
Hsp90	17AAG (25)
Ras/Raf/MEK/ERK	BAY-43-9006, PD184352
mTOR	CC1779, RAD001 (26)
VEGF receptor tyrosine kinase	SU5416, bevacizumab (27)
HDAC	Phenylbutyrate, depsipeptide, MS-27-275, SAHA (28)
CDK	Flavopiridol, UCN-01 (29), CYC202 (30)

EGF, epidermal growth factor, VEGF, vascular endothelial growth factor.

neered conditional transgenic mice to overexpress the c-*myc* oncogene, which resulted in the formation of malignant osteosarcomas. When c-*myc* overexpression was transiently stopped, the sarcomas differentiated into mature osteocytes that formed normal bone. Furthermore, restoration of c-*myc* expression resulted in apoptosis of the osteocytes rather than the predicted reversion to malignant growth. Several other examples illustrate how cancer cells appear physiologically dependent on the continued activation of certain oncogenes. When these oncogenes are switched off or expression is reduced, for example by antisense oligonucleotides, the cancer cells frequently die by apoptosis. Transgenic mice overexpressing *H-ras* or *BCR-ABL* genes developed melanoma and erythroleukemia, respectively, and when the expression of these genes was switched off the malignant cells subsequently died by apoptosis and tumors regressed (35,36). Treatment of human cancer cell lines constitutively overexpressing the HER/Neu2 or cyclin D1 oncogene products with antisense oligonucleotides against these targets resulted in inhibition of growth or tumorigenicity in mice, whereas cell lines not constitutively overexpressing HER/Neu2 or cyclin D1 were unaffected (37,38). These kinds of experiments have led to the hypothesis of "oncogene addiction" (38), which proposes that the multiple redundant signaling pathways in normal cells are lost in cancer cells through selection for key oncogenic pathways and genomic instability. Data of this type support the concept of interfering therapeutically with oncogene function. As a result of oncogene addiction, such agents should selectivity affect malignant cells, whereas normal cells should remain relatively unharmed. Furthermore, these data again emphasize the necessity of knowing which pathways are active in individual tumors.

We have preliminary data showing that overexpression of phosphatidyl inositol 3-kinase (PI3K) isoforms sensitizes cancer cells to small-molecule inhibitors targeting the PI3K pathway. In contrast, cells expressing low levels of the PI3K isoforms are relatively insensitive to inhibition of this pathway. Similar results were obtained with the rapamycin analogue CCI-779, an inhibitor of mTOR, which is a downstream target of the PTEN/PI3K/Akt pathway. PTEN is the phosphatase that negatively regulates PI3K signaling. *In vitro* and *in vivo* studies with PTEN+/+ and isogenic PTEN−/− mouse and human cancer cells showed that growth of PTEN−/− cells, which have increased PI3K signaling, was preferentially blocked by treatment with CCI-779, and the enhanced tumor growth of PTEN−/− cells in xenograft models was reversed by the drug (39).

MODERN GENOMIC APPROACHES TO IDENTIFY CANCER GENES

In the past, various methods have been used to identify oncogenes and tumor suppressors. Many were found by positional cloning of genes in regions of chromosomal gain or loss (e.g., *erbB2, PTEN*) or chromosomal translocations (e.g., *BCR* and *ABL*). Many oncogenes, such as *ras* and *myc,* were identified as the human homologs of viral transforming genes. Others were found through linkage analysis of families with inherited predisposition to cancer [e.g., *BRCA2* (40)]. Studies in model organisms such as yeast, fly, mouse, and worm have identified yet others; e.g., the identification of the MMR gene, *hMLH1*, as the human homologue of the bacterial *mutL* gene (41).

It is likely that most of the genes that can be identified with these traditional methods, particularly the analysis of chromosomal amplifications, deletions, and translocations, have now been discovered. At the very least the rate of discovery of new cancer genes by these approaches will decline, since the "low-hanging fruit" have already been harvested (42). Furthermore, point mutations resulting in amino acid substitution are even harder to find.

With the advance of the human genome project (3) (see Table 8.3 for information regarding useful genome and microarray Web sites) and the concomitant development of high-throughput sequencing technology (4), sequencing of genomic libraries constructed from cancer genomes and comparison with the normal human genomic sequence is now feasible and represents the most comprehensive and systematic way of identifying most of the remaining cancer genes (43). There is surprisingly little cancer sequence publicly available, the largest amount coming from the US-based Cancer Genome Anatomy Project (http:www.ncbi.nlm.nih.goc.CGAP).

The UK-based Cancer Genome Project at the Sanger Centre (Hinxton, UK) has started the enormous task of systematic genome-wide mutation screening of human cancers (42,43). Multiple genetic abnormalities frequently occur in important oncogenic pathways, although a given tumor will normally exhibit only a single defect in a particular pathway. A good example of this is the p53/p14ARF pathway with multiple reported abnormalities and mutations occurring in the *p53*, *MDM2*, and *p14ARF* genes. The project has therefore begun sequencing genes in pathways for which at least one gene is already known to be mutated. The Cancer Genome Project has recently identified the *BRAF* gene as an oncogene mutated in 66% of malignant melanomas and a lower frequency of mutations in a variety of other human cancers (44).

TABLE 8.3. *Useful genome and microarray Web sites*

Description	Web site
Sanger Centre	http://www.sanger.ac.uk
Cancer Genome Project	http://www.sanger.ac.uk/CGP/
Human genome annotation	http://genome.ucsc.edu
Human genome annotation	http://www.ensembl.org
UniGene gene clustering	http://www.ncbi.nlm.nih.gov/UniGene
The SNP Consortium	http://snp.cshl.org/
The Institute for Genomic Research	http://www.tigr.org/tdb/
Whitehead Genome Center	http://www.genome.wi.mit.edu
European Bioinformatic Institute	http://www.ebi.ac.uk
Cancer Genetics Branch, National Human Genome Research Institute	http://research.nhgri.nih.gov/microarray/main
Brown laboratory	http://cmgm.stanford.edu/pbrown/
European Bioinformatic Institute—microarray site	http://www.ebi.ac.uk/microarray/
National Cancer Institute, Bioinformatics	http://discover.nci.nih.gov/
Microarray gene-expression database group	http://www.mged.org
Microarray protocols and software	http://www.microarrays.org/
Affymetrix	http://www.affymetrix.com/
Agilent Technologies	http://www.chem.agilent.com/
Illumina	http://www.illumina.com

Identifying a drug target at such an early stage bodes well for discovering additional cancer genes in the course of the project. It should be noted that not all potential targets are equally tractable or "druggable." It is therefore appropriate that some emphasis has been placed on this in the initial selection of potential cancer genes. Kinases, such as B-Raf, represent particularly good candidates for drug development.

A possible next step could be to sequence kinase genes on a genome-wide basis, given that a large number of oncogenes identified to date are kinases and the fact that kinases represent tractable targets for small-molecule inhibitors and, in some cases, antibody-based approaches.

The publication of the human genomic sequence has greatly facilitated the identification of a large number of open reading frames of hitherto unknown genes. As the sequence of genes contains information on their likely function by encoding for functional domains, it is possible to search the human genome sequence for areas of homology to such functional domains, thus identifying genes with a probable biological activity. It should be noted, however, that analysis of the draft human genome sequence failed to identify any novel oncogenes based on close homology with the sequence of known cancer genes (42). This is because cancer genes have relatively little homology with each other, but rather disrupt common "mission critical" pathways (45) using different functional mechanisms.

A less comprehensive way of identifying cancer genes, but one which is rapid and amenable to high-throughput, involves the use of genome-wide expression profiling and comparative genomic hybridization (CGH) on microarrays. CGH with bacterial artificial chromosomes (BAC) DNA on microarrays can be used to identify regions of loss or gain on human chromosomes (46). This approach is faster and more powerful than using classical cytogenetic methods. The identified regions of gains and loss can then be further examined to identify which particular genes are amplified by using CGH on cDNA sequences (47,48). Gene-expression profiling can be used to verify whether amplification of these genes results in overexpression of the amplified genes, giving an indication as to which of the amplified genes is functionally important (47,48). Furthermore, in the absence of genomic amplifications, expression profiling can be used to identify overexpressed oncogenes or the absence of message for tumor suppressors, by comparing expression profiles of cancers to those of normal tissue (49).

As mentioned before, epigenetic gene silencing plays an important role in the malignant process. Epigenetic mechanisms of gene inactivation include DNA methylation and histone modification, including histone methylation and acetylation. Early studies to identify genes with aberrant methylation of CpG islands in human cancer have used a candidate gene approach, selecting the CpG islands to be analyzed. Although this methodology has already identified numerous methylation-silenced genes, to establish the full extent of DNA methylation in human cancer a genome-wide, unbiased approach is required. Two recently established methods are now available to start genome-wide screening of CpG islands.

Costello et al. (50) have developed restriction landmark genomic scanning, a technique based on end-labeling methylation-sensitive restriction sites and resolving the labeled products using two-dimensional gel electrophoresis. Analysis of the methylation status of 1,184 unselected CpG islands in 98 primary human tumors identified patterns of CpG island methylation that were shared within each tumor type, together with patterns and genes that displayed distinct tumor type specificity (50). The second approach, differential methylation hybridization, is based on a combination of methylation-sensitive DNA digestion and DNA microarrays. Using these microarray technologies, thousands of CpG islands can be screened simultaneously. Screening by differential methylation hybridization of paired primary breast tumor and normal samples revealed extensive hypermethylation in the majority of breast tumors relative to their normal controls, whereas other tumors had little or no detectable changes. Hypermethylation was associated with poorly differentiated tumors compared to moderately or well-differentiated tumors (51). Hierarchical clustering of the methylation patterns allowed segregation of the tumors and identified a methylation pattern that corresponded to the hormone-receptor status of the tumor (52). Using the same method to classify ovarian tumors identified two groups of patients with distinct methylation profiles. Progression-free survival after chemotherapy was significantly shorter for patients in the group with extensive methylation. In addition, a select group of CpG island loci was identified that could potentially be used as epigenetic markers for predicting treatment outcome in ovarian cancer patients (53).

Reversing epigenetic inactivation of genes often results in the suppression of tumor growth or sensitization to other anticancer drugs; e.g., by increased expression of MMR genes (15). Gene transcription is regulated by the local chromatin structure, which in turn is regulated by a complex interplay of DNA methylation and histone modification, including methylation and acetylation. Reversing epigenetic silencing has a distinct advantage over reversing mutational inactivation of genes, as the latter usually requires gene therapy delivery of the wild-type gene. Compounds that reverse epigenetic silencing have already been identified, including DNA methyltransferase inhibitors such as decitabine and histone deacetylase inhibitors such as suberoylanilide hydroxamic acid (SAHA) (15). Combinations of such agents appear to show particularly good reactivation of epigenetically silenced genes. Inhibitors of chromatin-modifying genes are also of particular pharmacological significance.

TARGET VALIDATION AND SELECTION

Having identified a cancer gene that could be a potential drug target, some form of target validation is required before the considerable resources required to develop therapeutic agents are allocated (1,2). As mentioned previously, not all cancer genes or gene products are easily amenable to therapeutic intervention. Hence, it is useful to have some criteria for target validation, in particular to help assess the technical risk and the potential value of the agents that will emerge from a drug discovery program. Table 8.4 lists criteria that are frequently used in target validation and selection. It should be noted that the criteria in the list are not prescriptive but rather can be used as general guidelines to help select an appropriate target. Any given target may not fulfill all the criteria, and there is a considerable amount of judgment involved in target selection. The criteria are useful for balancing risk, time, cost, and value across a portfolio of potential targets. This is particularly important at a time when our rapidly growing knowledge of the molecular pathology of cancer, accelerated by genomics, has led to the discovery of many more cancer genes and potential drug targets than can be handled by any one drug development organization.

Evidence that the potential target plays a role in the malignant process can be obtained by screening human tumor cell lines and tumor samples for mutations, deletions, amplifications, or overexpression. When activation or inactivation of a given gene is caused by a point mutation, primers spanning the exons can be designed based on the human genome sequence and the cDNA sequence; using high-throughput sequencing techniques, hundreds of samples can be screened relatively quickly. Determining expression levels or DNA copy number of target genes can also be assessed relatively easily by real-time polymerase chain reaction (PCR) assays.

The frequency of the abnormality (e.g., mutation or deregulated expression) can provide information about whether the target plays an important role in malignant progression, and can also give an indication as to the number of patients likely to benefit from therapy based on the target. The type of cancers likely to respond can also be predicted. Demonstrating that modulation of the target or the pathway in which the cancer gene operates can reverse the malignant phenotype gives a strong indication that the appropriate drugs, once developed, could prove useful therapy in patients that exhibit deregulation of the target. The recent advance of ribonucleic acid interference methodology (RNAi) is proving extremely useful in

TABLE 8.4. *Useful criteria for target validation and selection*

Guidelines	Methods
Evidence that the target gene or cognate pathway contributes to malignant phenotype	Molecular analysis of clinical samples, tumor cell lines, or engineered model systems
Frequency of abnormality or deregulation of a pathway in human cancer	High-throughput sequencing of target gene or expression level by real-time PCR
Evidence of reversal of the malignant phenotype when the target is inhibited	Gene knockouts
	Transfection of dominant negative protein or gene construct, antisense oligonucleotides, ribozymes, or inhibitors (RNAi)
Practical feasibility or tractability of modulating the target	Inhibiting enzyme function is pharmacologically more attractive and tractable than either protein–protein or protein–DNA interactions
Availability of a robust, efficient, and informative biological test cascade	Assays to measure target inhibition or inhibition of downstream effectors
Availability of structure-based drug design approach	Molecular structure of the target
Potential for the use of molecular diagnostics/prognostic markers and pharmacodynamic endpoints	Assays to measure target inhibition *in vitro* and *in vivo,* identification of genes conferring sensitivity/resistance to target inhibition

PCR, polymerase chain reaction, RNAi, ribonucleic acid interference methodology.

this respect. RNAi is based on a conserved biological response to double-stranded RNA (dsRNA). Cells respond to the introduction of dsRNA by silencing homologous genes (54). This response can be triggered in many different ways, ranging from experimental introduction of synthetic dsRNA to the transcription of endogenous RNAs that regulate gene expression (54). Although we are only just beginning to appreciate the mechanistic complexity of this response, RNAi has already been developed as a means to manipulate gene expression experimentally and to probe gene function on a whole-genome scale, as in *C. elegans* (55). Because of the discriminating selectivity of RNAi, it is conceivable to knockout a mutated oncogene without affecting the expression of wild-type alleles, and it may also be possible to apply this approach in virus-delivered therapy in the future. A recent example can be used to illustrate the utility of RNAi technology for target validation. Transfection of dsRNA specific for the *BCR-ABL* fusion messenger RNA (mRNA) into K562 leukemia cells depleted both the corresponding mRNA and the cognate *BCR/ABL* oncoprotein, and was accompanied by a strong induction of apoptosis. In contrast, cells not carrying the *BCR-ABL* translocation were unaffected. Furthermore, the same dsRNA with two point mutations in the central region abolished both the ability to deplete *BCR-ABL* and the induction of apoptosis (56). This demonstrates the selectivity of the RNAi mechanism.

THE DRUG DEVELOPMENT PROCESS

For target-based drug discovery, a biological test cascade is essential (57), in particular the use of biological endpoints of target inhibition. The test cascade is a continuous, hierarchically arranged series of biological assays. The assays must be reproducible, efficient, informative, and relevant to the disease target. The screen usually starts with the recombinant protein, often produced in baculovirus, and proceeds through cell-based assays and xenograft models. Mechanism-based drug discovery projects (1,57,58) usually work towards the desired profile of a clinical candidate, which encompasses the necessary potency, selectivity, and therapeutic index together with the likely route of delivery and administration schedule. Progress of the compounds in the test cascade is measured against this profile. Results from the biological assays are then used to modify and optimize the compounds in an iterative process based on readouts of biological activity.

Molecular Mechanism of Action

Molecular mechanism of action assays are essential to confirm that compounds being evaluated in the test cascade are exerting their anticancer effect through the desired target, or in the case of cell-based screens, to aid the identification of the cellular target. Such assays can also provide valuable pharmacodynamic endpoints for use in animal studies and subsequent clinical trials.

Compounds from cell-based screens can be submitted to be profiled across the National Cancer Institute (NCI) panel of 60 human cancer cell lines (http://dtp. nci.nih.gov). Activity in the panel can be correlated with data on the expression of particular molecular targets, in order to generate hypotheses on the potential mechanism of action (59). A more comprehensive way of identifying targets from cell-based screens is to use genome-wide expression profiling. Gene-expression profiling and proteomics are increasingly powerful methods for determining mechanism of action and identifying biomarkers of response (60). Correlation of the sensitivity of compounds in the NCI panel with constitutive gene-expression profiles has already proved useful (61). We have taken the approach of compiling a database of gene-expression profiles of signal-transduction inhibitors and classical anticancer agents. New compounds from our drug discovery projects are profiled for pharmacological, compound-induced expression changes. These profiles can consequently be compared to the profiles in the database using cluster analysis (see later section on data mining). This can indicate the likely mechanism of action of the new compound or can be used to determine whether the compound hits additional cellular targets. It can also identify biomarkers of cellular response.

When no inhibitors of a pathway are available for a given genomic target, molecular biological techniques can be used to modulate the target in tandem with gene-expression profiling. For example, the target can be ectopically expressed and subsequent expression changes can be assessed by microarray analysis. Inhibition of the target can reasonably be expected to reverse the changes seen with overexpression of the target or other components of the pathway. Approaches that can be used to mimic the pharmacological inhibition of the target include the construction of knockouts, transfection of dominant negative constructs, the use of antisense constructs, antisense oligonucleotides and ribozymes, or the microinjection of dominant negative proteins or neutralizing antibodies. The recent advance of RNAi technology may be particularly useful in this respect. Unique RNAi oligos can quickly be designed and screened and should provide a profile of selective inhibition of the target that can readily be compared to the profile of compounds in the test cascade.

Studies in which gene-expression microarrays have been used to profile the effects of drugs are beginning to emerge into the literature (5). In one of the first of such studies, our laboratory used this global approach to investigate the genes that showed increased or decreased expression in response to the Hsp90 inhibitor 17AAG (60). In a complimentary collaborative study, we also performed a proteomic analysis, using two-dimensional electrophoresis and matrix-assisted laser desorption ionization mass spectrometry, to identify changes in expression at the protein level (62). Changes observed were validated or confirmed using Western blotting. In the gene-expression microarray analysis, genes encoding Hsp90β, Hsp70, keratin 8, keratin 18, and caveolin-1 showed altered expression at the mRNA level in human colon cancer cell lines. All of these changes were validated at the protein level. Increased expression of Hsp90β is important because this is a target of the drug. Enhanced expression of Hsp70 is also of note because this may have an antiapoptotic effect. Changes in caveolin-1 and the keratin genes may reflect the known inhibitory effects of 17AAG on the Ras/Raf/ERK1/2 and PTEN/PI3K/AKT signal transduction pathways. With the exception of casein kinase, genes encoding "client proteins" for Hsp90 were not affected at the mRNA level but rather the proteins were depleted via the ubiquitin proteasome pathway. In addition to a number of consistent changes, some differences in gene-expression profiles were observed when different cell lines were compared.

In the complimentary proteomic analysis, we identified the novel gene product Aha1, a previously unknown cochaperone that activates the adenosine triphosphatase activity of Hsp90, as being subject to upregulation in tumor cells after 17AAG treatment (62). Reanalysis of the microarray data showed that *AHA1* gene expression is also upregulated at the mRNA level. Upregulation of an activating cochaperone, particularly alongside the Hsp90 molecular target itself, could clearly be of pharmacological significance.

Using the combination of gene-expression microarrays, proteomics, Western blotting, and enzyme-linked immunosorbent assay methodology, we defined a molecular signature or fingerprint that is diagnostic of Hsp90 inhibition in human cancer cell lines, tumor xenografts, and peripheral blood lymphocytes (63). This consists of a decrease in client proteins such as Raf-1, CDK4, and ErbB2, together with an increase in Hsp70. The molecular signature is specific for Hsp90 inhibition because it is shared with other active Hsp90 inhibitors of the same or different structural class, but is not seen with inactive analogues or cytotoxic agents such as paclitaxel. We are now using this gene-expression signature in clinical trials to demonstrate inhibition of Hsp90 in peripheral blood lymphocytes and tumor biopsy specimens from patients treated with 17AAG (63). In addition, we are using the molecular fingerprint to examine structure/activity relationships across established and novel Hsp90 inhibitors in order to identify on-target and off-target effects.

These studies with Hsp90 inhibitors illustrate the power of global genomic approaches of gene-expression and proteomic profiling. They show the utility of the approach in studying mechanism of action, discovering genes involved in sensitivity and resistance, and identifying pharmacodynamic markers of drug action for use in preclinical drug development and early clinical trials.

Example of the Use of Gene-expression Profiling to Predict Drug Sensitivity

Once a target is identified and small-molecule inhibitors have been developed, the next step in the drug development process is to define those cancers for which the drug is most likely to be active. Sensitivity and resistance to anticancer drugs is determined by the biology of the cell, which in turn is largely controlled by the expression of genes in that cell. Microarrays provide a very powerful tool to look at genome-wide gene expression in this context. We have used the global gene-expression profiling approach to establish a dataset of constitutive cell line expression patterns. The 40-cell-line panel comprises all four major human cancers—breast, lung, colon, and prostate—together with brain, melanoma, and ovarian cancer. Cells are harvested in midlog phase and mRNA is isolated from individual cell lines (see also http:www.icr.ac.uk/array/array). A reference sample is made by mixing equal amounts of mRNA from the individual cell lines. The reference sample and the individual cell line samples are labeled with Cy3-and Cy-5 dCTP respectively, and cohybridized on DNA microarrays (Fig. 8.1), thereby allowing assessment of the relative expression for each gene on the array for each cell line. The microarrays contain 30,000 sequence verified IMAGE clones from the Unigene II set, encompassing all known genes, and genes classified by the HUGO Gene Nomenclature Committee (HGNC). These are supplemented with novel expressed sequence tags (ESTs) to provide an even coverage of the genome.

Sensitivity data for drugs under development at the Cancer Research UK Centre for Cancer Therapeutics are obtained by assessing IC_{50} (50% inhibition/inhibitory concentration) data at 96 hours in the cell line panel by the MTT assay. The sensitivity data are used to separate the cell lines into sensitive and resistant groups for each particular drug. The gene-expression dataset is also divided into the two relevant sets. Software can then be used to find the genes that most contribute to the identity of each class, sensitive or resistant, thus identifying genes that will correlate with sensitivity or resistance to a particular drug. The same methodology using oligonucleotide arrays containing only 6,800 genes has successfully been used to predict sensitivity to 88 of 232 compounds investigated (64).

Of particular use in this instance is marker selection/neighborhood analysis (http://www-genome.wi.mit.edu/, see also data-mining section). Combining these predictor sets with drug-induced pharmacological expression profiles will identify genes that are both predictive of sensitivity or resistance and that can be used as pharmacodynamic markers of drug action. This strategy may be used to profile pretreatment biopsy material and predict whether a given patient is likely to respond to the drug. Obtaining biopsy material remains difficult because of the invasiveness of the procedure, and it may not be possible to obtain enough material to carry out microarray analysis. The power of the class prediction software is that it will identify genes that will contribute most to the difference between the two classes, and using that small set of genes can be just as accurate in predicting class as a much larger group. Using such a small marker set to define sensitive cancers makes it possible to apply reverse-transcription PCR or TAQman assays to predict whether a particular tumor is likely to be sensitive to a particular drug. Much smaller quantities of tissues are required with these methods because of the sensitivity of the assays.

Molecular Toxicology

The increasing emphasis in drug development is on finding small-molecule inhibitors to block essential oncogenic pathways in human cancers. Treatment with such agents can result in cell death and regression of tumors. However, they are more likely to produce cytostatic effects, resulting in containment rather than cure of the tumor. Therefore, the new generation of molecular therapeutics will most likely be used to treat cancer as a chronic disease. Patients will have to be treated for prolonged periods of time, thus requiring drugs that are generally nontoxic. Detailed toxicology assessment of potential drugs is a costly exercise and is therefore usually reserved for lead compounds at an advanced stage of the development process. When a compound fails at this stage, considerable resources will have already been spent.

Gene-expression microarrays have great potential not only for determining whether a drug or lead compound exerts the desired mechanism of action, but also for identifying "off target" effects, including

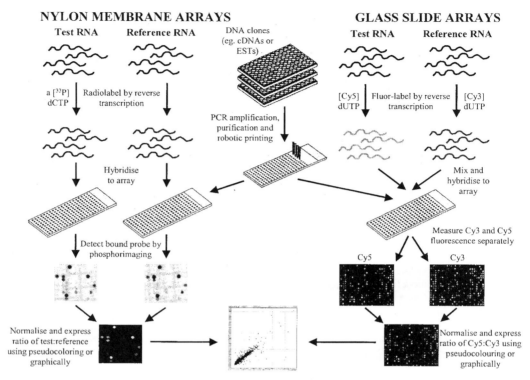

FIG. 8.1. Schematic of the various steps in a microarray experiment. Plasmid clones are propagated in bacteria, and the cloned inserts are amplified by polymerase chain reaction (PCR) and then purified. The purified PCR products are then robotically printed onto glass or nylon solid supports. Modifications of this approach include the use of oligonucleotides instead of PCR products or the *in situ* synthesis of oligonucleotides directly onto the glass support using photolithographic or other techniques. Separate nylon-based arrays are hybridized with 33P-radiolabeled cDNA prepared from the test and reference sample, whereas glass slide arrays are hybridized simultaneously with Cy5 and Cy3 fluorescently labeled test and reference samples, respectively. Following stringency washes, hybridization to nylon arrays is detected by phosphorimaging. Hybridization to glass slides is detected by excitation of the two fluors at the relevant wavelength and the fluorescent emission collected with a charge-coupled device. The test and reference images are overlaid using specialist software and can be displayed in a number of ways, including as a scatter plot of the ratio of test:reference gene expression. Modified with permission from Clarke PA, tePoele R, Wooster, R, et al. Gene-expression microarray analysis in cancer biology, pharmacology, and drug development: progress and potential. *Biochem Pharmacol* 2001;62:1311–1336.

molecular signatures that may be predictive of various types of toxicity. Although the use of microarrays will not be foolproof in determining whether a compound will have particular toxic features in the clinic, it will give clear indications as to the presence of undesirable gene-expression changes that are indicative of adverse effects. Because microarrays are relatively inexpensive compared to the extensive use of animals, they can be used to profile compounds emerging from the chemical optimization process, and undesirable gene-expression signatures can be flagged at an early stage and dealt with appropriately. Many pharmaceutical companies are now using expression profiling to weed out compounds that may cause unacceptable side effects, such as hepatotoxicity.

There is an increasing body of evidence that abnormalities in, and deregulation of, the PI3K pathway plays an active role in malignancy (65). The *PTEN* tumor-suppressor gene encodes a lipid phosphatase that hydrolyses the inositol lipid product (PIP3) of the PI3K reaction, thereby counteracting its oncogenic effects. In terms of the frequency of tumor-suppressor gene abnormalities, loss of *PTEN* function ranks second only to mutations and deletions in the *p53* gene (66). Activation of the PI3K pathway by loss of PTEN or other abnormalities contributes to the oncogenic phenotype and malignant progression by stimulating proliferation, survival, migration, invasion, angiogenesis, and metastasis, and may play a role in drug resistance. This makes inhibition of the PI3K pathway an attractive target for drug development. However, the PI3K pathway is also involved in insulin signaling. Thus, molecules targeting this particular pathway may disturb the balance of insulin metabolism, which may ultimately lead to diabetes. We have shown that LY294002, a broad-specificity PI3K inhibitor, does indeed affect components of the insulin-signaling pathway (67). However, the PI3K family consists of a large number of isoforms, and although no conclusive evidence has been published to date, indications are that certain components of this pathway are involved in insulin signaling whereas others are responsible for tumor progression (68). Targeting separate isoforms with inhibitors and profiling them using gene-expression microarrays may identify compounds that do not hit insulin signaling but retain the anticancer effects of LY294002, including apoptosis and growth inhibition. We are now using this approach to profile and identify compounds that may have differential effects on the specific PI3K isoforms. Another way to avoid hitting insulin metabolism is to look for "druggable" targets downstream of PI3K where the pathway has diverged into components responsible for survival, migration, proliferation, and insulin signaling. For example, we have followed the time course of gene-expression changes in response to LY294002 treatment to look for genes that are affected downstream of PI3K inhibition. Using this approach we have identified a number of mitotic genes that appear to be coregulated by the PI3K pathway, two of which have previously been implicated in cancer.

Metabolism and Pharmacokinetics

Pharmacokinetic behavior is commonly the rate-limiting step in the transition from compounds with activity in cell-based assays to those having activity in animal models. Prediction of pharmacokinetic behavior in the whole animal is difficult. Pharmacokinetic prioritization screens and the use of cassette dosing can increase the speed and efficiency of the transition from in vitro to whole-animal models (69). Pharmacokinetic behavior is very often controlled by metabolism of the compound, and knowledge of metabolic routes and rates of metabolism can be helpful in selecting compounds. A particular property to avoid in a clinical candidate is metabolism by polymorphic enzymes (see also the section on single nucleotide polymorphisms), such as cytochrome P450 3A4. This can lead to extensive variability in metabolism and pharmacokinetics. Inhibition of cytochrome P450s should also be avoided, since this may lead to unwanted drug–drug interactions. Measurement of metabolism by, and inhibition of,

recombinant P450 enzymes can be very useful at this stage. Assessment of the induction or repression of drug-metabolism genes can also provide valuable information.

CLINICAL TRIALS AND PATIENT SELECTION

The clinical trial is a critical stage of the drug development process. Studies of molecular mechanism of action alongside the more established toxicity and pharmacokinetic evaluation need to be a strong component in the early clinical testing of agents acting on new molecular targets. Cytotoxic drugs generally have a relatively nonspecific mechanism of action, and therefore may have a fairly broad spectrum of activity in human cancers. In contrast, with drugs targeting a particular oncogenic target or pathway, considerable emphasis has to be placed on patient selection. Even in the case of targeting pathways that are activated in a large percentage of patients and across a variety of different cancers, there will be a considerable number of patients with tumors in which these pathways are not activated and do not contribute to tumor progression. Treating such patients with the molecularly targeted drug would not have any therapeutic benefit; on the contrary, it may cause toxicity and additionally prevent treatment with other drugs that are more likely to be active against the tumor.

Gene-expression profiling is already beginning to rival classical pathology and immunohistochemistry in predicting clinical outcome in human cancers (70,71). The next step will be to use this technique to profile tumors before treatment to determine which oncogenic pathways are active within individual cancers. For example, platelet-derived growth factor receptor α and the ras/mitogen-activated protein kinase pathway were implicated in the progression from nonmetastatic to metastatic medulloblastoma using a class prediction algorithm to analyze DNA microarray data from 23 primary metastatic and non-metastatic medulloblastomas (49).

As emphasized throughout this chapter, oncogenic pathways are activated by a variety of means. All of these events result in changes in the mRNA pool within the cell, which can be mapped by using global gene-expression profiling. On the basis of such genome-wide analysis, a much more informed decision can be made as to which treatment would most likely be effective. When a new drug has a response rate of less then 20% in a phase 2 clinical trial, this would not normally be considered encouraging. However, if we can predict the 20% of patients who are likely to respond, this could be a very useful drug in that particular subset of patients. Exclusion of patients who are unlikely to respond but who might benefit from alternative treatment generates considerable pharmacoeconomic benefit.

As an example, the ability to more accurately predict prognosis in breast cancer patients would improve the selection of patients who might benefit from adjuvant therapy. Currently 70% to 80% of the patients receiving adjuvant therapy would have survived without it. Using a 70-gene classifier based on microarray expression data of 98 primary breast cancers, it was possible to correctly predict actual outcome in 83% of the cases. In a validation set of 19 tumors, only 2 were classified incorrectly, outperforming currently available clinical and histopathological prognostic factors. The power of the 70-gene prognosis profile was confirmed in a large follow-up study (70), where the mean overall survival in patients with a poor prognosis profile was 54.6%, whereas those with a good prognosis signature had a mean overall survival of 94.5%.

Zhan et al. (72) profiled bone marrow plasma cells (PC) from newly diagnosed patients with multiple myeloma (MM), monoclonal gammopathy, and healthy volunteers, together with MM cell lines. Using hierarchical clustering (see later for details of data mining methods), the normal and MM PC formed distinct clusters. Within the MM cluster four subgroups could be identified (MM1-MM4). The profile of MM1 PC most resembled that of normal and monoclonal gammopathy PC, whereas that of MM4 was similar to the profile of the MM cell lines. Poor prognosis was linked to class MM4 PCs. The study also identified 120 disease genes that discriminated between normal and malignant PCs. The MM4 PC exhibited a profile indicating a more proliferative and autonomous phenotype.

Two recent studies have used gene-expression profiling to successfully predict outcome in large B-cell lymphoma after chemotherapy (73,74). Both studies found molecularly distinct subgroups as described elsewhere (75) according to putative cell of origin, namely germinal-center B-cell–like or activated B-cell–like. Additionally, Rosenwald et al. (73) found a third subtype that did not express the genes associated with the other subtypes. Shipp et al. (74) used a weighted voting algorithm and cross-validating testing (http://www.genome.wi.mit.edu/MPR), to identify genes that distinguished between patients with cured versus fatal or refractory disease. Predictors containing 8 to 16 genes all resulted in statistically significant outcome predictions, and separated the patients into two groups with a median survival at 5 years of 70%

and 12%, respectively. The predictive gene-expression pattern was independent of the International Prognostic Index. The predictor genes encompassed those involved in B-cell receptor signaling, critical kinase cascades, and apoptosis. Rosenwald et al. (73) used a Cox proportional hazards model to identify genes correlated with outcome, and clustered these to group them into gene-expression signatures. The signatures fell into four biological groups, of which the most variable genes were chosen for the outcome predictor. The proliferation signature was the best predictor of an adverse outcome, whereas the signatures associated with a good outcome suggested that antigen presentation and the immune response might be critical determinants of outcome after chemotherapy.

Expression profiling in colorectal cancer (CRC) (76) revealed genes associated with Dukes classification, as well as genes linked to disease progression. Most of the expression changes occurred during the progression from normal to early-stage CRC, whereas far fewer genes were altered during the progression through the different Dukes stages. This suggested that the bulk of the changes occur at initiation and relatively few gene changes are required for malignant progression. Interestingly, the up- or down-regulated genes in CRC clustered to several distinct chromosomal locations, suggesting the possibility of some form of coregulation through common transcription factors, promoter methylation, or opening of the DNA duplex. These types of data suggest that a combination of expression profiling and CGH analysis on microarrays may prove even more powerful in classifying human cancers. CGH alone has already successfully been used to develop a molecular classifier to differentiate *BRCA1* mutation carriers from nonmutation carriers. Using this classifier, 84% of cases were correctly predicted in both the training set and the validation set of tumors (77).

SINGLE-NUCLEOTIDE POLYMORPHISMS

The term *pharmacogenetics* is used to describe studies of the variability of drug response due to inherited phenotypes in individuals. Unpredictable toxicity in clinical trials and after regulatory approval is the principal cause of attrition of candidate agents. For many years, pharmacogenetic studies have relied on the measurement of the status of drug-metabolizing enzymes to understand and predict the efficacy and toxicity of drugs in individuals. Inherited differences in DNA sequence contribute to phenotypic variation, influencing a given individual's risk of disease and also his or her reaction to the environment [e.g., adverse or therapeutic response to drug treatment (78)]. Most sequence variation in humans can be attributed to single-nucleotide polymorphisms (SNPs), specific locations in the human genome sequence where different individuals have different DNA bases. These can lead to a change in the protein sequence, and could consequently contribute to disease or adverse effects of drugs. With the publication of SNP maps and the rapid advance of high-throughput genotyping, statistical analysis, and bioinformatics, it is now possible to characterize disease genes and the response of individual patients to drugs, and to determine whether toxicity or efficacy is associated with a particular phenotype (78).

In February of 2001, a map of human genome sequence variation containing 1.42 million single SNPs was published (79). The publication was the culmination of the efforts of the SNP consortium (http://snp.cshl.org/) and the analysis of clone overlaps by the International Human Genome Sequencing Consortium (3). Genome-wide linkage analysis and positional cloning have been used to identify hundreds of human disease genes (http://www.ncbi.nlm.nih.gov/entrez/query.fcgi?db=OMIM). However, most of these are rare diseases in which the mutation of a single gene is sufficient to cause the condition. For common diseases, genome-wide linkage analysis has had little success, consistent with a more complex genetic pattern. With several individual loci contributing modestly to disease genetics or drug reactions, more powerful high-resolution techniques are required to identify susceptibility genes. Sequentially ordered, high-density SNP maps could provide such a technique to identify inherited profiles that are statistically associated with disease or drug response. SNPs are distributed throughout the human genome with an average density of 1 SNP every 1.9 kilobases (79). Global SNP analysis would therefore require genotyping millions of SNPs. However, SNP variants that are closely linked do not occur independently from each other, a phenomenon known as linkage disequilibrium (LD) between neighboring SNPs. Adjacent alleles are associated in a nonrandom manner reflecting "haplotypes" descended from single ancestral chromosomes (80). These haplotypes or LD blocks typically span 40 kb but can extend over a 800-kb range (81). The publication of a LD map of chromosome 22 (81) has shown that developing genome-wide LD maps is feasible. The next step is to use the great abundance of SNPs and their clustering in LD blocks in association type studies to identify disease genes and genes associated with drug efficacy or toxicity. The fact that the allelic variants that contribute to complex disease are often fixed in haplotype blocks, creating disease haplotypes, means that all of the SNPs in a block will show association with disease. It may therefore be possible to type one SNP per block to identify the location of a disease or drug-response gene, greatly reducing the amount of SNPs required to genotype individuals. If the haplotype blocks in a region are small (around 40 kb), as they commonly are, disease association implies a nearby susceptibility gene. Association based studies require markers that can capture LD between blocks and susceptibility genes, and therefore the intervals between SNPs must be between 40 to 100 kb (82). Linkage analysis relies on mapping recombinants in families and the frequency of recombination in humans results in a set of 350 markers throughout the genome at approximately 10-Mb intervals. Mapping SNPs in LD blocks requires genotyping between 30,000 to 100,000 SNPs per individual, and emphasizes the need for high-throughput genotyping assays. Several methods are under development, including those based on microarrays (78). Microarrays that are able to genotype a few thousand SNPs are commercially available (Affymetrix, Illumina; Table 8.3). However, for microarray-based genotyping to become the method of choice for the genetic analysis of complex disease and drug response, future SNP arrays will have to be genome-wide and use SNPs that capture variation in haplotype blocks. Nevertheless, the first experiments proving the power of association studies using high-density SNP maps have recently been published. For example, this approach was used to confirm that the apolipoprotein E allele is the susceptibility gene variant that is responsible for common, late-onset Alzheimer's disease (83), and also to identify the tumor necrosis factor α and HLA-B polymorphisms as susceptibility genes for hypersensitivity to abacavir, a reverse-transcriptase inhibitor used to treat human immunodeficiency virus (84). Applications of SNP technology to the development and use of anticancer agents can now be anticipated.

DATA MINING FOR
MICROARRAY ANALYSIS

A major advance of gene-expression profiling and related technologies is the genome-wide scale. However, this also creates a major challenge, that of bioinformatics and data mining. The easiest way to look at microarray data is simply to list the fold changes, rank them in order of magnitude, and then to inspect the list visually. This approach can sometimes be useful in identifying the most obvious changes. However, discerning more complex trends manually in such a manner quickly becomes impossible. Consider a relatively small experiment of 15 samples analyzed on a 30,000-gene array. This produces a data matrix containing 450,000 entries. The aim of data mining is to reduce the dimensionality of this matrix to allow visual inspection. Visualization is traditionally performed in two dimensions, and accordingly many of the methods allow reduction of a matrix of any size into just two dimensions. These methods include principal component analysis and clustering. We will briefly explain some of the methods and highlight the uses of the individual methods. For a more comprehensive introduction to the analy-

sis of microarray data, see reference 85 and the Web sites listed in Table 8.5 (85).

Normalization, Filtering, and Statistics

Samples to be analyzed have to be scaled or normalized, in order to ensure that the expression levels in the samples are directly comparable to those in the control. The first possibility is to include so-called housekeeping genes that are assumed to be constitutively expressed and relatively unchanged from experiment to experiment. These are then compared in the test and control sample, and the values in the test sample are then multiplied by a factor such that

TABLE 8.5. *Analysis software*

Software	Use	Web site
Cluster[a]	Clustering	http://rana.lbl.gov
GeneCluster[a]	Clustering, market selection/ neighborhood analysis	http://www-genome.wi.mit.edu
Expression Profiler[a]	Clustering, pattern discovery, ontology browsing	http://ep.ebi.ac.uk
ClustArray[a]	Clustering	http://www.cbs.dtu.dk/services/DNAarray
R package[a]	Clustering, correspondence analysis, PCA, classification, neural networks, statistical analysis	http://www.r-project.org
SAM[a]	Significance testing	http://www-stat.stanford.edu/~tibs/SAM/index.html
Promoter2.0[a]	PolII promoter search	http://www.cbs.dtu.dk/services/Promoter
Genesis	Clustering, PCA, classification	http://genome.tugraz.at/Software/GenesisCenter.html
Affymetrix Data Mining Tool	Statistical analysis, clustering	http://affymetrix.com
Affymetrix NetAffx	Database link	http://www.netaffx.com
Biomax Gene Expression Analysis Suite	Clustering, link with protein– protein database	http://www.biomax.de
GeneData Expressionist	Statistical analysis, clustering, promoter search	http://www.genedata.com
Informax Xpression NTI	Clustering	http://www.informaxinc.com
Lion Bioscience arraySCOUT	Statistical analysis, clustering, annotated database	http://www.lion-bioscience.com
Rosetta Resolver Gene Expression Data Analysis System	Statistical analysis, clustering, powerful database	http://www.rosettabio.com
Silicon Genetics GeneSpring	Statistical analysis, clustering, PCA	http://www.sigenetics.com
Spotfire	Clustering	http://www.spotfire.com
Axon Acuity	Clustering, PCA	http://www.axon.com/GN_Acuity.html

[a] Freely available.
PCA, principal component analysis.

the expression levels of the housekeeping genes are the same. Another method is to assume that the total amount of mRNA for each cell is constant; or that the overall ratio of expression between test and control averaged over the ratios for every gene on the array is one. The greater the number of genes on the array the more likely it is that this assumption will hold true.

Before proceeding with any kind of analysis, it is useful to filter the data set. Genes that do not change in any of the samples will not contribute to the variation and discrimination between samples. When possible, replicates of the experiment should be included, which allows the elimination of false positives through significance testing of the genes that are up- or down-regulated. If both the test and control sample are repeated, the *t* test can be used to determine whether a particular gene is significantly changed between sample and control. However, in most cases more then two conditions are tested and analysis of variance (ANOVA) should be used (see reference 86 and http://128.200.5.223/CyberT). Although most expression data are normally distributed and both the *t* test and ANOVA can cope with small deviations from normal distribution, in some cases the data will not be normally distributed and nonparametric testing should be used.

Principal Component Analysis

Principal component analysis (PCA) is useful for capturing as much variety in the expression data as possible in two dimensions. The principal components are constructed as the sums of the individual sample axes. The cloud that these genes will form is not spherical and will be extended in one direction according to expression in the samples, which is the first principal component. This component will not generally be one of the sample axes, but rather several samples that have projections on this axis. The second principal component captures the variation left in the data and is plotted perpendicular to the first axis. For example, PCA analysis was used to successfully classify central nervous system embryonal tumor subtypes (87).

Hierarchical Clustering

If the data are more complex, cluster analysis can be used. Hierarchical clustering treats each gene as a vector of N numbers, N being the number of samples. The algorithm then calculates the distance between two genes according to their respective expression in the different samples. This is done for all the genes and a distance matrix is formed. Genes that are closest together have similar expression in the samples and are grouped together. This can be combined with

grouping of the samples. The distance between the samples is calculated according to the expression of the individual genes. The samples are then grouped together according to the distance that separates them. This method can be used to identify genes whose expression is positively or negatively correlated to a group of samples.

K-means and Self-Organizing Maps

In K-means, clustering the distances between all the genes are not calculated. Rather, the experimenter decides how many clusters are required. The K-means algorithm then randomly assigns each gene to one of the K clusters. Next, the distance between each gene in a cluster and the center of that cluster (centroid) is calculated. When a gene is actually closer in distance to the centroid of a different cluster, it is then reassigned to that cluster. Following reassignment of all the genes to their closest cluster, the centroids are recalculated, and the distances of the genes can be reassessed. This process is repeated in an iterative fashion until the centroids remain unchanged.

Self-organizing maps (SOMs) are similar to K-means clustering. However, instead of the centroids changing to accommodate the gene-expression data as in K-means, they are confined to a two-dimensional grid specified by the user (e.g., 2×3, 3×3). The algorithm then organizes itself to best fit the data to this grid (88). K-means clustering and SOMs are fast algorithms and are useful for initial identification of expression patterns, but may not be powerful enough to distinguish subtle differences in expression between samples.

Classification

In order to classify, for example, cancer subtypes, nearest neighbor, neural networks, or support, vector machine analysis can be used. The simplest form is the nearest neighbor analysis method, which importantly can be used on a relatively small dataset (http://www.stat.berkeley.edu/tech-reports/index.html). For each sample the k most similar samples are calculated. Consequently, the sample is classified according to the class that the majority of the k nearest neighbors belong to. For example if k = 3 was chosen, for each sample the three closest samples would be calculated; if two of them belonged to class A and one to class B, the sample would be classified as class A (majority voting).

If the number of samples is high, the more advanced classification methods of neural networks and support vector machines can be used. Kahn et al. (89) used artificial neural networks (ANNs) to classify small round blue-cell tumors. The ANNs correctly classified all samples, including blind samples that were not included in the training set, and identified the genes most relevant to the classification. The support vector machine is particularly suitable to microarray data as it is designed to work with vectors and can therefore encompass the dimensionality of microarray data.

HISTORICAL CONTEXT AND HORIZON SCANNING

2003 is a landmark year for molecular biology and genomics, with the effective completion of the human genome sequence coinciding with the fiftieth anniversary of the publication of the double-helical structure of DNA (90,91). This iconic structure not only provided a beautiful physical explanation for the self-replication of the genome and the mechanism of heredity, but also paved the way for the development of recombinant DNA technology and indeed the biotechnology industry (92). The impact of the double helix and of recombinant DNA is impossible to overestimate. The ability to manipulate and analyze DNA in the way that we now do has revolutionized basic biological research and drug development; for example, by the cloning and expression of recombinant protein targets and the production of recombinant protein therapeutics.

Genomics is the next big thing to impact biomedical sciences, including drug development. Genomics is characterized by the ability to study normal biology and disease pathology on a genome-wide scale. Sequencing and PCR technologies transformed biology. The first methods to sequence DNA, developed in the early 1970s by Sanger (93) and Gilbert (94), allowed stretches of a few hundred DNA bases to be decoded and allowed the sequencing of the first viral genome of around 5,000 bases to be completed in about 12 months (95). The first partially automated DNA sequencers gave sequencing rates of about 250 bases per day and led, through the Human Genome Project, to the latest machines with sequencing rates of about 1.5 million bases per day (96).

Ongoing developments in automation, miniaturization, parallelization, and integration, together with microfluidics, microelectronics, and nanotechnology, will lead to a further jump in technology. For example, it has been predicted that with single DNA molecule sequencing, the complete genome of an individual could be decoded in 24 hours for less than US $10,000, as compared to an estimated cost of US $50 million today.

Genome sequencing can now be seen as only one, albeit important, component of the ability to take a new global approach to biology and medicine—analyzing and characterizing organisms and individuals in terms of genome sequence and the complete spectrum of expressed genes and proteins. This is leading, inexorably, to taking a systems approach to normal biology and pathology, including regulatory networks such as metabolite pathways (96).

The impact of genomics on the understanding of cancer and on new approaches to its treatment is already enormous, as this chapter has demonstrated. The ability to assess globally the multiple abnormalities present in the DNA, RNA, and proteins of cancer cells is a major advance. It has been speculated that the next step towards achieving a fully complete understanding will involve the development of a discipline of "mathematical oncology" that will provide descriptive and predictive models of the development and treatment of cancer (97).

The pace at which genomics will truly revolutionize medical treatment remains subject to lively debate (98,99). There seems, however, little doubt that clinical practice will be transformed across all therapeutic areas, including cancer, over the next few years and decades. Some advances will be quicker than others. There will be a new molecular and genomic taxonomy of human disease and a revolution in clinical practice based on the use of mechanism-based therapeutics, early diagnosis, and individualized treatment and prevention programs.

Oncology will be at the forefront of these developments. Genomic technologies already allow us to understand the molecular basis of many cancers, to diagnose and classify them more effectively, and to develop innovative treatments that target the precise molecular defects responsible for malignant progression. Success with Gleevec, Herceptin, and Iressa establish the precedent for genome-based therapeutics and individualized therapy.

CONCLUDING REMARKS

The process of new cancer drug development—from the identification of new targets through to the conduct of mechanism-driven preclinical and clinical development to the practice of individualized medicine—is being transformed by genomics. The development and use of new molecular reagents, including diagnostic and prognostic markers and also pharmacodynamic endpoints, is critically important. The application of genomics will open up an exciting new era of opportunities and challenges over the next 5 years, with prospects for major patient benefit.

The authors thank their colleagues for stimulating discussions. Cancer Research UK supported their research, and Paul Workman is a Cancer Research UK Life Fellow.

REFERENCES

1. Workman P, Kaye SB. Translating basic cancer research into new cancer therapeutics. *Trends Mol Med* 2002; 8:S1–S9.
2. Workman P. Scoring a bull's-eye against cancer genome targets. *Curr Opin Pharmacol* 2001;1: 342– 352.
3. The International Human Genome Sequencing Consortium. Initial sequencing and analysis of the human genome. *Nature* 2001;409:860–921.
4. Mullikin JC, McMurragy AA. Techview: DNA sequencing. Sequencing the genome, fast. *Science* 1999; 283:1867–1869.
5. Clarke PA, te Poele R, Wooster R, et al. Gene expression microarray analysis in cancer biology, pharmacology, and drug development: progress and potential. *Biochem Pharmacol* 2001;62:1311–1336.
6. Ponder BA. Cancer genetics. *Nature* 2001;411: 336–341.
7. Kinzler KW, Vogelstein B. Lessons from hereditary colorectal cancer. *Cell* 1996;87:159–170.
8. Hanahan D, Weinberg RA. The hallmarks of cancer. *Cell* 2000;100:57–70.
9. Morin PJ, Vogelstein B, Kinzler KW. Apoptosis and APC in colorectal tumorigenesis. *Proc Natl Acad Sci U S A* 1996;93:7950–7954.
10. Peltomaki P, Aaltonen LA, Sistonen P, et al. Genetic-mapping of a locus predisposing to human colorectal cancer. *Science* 1993;260:810–812.
11. Shibata D, Peinado MA, Ionov Y, et al. Genomic instability in repeated sequences is an early somatic event in colorectal tumorigenesis that persists after transformation. *Nat Genetics* 1994;6:273–281.
12. Weinberg RA. Oncogenes, antioncogenes, and the molecular-bases of multistep carcinogenesis. *Cancer Res* 1989;49:3713–3721.
13. Jones PA, Laird PW. Cancer epigenetics comes of age. *Nat Genet* 1999;21:163–167.
14. Baylin SB, Herman JG. DNA hypermethylation in tumorigenesis: epigenetics joins genetics. *Trends Genet* 2000;16:168–174.
15. Brown R, Strathdee G. Epigenomics and epigenetic therapy of cancer. *Trends Mol Med* 2002;8:S43–S48.
16. Esteller M, Herman JG. Cancer as an epigenetic disease: DNA methylation and chromatin alterations in human tumours. *J Pathol* 2002;196:1–7.
17. Baselga J, Averbuch SD. ZD1839 ('Iressa')(1,2) as an anticancer agent. *Drugs* 2000;60:33–40.
18. de Bono JS, Rowinsky EK. The ErbB receptor family: a therapeutic target for cancer. *Trends Mol Med* 2002;8: S19–S26.
19. Giaccone G, Johnson DH, Manegold C, et al. A phase III clinical trial of ZD1839 ('Iressa') in combination with gemcitabine and cisplatin in chemotherapy naive patients with advanced non-small-cell lung cancer (INTACT1) (Abstract 4O). *Ann Oncol* 2002;13:2.
20. Johnson DH, Herbst R, Giaccone G, et al. ZD1839 ('Iressa') in combination with paclitaxel & carboplatin in chemotherapy naive patients with advanced non-small-cell lung cancer (NSCLC): results from a phase III clinical trial (INTACT 2) (abstract 468O). *Ann Oncol* 2002;13:127.
21. Slamon DJ, Leyland-Jones B, Shak S, et al. Use of chemotherapy plus a monoclonal antibody against HER2 for metastatic breast cancer that overexpresses HER2. *N Engl J Med* 2001;344:783–792.
22. Esteva FJ, Valero V, Booser D, et al. Phase II study of weekly docetaxel and trastuzumab for patients with HER-2-overexpressing metastatic breast cancer. *J Clin Oncol* 2002;20:1800–1808.
23. Slamon D, Pegram M. Rationale for trastuzumab (Herceptin) in adjuvant breast cancer trials. *Semin Oncol* 2001;28:13–19.
24. Druker BJ. STI571 (Gleevec) as a paradigm for cancer therapy. *Trends Mol Med* 2002;8:S14–S18.
25. Neckers L. Hsp90 inhibitors as novel cancer chemotherapeutic agents. *Trends Mol Med* 2002;8 S55–S61.
26. Huang S, Houghton PJ. Inhibitors of mammalian target of rapamycin as novel antitumor agents: from bench to clinic. *Curr Opin Invest Drug* 2002;3:295–304.
27. Rosen LS. Clinical experience with angiogenesis signaling inhibitors: focus on vascular endothelial growth factor (VEGF) blockers. *Cancer Control* 2002;9: 36–44.
28. Johnstone RW. Histone-deacetylase inhibitors: novel drugs for the treatment of cancer. *Nat Rev Drug Discov* 2002;1:287–299.
29. Senderowicz AM. Small molecule modulators of cyclin-dependent kinases for cancer therapy. *Oncogene* 2000;19:6600–6606.
30. McClue SJ, Blake D, Clarke R, et al. In vitro and in vivo antitumor properties of the cyclin dependent kinase inhibitor CYC202 (R-roscovitine). *Int J Cancer* 2002; 102:463–468.
31. Kantarjian H, Sawyers C, Hochhaus A, et al. Hematologic and cytogenetic responses to imatinib mesylate in chronic myelogenous leukemia. *N Engl J Med* 2002; 346:645–652.
32. van Oosterom AT, Judson I, Verweij J, et al. Safety and efficacy of imatinib (STI571) in metastatic gastrointestinal stromal tumours: a phase I study. *Lancet* 2001; 358:1421–1423.
33. Demetri GD, von Mehren M, Blanke CD, et al. Efficacy and safety of imatinib mesylate in advanced gastrointestinal stromal tumors. *N Engl J Med* 2002;347:472–480.
34. Jain M, Arvanitis C, Chu K, et al. Sustained loss of a neoplastic phenotype by brief inactivation of MYC. *Science* 2002;297:102–104.
35. Chin L, Tam A, Pomerantz J, et al. A Essential role for oncogenic Ras in tumour maintenance. *Nature* 1999; 400:468–472.
36. Pelengaris S, Khan M, Evan GI. Suppression of Myc-induced apoptosis in beta cells exposes multiple oncogenic properties of Myc and triggers carcinogenic progression. *Cell* 2002;109:321–334.
37. Colomer R, Lupu R, Bacus SS, et al. erbB-2 antisense oligonucleotides inhibit the proliferation of breast carcinoma cells with erbB-2 oncogene amplification. *Br J Cancer* 1994;70:819–825.
38. Weinstein IB. Cancer. Addiction to oncogenes: the Achilles heal of cancer. *Science* 2002;297:63–64.
39. Neshat MS, Mellinghoff IK, Tran C, et al. Enhanced sensitivity of PTEN-deficient tumors to inhibition of FRAP/mTOR. *Proc Natl Acad Sci U S A* 2001;98: 10314–10319.
40. Wooster R, Bignell G, Lancaster J, et al. Identification of the breast-cancer susceptibility gene Brca2. *Nature* 1995;378:789–792.
41. Papadopoulos N, Nicolaides NC, Wei YF, et al. Mutation of a mutL homolog in hereditary colon cancer. *Science* 1994;263:1625–1629.
42. Futreal PA, Kasprzyk A, Birney E, et al. Cancer and genomics. *Nature* 2001;409:850–852.

43. Wooster R. Richard Wooster on cancer and the Human Genome Project (interview by Ezzie Hutchinson). *Lancet Oncol* 2001;2:176–178.

44. Davies H, Bignell GR, Cox C, et al Mutations of the BRAF gene in human cancer. *Nature* 2002;417:949–954.

45. Evan GI, Vousden KH. Proliferation, cell cycle and apoptosis in cancer. *Nature* 2001;411:342–348.

46. Cai WW, Mao JH, Chow CW, et al. Genome-wide detection of chromosomal imbalances in tumors using BAC microarrays. *Nat Biotechnol* 2002;20:393–396.

47. Fritz B, Schubert F, Wrobel G, et al. Microarray-based copy number and expression profiling in dedifferentiated and pleomorphic liposarcoma. *Cancer Res* 2002;62:2993–2998.

48. Pollack JR, Sorlie T, Perou CM, et al. Microarray analysis reveals a major direct role of DNA copy number alteration in the transcriptional program of human breast tumors. *Proc Natl Acad Sci U S A* 2002;99:12963–12968.

49. MacDonald TJ, Brown KM, LaFleur B, et al. Expression profiling of medulloblastoma: PDGFRA and the RAS/MAPK pathway as therapeutic targets for metastatic disease. *Nat Genet* 2001;29:143–152.

50. Costello JF, Fruhwald MC, Smiraglia DJ, et al. Aberrant CpG-island methylation has non-random and tumour-type-specific patterns. *Nat Genet* 2000;24:132–138.

51. Yan PS, Perry MR, Laux DE, et al. CpG island arrays: an application toward deciphering epigenetic signatures of breast cancer. *Clin Cancer Res* 2000;6:1432–1438.

52. Yan PS, Chen CM, Shi H, et al. Dissecting complex epigenetic alterations in breast cancer using CpG island microarrays. *Cancer Res* 2001;61:8375–8380.

53. Wei SH, Chen CM, Strathdee G, et al. Methylation microarray analysis of late-stage ovarian carcinomas distinguishes progression-free survival in patients and identifies candidate epigenetic markers. *Clin Cancer Res* 2002;8:2246–2252.

54. Hannon GJ. RNA interference. *Nature* 2002;418:244–251.

55. Kamath RS, Fraser AG, Dong Y, et al. Systematic functional analysis of the Caenorhabditis elegans genome using RNAi. *Nature* 2003;421:231–237.

56. Wilda M, Fuchs U, Wossmann W, et al. Killing of leukemic cells with a BCR/ABL fusion gene by RNA interference (RNAi). *Oncogene* 2002;21:5716–5724.

57. Aherne GW, McDonald E, Workman P. Finding the needle in the haystack: why high-throughput screening is good for your health. *Breast Cancer Res* 2002;4:148–154.

58. Workman P. Overview: changing times: developing cancer drugs in genomeland. *Curr Opin Invest Drugs*, 2001;2:1128–1135.

59. Weinstein JN, Myers TG, O'Connor PM, et al. An information-intensive approach to the molecular pharmacology of cancer. *Science* 1997;275:343–349.

60. Clarke PA, Hostein I, Banerji U, et al. Gene expression profiling of human colon cancer cells following inhibition of signal transduction by 17-allylamino-17-demethoxygeldanamycin, an inhibitor of the hsp90 molecular chaperone. *Oncogene* 2000;19:4125–4133.

61. Scherf U, Ross DT, Waltham M, et al. A gene expression database for the molecular pharmacology of cancer. *Nat Genet* 2000;24:236–244.

62. Panaretou B, Siligardi G, Meyer P, et al. Activation of the ATPase activity of hsp90 by the stress-regulated cochaperone aha1. *Mol Cell* 2002;10:1307–1318.

63. Banerji U, O'Donnell A, Scurr M, et al. A pharmacokinetically (PK) - pharmacodynamically (PD) driven phase I clinical trial of the HSP90 molecular chaperone inhibitor 17-allyamino17-demethoxygeldanamycin (17AAG) (abstract 1352). *Proc Am Assoc Cancer Res* 2002;43:72–73.

64. Staunton JE, Slonim DK, Coller HA, et al. Chemosensitivity prediction by transcriptional profiling. *Proc Natl Acad Sci U S A* 2001;98:10787–10792.

65. Vivanco I, Sawyers CL. The phosphatidylinositol 3-Kinase AKT pathway in human cancer. *Nat Rev Cancer* 2002;2:489–501.

66. Ali IU, Schriml LM, Dean M. Mutational spectra of PTEN/MMAC1 gene: a tumor suppressor with lipid phosphatase activity. *J Natl Cancer Inst* 1999;91:1922–1932.

67. te Poele R, Cattini N, Maillard K, et al. The gene expression profile of the phosphatidylinositol 3-kinase (PI3K) inhibitor LY294002 in human colon adenocarcinoma cells (abstract 1345). *Proc Am Assoc Cancer Res* 2002;43:271.

68. Roche S, Downward J, Raynal P, et al. A function for phosphatidylinositol 3-kinase beta (p85alpha-p110beta) in fibroblasts during mitogenesis: requirement for insulin- and lysophosphatidic acid-mediated signal transduction. *Mol Cell Biol* 1998;18:7119–7129.

69. Rodrigues AD. Preclinical drug metabolism in the age of high-throughput screening: an industrial perspective. *Pharm Res* 1997;14:1504–1510.

70. van de Vijver MJ, He YD, van't Veer LJ, et al. A gene-expression signature as a predictor of survival in breast cancer. *N Engl J Med* 2002;347:1999–2009.

71. van 't Veer LJ, Dai H, van de Vijver MJ, et al. Gene expression profiling predicts clinical outcome of breast cancer. *Nature* 2002;415:530–536.

72. Zhan F, Tian E, Bumm K, et al. Gene expression profiling of human plasma cell differentiation and classification of multiple myeloma based on similarities to distinct stages of late stage B-cell development. *Blood* 2002;101:1128–1140.

73. Rosenwald A, Wright G, Chan WC, et al. The use of molecular profiling to predict survival after chemotherapy for diffuse large-B-cell lymphoma. *N Engl J Med* 2002;346:1937–1947.

74. Shipp MA, Ross KN, Tamayo P, et al. Diffuse large B-cell lymphoma outcome prediction by gene-expression profiling and supervised machine learning. *Nat Med* 2002;8:68–74.

75. Alizadeh AA, Eisen MB, Davis RE, et al. Distinct types of diffuse large B-cell lymphoma identified by gene expression profiling. *Nature* 2000;403:503–511.

76. Birkenkamp-Demtroder K, Christensen LL, Olesen SH, et al. Gene expression in colorectal cancer. *Cancer Res* 2002;62:4352–4363.

77. Wessels LF, van Welsem T, Hart AA, et al. Molecular classification of breast carcinomas by comparative genomic hybridization: a specific somatic genetic profile for BRCA1 tumors. *Cancer Res* 2002;62:7110–7117.

78. Roses AD. Genome-based pharmacogenetics and the pharmaceutical industry. *Nat Rev Drug Discov* 2002;1:541–549.

79. Sachidanandam R, Weissman D, Schmidt SC, et al. A map of human genome sequence variation containing

1.42 million single nucleotide polymorphisms. *Nature* 2001;409:928–933.

80. Reich DE, Cargill M, Bolk S, et al. Linkage disequilibrium in the human genome. *Nature* 2001;411: 199–204.

81. Dawson E, Abecasis GR, Bumpstead S, et al. A first-generation linkage disequilibrium map of human chromosome 22. *Nature* 2002;418:544–548.

82. Cheung VG, Spielman RS. The genetics of variation in gene expression. *Nat Genet* 2002;32(Suppl):522–525.

83. Lai E, Riley J, Purvis I, et al. A 4-Mb high-density single nucleotide polymorphism-based map around human APOE. *Genomics* 1998;54:31–38.

84. Hetherington S, Hughes AR, Mosteller M, et al. Genetic variations in HLA-B region and hypersensitivity reactions to abacavir. *Lancet* 2002;359:1121–1122.

85. Knudsen S. *A biologist's guide to analysis of DNA microarray data.* New York: John Wiley & Sons, 2002.

86. Baldi P, Long AD. A Bayesian framework for the analysis of microarray expression data: regularized t -test and statistical inferences of gene changes. *Bioinformatics* 2001;17:509–519.

87. Pomeroy SL, Tamayo P, Gaasenbeek M, et al. Prediction of central nervous system embryonal tumour outcome based on gene expression. *Nature* 2002;415:436–442.

88. Kohonen T. *Self-organizing maps.* Berlin: Springer-Verlag, 1995.

89. Khan J, Wei JS, Ringner M, et al. Classification and diagnostic prediction of cancers using gene expression profiling and artificial neural networks. *Nat Med* 2001;7:673–679.

90. Watson JD, Crick FH. A structure for deoxyribose nucleic acid. *Nature* 1953;171:964–967.

91. Watson JD, Crick FH. A structure for deoxyribose nucleic acid. 1953. *Nature* 2003;421:396–398.

92. Russo E. Special report: the birth of biotechnology. *Nature* 2003;421:456–457.

93. Sanger F, Coulson AR. A rapid method for determining sequences in DNA by primed synthesis with DNA polymerase. *J Mol Biol* 1975;94: 441–448.

94. Maxam AM, Gilbert W. A new method for sequencing DNA. *Proc Natl Acad Sci U S A* 1977;74:560–564.

95. Sanger F, Air GM, Barrell BG, et al. Nucleotide sequence of bacteriophage phi X174 DNA. *Nature* 1977;265:687–695.

96. Hood L, Galas D. The digital code of DNA. *Nature* 2003;421:444–448.

97. Gatenby RA, Maini PK. Mathematical oncology: cancer summed up. *Nature* 2003;421: 321.

98. Ratain MJ, Relling MV. Gazing into a crystal ball-cancer therapy in the post-genomic era. *Nat Med* 2001;7:283–285.

99. Bell JI. The double helix in clinical practice. *Nature* 2003;421:414–416.

9

The Application of Proteomics to Drug Development

Lasantha R. Bandara and Sandy Kennedy

Oxford GlycoSciences (UK) Ltd, Abingdon, Oxon OX14 4RY, United Kingdom

The completion of the human genome map marked an important milestone in genetic research. The scientific community has access to a vast amount of genetic information; however, attention has now turned to alternative technologies that are part of the so-called "post-genomic era." It is clear that genome-based technologies will identify numerous new drug targets, although in some cases the supporting biological evidence may be limited. It is also probable that these approaches will yield a variety of diagnostic biomarkers, although again larger studies may be required to confirm the validity of the markers. We imagine that in the future, patients could be offered personalized medicines tailored to their individual genetic composition; however, this concept comes with many practical issues and it is likely that such options will not be available for some time.

It has become increasingly clear that genetic alterations will ultimately result in protein modifications and hence changes in protein function. Several studies have highlighted the discrepancy between genomic and protein regulation, intensifying interest in the direct study of proteins. The proteome is often used to describe the protein composition of a given cell or body compartment, although this is not a static image but rather a fluid entity (1,2). Therefore, it is important to realize that proteomic approaches capture "snapshots" of cellular processes. Generally speaking, the aim of proteomics is to separate complex mixtures of proteins and to identify those proteins participating in a given biological phenomenon. In some cases, however, unidentified proteins could also be of value if the protein profiles are predictive of a disease or a specific cellular process. One particular advantage of a proteomics approach is that proteins can be readily detected in body fluids such as blood and urine. In addition, protein markers can be developed into simple antibody-based assays that can be used to screen large numbers of samples.

Proteomics has a wide range of potential applications in drug discovery and drug development, and the term *pharmacoproteomics* has been coined to encompass these applications (3). For example, proteomics could be used to identify new markers of toxicity or drug efficacy. Alternatively, new diagnostic markers may be identified or markers indicating the suitability of a patient for a particular drug may be defined. In this chapter we will focus mainly on the contribution of proteomics to preclinical research, particularly its application to toxicology.

The potential toxicity of a new compound is traditionally assessed using a range of preclinical animal studies. In many cases, toxicity is quantitated by histopathological examination of tissues or using a range of biochemical techniques (4,5). However, many compounds are not successfully identified in these models, and there is a need to improve the predictability of preclinical testing. Proteomics can be used to identify individual proteins or groups of proteins associated with the properties of a single toxicant. These proteins or "signature" profiles may be reflective of a common mechanism of toxicity. New markers may be more sensitive and predictive than current markers, and therefore may be more appropriate for assessing the toxicity of new drugs. Examples of the applications of proteomics to study differing mechanisms of toxicity in preclinical models will be reviewed briefly. In addition, the utility of proteomics in aiding toxicology and drug development will also be discussed.

PROTEOMIC TECHNOLOGIES

Two-dimensional (2D) polyacrylamide gel electrophoresis (PAGE) is the most common technique employed for studying the proteome. Protein samples are initially separated by electric charge in the first dimension and by molecular weight in the second dimension, resulting in an array of protein spots or "features" (Fig. 9.1). Although 2D PAGE is considered a relatively "old" technology, automation of the process and the development of specialized software for data analysis have made a significant impact on the proteomics process. Several companies have developed additional techniques to enhance the methodology and simplify the data analysis. For example, Oxford GlycoSciences UK Ltd (OGS) has developed sensitive fluorescent dyes that can detect low-abundance proteins (6,7). A serum-enrichment technique has also been developed to remove high-abundance proteins such as immunoglobulins, haptoglobin, transferrins, and albumin from blood samples so that the lower-abundance proteins are revealed (8). Protein samples are typically separated across a pH range of 3 to 10; however, it is also pos-

sible to run smaller pH ranges (9), which enables the high-resolution separation of proteins with a similar pH and molecular weight (Fig. 9.1). By combining the images from smaller pH ranges, it is possible to detect several thousand protein features rather than the 2,000 that may be visualised using standard techniques. Last, the reproducibility of 2D PAGE process is essential for data interpretation as small fluctuations in gel compositions may in turn influence analysis. This problem can be circumvented by scanning each gel and producing a composite or "master gel" containing all the gel images. Specialized software packages have been developed to match the corresponding protein in each gel with each other in a process termed *gel warping* (6).

Because a large number of protein features are produced from a 2D gel image, additional software is necessary for mining and interpreting the information. Again, several groups have developed software specifically for this process. For example, OGS,

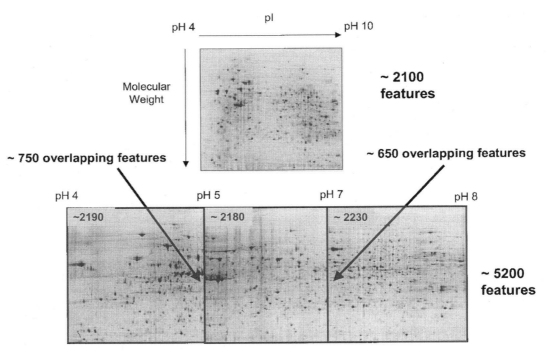

FIG. 9.1. Example of two-dimensional gel proteomics technology. Proteins are initially loaded onto an immobilized pH gradient (IPG) gel and separated by charge across a pH range of 3 to 10. The second dimension separates proteins by their molecular weight. Gels are treated with a fixative and stained using an appropriate protein dye. The resulting image is generated by scanning the gel using a high-resolution fluorescence scanner. A typical gel will generate approximately 2,000 protein features. Samples can also be separated using smaller pH ranges (e.g., 4–5, 5–7, and 7–8). Each method identifies approximately 2,000 proteins with a number of overlapping features. The combination of three smaller pH ranges results in the discovery of approximately 5,000 features from the sample.

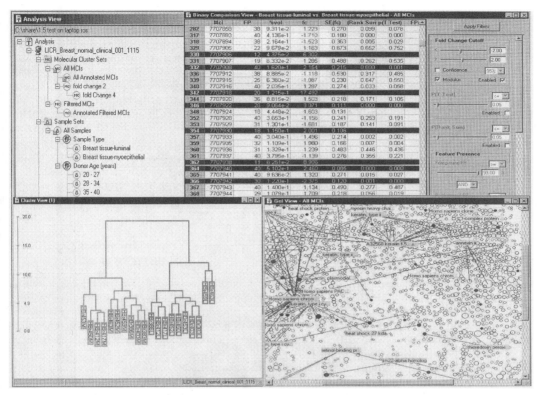

FIG. 9.2. Properties of specialised software for mining proteome data, Rosetta software (Oxford GlycoSciences). The database or "master group" (top left) contains all the protein or MCIs (molecular cluster indexes) identified. Information on the sample type and additional patient information (such as age) can be used to group samples together. A binary comparison can be performed on the grouped samples and further analyzed using parameters such as fold change and *t* test (top right). Also indicated is the feature presence (FP) in the samples, the volume of the protein spot represented as the percentage of the gel fluorescence (%vol). The fold change (fc) and other statistical parameters are also shown. The similarity of each sample can be assessed by a hierarchical cluster analysis tool, which compares the similarity of each spot on each gel and then separates based on the extent of that similarity. In the example shown, the clustering separates the luminal and myoepithelial samples (bottom left). The position of the protein on the composite gel can be determined, and if known, the protein's identity will also be shown (bottom right).

Large Scale Biology, and Scimagix have developed image-analysis platforms such as Rosetta (Oxford GlycoSciences), Kepler (Large Scale Biology) and ProteinMine (Scimagix). By using Rosetta software, for example (Fig. 9.2), data from several samples can be grouped together and analyzed using a variety of statistical parameters (6). The abundance and regulation of specific proteins can be plotted in different samples and the position of the spot(s) on the master gel can be visualized. Once a particular protein or group of proteins of interest have been selected, the identity can be determined by mass spectrometry (MS) analysis. The protein will be embedded in the gel matrix and must be excised and fragmented via protease digestion before analysis. In most cases,

MALDI-TOF (matrix-assisted laser desorption ionization/time of flight) is used to determine peptide sequences; however, more recently TOF-TOF-MS, which has a greater sensitivity and capacity, has also been used. Once a peptide sequence has been determined, it can be used to search a variety of sequence databases to identify the protein and predict its full sequence. For an in-depth and detailed review of 2D gel proteomics, the reader is referred to reference 10.

Several alternative proteomic technology platforms have been developed to complement the 2D gel approach. A number of protein chips have been developed to bind proteins directly or indirectly (11–14). Antibody-based chips have been developed to selectively capture and separate known proteins. In some cases the proteins must be labeled to facilitate detection. Alternatively, a dual-antibody strategy using one antibody to separate the protein and a second antibody to monitor the protein abundance has been suggested (12). The advantage of this kind of approach is the potential high-throughput analysis of samples that can be achieved using this technology, making it attractive for routine testing. However, major limitations include the requirement for the proteins to be known, characterized, and amenable to antibody production. Furthermore, as the number of antibodies used on a single chip increases, the likelihood of obtaining similar binding conditions for all antigen–antibody interactions is likely to decrease. Finally, a molecular chip of this type may become cumbersome if all protein variants and posttranslation modifications are included. Such a tool might contain 100,000 proteins, which would be both challenging to create and to interpret.

Ciphergen Biosystems has produced a protein chip format (ProteinChip) that uses a variety of affinity surfaces to bind proteins based on their chemical and physical characteristics (15). The chip requires small amounts of material and requires washing steps to remove nonspecific protein interactions. Using SELDI (surface-enhanced laser desorption ionization) TOF-MS, it is possible to quantitatively detect proteins from different samples. Although antibodies can be combined with this technology, it is not a prerequisite as binding to a range of different molecular surfaces has been achieved. Once the binding and wash conditions have been optimized data can be rapidly generated, which is advantageous. However, one drawback is the need to use alternative methods to identify protein sequences. Nevertheless, the system has already been used to identify markers of prostate and ovarian cancer and it could also be applied to the discovery of new toxicity markers (16,17). An ovarian marker study conducted by Petricoin et al. (17) raised an interesting question as to the use of protein profiles without the knowledge of the protein identity. One issue with this approach is the validation of such markers (discussed later in the chapter). Very large studies might be required to prove the specificity of the markers. In addition, many regulatory groups may be reluctant to use such information without a plausible biological link between the protein profile and the disease in question.

Another recent and exciting proteomic technology of note is the isotope-coded affinity tag (ICAT; a trademark of the University of Washington exclusively licensed to Applied Biosystems.) method (18). The technique uses a thiol-specific reactive group incorporating a stable isotope and an affinity tag for purification. By using two different isotopes, it is pos-

sible to label two different samples and to compare protein profiles in each sample in parallel. After labeling, the samples are pooled and digested with proteases to produce peptide fragments, which are analyzed by tandem MS. Since the ICAT approach is very rapid, it is possible to process several thousand peptides in a day. A particular advantage of this procedure is the ability to analyze membrane fractions that are difficult to resolve by 2D PAGE. This technique has already been used to study proteome changes in yeast and to specifically monitor changes in phosphorylation patterns (19,20). An analogous strategy could also be taken to monitor toxic effects of compounds with the aim of understanding the action of novel drugs.

APPLICATIONS OF PROTEOMICS IN TOXICOLOGY

Proteomics can be applied to two main areas of toxicology: investigative research and predictive toxicology. Proteomics can identify new toxic mechanisms through the discovery of new proteins and pathways, which in turn could result in a greater understanding of idiosyncratic toxicity. Although the contribution to research toxicology may be of great benefit, the role of proteomics in predictive toxicology may be more valuable. For example, proteomics can be used to identify new protein markers that could be used to predict the toxicity of a new compound. New markers may be more sensitive than existing tools and may monitor toxicity at lower doses than possible using conventional methods. The opportunity of detecting toxicity at an early stage may be crucial in a clinical setting and may also be very valuable during drug discovery. As with all new technologies it is important to compare proteomic data with conventional toxicology practices. It is also important that the data are carefully analyzed and put into context with the toxicity under evaluation (7,21,22).

Hepatotoxicity

The liver participates in the metabolism and detoxification of many compounds and is a common site for toxicity within the body. Consequently, liver function testing is a common component of the toxicological evaluation of any new compound. Furthermore, the liver is also a frequent site for adverse drug reactions (ADR) leading to the withdrawal of many drugs from the market (23). The proteomic liver toxicity database developed by Anderson et al. (24) represents an intriguing concept in predictive toxicology. Using a range of hepatotoxins, a series of protein toxicity profiles in the rat liver were generated. The database was used to identify and categorize a broad range of known hepatotoxins. The authors were also able to correlate the proteins identified with molecular pathways of toxicity confirming the value of the dataset. One might imagine that this database could be used to expose the potential hepatotoxicity of a new compound by comparing the proteomes after compound treatment. A similar profile to a known toxicant could serve as an early warning of toxicity for further studies. Unfortunately, this particular database contained limited doses and time points, and in some cases the data points might not have been relevant for the different toxicants. A more comprehensive collection of data points would be required to gain confidence of the predictive value of such a preclinical tool.

Another example of the value of proteomics in lead candidate selection is exemplified by the study by Cunningham et al. (25). The histamine H1 receptor antagonists pyrilamine and methapyrilene are both similar chemically, although methapyrilene is known to be a nongenotoxic carcinogen. Examination of the protein profiles from the livers of compound-treated animals revealed numerous changes with methapyrilene but not with pyrilamine. Interestingly, many of the proteins altered after methapyrilene treatment were also altered after treatment with the peroxisome proliferator WY14,643. Therefore, during lead optimization, knowledge of such protein profiles could allow compounds to be prioritized such that the most specific compounds are taken forward into development. The assumption is that the compounds with fewer proteomic changes are less likely to cause unexpected side effects, although this remains to be proven.

A number of other studies have also been performed using a range of known hepatotoxins. In each case, proteomic changes were noted and protein identification revealed a variety of proteins involved in different aspects of liver metabolism (26–29). Of interest is the combined genomic and proteomic study that was performed recently using paracetamol or acetaminophen (30). Although no direct correlation between gene expression and the corresponding protein levels was observed, the authors did note that similar pathways were regulated.

Renal Toxicity

The kidney is also a common site of toxicity because compounds are often concentrated or reabsorbed in the kidney as a part of normal renal function. Several proteomic studies have been performed to define changes in kidney tissues in response to damage. The aminoglycoside antibiotic gentamicin is a recognized renal toxin that damages the proximal tubules within the renal cortex. Two recently published studies examined protein changes induced by gentamicin treatment (31,32). Examination of kidney cortex samples revealed several treatment-specific changes that were related to changes in glucose and lipid metabolism and stress response, consistent with gentamicin-induced toxicity. In the second study a parallel tissue and serum analysis was performed. Similar proteins in the cortex were identified, and an examination of the serum samples revealed a protein that was overexpressed in all the gentamicin groups. The protein was identified as a component of the alternate pathway of complement activation and was shown to be regulated in a dose- and time-dependent fashion, returning to control levels during the recovery phase (8,31). Furthermore, this protein was detected at low doses and at early time points before changes were observed by routine clinical pathology, highlighting the sensitivity of proteomics. If conserved in humans, the value of this type of marker in a clinical setting is clear. Patients undergoing treatment with drugs known to cause nephrotoxicity could be monitored, and the appearance of a marker before cellular damage is evident would allow an alternative treatment to be pursued, thereby reducing the risk of fatality.

Lead is a potent neurotoxin and nephrotoxin in humans. Analysis of the rodent kidney after lead acetate treatment revealed a number of proteins that are regulated in the kidney cortex and medulla (33). Several proteins associated with oxidative stress and mitochondrial function were altered. In addition, the authors highlighted changes in calcium-binding proteins. A further study using the immunosuppressant cyclosporine A (CsA) also highlighted calcium binding, in particular the calcium-binding protein calbindin-D (34). Calbindin-D (28K) was determined to be a novel marker of renal toxicity and proceeding studies in a range of species indicated that the protein was regulated in rats and humans but not in monkeys and dogs. This pattern of regulation was also consistent with the species-specific cellular toxicity observed with CsA (35). The discovery of calbindin-D in CsA-mediated toxicity was exciting because it had not previously been associated with this pathway. The identification of this protein again emphasizes the role proteomics can play in providing essential information to understand mechanisms of toxicity.

Cardiovascular Toxicity

Cardiovascular toxicity represents a major concern during drug development, particularly because several therapeutic entities have been associated with this type of toxicity (36). Although the measurement of QT function in preclinical studies is used to monitor cardiac arrhythmias, a simple blood test would be more convenient and desirable (37). Serum markers such as cardiac troponins are considered by some to be an "ideal" marker, although their value in predicting cardiac damage has been questioned (38,39). Few cardiotoxicity studies utilizing proteomics have been reported in the literature; however, several reports have monitored protein changes in cardiovascular diseases (40–42). One recent report encompassed the anticancer drug doxorubicin, which is often used to treat childhood leukemias but is also known to induce dose-dependent cardiotoxicity (43). A rat model for doxorubicin cardiotoxicity has been used in conjugation with proteomic analysis (31). As a part of the study, specific groups also received the compound ICRF-187, which provides chemoprotection against the toxic effects of doxorubicin. Proteomic analysis of serum samples revealed a number of potential markers of cardiotoxicity, many of which were normalized in the ICRF-187 groups (44). Further validation was also obtained though identification of the proteins, which revealed several protein classes consistent with the chemoprotective effects of ICRF-187. Further proteome studies are in progress using the phosphodiesterase (PDE) inhibitor SKF 95654, which is known to induce vascular toxicity or vasculitis (45). As with cardiotoxicity, there are no reliable serum markers of vascular toxicity. In one study, dose-dependent markers of vasculitis were identified in two different rat strains (Fig. 9.3).

Carcinogenesis

Carcinogenicity safety studies usually require costly long-term animal studies. A more rapid assay predicting the carcinogenic potential of a compound would be very valuable provided that the assay was highly correlative. Numerous experiments have been performed to identify proteomic changes that occur as cells become cancerous (7,46,47). For example, Harris et al. (7) compared the proteomes of several breast cancer cell lines and were able to classify the most tumorigenic lines based on the proteome profile. Furthermore, a smaller subset of proteins that were specifically altered in the tumor-forming lines was identified. If a compound under development was found to affect these particular proteins or was capable of producing protein profiles similar to the tumor cell lines, there may be concern as to its oncogenic potential. This concept is also emphasised by the methapyrilene study discussed previously (in Hepatotoxicity) and by other studies that have used peroxisomes proliferators (25,48). Similar studies have also been performed using material from ovarian tumors rather than cell lines (49) and Verma et al. (50) recently highlighted the value of using multiple proteomic technologies in the search for new cancer biomarkers.

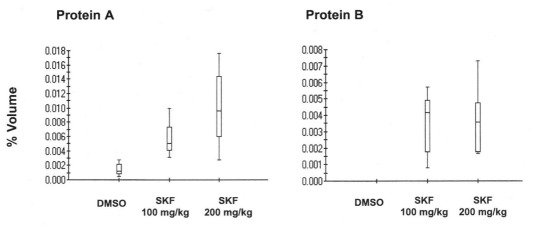

FIG. 9.3. Examples of rat plasma markers of vasculitis induced by SKF 95654. Blood samples from rats treated with 100 and 200 mg/kg SKF 95654 were analyzed by two-dimensional gel proteomics. The resulting graphs indicate the regulation of two potential protein markers. The percent volume indicates the protein density in each group as a percentage of the total gel fluorescence. Both proteins are present at low levels in the control dimethyl sulfoxide–treated group and are induced in the SKF 95654–treated groups. Note protein A shows a clear dose-dependent change consistent with vascular toxicity.

To complement these approaches, the US National Cancer Institute has been collating a vast array of information on the growth inhibitory effects of compounds on cell lines. This information has been combined with protein-expression data to create a database linking protein expression changes with growth inhibitory effects (51,52) Again, this large reference dataset could prove very valuable for future compounds if protein signature patterns can be used to predict carcinogenicity or antitumor efficacy.

BIOMARKER VALIDATION

The extent of validation required for any biomarker is closely linked to its intended use. Research tools for lead candidate selection or surrogate markers used in clinical trials for efficacy studies will require different validation strategies to diagnostic markers used to make crucial clinical decisions. Furthermore, diagnostic markers will ultimately require approval by regulatory bodies before use. Several authors have described the properties of an ideal biomarker (53,54), which are briefly discussed in the next section.

Clinical Relevance

Potential markers should measure the physiological or pathological process. There should be a mechanistic rationale for the activity of the marker correlating with a clinical endpoint.

Sensitivity and Specificity

The marker should be specific for a given disease or treatment and detectable within the target population at the appropriate time. The magnitude of the marker change should correlate with the severity of the disease.

Reliability and Consistency

The biomarker should ideally be reproducible in its effect, measurable, accurate, precise, and robust enough to monitor in a clinical setting.

Practicality and Simplicity

Ideally, it should be possible to monitor the biomarker by noninvasive methods without posing a significant risk to patient health. A simple low-cost routine assay with an uncomplicated read out is also desirable.

At present, it is clear that many of the markers identified by proteomics do not fulfil these criteria; however, it should be emphasised that both the scientific and regulatory communities are evolving in their in-

terpretation of these techniques. As new potential biomarkers are published in scientific journals, it is likely they will be initially utilized as research tools and may ultimately be validated over time. It is also possible in the future that complex biomarkers patterns identified using proteomics may be used in the absence of fulfilling these criteria if the profile can be reduced to simple assay and read out.

THE ROLE OF PROTEOMICS IN DRUG DEVELOPMENT

Proteomics can impact a number of processes in drug discovery and development (Fig. 9.4). For example, proteomics can be used to identify and validate drug targets, and in addition *in vitro* efficacy and toxicity profiles could be very valuable in selecting lead candidates for development. Extensive data have also been collected on the effects of toxicants in preclinical and *in vitro* models; therefore, it may be possible to use these data to predict toxicity. For example, the information could be combined into a reference "proteomic library" as suggested by Anderson et al. (24) for comparison with new drug candidates. As discussed previously, a positive correlation with a known toxicant may serve as a warning for further studies or aid in the prioritization of candidates for development. For such a library to be of value, it would need to contain data generated from a large number of compounds with a variety of different mechanistic activities. Furthermore it would be necessary to have data from a range of time points and doses. Preclinical models could also be used to identify markers of drug efficacy or the mode of action of a compound. Surrogate markers of response may be identified from animal models, which could also be used in subsequent clinical trials. The value of surrogate markers in the development of anticancer drugs has recently been reviewed and was highlighted as an essential requirement for determining optimal dosing in clinical trials (55).

Toxicoproteomic profiles or isolated markers discovered in preclinical models could also be used in a clinical setting. In this case the marker(s) identified would also need to be relevant in human toxicity. Alternatively, analyzing samples from patients undergoing treatment with drugs known to cause toxicity could identify human-specific toxicity markers. The study could be designed such that a large number of samples are collected initially during the course of treatment. A subset of samples from patients that showed signs of toxicity could then be analyzed to discover markers expressed before clinical manifestations were evident. If the marker is expressed before traditional markers are detected, alternative treat-

Drug Discovery	Preclinical Research	Clinical Development	Therapeutic Population
Target discovery/ validation	Efficacy studies	Surrogate markers	Diagnosis
Lead selection	Toxicology	Patient selection	Drug efficacy
Mode of action studies	Mode of action studies	Disease sub-typing	Patient selection
		Toxicology	Toxicology

FIG. 9.4. Proteomic applications to the drug discovery and development pipeline. The drug discovery process is summarized from target discovery to clinical application. Key stages of the process are separated to highlight the influence of proteomics at each stage.

ment regimes could be utilized to avoid future complications.

Although ADRs generally occur at low frequencies in hospitals, it is clear that this type of reaction presents a major problem in the clinic (56,57). An exciting and challenging application of proteomics could be in identifying markers of an ADR or possibly markers that predispose a patient to the event. Again, it will be necessary to collect large numbers of samples with the intention of specifically examining the samples in which an ADR has occurred. The appearance of the marker during treatment would act as warning to halt further treatment. Individuals who may be predisposed to an ADR could be selected to receive an alternative drug treatment, thereby avoiding complications. A similar approach could also be taken to identify patients who respond favorably or unfavorably to a given drug.

It is unlikely that proteomics will be used in isolation; rather, it is likely to complement other new technologies and traditional methods. A vast amount of information has been collated using gene expression profiling techniques to monitor messenger RNA changes altered in response to xenobiotic exposure (58–60). Although predictive in many cases, some authors have noted that messenger RNA data are too variable to be used in this manner (61). Many companies and research groups are also cataloging substantial numbers of single-nucleotide polymorphisms within the genome, some of which are known to affect drug-metabolizing enzymes (62,63). Although highly challenging, the combination and integration of these

approaches will no doubt have a significant impact on toxicology. Unfortunately, for the end user of these tools (i.e., the clinical or research scientist), a simple answer to a complex question is unlikely and an attempt to provide this information in one unified format may not be possible.

CONCLUSIONS

The combination of proteomics and other 'omic' technologies is already making an impact on drug discovery and development. The opportunity of identifying markers of drug efficacy or drug suitability as well as markers of toxicity and disease will potentially revolutionize patient care in the future. One of the key features of the proteomics approach is that protein markers are present in body fluids. Therefore, samples can be acquired by simple noninvasive methodologies and potentially converted into standard immunoassays for routine screening. One imagines that proteomics will significantly reduce the investment of time and money required to develop new drugs (64). Specifically, proteomics will allow the rapid selection of the most promising drug candidates for further development, as well as allow candidates with poor efficacy or excessive toxicity to be eliminated earlier in development.

The authors thank Glenn Malpass for the Rosetta software images and Caroline Buckland for technical assistance.

REFERENCES

1. Anderson NG, Anderson NL. Proteome and proteomics: new technologies, new concepts, and new words. *Electrophoresis* 1998;19:1853–1861.
2. Blackstock WP, Weir MP. Proteomics: quantitative and physical mapping of cellular proteins. *Trends Biotechnol* 1999;17:121–127.
3. Moyses C. Pharmacogenetics, genomics, proteomics: the new frontiers in drug development. *Int J Pharm Med* 1999;13:197–202.
4. Evans GO, Davis DT, eds. *Animal clinical chemistry*. London: Taylor and Francis, 1996:1–19.
5. Trimbrell J. *Introduction to toxicolgy*, 3rd ed. London: Taylor and Francis, 2002.
6. Page MJ, Amess B, Townsend RR, et al. Proteomic definition of normal human luminal and myoepithelial breast cells purified from reduction mammoplasties. *Proc Natl Acad Sci U S A* 1999;96:12589–12594.
7. Harris RA, Yang A, Stein RC, et al. Cluster analysis of an extensive human breast cancer cell line protein expression map database. *Proteomics* 2002;2:212–223.
8. Kennedy S. Proteomic profiling from human samples: the body fluid alternative. *Toxicol Lett* 2001;120:379–384.
9. Hanash SM, Madoz-Gurpide J, Misek DE. Identification of novel targets for cancer therapy using expression proteomics. *Leukemia* 2002;16:478–485.
10. Link AJ, ed. *2-D proteome analysis protocols*. New Jersey: Humana Press, 1999.
11. Templin MF, Stoll D, Schrenk M, et al. Protein microarray technology. *Drug Discov Today* 2002;7: 815–822.
12. Cahill DJ. Protein and antibody arrays and their medical applications. *J Immunol Methods* 2001;250:81–91.
13. Jenkins RE, Pennington SR. Arrays for protein expression profiling: towards a viable alternative to two-dimensional gel electrophoresis. *Proteomics* 2000;1:13–29.
14. Kodadek T. Development of protein detecting microarrays and related devices. *Trends Biochem Sci* 2002; 27:295–300.
15. Davies HA. The ProteinChip System from Ciphergen: a new technique for rapid, micro-scale protein biology. *J Mol Med* 2000;78:B29.
16. Wright GL, Cazares LH, Leung SM, et al. ProteinChip surface enhanced laser desorption/ionisation (SELDI) mass spectrometry: a novel protein biochip technology for detection of prostate cancer biomarkers in complex protein mixtures. *Prostate Cancer Prostatic Dis* 2000;2:264–276.
17. Petricoin EF, Ardekani AM, Hitt BA, et al. Use of proteomic patterns in serum to identify ovarian cancer. *Lancet* 2002;359:572–577.
18. Gygi SP, Rist B, Gerber SA, et al. Quantitative analysis of complex protein mixtures using isotope-coded affinity tags. *Nat Biotechnol* 1999;17:994–999.
19. Ideker T, Thorsson V, Rannish JA, et al. Integrated genomic and proteomic analyses of a systematically perturbed metabolic network. *Science* 2001;292:929–934.
20. Goshe MB, Veenstra TD, Panisko EA, et al. Phosphoprotein isotope-coded affinity tags: application to the enrichment and identification of low-abundance phosphoproteins. *Anal Chem* 2002;74:607–616.
21. Pennie WD, Tugwood, JD, Oliver GJA, et al. (2000) The principles and practice of toxicogenomics: applications and opportunities. *Toxicol Sci* 2000;54:277–283.
22. Smith LL. Key challenges for toxicologists in the 21st century. *Trends Pharmacol Sci* 2001;22:281–285.
23. Park BK, Kitteringham NR, Powell H, et al. Advances in molecular toxicology–towards understanding idiosyncratic drug toxicity. *Toxicology* 2000;153:39–60.
24. Anderson NL, Taylor J, Hofmann J-P, et al. Simultaneous measurement of hundreds of liver proteins: application in assessment of liver function. *Toxicol Pathol* 1996;24:72–76.
25. Cunningham ML, Pippin LL, Anderson NL, et al. The hepatocarcinogen methapyrilene but not the analogue pyrilamine induces sustained hepatocellular replication and protein alterations in F344 rats in a 13 week feed study. *Toxicol Appl Pharmacol* 1995;131:216—222.
26. Anderson NL, Esquer-Blasco R, Richardson F, et al. The effects of peroxisome proliferators on protein abundances in mouse liver. *Toxicol Appl Pharmacol* 1996;137:75–89.
27. Edvardsson U, Alexandersson M, von Löwenhielm HB, et al. A proteome analysis of livers from obese (ob/ob) mice treated with the peroxisome proliferator WY 14,643. *Electrophoresis* 1999;20:935–942.
28. Fountoulakis M, Berndt P, Boelstreli, et al. Two-dimensional database of mouse liver proteins: changes in hepatic protein levels following treatment with acetaminophen or its nontoxic regioisomer 3-acetamidophenol. *Electrophoresis* 2000;21:2148–2161.
29. Steiner S, Gatlin CL, Lennon JJ, et al. Proteomics to display lovastatin-induced protein and pathway regulation in rat liver. *Electrophoresis* 2000;21:2129–2137.
30. Ruepp SU, Tonge RP, Shaw J, et al. Genomics and proteomics analysis of acetaminophen toxicity in mouse liver. *Toxicol Sci* 2002;65:135–150.
31. Kennedy S. The role of proteomics in toxicology: identification of biomarkers of toxicity by protein expression analysis. *Biomarkers* 2002;7:1–22.
32. Charlwood J, Skehel M, King N, et al. Proteomic analysis of rat kidney cortex following treatment with gentamicin. *J Proteome Res* 2002;1:73–82.
33. Witzmann FA, Fultz CD, Grant RA, et al. Regional protein alterations in rat kidneys induced by lead exposure. *Electrophoresis* 1999;20:943–951.
34. Steiner S, Aicher L, Raymackers J, et al. Cyclosporine A decreases the protein level of the calcium binding protein calbindin-D 28kDa in rat kidney. *Biochem Pharmacol* 1996;51:253–258.
35. Aicher L, Arce A, Grenet O, et al. New insights into cyclosporine A nephrotoxicity by proteome analysis. *Electrophoresis* 1998;19:1998–2003.
36. Pai VB, Nahata MC. Cardiotoxicity of chemotherapeutic agents: incidence, treatment and prevention. *Drug Saf* 2000;22:263–302.
37. Malik M, Camm AJ. Evaluation of drug-induced QT interval prolongation. *Drug Saf* 2001;24:323–351.
38. Collinson PO, Boa FG, Gaze DC. Measurement of cardiac troponins *Ann Clin Biochem* 2001;38:423–449.
39. Sparano JA, Brown DL, Wolff AC. Predicting cancer therapy-induced cardiotoxicity. *Drug Saf* 2002;25:301–311.
40. Heinke MY, Wheeler CH, Chang D, et al. Protein changes observed in pacing-induced heart failure using two-dimensional electrophoresis. *Electrophoresis* 1998;19:2021–2030.

41. Van Eyk JE Proteomics: unraveling the complexity of heart disease and striving to change cardiology. *Curr Opin Mol Ther* 2001;3:546–553.

42. Sironi L, Tremoli E, Miller I, et al. Acute-phase proteins before cerebral ischemia in stroke-prone rats: identification by proteomics. *Stroke* 2001;32:753–760.

43. Wojtacki J, Lewicka-Nowak, E, Lesniewski-Kmak K. Anthracycline-induced cardiotoxicity: clinical course, risk factors, pathogenesis, detection and prevention-review of the literature. *Med Sci Monit* 2000;6:411–420.

44. Bandara LR, Kennedy S. Toxicoproteomics: a new preclinical tool. *Drug Discov Today* 2002;7:411–418.

45. Zhang J, Herman EH, Knapton A, et al. SK&F 95654-induced acute cardiovascular toxicity in Sprague-Dawley rats: histopathologic, electron microscopic, and immunohistochemical studies. *Toxicol Pathol* 2002;30:28–40.

46. Pucci-Minafra I, Fontana S, Cancemi P, et al. Proteomic patterns of cultured breast cancer cells and epithelial mammary cells. *Ann N Y Acad Sci* 2002;963:122–139.

47. Wu W, Tang X, Hu W, et al. Identification and validation of metastasis-associated proteins in head and neck cancer cell lines by two-dimensional electrophoresis and mass spectrometry. *Clin Exp Metastasis* 2002;19:319–326.

48. Chevalier S, Macdonald N, Tonge, et al. Proteomic analysis of differential protein expression in primary hepatocytes induced by EGF, tumour necrosis factor alpha or the peroxisome proliferator nafenopin. *Eur J Biochem* 2000;267:4624–4634.

49. Alaiya AA, Franzen B, Hagman A, et al. Molecular classification of borderline ovarian tumors using hierarchical cluster analysis of protein expression profiles. *Int J Cancer* 2002;98:895–899.

50. Verma M, Wright GL Jr, Hamash SM. Preoteomic approaches within the NCI early detection research network for the discovery and identification of cancer biomarkers. *Ann N Y Acad Sci* 2002;945:103–115

51. Myers TG, Anderson NL, Waltham M, et al. A protein expression database for the molecular pharmacology of cancer. *Electrophoresis* 1997;18:647–653.

52. Weinstein JN, Myers TG, O'Connor PM, et al. An information-intensive approach to the molecular pharmacology of cancer. *Science* 1997;275,343–349.

53. Lesko LJ, Atkinson AJ Jr. Use of biomarkers and surrogate endpoints in drug development and regulatory decision making: Criteria, validation, strategies. *Annu Rev Pharmacol Toxicol* 2001;41:347–366.

54. Hill AB. The Environment and Disease: association or Causation? *Proc R Soc Med* 1965;58:295–300.

55. Sikora K. Surrogate endpoints in cancer drug development. *Drug Discov Today* 2002;7:951–956.

56. Jefferys DB, Leakey D, Lewis JA, et al. New active substances authorized in the United Kingdom between 1972 and 1994. *Br J. Clin. Pharmacol* 1998;45:151–156.

57. Lazarou J, Pomeranz BH, Corey PN. Incidence of adverse drug reactions in hospitalised patients. *JAMA* 1998;279:1200–1205.

58. Thomas RS, Rank DR, Penn SG, et al. Identification of toxicologically predictive gene sets using cDNA microarrays. *Mol Pharmacol* 2001;60:1189–1194.

59. Bulera SJ, Eddy SM, Ferguson E, et al. RNA expression in the early characterization of hepatotoxicants in Wistar rats by high-density DNA microarrays. *Hepatology* 2001;33:1239–1258.

60. Pennie WD, Woodyatt NJ, Aldridge TC, et al. Application of genomics to the definition of the molecular basis for toxicity. *Toxicol Lett* 2001;120:353–358.

61. Burczynski ME, McMillian M, Ciervo J, et al. Toxicogenomics-based discrimination of toxic mechanism in HepG2 human hepatoma cells. *Toxicol Sci* 2000;58:399–415

62. Ulrich CM, Robien K, Sparks R. Pharmacogenetics and folate metabolism- a promising direction. *Pharmacogenomics* 2002;3:299–313.

63. Howard LA, Seller EM, Tyndale RF. The role of pharmacogenetically variable cytochrome P450 enzymes. *Pharmacogenomics* 2002;3:185–199.

64. Flamenbaum M. Business strategy for implementation of biomarkers in drug development. *Drug Discov World* 2002;3:9–18.

PART 3

Preclinical Models

10

The Role of *In Vitro* Cell Line, Human Xenograft, and Mouse Allograft Models in Cancer Drug Development

Theodora Voskoglou-Nomikos, Stefan D. Baral, and Lesley K. Seymour

National Cancer Institute of Canada Clinical Trials Group, Queen's University, Kingston, Ontario K7L 3N6, Canada

In the initial stages of cancer drug development, drug candidates are tested in cancer models in the laboratory (Fig. 10.1). The agents that are found to be "active" or "promising" (by a set of predetermined criteria) in such models enter early (phase 1/2) clinical trials, based on the assumption that anticancer activity in the laboratory will ultimately correspond to efficacy in human cancers.

The screening of new agents for efficacy in the laboratory prior to initiating clinical studies is attractive for a number of reasons (Table 10.1). Ideally, these investigations would allow decisions to be made about selecting compounds to test in the clinic (based on demonstration of superior efficacy compared to similar compounds or standard treatments) and which tumor types to target. Preclinical studies that could predict which compounds would be successful in the clinic (or which would fail in the clinic) would allow significant savings in resources and costs, and minimize the exposure of patients to ineffective (and potentially toxic) agents.

Although preclinical models are clearly attractive, there are some caveats worth considering. Much of the work performed to date, using preclinical models to evaluate efficacy, has been done testing traditional cytotoxic drugs; these results may not be relevant when testing drugs that have a different mechanism of action, such as signal-transduction inhibitors. Further, reviews of work done to date suffer from inherent bias, as drug candidates that are abandoned early in development have no clinical data to evaluate.

The success of any preclinical screening program, consisting of a chosen category and kind of experimental model under a certain testing strategy, depends on its predictive value for efficacy in later clinical studies. Although the gold standard of efficacy in clinical studies is an improvement in survival demonstrated in a randomized controlled trial, an accepted surrogate of efficacy is objective response in the phase 2 setting (1–4). Standard criteria (World Health Organization) define an objective response as one when all measurable lesions collectively decrease by 50% or more in cross-sectional area compared to their size prior to treatment, and when this decrease lasts for at least 4 weeks (5). A "complete response" (CR) is defined as the complete disappearance of all measurable lesions, whereas all other responses are termed "partial" (PR). The Response Evaluation Criteria in Solid Tumors (RECIST) criteria (6) recently updated and simplified these principles using unidimensional rather than bidimensional measurements. To date, few published phase 2 trials have reported their results using the RECIST criteria. Generally, a response rate of 20% or more (CR plus PR) has been considered as an indicator of drug activity in phase 2 clinical trials of nonhematologic tumor types (7), but does vary from tumor type to tumor type dependent on the level of response anticipated.

LABORATORY MODELS

There are three well-described categories of laboratory models used for the preclinical testing of drug candidates. These include both *in vivo* (using live animals, allograft and xenograft models) and *in vitro* (using cell lines in culture) models. Within each category a number of different kinds of models exist, usually dependent on the histologic origin of the tumor (site of origin, grade of differentiation), as well as (for *in vivo* models) different sites of implantation (subcutaneous

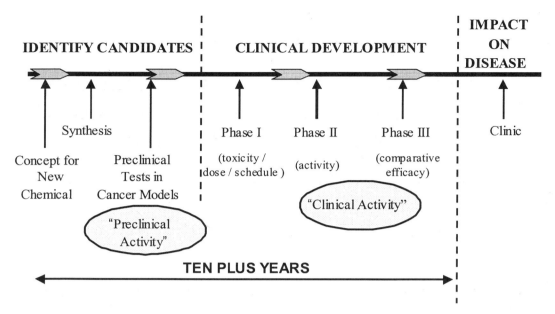

FIG. 10.1. Simplified schematic of the drug discovery process.

versus orthotopic) (8–14) and whether the tumor is metastatic. In addition, the timing of administration of the therapeutic (before implantation, at implantation, established tumors of a predefined size) may affect the conclusions that can be drawn from different models.

Considerations such as tumor types, histology, and how many lines from each kind of cancer to use to build an effective mouse cancer model or tumor cell line screen define the "strategy," or rationale, for using a particular preclinical cancer model. Either compound-oriented or disease-oriented strategies can be used (15). The compound-oriented strategy theo-

rizes that cancer is a complex and diverse group of diseases sharing the same fundamental characteristics that define malignancy. In contrast, the disease-oriented approach adopts the position that cancer is a group of diseases that are collectively associated with malignancy, but that possess distinct biological features and different behaviors and that respond differently to therapeutics. Using the compound-oriented strategy, a drug candidate is screened in only one type of cancer and the results are generalized to all human cancers (Fig. 10.2A). In the case of the disease-oriented approach, multiple tumor types are tested in

TABLE 10.1. *Laboratory models: objectives and required observations*

Objective	Relevant observation
Make decisions about which compounds to select when multiple candidates exist	Demonstration that a drug is better than another candidate and existing standard drugs
Select tumor types for clinical studies	Activity in preclinical models, especially if superior to the effect obtained with standard treatment
Go/No Go decisions: is a drug interesting enough to take forward into development	Demonstration of efficacy superior to standard therapy, or demonstration of a superior therapeutic index (similar efficacy but reduced toxicity)
Evaluate combinations with other agents	Provide information about synergistic, additive, or antagonistic combinations, interactions, and toxicity profiles of combinations

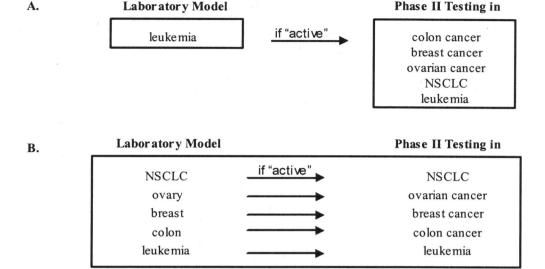

FIG. 10.2. Hypothetical example illustrating the compound-oriented **(A)** and disease-oriented **(B)** strategies.

the laboratory and results are extrapolated to the same human tumor type (Fig. 10.2B).

In Vivo Models

The mouse has been extensively developed as a tumor-bearing animal in the last 40 years and remains the animal of choice for cancer models. Initially, in the 1950s, spontaneously arising or chemically induced tumors of mice were used. However, with the development of technologies for creating immunocompromised mice and, especially, with the discovery of the nude mouse, the transplantation of human tumors in mice became possible (8,9,16). The first such "human xenograft" was created in 1969 (17), and the subsequent years have seen the development and establishment of many human xenografts representing tumors of almost all known types and histologies. The majority of studies to date with the two kinds (murine or human) of mouse models have involved ectopic transplantation of tumor cells; i.e., implantation at a site different from the organ or tissue of tumor origin.

Most commonly, testing of drugs candidates in the ectopic murine allograft or human xenograft models involves the implantation of a prespecified number of cultured tumor cells into a group of animals (usually 10–20) to be used for screening. When the tumor has grown to a small but measurable size, the mice are divided into control and treatment groups (usually of 5–10 animals each), with each group having the same average tumor volume. Animals in the treatment

group are injected with the experimental agent while the control group receives saline or the corresponding drug vehicle. The effect of treatment is then evaluated by scoring drug-induced differences between the two groups over time (8,9,16,18,19).

Studies using the murine allograft and human xenograft models measure one of two parameters of efficacy: tumor size or animal survival (8,18). Differences in tumor size between treated (T) and control (C) groups of animals are most commonly expressed by the percent change in tumor size (T/C%) or by the tumor growth delay/specific growth delay. The measure used to denote differences in survival is the percent increase in life span (ILS%).

Figure 10.3 demonstrates a typical pattern of the tumor and control growth curves in an *in vivo* preclinical model. The percent change in tumor size at a time (t) relative to the start of exposure to drug is defined as T/C% = [(RV$_{treated}$)/(RV$_{control}$)] × 100%, where RV$_{treated}$ and RV$_{control}$ are the relative tumor volumes in the treated and control groups, respectively. The relative tumor volume, RV, in a group at time t is calculated by dividing the average tumor volume of the group at time t with the average tumor volume of the group at the start of treatment. Some investigators prefer to measure growth inhibition (GI%), which is the reverse of T/C% (i.e., T/C% = 100% − GI%) and is arrived at in a similar fashion.

The tumor growth delay (T − C) is defined based on a clinically relative multiple of the initial relative tumor volume. This multiple is most commonly set

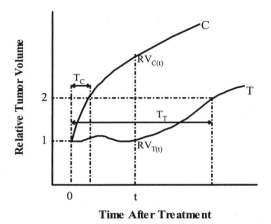

FIG. 10.3. Typical pattern of the tumor growth curve of a mouse xenograft. C, control; T, treated; RV, relative volume; T_C and T_T, time taken by the control and treatment group, respectively.

at 2, as in Figure 10.3, or, less often, at 10. The tumor growth delay is defined as $(T - C) = T_{treated} - T_{control}$, where $T_{treated}$ is the time taken by the treated group to double its initial relative tumor volume and $T_{control}$ is the corresponding time taken by the control group (Fig. 10.3). The specific growth delay (SGD) is a standardized version of the growth delay and is given by the formula $SGD = (T_{treated} - T_{control})/T_{control}$. In practical terms, the SGD is the number of volume doublings that mice in the treated group were spared because of the drug.

The percent increase in life span (ILS%) is defined as the percent increase in the mean time to death of treated animals over the corresponding time to death for untreated mice and is given by the formula $ILS\% = [(\text{mean time to death for treated})/(\text{mean time to death for controls})] - 100\%$.

The criteria for activity in murine allografts and human xenografts are not standardized. Some investigators choose not to set specific rules for activity and to view instead the whole range of measurement values as informative of different degrees of a drug's effectiveness. The majority, however, arbitrarily specify cut-off values and a drug is considered active only when its measure of efficacy falls within these values. In general, and depending on which measure is employed, most investigators consider an experimental drug active in a mouse tumor when the T/C% is less than or equal to 42% (the GI% is at least 58%), the ILS% is at least 25%, or the SGD at least 2 (8). The relevance of these criteria to cytotoxic drug tumor activity in phase 2 clinical trials is unclear.

The main advantage of using murine allografts or human xenografts as cancer models is that the response of a tumor to an experimental drug is studied in the context of a living organism with a fully functional metabolic system and the potential to exhibit possible drug-related toxic effects. For human xenografts in particular, the transplanted tumor generally maintains characteristics of its origin, such as the human histological differentiation, karyotype, cellular DNA content, and isoenzymes (8,9,18). However, a major limitation is that tumor growth and progression in ectopic human xenografts do not match those in humans: subcutaneously xenografted tumors grow as well-circumscribed nodules at the site of transplantation, have stromal tissues that are derived from the host, and they only rarely infiltrate the surrounding tissue and metastasize to other sites (8,9,13). Even orthotopic models, where cells are implanted into the same organ site as origin of the cell line (i.e., pancreas, lung), rarely have the same growth and metastatic potential as in humans. Additionally, tumor-doubling times are considerably faster in mice than in humans (8,14,18).

In Vitro Models

In vitro models are an attractive option for screening purposes due to the relative ease of establishment and maintenance. They allow a large number of drug candidates to be tested in a fraction of the time and for a fraction of the cost of *in vivo* models. Two approaches, resulting in two different kinds of models, are commonly used to test new cancer therapeutics: growth in culture of tumor cells freshly extracted from patients [with the human tumor colony-forming assay (HTCFA) being the most successful of these efforts (20)] and establishment and long-term maintenance of immortalized human tumor cell lines. The HTCFA can be associated with technical difficulties and poor growth rates (15,21–23) and is not currently widely used in drug development, although it is not infrequently used to select therapy for individual patients. In contrast, the establishment and long-term maintenance of human cell lines from all types of cancers has proven more straightforward. Multiple cell lines have now been created and characterized. When used for drug screening, human cancer cell lines are grown in culture, treated with experimental drugs, and observed for drug-induced effects relative to untreated controls.

The main disadvantage of *in vitro* cancer models is their inability to identify useful cancer drugs that require metabolic activation, or conversely to identify compounds that would be rendered inactive by the host's metabolic machinery (24). Additionally, *in vitro* cancer models cannot provide any toxicologic information. Immortalized cell lines in particular have the disadvantage that, by virtue of the process used for their establishment, they are not representative of an *in situ* tumor cell population. Also, the doubling times of human tumor cell lines are much faster than tumors in humans.

The most widely employed parameter of drug effect in *in vitro* cell lines is the GI_{50}, defined as the drug concentration that causes a 50% reduction in cell number in test plates relative to control plates. The GI_{50} is a dose–response related measure (i.e., a dose–response curve is constructed in order to obtain it experimentally) and evaluates a test drug's ability to cause growth inhibition.

The criteria for activity in cell line screens are probably the hardest to define. The difficulty lies with the fact that the measures of drug efficacy in use for cell lines are basically pharmacological measures of potency and the degree of potency of a compound in cultured cells might or might not be related to the extent of its therapeutic value for human tumors. Therefore, most investigators tend to simply look at whether a compound under study can elicit growth inhibition at a reasonably low concentration and the actual drug potency as shown by the specific value of the GI_{50} is considered only secondarily to the observation of a drug effect.

PRECLINICAL CANCER SCREENING PROGRAMS AT THE NATIONAL CANCER INSTITUTE: A HISTORICAL PERSPECTIVE

In the mid-1950s, the discovery that antifolates had activity against leukemia and the reluctance of pharmaceutical companies to commit resources to cancer drug development, led the US Congress to mandate responsibility for cancer drug research to the National Cancer Institute (NCI) (25). As a result, the NCI developed the first comprehensive cancer drug screening program, led the way in cancer drug development from 1955 into the early 1990s, and is responsible for generating much of the knowledge we have today about preclinical cancer models.

Between 1955 and 1969 the only available cancer model was the murine allograft. Although other murine allograft tumor types had been developed, leukemia tumors, especially L1210 and P388, were fast growing and thus both easily handled and cost-effective. In addition, the strategic approach of the time was compound oriented. As a result, the NCI screening programs between 1955 and 1975 used one to three murine allografts, with at least one of them being L1210 or P388 leukemia (25,26) (Table 10.2).

TABLE 10.2. *Historical evolution of* in vivo *screening programs at the National Cancer Institute before 1975*

Year	Screening program
1955	Leukemia L1210, sarcoma 180, carcinoma 755
1960	Leukemia L1210 plus two models from a pool of 21
1965	Leukemia L1210 plus Walker carcinoma 256
1968	Leukemia L1210 and leukemia P388
1972	Leukemia L1210 and leukemia P388; B16 melanoma and Lewis lung carcinoma for special testing

Modified from Staquet MJ, Byar DP, Green SB, et al. Clinical predictivity of transplantable tumor systems in the selection of new drugs for solid tumors: rationale for a three-stage strategy. *Cancer Treat Rep* 1983; 67:753–765.

By 1973 it had become clear that these leukemia-based, compound-oriented preclinical screening programs predominantly identified drugs with activity on human leukemias and lymphomas, while the most prevalent solid tumors (colon, lung, breast, ovary, melanoma) were essentially unresponsive to the new therapies (27,28). In 1975, the NCI cancer drug screening program was redesigned (29,30) to include a panel of murine allografts of slower-growing solid tumors in addition to the leukemias in order to move towards a more disease-oriented approach. It also incorporated a second model, the human xenograft, which had recently been developed (17) (Fig. 10.4). Cost and time considerations necessitated two strategies: a prescreen to narrow down the number of compounds tested in the panel of eight xenografts/allografts and, that, for most tumors, only one experimental tumor per tumor type per model could be used in the panel (Fig. 10.4). As P388 leukemia was selected as the prescreen and activity in any one of the xenografts in the panel advanced a test compound to phase 2 testing in all five types of cancer, the NCI screening program implemented in 1975 remained essentially compound-oriented.

In the late 1980s, in search of a truly disease-oriented screen, the NCI turned its attention to the faster and cheaper *in vitro* test systems. The intent was to use such systems in the place of the P388 screen so as to select truly disease-specific compounds for further testing in human xenografts. The HTCFA, first developed in 1977, was initially considered. It involved the collection of tumor samples from cancer patients and their disassociation into single cell suspensions that were treated either with the drug under study or with drug vehicle. Plating an equal number of the treated and control cells in suspension in two separate plates of soft agar and comparing the number of colonies formed in those plates then tested drug sensitivity. The HTCFA was deemed a good candidate for drug screening because the colonies formed on soft agar retained the morphological and histochemical characteristics of the tumor of origin (31) and because studies showed that there was a high degree of correlation (overall 69% true-positive and 91% true-negative rate) between drug sensitivity and resistance patterns in the HTCFA and the original tumor in patients (21,23,32,33). In addition, it was found that the HTCFA was able to categorize most standard cancer drugs as active and 97% of clinically ineffective compounds as inactive. However, the assay showed serious technical limitations with wide variability among tumor types in their colony-forming efficiency. Thus, despite other reports showing the HTCFA to have a high predictive value (34), immortalized human tumor cell lines were pursued instead as an *in vitro*, disease-oriented screening system.

To facilitate the development of a human tumor cell line screen, the NCI first collected over 100 cell lines from all major human tumor types and from different representative histologies within each tumor type (35). These lines were tested for their growth characteristics, their ability to produce tumors of the appropriate histology when transplanted into nude mice, and for the degree to which they had retained the important characteristics of their tumor of origin. Next, three possible detection assays (the MTT, XTT, and SRB assays) suited to high-volume cell line screening were investigated (36,37), and a technical feasibility study was conducted (1). Finally the NCI

DTP human tumor cell line screen was implemented in 1990 (38) and remains in use until today.

As part of the screen, the NCI maintains in excess of 80 different human cell lines from the most common adult tumors of leukemia, breast, lung, colon, brain, ovary, prostate, kidney, and melanoma. In this collection, there are 2 to 12 cell lines from each tumor type, selected to represent different histologies and common drug resistance profiles. Each drug that enters the screen is tested on a panel of 60 to 75 cell lines; the particular selection varies from time to time. The screening protocol (39) (Fig. 10.5) involves plating the cell lines in 96-well plates for 24 hours and then treating them with drug (treatment plates), added in five 10-fold dilutions (usual starting range is 10^{-8}–10^{-4} mol/L), or vehicle (control plates). After 48 hours of drug exposure, the cells are washed and the protein content in each plate is determined by the SRB assay. This involves fixing and staining of the cells and measurement of optical density of fluid in wells. Absorbance densities of the treated and control plates are finally used to construct dose–response curves for each cell line, which allow the determination of GI_{50} values. The assay is automated and computerized and has the capacity to screen 10,000 to 15,000 compounds a year. The screen has been shown to be reproducible over several passages of cell lines and different drug preparations (38,39).

To meet the main objective of identifying drug leads with selective activity against particular tumor types, investigators at the NCI devised the "mean graph" (40). Simply, the mean graph of a test compound is a bar graph presentation of the 60 to 75 GI_{50} values obtained from testing that compound in the cell

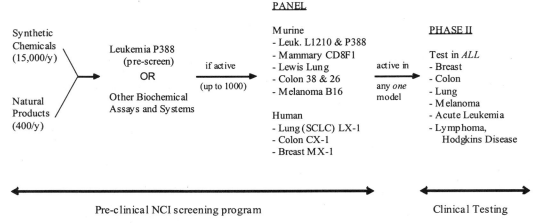

FIG. 10.4. National Cancer Institute screen 1975–1983. Modified from Venditti JM. Preclinical drug development: rationale and methods. *Semin Oncol* 1981; 8:349–353.

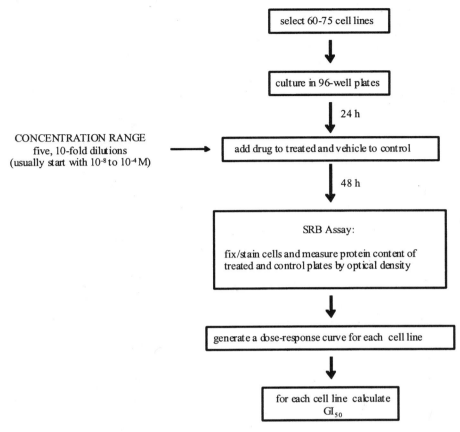

CONCENTRATION RANGE
five, 10-fold dilutions
(usually start with 10^{-8} to 10^{-4} M)

select 60-75 cell lines

culture in 96-well plates

24 h

add drug to treated and vehicle to control

48 h

SRB Assay:

fix/stain cells and measure protein content of treated and control plates by optical density

generate a dose-response curve for each cell line

for each cell line calculate GI_{50}

FIG. 10.5. National Cancer Institute *in vitro* cell line screen protocol.

line panel of the NCI, with the specific feature being that it relates the magnitude of every individual cell line GI_{50} to the mean GI_{50} for all the cell lines (Fig. 10.6). To construct such a graph, all the GI_{50}s resulting from the tumor cell line screen of a compound are first converted to log(10) values and then averaged. The magnitude of the log(10) of each GI_{50} is then plotted as a bar to the right or the left of a vertical line, which represents the log(10) of the average GI_{50} value over all the cell lines. Bars on the right and the left of the vertical line denote cell lines more or less sensitive than average, respectively, to the test drug. In the example of the GI_{50} mean graph of menogaril shown in Figure 10.6, two patterns of tumor selectivity are readily obvious: the drug is selectively active against leukemia (five out of six cell lines tested are more sensitive than average) and selectively inactive against colon tumors (seven out of nine cell lines tested are less sensitive than average).

CLINICAL PREDICTIVE VALUE OF PRECLINICAL CANCER MODELS

NCI Screening Programs

The parameters measured and criteria used for activity in the 1975 NCI screening program (Fig. 10.4) are shown in detail in Table 10.3 (30). Using these definitions of preclinical antitumor activity and the standard phase 2 trial response criteria, four studies investigated the predictive value of the NCI preclinical program implemented in 1975. Goldin et al. (41) examined the performance of the screen as of 1980 and concluded that drugs with high preclinical activity in a variety of experimental tumor types usually had at least minimal activity in the clinic for one or more human cancers. Overall, the murine allografts were more likely to declare a compound active than the human xenografts. Human xenografts in the panel were relatively resistant to drugs, similar to

GI₅₀ Mean Graph for Compound S269148 Results from the National Cancer Institute Human Tumor Cell Line Screen

GI_{50} Mean Graph for Compound S269148 Results from the National Cancer Institute Human Tumor Cell Line Screen

These results provided by the Developmental Therapeutics Program, DCTD, NCI

Highest concentration tested is 1.0E-04 M; Average GI_{50} over all cell lines is 7.7E-07 M

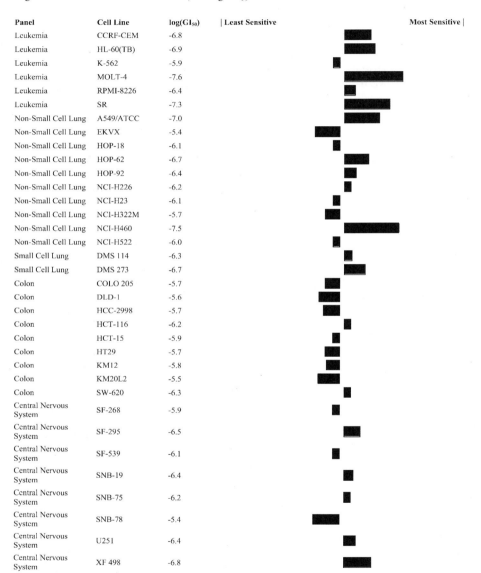

Panel	Cell Line	log(GI_{50})		Least Sensitive	Most Sensitive	
Leukemia	CCRF-CEM	-6.8	
Leukemia	HL-60(TB)	-6.9	
Leukemia	K-562	-5.9	
Leukemia	MOLT-4	-7.6	
Leukemia	RPMI-8226	-6.4	
Leukemia	SR	-7.3	
Non-Small Cell Lung	A549/ATCC	-7.0	
Non-Small Cell Lung	EKVX	-5.4	
Non-Small Cell Lung	HOP-18	-6.1	
Non-Small Cell Lung	HOP-62	-6.7	
Non-Small Cell Lung	HOP-92	-6.4	
Non-Small Cell Lung	NCI-H226	-6.2	
Non-Small Cell Lung	NCI-H23	-6.1	
Non-Small Cell Lung	NCI-H322M	-5.7	
Non-Small Cell Lung	NCI-H460	-7.5	
Non-Small Cell Lung	NCI-H522	-6.0	
Small Cell Lung	DMS 114	-6.3	
Small Cell Lung	DMS 273	-6.7	
Colon	COLO 205	-5.7	
Colon	DLD-1	-5.6	
Colon	HCC-2998	-5.7	
Colon	HCT-116	-6.2	
Colon	HCT-15	-5.9	
Colon	HT29	-5.7	
Colon	KM12	-5.8	
Colon	KM20L2	-5.5	
Colon	SW-620	-6.3	
Central Nervous System	SF-268	-5.9	
Central Nervous System	SF-295	-6.5	
Central Nervous System	SF-539	-6.1	
Central Nervous System	SNB-19	-6.4	
Central Nervous System	SNB-75	-6.2	
Central Nervous System	SNB-78	-5.4	
Central Nervous System	U251	-6.4	
Central Nervous System	XF 498	-6.8	

FIG. 10.6. GI_{50} (the drug concentration that causes a 50% reduction in cell number in test plates relative to control plates) mean graph for menogaril (10^{-8}–10^{-4} mol/L). Only 35 of the 71 cell lines tested are shown.

what is generally observed in the clinic, and murine allografts yielded many false-positive compounds. In addition, there was a "partial correspondence of activity" between xenografts and human patients of the same tumor type. A small study by Marsoni and Wittes (42) examined 13 drugs for which experimental and clinical data were available and concluded that most of the murine allografts and human xenografts of the NCI panel were reliable at predicting true-negative results, but had very low probabil-

TABLE 10.3. *Parameters and criteria of activity for the xenografts/allografts in the 1975 National Cancer Institute screening programs*

Tumor	Parameter		Criteria for activity	
			Low	High
Leukemia P388	Survival	ILS%:	20	75
Leukemia L1210	Survival	ILS%:	25	50
Melanoma B16	Survival	ILS%:	25	50
Lewis lung	Survival	ILS%:	25	50
Mammary CD8F1	Tumor volume	T/C%:	≤42	≤10
Colon 38	Tumor volume	T/C%:	≤42	≤10
Breast MX-1	Tumor volume	T/C%:	≤20	≤10
Colon CX-1	Tumor volume	T/C%:	≤20	≤10
Lung LX-1	Tumor volume	T/C%:	≤20	≤10

ILS%, percent increase in life span; T/C%, percent change in tumor size between treatment and control groups.
Modified from Venditti JM. Preclinial drug development: rationale and methods. *Semin Oncol* 1981;8:349–353.

ity of determining true-positive compounds. An internal evaluation conducted by the NCI in 1983 (43,44) showed that leukemia P388 had performed satisfactorily as a prescreen, but that many of the tumors in the panel of xenografts were redundant. A non-NCI team of investigators (45) reached a similar conclusion, and additionally noted that the screen's predictive value was low. A new version of the screen, including a modified panel of xenografts and an additional secondary screening step, was thus proposed (43–45) (Fig. 10.7).

In addition to its clinical predictive value, the 1975 preclinical cancer drug screening program of the NCI was evaluated for its yield of antitumor drugs. An analysis of phase 2 clinical trials conducted between 1970 and 1985 showed that among the 75 drugs selected by the NCI for phase 2 testing, only 24 had activity in humans (46). More importantly, it was shown that among the active agents, 74% targeted lymphoma and 35% targeted leukemia, and that even for the most responsive solid tumors, such as breast and small cell lung cancer (SCLC), the number of active drugs was small. Thus, it appeared that the 1975 multitumor type, murine allograft/human xenograft screen did not improve the preferential discovery of drugs active against leukemias and lymphomas.

The most recent study regarding the predictive value of NCI preclinical cancer models was reported

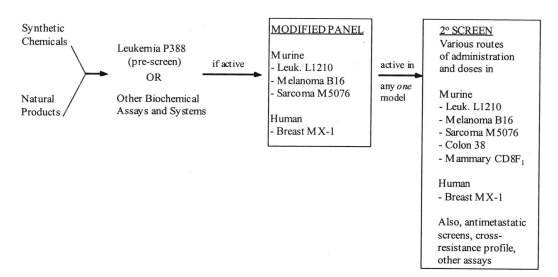

FIG. 10.7. National Cancer Institute screen, 1983–1990.

TABLE 10.4. *Summary of National Cancer Institute screening programs*

Years in use	Description of screen	Advantages	Shortcomings	Reference(s)
Pre-1975	One to three murine allografts, at least one leukemia	Few, fast growing, test tumors— easy to handle, low cost. Animal models— allowed examination of metabolic effect and toxicity profile of test compounds	Preferential selection of compounds with activity in hematologic tumors	25–28
1975–1983	P388 leukemia pre screen. Panel of five murine allografts and three human xenografts	Solid tumor types and leukemia. Human tumors included. Animal models	Low predictive value yielded many false positives; low probability of identifying true positives. Preferential selection of compounds with activity in hematologic tumors	29,30, 41–45
1983–1990	P388 leukemia pre-screen. Modified panel of three murine allografts and one human xenograft. Secondary screen: panel of five murine allografts and one human xenograft plus other assays	Exclusion of "redundant" allografts/xenografts. Earlier elimination of inactive compounds (modified panel). More extensive preclinical testing on active agents (secondary screen). Animal models	Similar to the 1975–1983 screen	43–45
1990 to date	*In vitro* human tumor cell line screen used as a pre-screen to select compounds for further testing (human xenografts, hollow fiber assay, other assays)	Truly disease oriented. Rapid, high-throughput, and cost-effective. Compounds can be compared based on their mean graph patterns	Metabolic/toxic effects cannot be studied in the *in vitro* pre-screen	35–40

by Johnson et al. (47). A complex series of correlations was examined. Of interest to this chapter, activity in the *in vitro* cell line screen was correlated with activity in human xenografts (using chi-square tests) and activity in human xenografts was correlated with activity of phase 2 clinical trials (using Spearman rank correlation coefficients). In phase 2 clinical trials, activity was defined as a response rate greater than 20%. In human xenografts of solid tumors two levels of activity were considered, T/C% less than 40% and T/C% less than 10%. Finally, for the *in vitro* cell line screen activity was considered in relation to the number of cell lines within a tumor-specific panel that were "selectively" active; i.e., that had a smaller GI_{50}

than the mean GI_{50} across all cell lines in the screen. With the exception of non–small cell lung cancer (NSCLC), preclinical activity in human xenografts of a particular tumor type did not correlate significantly with phase 2 activity in the same kind of tumor; with the exception of breast and colon tumors, human xenografts did not significantly predict phase 2 clinical activity in other cancers types. Compounds that were active in at least one third of all tested human xenografts were likely to have at least some activity in phase 2 clinical trials. Finally, for lung and breast cancers only, the greater the number of cell lines in the *in vitro* human cell line screen for which a compound was selectively active the greater the likelihood that this compound would be found active in the corresponding human xenograft models.

A summary of NCI preclinical screening programs together with their advantages and shortcomings is provided in Table 10.4.

Other Studies of the Clinical Predictive Value of Preclinical Models

Studies on the clinical predictive value of *in vivo* preclinical cancer models conducted outside of the auspices of the NCI are relatively limited (Table 10.5).

In 1979, Bellet et al. (48) used a panel of seven subcutaneously implanted human melanoma xenografts to evaluate the activity of four agents of known clinical profiles. Volume was measured as the parameter of efficacy, but none of the usual volume measures

(e.g., T/C%, GI%) was employed. Instead, tumor volumes for treated and control animals were measured every week, a comparison was made between the two groups using a *t* test, and a drug was considered active if a statistically significant difference was found. The authors observed that four and one of the seven melanoma tumors were sensitive to the drugs DTIC and BCNU, respectively, which had shown promise in the clinic, while no xenograft responded to the clinically ineffective drugs adriamycin and 5-azacytidine. They concluded that the human xenograft model was a potentially predictive screen and argued that the model should be used in the form of a panel of tumors from each tumor type. However, DTIC and BCNU have not proven particularly useful in melanoma in subsequent study; therefore, the conclusions of Bellet et al. may have been flawed.

TABLE 10.5. *Studies on the clinical predictive value of the human xenograft model 1979–1994 (non–National Cancer Institute)*

Year	Study	Findings	Reference(s)
1979	Evaluated four drugs of known clinical profile in melanoma against a panel of seven melanoma xenografts	Promising trends	48
1980	Evaluated six drugs and two drug combinations of known clinical activity in breast cancer against a panel of five breast xenografts	Some of the preclinical results were in agreement with clinical findings	49
1983	Evaluated 17 drugs with known clinical activity in breast cancer against the breast xenograft MX-1	The model correctly identified as active seven out of eight clinically useful drugs; it incorrectly identified as active five out of eight drugs with no efficacy in humans	50
1983	Looked at the three most clinically active drugs in six different cancers; for each tumor, compared mean response rates in phase 2 clinical trials to mean preclinical activity in a panel of xenografts	Very good correspondence between preclinical and clinical results	18
1987	Evaluated 10 established cancer drugs against seven melanoma and three ovarian xenografts	Correspondence between preclinical and clinical activity was poor for melanoma and moderate for ovarian cancer	51
1988	Compared "response rate in xenografts" with response rate in phase 2 clinical trials for various cancer types	Generally a good correspondence; xenografts tended to overestimate clinical efficacy	8
1988–1994	Tested seven drugs in disease-specific panels of xenografts; compared with clinical experience	Inconclusive	52–54

Bailey et al. (49) tested a panel of five human breast xenografts of different histologies with six drugs and two drug combinations. They measured SGD as the endpoint, but avoided setting specific criteria for activity. Instead, they recorded all the individual SGD values and, for each tested drug, calculated a mean SDG over all the five xenografts under study. They found that in human breast xenografts, as in the clinic, combination chemotherapy was more active than single agents. Also in agreement with clinical experience was the observation of considerable variation in the responsiveness of the five experimental tumors. However, melphalan was the most active single agent among the ones tested (adriamycin, cyclophosphamide, fluorouracil, vincristine and methotrexate) in xenografts.

In contrast to Bellet and Bailey, Inoue et al. (50) investigated the preclinical/clinical correlation afforded by a single human xenograft rather than a panel. They used the breast xenograft MX-1 to test 17 drugs of known clinical activity. Of the eight drugs with very good clinical activity in breast cancer (phase 2 single-agent response rates of 20%–37%), five showed a very high growth inhibition (i.e., G.I.% more than 90%) in MX-1, two exhibited moderate inhibition of about 75%, and one was inactive.

Steel et al. (18) reviewed the results obtained with human xenografts of several tumor types prior to 1983 in the Institute of Cancer Research in Sutton, United Kingdom, and attempted to correlate them with published clinical results. Specifically, they calculated the SGD values of a few clinically useful cancer drugs for every one of six tumor types, represented by more than one xenograft line (three to ten) each. Based on these results, the three most effective single agents were selected in every tumor type and the corresponding three SGD values were averaged. Thus, six average SGD values, one for each of the tumors types studied in the human xenograft model, were obtained. They were then compared with published averaged complete response rates (thought to reflect general clinical experience) from clinical trials. The agreement was very good: testicular teratoma, SCLC, and breast cancer, which had the three highest average SGDs in human xenografts (5.7, 4.2, and 1.9, respectively), also had the three highest clinical response rates, which followed the same rank order (70%, 31%, and 15.3%, respectively). In contrast, melanoma, colorectal cancer, and NSCLC, which had the three lowest SGD values (1.0, 0.76, and 0.54, respectively), had three equally low clinical response rates (4%, 3%, and 5%, respectively).

Taetle et al. (51) looked at the response of seven human melanoma and three human ovarian xenografts to 10 established cancer drugs. They employed the rather unusual measure of "growth delay index," which was calculated based on the regression lines fitted to tumor growth curves and quantitated a drug's effect over the entire length of treatment. They found that the results obtained with the seven melanoma xenografts did not correlate well with clinical experience. In contrast, the three human ovarian xenografts correctly identified three clinically active drugs in ovarian cancer (melphalan, doxorubicin, and cisplatin).

Mattern (8) reviewed the results of multiple drugs in many different human xenografts of various cancer types and tabulated them alongside results from clinical trials on the corresponding disease populations. Activity in xenografts was based on the criteria of T/C% equal to or less than 42% (GI is equal to or more than 58%), ILS% equal to or more than 25%, or SGD equal to or more than 2. Then he devised the concept of "response rate in xenografts," defined as the number of xenografts of a given tumor type in which a drug was active (by the previous criteria) over the total number of human xenografts of that tumor type the drug was tested on. He noted that there was a generally "good" correspondence by tumor type between published response rates in patients and in human xenografts, despite the fact that xenografts tended to overestimate the actual numerical values of clinical response rates. It should be noted, however, that no formal statistical methods were used.

Finally, a European prospective study, carried out by the European Organization for Research on the Treatment of Cancer, looked at the clinical predictive value of the human xenograft model using a disease-oriented approach (52–54). The study involved testing a handful of drugs on a panel of human xenografts, selected to include four to eight different histologies from each of seven types of cancer, namely, breast, colon, head and neck, NSCLC, SCLC, melanoma, and ovarian cancer. The T/C% and SGD were used for measuring activity in xenografts and the criteria were T/C% greater than or equal to 50 or SGD less than or equal to 1 for "inactive," T/C% greater than or equal to 25 and less than 50 or SGD greater than 1 and less than or equal to 2 for "active," T/C% less than 25 or SGD greater than 2 for "very active," and complete remissions for "highly active." No formal criteria of clinical activity or statistical methods were employed in the assessment of correlations. The authors referred to a drug's "known activity" or "lack of activity" in the clinic, as gleaned from review articles. Human xenograft panel profiles of doxorubicin and amsacrine were found to be predictive of their clinical behavior. For cisplatin, xenografts were only "reasonably" predictive of clinical activity while diaziquone (AZQ) was much more active in the panel of xenografts than it proved to be in patients. Four other compounds that were in early clinical development at the time of the study were also tested in the xenograft panel (brequinar sodium, datelliptium, pazelliptine, and retelliptine), but no further information was provided.

Recent Studies Examining the Clinical Predictive Value of NCI and Other Preclinical Models

The majority of studies to date, both within and outside the NCI, have based their conclusions on the observation of trends rather than the use of statistical methods, and have utilized dichotomous definitions of preclinical and/or clinical activity based on largely unvalidated "cut-off" values of measures of activity: a 20% response rate in phase 2 clinical trials and (most commonly) a 42% T/C% in human xenografts and mouse allografts. Two important questions have not been addressed clearly by previous studies: the clinical predictive value of the *in vitro* cell line as a preclinical model in its own right and the relative clinical usefulness of the different preclinical cancer models in use today.

We recently reported a study comparing the clinical phase 2 predictive value of the *in vitro* human cell line, the mouse allograft, and the human xenograft (55) using quantitative measures of both clinical and preclinical activity and formal statistical methods. We considered three relevant questions: the clinical predictive value of the three models within the same tumor type (disease-oriented approach), the clinical predictive value of the three models when one preclinical tumor type is used as a predictor of overall clinical activity in all other tumor types (compound-oriented approach), and the clinical predictive value of the three models when overall preclinical and clinical activity in all tumor types combined is considered.

A group of cancer drugs that had undergone phase 1 clinical testing in 1991 or 1992 was identified. Data relating to phase 2 trials, human xenograft, and mouse allograft studies in breast, NSCLC, ovary, and colon cancers were obtained from the literature. For each drug, clinical activity was scored as the response rate across all phase 2 trials of the same tumor type and preclinical activity as the mean T/C% across all xenografts/allografts of the same disease site. Publicly available data from the NCI human tumor cell line screen (mean graphs) were used to calculate two measures of drug *in vitro* preclinical activity for each of the four cancer types: the mean $Log10GI_{50}$, computed by averaging the $Log10GI_{50}$ values from all the cell lines of that tumor type in the mean graph and a measure we termed the "activity fraction," arbitrarily defined as the number of cell lines of a given tumor type that were more sensitive than average to the drug over the total number of cell lines from that tumor type in the mean graph. Overall phase 2 and preclinical activities were also calculated (for NSCLC, breast, colon, and/or ovary combined) by averaging the individual tumor type activities.

For each preclinical cancer model, nine phase 2 versus preclinical activity relationships were examined, for a total of 27: relationships by tumor type (disease-oriented approach, four relationships per model), predictive ability of one tumor type for the other three tumor types combined (compound-oriented approach, four relationships per model), and general predictive ability for all four tumor types combined (one relationship per model). Depending on preclinical and clinical data availability for each tumor type, correlations were examined for between five and 17 drugs.

In the *in vitro* cell line model, when the mean $Log10GI_{50}$ was used as the measure of preclinical activity, significant negative correlations were found for NSCLC, for breast or ovarian cell lines versus overall phase 2 activity in the other three tumor types and for preclinical activity versus phase 2 activity in all four tumor types. No significant correlations were obtained when the activity fraction was employed as a preclinical activity measure.

No significant correlations between preclinical and clinical activity were observed for the human xenograft model. However, when the relationships were reanalyzed to include only the drugs for which preclinical information on *panels* of human xenografts was available, the activity relationship for NSCLC became statistically significant and a highly significant correlation was seen for ovarian cancer. A near-significant correlation was obtained when ovarian human xenograft panels were used to predict clinical activity in the other three tumor types combined. No significant correlations between preclinical and clinical activity were observed for any of the relationships examined for the murine allograft model.

In regard to the human xenograft model, a more detailed examination of the NSCLC and ovarian xenograft panels was conducted. As seen in Figures 10.8A and 10.9A, panels of NSCLC and ovarian human xenografts that were used to test each of six and seven different compounds, respectively, showed no similarities in numbers or content. Detailed analysis of ovarian panels by histology/grade was hindered by lack of detailed information for many of the xenografts (Fig. 10.8B, "unspecified"),

A.

NAME	HISTOLOGY / GRADE	DATA POINTS (DRUGS)					
		EPIRUBICIN	FOSQUIDONE	GEMCITABINE	MENOGARIL	TAXOTERE	PACLITAXEL
MRI-H-207	undifferentiated	+	+		+	+	
A2780	undifferentiated	+		+	+		+
Ov.He	mod. diff, mucinous	+	+	+	+		
Ov.Me	carcinosarcoma	+	+		+		
OvRiC	mod. diff, serous	+	+	+	+		
Fma	poorly diff., mucinous	+	+		+	+	
Ov.Pe	mod. diff, mucinous	+	+	+	+	+	
Fco	clear cell sarcoma	+	+		+		
T17	cystoadenocarcinoma	+					
T385	adenocarcinoma	+					
OvGR	mod. diff, mucinous		+				
Fko	mod. diff, serous		+	+		+	
OvG1	poorly diff., serous		+				
OVCAR-3	adenocarcinoma			+		+	+
A121a	?					+	+
HOC18	poorly diff., serous					+	+
HOC22	poorly diff., serous					+	+
A2780/DDP	undifferentiated						+
A2780/DX	undifferentiated						+
SKOV-3	adenocarcinoma						+
1° ovary 1	cystoadenocarcinoma						+
1° ovary 2	dediff. serous adenoc.						+
IGROV 1	moderately diff.						+
OVCAR-8	Poor;y diff. adenoc.						+
OVCAR-5	adenocarcinoma						+
OvSh	poorly diff., serous					+	
HOC22-S	poorly diff., serous					+	
TOTAL NO.		10	10	6	8	10	13

B.

HISTOLOGY/GRADE FREQUENCIES IN HUMAN OVARIAN XENOGRAFT PANELS						
HISTOLOGY / GRADE	EPIRUBICIN NO. (%)	FOSQUIDONE NO. (%)	GEMCITABINE NO. (%)	MENOGARIL NO. (%)	TAXOTERE NO. (%)	PACLITAXEL NO. (%)
undifferentiated	2 (20)	1 (10)	1 (17)	2 (25)	1 (10)	3 (23)
mod. diff, mucinous	2 (20)	3 (30)	2 (33)	2 (25)	1 (10)	0 (0)
mod. diff, serous	1 (10)	2 (20)	2 (33)	1 (13)	1 (10)	0 (0)
poorly diff., mucinous	1 (10)	1 (10)	0 (0)	1 (13)	1 (10)	0 (0)
poorly diff., serous	0 (0)	1 (10)	0 (0)	0 (0)	4 (40)	2 (15)
unspecified	4 (40)	2 (20)	1 (17)	2 (25)	2 (20)	8 (62)
TOTAL	10 (100)	10 (100)	6 (100)	8 (100)	10 (100)	13 (100)

FIG. 10.8. Human ovarian xenograft panels for the six data points (drugs) included in the phase 2 versus preclinical activity correlation analysis for ovarian cancer (55). **A:** Names and histologies/grades ("?" indicates unknown; mod. diff., moderately differentiated; poorly diff., poorly differentiated; dediff., dedifferentiated; adenoc., adenocarcinoma) of all the xenografts tested. Inclusion of a xenograft in one of the panels is shown by a "+" sign in the corresponding row and under the appropriate drug column. **B:** Histology/grade frequencies in the human ovarian xenograft panels, by number and percentage ('unspecified" refers to xenografts for which histology and/or grade was not available).

A.

XEN. NAME	XENOGRAFT HISTOLOGY	DRUGS						
		EPI	FAZ	GEM	IRINO	PACLIT	TOPO	VINRLB
T222	epidermoid carc.	+						
T291	adenocarcinoma	+						
UCLA-P3	adenocarcinoma		+					
ACCOLU-78	squamous cell		+					
NCI-H460	large cell			+	+	+	+	+
A549	adenocarcinoma			+	+	+	+	+
CaLu-6	adenocarcinoma			+				
H-74	?			+				
LC-376	?			+				
QG-56	squamous cell				+			+
NCI-H23	adenocarcinoma				+	+		
NCI-H226	squamous cell				+	+	+	
MV-522	adenocarcinoma					+		
CaLu-3	adenocarcinoma					+		
1° NSCLC	adenocarcinoma					+		
L2987	adenocarcinoma					+		
L-27	adenocarcinoma							+
LC-06	large cell							+
LU-65	large cell							+
PC-12	adenocarcinoma							+
LU-99	large cell							+
TOTAL NO.		2	2	5	5	8	3	8

B.

HISTOLOGY FREQUENCY IN HUMAN NSCLC XENOGRAFT PANELS							
HISTOLOGY	EPI NO. (%)	FAZ NO. (%)	GEM NO. (%)	IRINO NO. (%)	PACLIT NO. (%)	TOPO NO. (%)	VINORLB NO. (%)
adenocarcinoma	1 (50)	1 (50)	2 (40)	2 (40)	6 (75)	1 (33)	3 (37.5)
large cell	0 (0)	0 (0)	1 (20)	1 (20)	1 (12.5)	1 (33)	4 (50)
squamous cell	1 (50)	1 (50)	0 (0)	2 (40)	1 (12.5)	1 (33)	1 (12.5)
unknown				2 (40)			
TOTAL	2 (100)	2 (100)	5 (100)	5 (100)	8 (100)	3 (100)	8 (100)

C. NSCLC VS NSCLC (ADDITIONAL DATA)

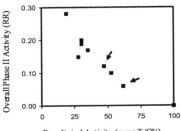

FIG. 10.9. Human non–small cell lung cancer (NSCLC) xenograft panels for the seven data points (drugs) included in the phase 2 versus preclinical activity correlation analysis for NSCLC (55). **A:** Drug names (EPI, epirubicin; FAZ, fazarabine; GEM, gemcitabine; IRINO, irinotecan; PACLIT, paclitaxel; TOPO, topotecan; VINRLB, vinorelbine) and histologies ("?" indicates unknown) of all the xenografts tested. Inclusion of a xenograft in one of the panels is shown by a "+" sign in the corresponding row and under the appropriate drug column. **B:** Histologic frequency in the human NSCLC xenograft panels, by number and percentage. **C:** Scatter plot and correlation analysis for the clinical vs. preclinical activity relationship in NSCLC, including the seven original data points (55) plus two additional agents, doxorubicin and amsacrine (arrows) with known activities in phase 2 trials and NSCLC xenograft panels. The star indicates statistical significance at the 5% level.

A.

	DRUG	PHASE II RESPONSE RATE	HUMAN OVARIAN XENOGRAFT MEAN T/C%
STUDY DRUGS	EPIRUBICIN	0.20	42
	FOSQUIDONE	0.00	72
	GEMCITABINE	0.16	36
	MENOGARIL	0.12	58
	PACLITAXEL	0.26	30
	TAXOTERE	0.27	13
ADDITIONAL DRUGS	DOXORUBICIN	0.19 [58–61]	47
	AMSACRINE	0.05 [62]	75
	CISPLATIN	0.25 [63,64]	41
	HEXAMETHYL-MELAMINE	0.19 [65–70]	28
	METHOTREXATE	0.09 [71,72]	76
	5-FU	0.10 [73–82]	71

B.

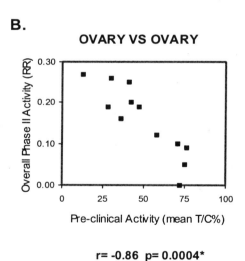

r= -0.86 p= 0.0004*

FIG. 10.10. **A:** Preclinical and phase 2 clinical activity data for ovarian cancer, including the six drugs from the original analysis ("study drugs") as well as an additional six drugs ("additional drugs") with known ovarian phase 2 and human xenograft activities (55). Literature references for phase 2 response rates are shown in superscript font next to the corresponding response rates. **B:** Scatter plots and correlation analysis for the clinical versus preclinical activity relationship in ovarian cancer based on the data in A. The star indicates statistical significance at the 5% level.

but, in general, all panels contained 10% to 20% undifferentiated tumors. Additionally, all panels included both poorly differentiated and moderately differentiated subtypes (Figs. 10.8A and 10.8B). For NSCLC panels, common characteristics included that the majority contained adenocarcinoma, large cell and squamous cell carcinoma histologies, and that the adenocarcinoma content was higher than 30% in all cases (Fig. 10.9B).

In order to see whether panels of xenografts with the previously discussed characteristics could provide clinically predictive results for drugs other than the ones used in this study, the literature was reviewed for additional data. Six more agents with known overall phase 2 response rates in patients with ovarian cancer were found. All had been tested in panels of human ovarian xenografts with similar characteristics as the ones shown in Figure 10.8B. For NSCLC, phase 2 activity and preclinical results in panels conforming to the common characteristics described above were obtained on two additional agents, amsacrine and doxorubicin (53,62,83). As shown in Figures 10.9C and 10.10B, significant correlations were maintained in both cancer types when these additional data points were included in the analysis.

CONCLUSIONS

The work that has been done to date on the clinical predictive value of preclinical cancer models has only partially substantiated the widely held assumption that drug activity in the laboratory is predictive of activity in phase 2 clinical trials. Nonetheless, it seems that *in vitro* cell line and human xenograft models (when used as panels) can be useful in predicting the phase 2 clinical trial performance of cancer drugs.

Published data suggest that the murine allograft model is not predictive of clinical performance and that its continued use in drug development (at least for cytotoxic agents) may not be justified. Further, the NCI's experience with its cancer drug screening programs from 1955 to 1990 as well as recent evidence suggest that leukemia laboratory models are not reliable predictors of activity in solid tumors, although they are efficient in selecting drugs active in hematologic malignancies. Nonetheless, as demonstrated by the results of Johnson et al. and our own data, the compound-oriented approach can be successful when applied within the context of solid tumors.

The ectopic human xenograft model appears to be of clinical relevance for some but not all cancer types. Panels of xenografts with specific characteristics appear to enhance the predictive value of this model for NSCLC and ovarian cancers and recent data suggest that such "appropriate" panels should be explored for other tumor types.

The emerging role of the *in vitro* cell line model, in the context of the NCI *in vitro* human cell line screen, is intriguing. The *in vitro* human tumor cell line screen can be a successful prescreen for some tumor types. Results suggest that this model could also be used as a preclinical cancer model in its own right with predictive value at least as good as the one afforded by the human xenograft.

Preclinical models clearly have utility in cancer drug development and can assist in selecting drugs for development and tumor types to target in the clinic with some success. Unfortunately, no data are yet available regarding the utility of these models in the preclinical testing of novel agents such as the signal transduction inhibitors, and their use in these settings should be carefully evaluated.

REFERENCES

1. Pazdur R. Response rates, survival, and chemotherapy. *J Natl Cancer Inst* 2000;92:1552–1553.
2. Chen TT, Chute JP, Feigal E, et al. A model to select chemotherapy regimens for phase III trials for extensive-stage small-cell lung cancer. *J Natl Cancer Inst* 2000;92:1601–1607.
3. Markman M. Why does a higher response rate to chemotherapy correlate poorly with improved survival. *J Cancer Res Clin Oncol* 1993;119:700–701.
4. Buyse M, Thirion P, Carlson RW, et al. Relation between tumor response to first-line chemotherapy and survival in colorectal cancer: a meta-analysis. *Lancet* 2000;356:373–378.
5. Miller AB, Hoogstraten B, Staquet M, et al. Reporting results of cancer treatment. *Cancer* 1981;47:207–214.
6. Therasse P, Arbuck SG, Eisenhauer EA, et al. New guidelines to evaluate the response to treatment in solid tumors. *J Natl Cancer Inst* 2000;92:205–216.
7. ten Bokkel Huinink W. Anticancer drug evaluation: continuing progress from existing methodology. *Eur J Cancer* 1997; 33[Suppl 2]:S8–S10.
8. Mattern J, Bak M, Hahn EW, et al. Human tumor xenografts as models for drug testing. *Cancer Metastasis Rev* 1988;7:263–284.
9. Ovejera AA, Houchens DP. Human tumor xenografts in athymic nude mice as a preclinical screen for anticancer agents. *Semin Oncol* 1981;8:386–393.
10. Wilmanns C, Fan D, O' Brian CA, et al. Orthotopic and ectopic organ environments differentially influence the sensitivity of murine colon carcinoma cells to

doxorubicin and 5-fluorouracil. *Int J Cancer* 1992; 52:98–104.

11. Wilmanns C, Fan D, O' Brian CA, et al. Modulation of doxorubicin sensitivity and level of P-glycoprotein expression in human colon carcinoma cells by ectopic and orthotopic environments in nude mice. *Int J Cancer* 1993;53:412–422.

12. Radinsky R. Modulation of tumor cell gene expression and phenotype by the organ-specific metastatic environment. *Cancer Metastasis Rev* 1995;14:323–338.

13. Killion JJ, Radinsky R, Fidler IJ. Orthotopic models are necessary to predict therapy of transplantable tumors in mice. *Cancer Metastasis Rev* 1999;17:279–284.

14. Kerbel RS. What is the optimal rodent model for antitumor drug testing? *Cancer Metastasis Rev* 1999;17: 301–304.

15. Roth JA, Ruckdeschel JC, Weisenburger TH, eds. *Thoracic oncology*. Philadelphia: WB Saunders, 1989.

16. Winograd B, Boven E, Lobbezoo MW, et al. Human tumor xenografts in the nude mouse and their value as test models in anticancer drug development. *In Vivo* 1987;1:1–14.

17. Rygaard J, Povlsen CO. Heterotransplantation of a human malignant tumor to nude mice. *Acta Pathol Microbiol Scand* 1969;77:758–760.

18. Steel GG, Courtenay VD, Peckhan MJ. The response to chemotherapy of a variety of human tumor xenografts. *Br J Cancer* 1983;47:1–13.

19. Kraemer HP, Sedlacek HH. Human tumor test systems: a new screening approach. *Behring Inst Mitt* 1986;80: 103–112.

20. Hamburger AW, Salmon SE. Primary bioassay of human tumor stem cells. *Science* 1977;197:461–463.

21. Von Hoff DD, Clark GM, Stogdill BJ, et al. Prospective clinical trial of a human tumor cloning system. *Cancer Res* 1983;43:1926–1931.

22. Shoemaker RH, Wolpert-DeFilippes MK, Kern DH, et al. Applications of a human tumor colony forming assay to new drug screening. *Cancer Res* 1985;45:2145–2153.

23. Hoff DD. Human tumor cloning assays: applications in clinical oncology and new antineoplastic agent development. *Cancer Metastasis Rev* 1988; 7:357–371.

24. Robert J. Role des modeles in vitro dans l'evaluaton preclinique des medicaments anticancereux. *Bull Cancer* 1996;83:801–808.

25. Curt GA. The use of animal models in cancer drug discovery and development. *Stem Cells* 1994;12:23–29.

26. Goldin A, Serpick AA, Mantel N. Experimental screening procedures and clinical predictability value. *Cancer Chemother Rep* 1966;50:173–218.

27. De Vita VT, Schein PS. The use of drugs in combination for the treatment of cancer. *N Engl J Med* 1973; 288: 998–1006.

28. Zubrod CG. Chemical control of cancer. *Proc Natl Acad Sci U S A* 1972;69:1042–1047.

29. Venditti JM. Drug evaluation branch program: report to screening contractors. *Cancer Chemother Rep* 1975; 5(Part 2):1–4.

30. Venditti JM. Preclinical drug development: rationale and methods. *Semin Oncol* 1981; 8:349–353.

31. Hamburger AW, Salmon SE, Kim MB, et al. Direct cloning of human ovarian carcinoma cells in agar. *Cancer Res* 1978;38:3438–3444.

32. Salmon SE, Hamburger AW, Soehnlen BJ, et al. Quantitation of differential sensitivity of human-tumor stem cells to anticancer drugs. *N Engl J Med* 1977;298: 1321–1328.

33. Alberts DS, Salmon SE, Chen HSG, et al. *In vitro* detection of cross-resistance and sensitivity in relapsing ovarian cancer with the human tumor stem cell assay. *Proc Am Assoc Cancer Res* 1980;21: 181(abstr 725).

34. Staquet M, Brown BW, Rozencweig M, et al. Validation of the clinical predictive values of the *in vitro* Phase II clonogenic assay in cancer of the breast and ovary. *Am J Clin Oncol* 1987;10:485–490.

35. Shoemaker RH, Monks A, Alley MC, et al. *Development of human tumor cell line panels for use in disease-oriented drug screening. Prediction of response to cancer therapy.* New York: Alan R. Liss, 1988.

36. Skehan P, Storeng R, Scudiero D, et al. New colorimetric cytotoxicity assay for anticancer drug screening. *J Natl Cancer Inst* 1990; 82:1107–1112.

37. Rubinstein LV, Shoemaker RH, Paull KD, et al. Comparison of *in vitro* anticancer drug screening data generated with a tetrazolium assay versus a protein assay against a diverse panel of human tumor cell lines. *J Natl Cancer Inst* 1990;82:1113–1118.

38. Alley MC, Scudiero D, Monks A, et al. Feasibility of drug screening with panels of human tumor Cell lines using a microculture tetrazolium assay. *Cancer Res* 1988; 48:589–601.

39. Monks A, Scudiero D, Skehan P, et al. Feasibility of a high-flux anticancer drug screen using a diverse panel of cultured human tumor cell lines. *J Natl Cancer Inst* 1990; 83:757–766.

40. Paull KD, Shoemaker RH, Hodes L, et al. Display and analysis of patterns of differential activities of drugs against human tumor cell lines: development of mean graph and COMPARE algorithm. *J Natl Cancer Inst* 1989; 81:1088–1092.

41. Goldin A, Venditti JM, MacDonald JS, et al. Current results of the screening program at the division of cancer treatment, National Cancer Institute. *Eur J Cancer* 1981;17:129–142.

42. Marsoni S, Wittes R. Clinical development of anticancer agents: a National Cancer Institute perspective. *Cancer Treat Rep* 1983; 68:77–85.

43. Venditti JM, Wesley RA, Plowman J. Current NCI preclinical antitumor screening *in vivo*: results of tumor panel screening. 1976–1982 and future directions. *Adv Pharmacol Chemother* 1984; 20:1–19.

44. Venditti JM. The National Cancer Institute antitumor drug discovery program, current and future perspectives: a commentary. *Cancer Treat Rep* 1983; 67: 767–772.

45. Staquet MJ, Byar DP, Green SB, et al. Clinical predictivity of transplantable tumor systems in the selection of new drugs for solid tumors: rationale for a three-stage strategy. *Cancer Treat Rep* 1983;67:753–765.

46. Marsoni S, Hoth D, Simon R, et al. Clinical drug development: an analysis of phase II trials, 1970–1985. *Cancer Treat Rep* 1987;71:71–80.

47. Johnson JI, Decker S, Zaharevitz D, et al. Relationship between drug activity in NCI preclinical in vitro and *in vivo* models and early clinical trials. *Br J Cancer* 2001; 84:1424–1431.

48. Bellet RE, Danna V, Mastrangelo MJ, et al. Evaluation of a "nude" mouse-human tumor panel as a predictive secondary screen for cancer Chemotherapy agents. *J Natl Cancer Inst* 1979;63:1185–1187.

49. Bailey MJ, Gazet J-C, Smith IE, et al. Chemotherapy of human breast-carcinoma xenografts. *Br J Cancer* 1980; 42:530–536.

50. Inoue K, Fujimote S, Ogawa M. Antitumor efficacy of seventeen anticancer drugs in human breast cancer xenograft (MX-1) transplanted in nude mice. *Cancer Chemother Pharmacol* 1983;10:182–186.

51. Taetle R, Rosen F, Abramson I, et al. Use of nude mouse xenografts as preclinical drug screens: *in vivo* activity of established chemotherapeutic agents against melanoma and ovarian carcinoma xenografts. *Cancer Treat Rep* 1987; 71:297–304.

52. Boven E, Winograd B, Fodstad O, et al. Preclinical phase II studies in human tumor lines: a European multicenter study. *Eur J Cancer* 1988; 24:567–573.

53. Boven E, Winograd B, Berger DP, et al. Phase II preclinical drug screening in human tumor xenografts: a first European multicenter collaborative study. *Cancer Res* 1992;52:5940–5947.

54. Langdon S, Hendriks HR, Braakhuis BJM, et al. Preclinical phase II studies in human tumor xenografts: a European multicenter follow-up study. *Ann Oncol* 1994;5:415–422.

55. Voskoglou-Nomikos T, Pater J, Seymour L. Clinical predictive value of the *in vitro* cell line, human xenograft and mouse allograft preclinical cancer models. *Proc Am Soc Clin Oncol* 2001; 21:360(abst).

56. Louie AC, Issell BF. Amsacrine (AMSA): a clinical review. *J Clin Oncol* 1985;3:562–592.

57. Minna JD, Pass H, Glatsein E, et al, eds. *Cancer principles and practice of oncology*. Philadelphia: JB Lippincott Co, 1989.

58. Gordon A.N, Granai CO, Rose PG, et al. Phase II study of liposomal doxorubicin in platinum- and paclitaxel-refractory epithelial ovarian cancer. *Clin Oncol* 2000;18: 3093–3100.

59. Israel VP, Garcia AA, Roman L, et al. Phase II study of liposomal doxorubicin in advanced gynecologic cancers. *Gynecol Oncol* 2000;78:143–147.

60. Muggia FM, Hainsworth JD, Jeffers S, et al. Phase II study of liposomal doxorubicin in refractory ovarian cancer: antitumor activity and toxicity modification by liposomal encapsulation. *J Clin Oncol* 1997;15:987–993.

61. Blum RH, Carter SK. Adriamycin. A new anticancer drug with significant clinical activity. *Ann Intern Med* 1974;80:249–259.

62. Louie AC, Issell BF. Amsacrine (AMSA)-a clinical review. *J Clin Oncol* 1985;3:562–592.

63. Thigpen JT, Lagasse L, Homesley H, et al. Cis-platinum in the treatment of advanced or recurrent adenocarcinoma of the ovary. A phase II study of the Gynecologic Oncology Group. *Am J Clin Oncol* 1983;6:431–435.

64. Wiltshaw E, Kroner T. Phase II study of cis-dichlorodiammineplatinum(II) (NSC-119875) in advanced adenocarcinoma of the ovary. *Cancer Treatment Reports* 1976;60:55–60.

65. Bonomi PD, Mladineo J, Morrin B, et al. Phase II trial of hexamethylmelamine in ovarian carcinoma resistant to alkylating agents. *Cancer Treatment Reports* 1979;3: 137–138.

66. Johnson BL, Fisher RI, Bender RA, et al. Hexamethylmelamine in alkylating agent-resistant ovarian carcinoma. *Cancer* 1978;42:2157–2161.

67. Omura GA, Blessing JA, Morrow CP, et al. Follow-up on a randomized trial of melphalan (M) vs. melphalan plus hexamethylamine (M+H) vs adriamycin plus cyclophosphamide (A+C) in advanced ovarian carcinoma. *Proc Annual Meeting Am Assoc Cancer Res* 1981;22:470, AC-537.

68. Bolis G, D'Incalci M, Belloni C, et al. Hexamethylmelamine in ovarian cancer resistant to cyclophosphamide and adriamycin. *Cancer Treatment Reports* 1979;63: 1375–1377.

69. Manetta A, MacNeill C, Lyter JA, et al. Hexamethylmelamine as a single second-line agent in ovarian cancer. *Gynecol Oncol* 1990;36:93–96.

70. Rosen GF, Lurain JR, Newton M. Hexamethylmelamine in ovarian cancer after failure of cisplatin-based multiple-agent chemotherapy. *Gynecol Oncol* 1987;27: 173–179.

71. Parker LM, Griffiths CT, Yankee RA, et al. High-dose methotrexate with leucovorin rescue in ovarian cancer: a phase II study. *Cancer Treatment Reports* 1979;63: 275–279.

72. Barlow JJ, Piver MS. Methotrexate (NSC-740) with citrovorum factor (NSC-3590) rescue, alone and in combination with cyclophosphamide (NSC-26271), in ovarian cancer. *Cancer Treatment Reports* 1976;60: 527–533.

73. Morgan RJ Jr, Speyer J, Doroshow JH, et al. Modulation of 5-fluorouracil with high-dose leucovorin calcium: activity in ovarian cancer and correlation with CA-125 levels. *Gynecol Oncol* 1995;58:79–85.

74. Markman M, Reichman B, Hakes T, et al. Intraperitoneal chemotherapy as treatment for ovarian carcinoma and gastrointestinal malignancies: the Memorial Sloan-Kettering Cancer Center experience). *Acta Med Aust* 1989;16:65–67.

75. Prefontaine M, Donovan JT, Powell JL, Buley L. Treatment of refractory ovarian cancer with 5-fluorouracil and leucovorin. *Gynecol Oncol* 1996;61:249–252.

76. Kamphuis JT, Huider MC, Ras GJ. et al. High-dose 5-fluorouracil and leucovorin as second-line chemotherapy in patients with platinum-resistant epithelial ovarian cancer. *Cancer Chemother Pharmacol* 1995;37:190–192.

77. Burnett AF, Barter JF, Potkul RK, et al. Ineffectiveness of continuous 5-fluorouracil as salvage therapy for ovarian cancer. *Am J Clin Oncol* 1994;7:490–493.

78. Reed E, Jacob J, Ozols RF, et al. 5-Fluorouracil (5-FU) and leucovorin in platinum-refractory advanced stage ovarian carcinoma. *Gynecol Oncol* 1992;46:326–329.

79. Ozols RF, Speyer JL, Jenkins J, et al. Phase II trial of 5-FU administered Ip to patients with refractory ovarian cancer. *Cancer Treatment Reports* 1984;68:1229–1232.

80. Long HJ 3rd, Nelimark RA, Su JQ, et al. Phase II evaluation of 5-fluorouracil and low-dose leucovorin in cisplatin-refractory advanced ovarian carcinoma. *Gynecol Oncol* 1994;54:180–183.

81. Look KY, Muss HB, Blessing JA, et al. A phase II trial of 5-fluorouracil and high-dose leucovorin in recurrent epithelial ovarian carcinoma. A Gynecologic Oncology Group Study. *Am J Clin Oncol* 1995;18:19–22.

82. de Graeff A, van Hoef ME, Tjia P, et al. Continuous infusion of 5-fluorouracil in ovarian cancer patients refractory to cisplatin and carboplatin. *Ann Oncol* 1991;2:691–692.

83. Minna JD, Pass H, Glatstein E, et al. Cancer of the lung. In: DeVita VT, Hellman S, Rosenberg SA, eds. *Cancer principles and practice in oncology*. Philadelphia: JB Lippincott, 1989:660.

11

Drug-Drug Interaction Studies During Early Clinical Drug Development

Jochen Kuhlmann and Christoph Wandel

Institute of Clinical Pharmacology, Bayer AG, Pharma-Research-Center, Wuppertal, Germany

Drug–drug interactions in patients receiving multiple drug regimens are a constant concern for the clinician. Fatal adverse drug effects rank between the fourth and sixth leading causes of death in the United States (1). As many as 20% to 30 % of all adverse drug reactions are assumed to be caused by a drug—drug interaction (DDI) (2,3). Adverse events related to DDI contributed to the market withdrawal of four drugs (terfenadine, mibefradil, cisapride, and astemizole) between 1997 and 2000. Incidence estimates for clinically significant DDIs range from 4.7% in general patient populations to as many as 88% in geriatric patients, of which 22% were regarded as serious or life-threatening (4–6). Reviews of hospital and outpatient prescribing practices suggest that when a DDI-related adverse event is reported, the patient is taking an average of four to eight drugs at that time (7). In another study, the number of adverse drug reactions observed in an elderly patient population decreased from 24% to 7% when the average number of drugs was decreased by one medication (8).

Therefore, the study of DDIs is an important aspect in the development process of new drugs. The growing understanding of principles that are involved in the mechanism of DDI provides the opportunity to estimate and to follow up a DDI potential before a drug is marketed. Principally, the cardinal logic behind serially conducted studies of a medicinal product in clinical development is that the results of prior studies should influence the planning of later studies (9), particularly for DDI studies in the early stages of drug development. Optimally, a sequence of studies is planned, moving from *in vitro* studies to early exploratory studies, to later more definitive studies, employing special study designs and methodology where necessary and appropriate. The goal is the prevention of (i) adverse events due to DDIs and (ii) any misinterpretation of the results from phase 2 and 3 trials because of not-yet-identified DDIs.

It should be noted that this chapter does not include a review of pharmacogenetics, even though the relevance of this field to drug efficacy and DDI has been established and is becoming increasingly apparent. The reader is referred to some selected, introductory reviews of pharmacogenetics (10–13).

TYPES OF DRUG–DRUG INTERACTIONS

Making distinctions among pharmaceutical, pharmacokinetic, and pharmacodynamic DDIs gives a rationale for analyzing the DDI potential of a new drug candidate. Pharmacokinetic DDIs are further differentiated according to the traditional scheme of ADME (absorption, distribution, metabolism, and excretion). There is an increasing body of knowledge about the underlying mechanisms of metabolic and transporter-mediated DDIs. Such knowledge supports the goals of DDI studies in early drug development (i.e., to better understand and predict the variability among patients' responses to a drug as well as to a combination of drugs from both a safety and efficacy point of view). It should be noted that these more mechanistic approaches overlap with the classic ADME approach. For instance, a change in the metabolic CYP3A activities at specific gut and liver sites not only alters the metabolism of a drug, but simultaneously changes absorption and excretion.

Although the differentiation among pharmaceutical, pharmacokinetic, and pharmacodynamic interactions is helpful, if not essential, to analyze a new drug's DDI potential and to reasonably structure the strategy on how to carefully investigate such an interaction potential in humans, it is clear that the various types of

DDIs have to be determined and discussed as a whole to assess the clinical relevance of a DDI.

Pharmaceutical Drug–Drug Interactions

Pharmaceutical DDIs occur when two molecules interact through their physicochemical properties, without involvement of any host-bound mediator–like enzyme or transporter. Pharmaceutical DDIs also include such interactions that are caused by the direct interaction of the excipients of one drug with the coadministered drug molecule. Examples of pharmaceutical DDIs are the chelate-complex building of certain bivalent cations with some antibiotics (14,15) and the entrapment of paclitaxel and epirubicin by Cremophor EL (16–19). However, pharmaceutical DDIs are in most cases foreseeable by means of *in vitro* investigations, and it should be possible to avoid them in clinical practice (20).

Pharmacokinetic Drug–Drug Interactions

Metabolic Drug–Drug Interactions

During preclinical development, the metabolism of a new drug is investigated *in vitro*. A typical drug-metabolism pathway is the oxidation of the parent drug (phase I oxidation), followed by conjugation of the oxidized moiety with highly polar molecules, such as glucose, sulfate, methionine, cysteine or glutathione (phase II conjugation). The key enzymes for phase I oxidation are the isoforms of cytochrome P450 (CYP), flavine mono-oxygenases (FMO), and N-acetyltransferases (NAT). The key phase II enzymes include UGP-dependent glucuronosyl transferase (UGT), phenol sulfotransferase (PST), estrogen sulfotransferase (EST), and glutathione S-transferase (GST). With the exception of UGT, phase II enzymes are cytosolic and are, therefore, absent from the liver microsomes. Phase I and II enzymes build the metabolic clearance of a drug. Pending on the contribution of the metabolic to the total clearance, these enzyme activities determine the plasma concentrations of their drug substrates.

One of the major important metabolic phase I enzymes frequently involved in drug metabolism is CYP3A4. This enzyme participates in the metabolism of many drugs, including anticancer drugs like cyclophosphamide, ifosfamide, docetaxel, paclitaxel, doxorubicin, etoposide, teniposide, vinblastine, and vindesine (21,22). Some of the anticancer agents are metabolized by various enzymes, including CYP enzymes. Thus, inhibition of CYP3A4 may result in a shift of the metabolite pattern of a drug. In the case of cyclophosphamide, a decrease in CYP3A4 activity results in a higher concentration of the active metabolite produced by CYP2B6, and alternatively, 4-hydroxy-cyclophosphamide is formed (23,24). In contrast, in the case of ifosfamide, an inhibition of CYP3A4 leads to a higher concentration of the neurotoxic metabolite dechloroethylifosfamide, which has no antitumor activity (25). The induction of CYP3A4 by methyl-prednisolone resulting in an increased production of 3-p-hydroxypaclitaxel reflects the role of CYP3A4 activity in the *in vivo* disposition of paclitaxel (26).

The metabolism of xenobiotics is mainly located in the liver, where the phase I and II enzymes contribute to the metabolic clearance of a drug from plasma as well as to the first pass elimination after oral drug administration. However, CYP3A4 is not only expressed in the liver, but it is also the most abundant CYP enzyme in the intestinal mucosa (27,28). After oral administration, the drug fraction exposed to CYP3A4 is therefore enlarged compared to the intravenous route; hence, intestinal CYP3A4 activity can significantly influence the oral bioavailability of its substrates. Indeed, after oral administration the plasma concentrations of the prototypical CYP3A4 substrate midazolam are more closely related to the intestinal activity than to hepatic CYP3A activity (29–31).

The clinical consequences of the outstanding role of metabolism in general and of CYP3A4 in particular in anticancer drug therapy are demonstrated by the analysis showing that the coadministration of anticonvulsant therapy resulted in a lower efficacy of chemotherapy among patients with B-lineage acute lymphoblastic leukemia (ALL). This is explained by the CYP3A4-inducing effect of anticonvulsant therapy and the subsequent increase in metabolic clearance and decrease in the plasma concentrations of several antileukemic agents (32). Similarly, it is recommended that children who are receiving the CYP3A substrate irinotecan (33,34) are treated with alternative anticonvulsants such as gabapentin that do not induce drug-metabolizing enzymes (35).

Other metabolic DDIs besides those mediated by CYP3A4 can also gain high clinical relevance. For example, the antiviral drug sorivudine was withdrawn from the Japanese market by its manufacturer within 1 year of its introduction because of the fatal result of its interaction with fluorouracil (5-FU) prodrugs. Data obtained by *in vivo* and *in vitro* studies strongly suggest that a metabolite generated from sorivudine by gut flora was reduced in the presence of the reduced form of nicotinamide adenine dinucleotide phosphate (NADPH) to a reactive form by hepatic dihydropyrimidine dehydrogenase (DPD), a key enzyme determining the tissue 5-FU levels, bound covalently to DPD as a suicide inhibitor, and markedly retarded the catabolism of 5-FU (36).

Transporter-related Drug–Drug Interactions

Drug transporters have now been recognized as a significant determinant of disposition in humans for several drugs. Probably the most detailed described transporter to date is P-glycoprotein (Pgp), a cellular efflux transporter of the ABC transporter family. Primarily discovered as the cause of multidrug resistance by pumping anticancer agents out of the tumor cells, its relevance to drug disposition was shown in 1994 by using Pgp knockout mice (37). Pgp expressed in the intestinal epithelium pumps its substrates into the gut lumen, whereas Pgp expressed in the liver and kidney pumps its substrates into the bile and urine. Thus, Pgp activity limits the oral bioavailability and pushes the hepatic and renal excretion of its drug substrates. Thus, on both fronts—the absorption site and the excretion site—inhibition of Pgp increases the plasma concentrations of its substrates. Importantly, Pgp expressed in endothelial cells of the blood–brain barrier limits the entry of its substrates into the central nervous system. For example, the brain levels of loperamide, ondansetron, and vinblastine were increased by factors 13.5, 4.0, and 22.4, respectively, while the brain:plasma concentration ratio increased by about sixfold, fourfold, and ninefold (37,38).

Thinking about the interaction of a drug with Pgp is important from various points of view. First, inhibition of Pgp may serve as a pharmaceutical target to circumvent multidrug resistance in cancer patients. It affects the *in vivo* disposition of its drug substrates like cyclosporine, tacrolimus, digoxin, loperamide, and human immunodeficiency virus protease inhibitors. Several anticancer drugs like vinca alkaloids, anthracyclines, epipodophyllotoxins, and taxanes have also been shown to be substrates of Pgp. In Pgp knockout mice, the biodistribution including the intestinal transport of paclitaxel is markedly changed compared to wild-type mice (39). Human studies revealed that the coadministration of the Pgp inhibitor PSC833 requires dosage reductions of the Pgp substrate doxorubicin because of elevated plasma concentrations and associated toxicity (40,41). The coadministration of the Pgp inhibitor GF120918 resulted in an approximately sevenfold increase in the oral bioavailability of paclitaxel (42). Because of the occurrence of unacceptable systemic toxicity, dose reductions were recommended for the CYP3A-plus-Pgp substrates paclitaxel (43), etoposide (44), and vinblastine (45) when combined with PSC833. Also, Pgp-mediated DDIs might have caused the increased risk of cardiotoxicity of epirubicin and doxorubicin that was observed when these agents were administered together with paclitaxel (46,47). It

should be noted that not only molecules specifically designed to inhibit Pgp may exert DDIs, but unexpectedly, formulation excipients may also contribute to Pgp-mediated DDIs. Cremophor EL not only has the potential of pharmaceutical interactions, but through its inhibitory effects on Pgp activity it reduces the elimination of the Pgp substrates epirubicin, epirubicinol, and doxorubicin (48,49).

Second, there is a marked overlap between CYP3A and Pgp in terms of expression sites, substrates, inducers, and inhibitors potentially amplifying the risk of DDI (Fig. 11.1). Several drugs, including anticancer drugs like paclitaxel, vinblastine, and vincristine, are not only substrates of CYP3A, but also of Pgp. Thus, oral bioavailability and hepatic elimination can be altered through metabolic and distributional mechanisms that both affect plasma concentrations in the same direction (e.g., inhibition leads to increased plasma concentrations). Several drugs inhibit both CYP3A and Pgp (50), even though there is no significant correlation between CYP3A-inhibiting and Pgp-inhibiting potencies (51). Interestingly, the effects of CYP3A− and Pgp− inhibition can be also used in a beneficial way. For example, the CYP3A and Pgp inhibitor cyclosporine increased the oral bioavailability of the CYP3A− and Pgp− substrate paclitaxel in such a way that therapeutically effective plasma concentrations were achieved (52–54). The overlap between CYP3A and Pgp also includes the mode of induction of their activities (55–58). For example, rifampicin induces both proteins through activation of the nuclear pregnane X receptor (PXR), decreasing the plasma concentrations of CYP3A−/Pgp− substrates. It is worthy to note that the nuclear receptor PXR, which can activate both CYP3A4 and Pgp, has interspecies differences in the pattern of induction (59–61). Unfortunately, no *in vivo* method has been established to differentiate between Pgp and CYP3A contributions to a DDI between a drug that potentially inhibits both proteins and one that is a substrate of both proteins.

Third, while the clinical relevance has yet to be proven, several lines of evidence indicate an association between apoptosis and Pgp activity. The Pgp inhibitor PSC833 has been shown to stimulate caspase-dependent apoptosis (62). It has been hypothesized that within the cell membrane, Pgp shifts the substrates of the sphingomyelinases away from the enzymes. When Pgp activity is inhibited, the intracellular concentration of ceramide that is produced by sphingomyelinases increases. Ceramide itself induces apoptosis (63,64).

Altogether, when determining the clinical effects of Pgp inhibition, one has to consider (i) circumvention

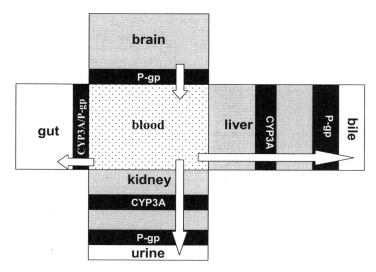

FIG. 11.1. The influence of cytochrome P450 3A (CYP3A) and P-glycoprotein (Pgp) on plasma concentrations. Both CYP3A and Pgp prevent the absorption of their drug substrates from the intestine, and both eliminate their drug substrates from the blood compartment by metabolism and excretion into the bile and urine, respectively. Pgp expressed at the blood–brain barrier prevents the uptake of its drug substrates by the central nervous system.

of multidrug resistance and subsequent intratumor accumulation of cytostatic agents, (ii) systemic pharmacokinetic DDI, and (iii) an alteration of the apoptotic response of tumor cells due to Pgp inhibition.

Transporters other than Pgp are thought to be meaningful for the *in vivo* disposition of their drug substrates. Members of the multidrug resistance protein (MRP) family, MRP1 and MRP2, affect the *in vivo* pharmacokinetics of a range of drugs (65–68). Interestingly, it has been shown that MRP transporters are also inducible by rifampin (69). No clinically applicable modulation of MRP activity is currently available. Besides cellular efflux transporters, drug transporters may also mediate the cellular uptake of drugs. The cellular uptake transporter organ anion transporting polypeptide (OATP), also expressed at the luminal intestinal site, affects the *in vivo* disposition of the antihistaminic drug fexofenadine, which is a substrate of not only Pgp, but also of OATP. Grapefruit juice inhibits OATP *in vitro* and decreases the plasma concentrations of fexofenadine in humans, probably by a reduction in its oral bioavailability by OATP inhibition (70,71).

In conclusion, drug transporters have increasingly been shown to be a possible cause of DDIs, and such DDIs should be considered when setting up a DDI-studies program during the early stages of clinical drug development.

Pharmacodynamic Drug–Drug Interactions

Pharmacodynamic DDIs occur when drugs share a common mode of pharmacologic and toxicologic action, respectively. Even when the respective pathomechanism cannot be identified, sharing an adverse event pattern also indicates the possibility of a pharmacodynamic DDI.

Compared to the number of principles that are currently known to cause pharmacokinetic DDIs, the possibilities of pharmacodynamic DDIs appear to be innumerable. To mention only a few, inhalational agents such as isoflurane and sevoflurane increase the potency of nondepolarizing muscle relaxants (72,73). The coadministration of statins with fibrates increases the incidence of myopathias (74). In cancer drug development, the use of drug combinations significantly increases the number and duration of complete remissions. The overriding rationale for the use of combination chemotherapy is to overcome drug resistance to individual agents. Combination chemotherapy also may prevent or delay the development of acquired resistance in initially responsive tumors. A combination regimen normally includes drugs that are non–cross-resistant to overlap drug-resistant subpopulations of tumor cells, drugs with nonantagonistic and preferably additive or synergistic mechanisms of action, and drugs with nonoverlapping toxicity profiles, allowing each agent to be administered at its optimal dose and schedule. Drug combinations also have been designed to take advantage of biochemical interactions (synergism). The active folate leucovorin does not have inherent antitumor activity, but when administered with 5-FU, it can markedly increase the cytotoxic effect of 5-FU by enhancing the binding of an active intracellular metabolite of 5-FU to its target enzyme, thymidylate synthase. The combination of leucovorin and 5-FU has shown a higher response rate than 5-FU alone against a variety of epithelial tumors, principally colorectal cancer (75).

More generally speaking, any multiple-drug regimen proven be more beneficial or detrimental for any given treatment and that does not change the drug's concentration in blood and tissues, respectively, may be regarded a pharmacodynamic DDI. Clearly, it depends on the pharmacodynamic parameter chosen to describe and analyze a pharmacodynamic DDI. Whenever possible, pharmacodynamic parameters should be related to fluid/tissue concentration to allow pharmacokinetic simulation and to deduce a pharmacokinetic–pharmacodynamic interrelationship that may change because of a pharmacodynamic DDI.

A pharmacodynamic DDI is to be described as antagonistic, additive, or more than additive (synergistic). It has been suggested that only when the combined effects of the interacting drugs are greater or less than the arithmetic sum of their individual actions can the interaction be considered a true interaction (4,7,76). However, with respect to the clinical relevance and the necessity to provide recommendations for dosing adjustments, pharmacodynamically based DDI studies are to be conducted even if only an additive effect is expected.

Whereas the demonstration of the benefit of a multiple-drug regimen in cancer therapy is pursued in phase 2 and 3 trials, the objectives of pharmacodynamically related DDIs considered in early clinical drug development include:

- To explore the toxicity of a combination therapy in dependency of various dosing regimens acknowledging that features such as myelosuppression and gastrointestinal toxicity are shared by most cytostatic agents.
- To explore the effect of a combination therapy on a biomarker that is thought to indicate toxicity or efficacy. For instance, the effects of growth hormone receptors can be blocked at various steps of signaling, and combining multiple targets may positively interact on biomarkers downstream of the growth receptor.

Like pharmaceutical and pharmacokinetic DDIs, pharmacodynamic DDIs should be, whenever possible, first adequately explored *in vitro* and in animals to define the most sensitive and the most relevant parameter of pharmacodynamic interaction, the dosing regimen that is most suitable to explore this interaction, and the pharmacokinetic–pharmacodynamic relationship for the parameter selected. With regard to safety issues, preclinical investigations should be extensive when the toxicity in question cannot be easily monitored and has the potential to be severe and irreversible.

METHODS OF DRUG–DRUG INTERACTION STUDIES

Design

Drug–drug interactions can either be investigated in formal studies or by subanalyses of patients from phase 2 or 3 trials applying population pharmacokinetics (Fig. 11.2). In general, formal DDI studies are conducted using a crossover design. In crossover studies, it is absolutely necessary to keep a washout period of at least four to five half-lives between the single study periods. Particularly for pharmacodynamic DDI studies, a design is beneficial that allows the drugs in question to reach steady-state conditions. Multiple dosing may be also considered when a DDI is based on enzyme/transporter induction or the metabolites of the drug in question are likely to contribute to this DDI. When attainment of steady state is important and either the substrate or interacting drugs and/or their metabolites exhibit long half-lives, special approaches can be considered, including the use of a loading dose to achieve steady-state conditions more rapidly. However, with respect to pharmacodynamic DDIs, the loading-dose phase may not allow relevant conclusions due to the artificial dosing regimen, which does not reflect the clinical situation. Another alternative approach is the one-sequence crossover, where pretreatment and posttreatment control are used (i.e., each subject serves as his or her own control). This approach provides the chance to study patients who may require continuous administration of the test drug to control their disease. However, the one-sequence design has inherently the risk of a non–drug-related period effect that cannot be distinguished from a drug effect. Finally, a parallel-group design will also be acceptable when a crossover design is not practical (77).

Analyses of population pharmacokinetics of data obtained from blood samples collected infrequently (sparse sampling) in phase 2 and 3 trials can be valuable in characterizing the clinical impact of known or newly identified interactions, and in making recommendations

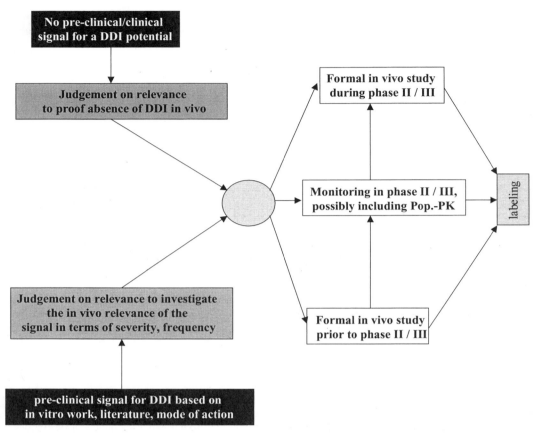

FIG. 11.2. Main factors in the prioritization process in setting up a drug–drug interaction (DDI) studies plan together with the various approaches on when and how to address the potential of DDIs during clinical development.

for dosage modifications. Sometimes, a combination of DDI studies during early clinical drug development and population pharmacokinetics in phase 2 and 3 studies is favorable (4). It is possible that analysis or skillful examinations of such data could detect unsuspected DDIs. Population pharmacokinetic data can also provide further evidence of the absence of a pharmacokinetic DDI when this is suggested by *in vitro* studies. For drugs that are frequently co-administered in the target population, but based on *in vitro* screening and theoretical thoughts on possible physicochemical characteristics, are unlikely to produce clinically relevant interactions with a new drug, an initial screen for pharmacokinetic and/or pharmacodynamic (efficacy and safety) related DDI during phase 2 or 3 clinical trials with plasma concentration measurements and a possible concentration/effect relationship might be sufficient. On the basis of these data, it should be critically estimated whether the screening itself is sufficient for an estimation of risk/benefit or if an additional formal study is necessary.

The power of a sparse sampling strategy to detect DDI is not yet well established; thus, it is unlikely that population analysis can be used to prove the absence of an interaction that is strongly suggested by findings of *in vitro* or *in vivo* studies specifically designed to assess a DDI (78).

Blinding

Studies can usually be open label (unblinded), unless pharmacodynamic endpoints (e.g., adverse events that are subject to bias) are part of the assessment of the interaction (77).

Selection of an *In Vivo* Probe

The understanding of some of the major principles in pharmacokinetic DDIs resulted in the search and agreement that some substrates, in particular those of individual CYP enzymes, are considered suitable probes to assess the enzyme activity in humans. If an initial, formal clinical DDI study is positive for inhibitory effects of the new drug candidate, further studies of other substrates may be useful, representing a range of substrates based on the likelihood of coadministration. However, if findings of such an initial study using the most sensitive substrate are negative, it can be presumed that less sensitive substrates will also be unaffected. In turn, if the drug candidate is a CYP3A4 substrate and if the DDI study results using a strong inhibitor (e.g., ketoconazole) and inducer (e.g., rifampin), respectively are negative, then absence of a clinically important DDI for the metabolic pathway could be assumed. However, if the clinical study of the most potent specific inhibitor or inducer is positive and the sponsor (drug manufacturer) wishes to claim the absence of an interaction between the test drug and other less potent, specific inhibitors or to give advice on dosage adjustment, further clinical studies would generally be recommended (77).

With regard to transporter-related DDIs, no guidance has been provided by health authorities thus far. Digoxin and fexofenadine are two drugs that have been used as *in vivo* probes of Pgp. The advantage of using fexofenadine over digoxin as a Pgp probe is its lower oral bioavailability, which allows a clearer demonstration of any effects of a potential Pgp inhibitor on oral bioavailability. However, fexofenadine is also a substrate of OATP (70,71), and prior to a formal DDI study in humans, any modulating effects of a new drug on OATP must be excluded *in vitro* to adequately assess its effects on Pgp activity when using fexofenadine as a Pgp *in vivo* probe.

Selection of Subjects

In view of their greater clinical relevance, DDI studies in the target population are in principle to be preferred. This includes the opportunity to study pharmacodynamic endpoints not present in healthy subjects (77). Studies in patients who need basic treatment have to be performed without using washout periods between the study periods. Here, a run-in phase to obtain steady state of basic treatment will be followed by a period to estimate the pharmacokinetics and pharmacodynamics of basic treatment and, subsequently, of combination therapy. In addition, safety considerations may preclude the inclusion of healthy subjects. If such considerations do not apply, DDI studies are frequently conducted in healthy subjects for practical reasons. When the DDI studies are conducted in healthy subjects, the assumption is that the findings in this population should predict findings in the patient population for which the drug is intended.

Study Endpoints

Pharmacokinetic endpoints include area under the curve (AUC), maximum concentration of drug (C_{max}), time of occurrence for maximum drug concentration (t_{max}), and other measures such as volumes of distribution, half-lives, and clearance, as appropriate. When a DDI is clearly present (e.g., comparisons indicate twofold or greater increments in systemic exposure measures for combination of a protein inhibitor with a protein substrate compared to protein substrate alone), the clinical significance of the interaction based on what is known about the dose—response relationship for the investigational agent or the approved drugs used in the study should be evaluated. This information should form the basis making recommendations with respect to the dose, dosing regimen adjustments, precautions, warnings, or contraindications of the investigational or approved drug (77).

Pharmacodynamic interactions are more complex and more complicated to investigate. Both drugs under consideration should be dosed so that they produce pharmacodynamic effects when given alone, but are safe when given in combination. Clearly, the dosing regimen chosen for pharmacodynamic DDI needs to consider the dose–response curve of the individual players. In some cases, the pharmacodynamic DDI will be first evaluated in an animal model so that the data provided can be used to design the pharmacodynamic DDI study in humans.

Sample-size Estimation

The number of subjects involved in such DDI studies depends on (i) the study design, (ii) variability of pharmacodynamic and pharmacokinetic parameters, (iii) criteria to assess a clinically relevant difference, and (iv) additional ethical considerations or limitations (4). A problem of the sample-size estimation for DDI studies is the fact that in most cases, clearly defined criteria to assess a clinically relevant interaction do not exist (79). For these reasons, the *in vivo* evaluation of a pharmacodynamically based DDI may be pursued in two steps, where an exploratory study is required first so that a subsequent study that allows the judgment of the clinical relevance of that DDI can be appropriately designed.

Biostatistical Evaluation

From a statistical viewpoint, considering different drug treatments in a DDI study, "lack of relevant interaction" can be demonstrated by proving "equivalence" using the confidence-interval approach established for bioequivalence studies. A lack of relevant interaction is concluded if the 90 % confidence interval for the ratio of the combined treatment of both drugs divided by the reference (mono-) treatment is entirely within the equivalence range (range of clinically acceptable variation). This ratio can be calculated for AUC, C_{max}, or any other parameter of intent. This decision procedure ensures that the consumer risk, incorrectly concluding "no interaction," is limited to 5% (80). However, in standard hypothesis testing for differences between treatments, the consumer risk is not controlled because a nonsignificant result does not imply that there is no interaction and a significant result does not imply a clinically relevant interaction. For DDI, the equivalence range may be wider or narrower depending on the therapeutic range of the drug and the pharmacokinetic and pharmacodynamic variability of the affected drug. According to the limits for analysis, the contraindication for a combination must be defined early. Otherwise, the clinical relevance of possible interactions has to be investigated in additional, nonformal clinical studies in patients (4).

TIMING OF *IN VIVO* DRUG–DRUG INTERACTION STUDIES

The DDI potential of a new compound has to be assessed in detail, starting with preclinical *in vitro* and animal studies at candidate selection and continuously supplemented during ongoing preclinical and clinical development. Because it is not practical to examine all thinkable DDIs by *in vivo* studies during early clinical development, a careful selection of a limited number of drug combinations to be investigated during this development phase is indicated. Here, the prioritization process will be guided by the likelihood and the expected severity of a DDI (7). Subsequent to the scientific progress made in the areas of pharmacokinetics and pharmacodynamics, the focus of DDI studies has changed from *ad hoc* observational studies to rationally designed studies (77,81).

Various lines have the potential to provide a scientific rationale for conducting a formal *in vivo* DDI study at an early stage of clinical development, before that drug combination is released for phase 2 and 3 trials. This is for safety reasons and to reduce the variability in the results for efficacy. When the possibility of a pharmaceutical, pharmacokinetic and pharmacodynamic DDI is raised by experimental preclinical *in vitro* and animal work, an *in vivo* DDI study should be conducted before the to-be-coadministered drug in question is released for phase 2 and 3 studies. Several attempts have been made to extrapolate the clinical

relevance of a DDI from *in vitro* data. Although there is no general method allowing quantitative assessments, several factors have been worked out that help at least to estimate the *in vivo* risk of a relevant DDI seen *in vitro*.

A steep course of the dose–response curve of a drug indicates that its pharmacodynamic effects are sensitive to even a slight change in its pharmacokinetics. It may be argued that a steep dose–response curve is also prone for pure pharmacodynamic DDIs. Chemotherapeutic drugs frequently have a steep dose–response curve with regard to efficacy and toxicity (82,83).

Another issue related to the consideration of the dose–response curve deals with the release of narrow therapeutic index drugs such as warfarin and digoxin in phase 2 and 3 trials. Although CYP2C9/protein binding and Pgp are identified as the major players in DDIs with warfarin and digoxin, respectively, it still may be wise to conduct formal *in vivo* DDI studies prior to their release in clinical efficacy trials, even when *in vitro* work does not indicate any DDI potential for a new drug candidate. This precaution should be taken not only because warfarin and digoxin are narrow therapeutic index drugs, but also because of the severity of adverse events that are eventually associated with a DDI with warfarin or digoxin. In case a warfarin-associated or digoxin-associated adverse event occurs in phase 2 or 3 trials during coadministration with the investigational new drug, the absence of any *in vitro* signals for a DDI potential on the one hand competes with the clinical observation of a timely coincidence of the adverse event with the coadministration with the new drug on the other hand. In this situation, data from a specific DDI *in vivo* study excluding a relevant interaction between drugs *in vivo* will be helpful to determine the correct relationship of this adverse event to drug intake. This approach also acknowledges the fact that there is always some risk that new players that mediate DDI will be discovered and that narrow therapeutic drugs are, by definition, sensitive to DDI.

Additional factors can be identified that increase the risk of a clinically relevant DDI, including (i) problematic pharmacokinetics, (ii) necessity of long-term therapy with different drugs (this is a concern not only because the duration of treatment itself is an independent risk factor, but also because several drugs exert adverse reactions only after weeks and months of treatment), (iii) likelihood of simultaneous prescription of several drugs by different physicians, and (iv) likelihood of self-medication by the patient, with (iii) and (iv) being less unlikely in a hospital setting compared with an outpatient setting.

Information on DDIs from other drugs of the same class also provides an estimate on the severity and incidence of DDI of a new drug candidate. Examples include:

- β-Lactam antibiotics may induce allergic reactions including such of the immediate type
- Vinca-alkaloids and anthracyclines are often substrates of Pgp and, subsequently, put patients at risk for Pgp-mediated DDI
- Most of the cytostatic agents cause myelosuppression

Obviously, classes of drugs should not only be defined by their chemical structure, but also by their pharmacokinetic characteristics and modes of biological action. It becomes evident that if a single drug is grouped together with other drugs according to one given characteristic, this grouping does not necessarily hold true for a different aspect.

Preclinical Signals for Pharmacokinetic DDIs

Due to the frequency and potential severity of metabolic DDIs, a significant amount of effort has been undertaken to predict the magnitude of DDI *in vivo* from *in vitro* data. All models proposed have limitations. Thus, *in vitro* data may result in semiquantitative statements rather than be accepted as reliable means by which to predict the change in plasma concentrations of a drug after a metabolic interaction with another drug. Recently, a consensus conference proposed an algorithm for evaluating DDI focussing on *in vitro* signals for metabolism/transporter-driven DDIs (83). This algorithm confirms that *in vivo* studies investigating any inhibitory or inducing effect of a drug candidate on an enzyme or transporter's activity, the most sensitive *in vivo* probe of that enzyme or transporter should be elected. In turn, DDI studies investigating the effect of enzyme or transporter activity modulation on the pharmacokinetics of a drug candidate, an established strong inhibitor and inducer, respectively, should be chosen.

Although the *in vitro* experiments are not sufficient to quantify the change in plasma concentrations of a drug *in vivo*, work with various models (84,85) has revealed several aspects that help to prioritize among the DDI studies to be conducted during early clinical development.

For low-clearance drugs (limited enzyme activity, hepatic extraction ratio less than 0.5), a decrease in Cl_{intr} (as obtained *in vitro*) caused by enzyme inhibition yields an almost proportional increase in the AUC regardless of the route of administration or the choice of hepatic models. In contrast, a reduction of the Cl_{intr} has little effect on the AUC of high-clearance drugs (limited hepatic flow, hepatic extraction ratio greater than 0.9) after intravenous administration. Changes in the AUC of high-clearance drugs are more profound after oral administration than after intravenous administration (86).

Several extrapolations from *in vitro* to *in vivo* data focussed on the metabolic fraction of a drug's metabolism that is catalyzed by the enzyme in question (87,88). It has been estimated that this fraction has to be at least 50% in order to suggest that enzyme inhibition shown *in vitro* will also be relevant *in vivo*. When $f_{m,E}$ is larger than 0.7, in the presence of the inhibitor in question, the AUC ratios of the substrate would increase at least 50% with $[I]/K_i$ of 1, and 275% with $[I]/K_i$ of 10, and if the overall fraction of drug clearance catalyzed by a single enzyme is larger than 50%, the AUC ratio would be larger than 1.3, assuming $[I]/K_i = 1$. In contrast, if metabolism of a drug is mediated by several enzymes and no enzyme exhibits an $f_{m,E}$ larger than 20%, the consequence of coadministration of an inhibitor of a single enzyme is unlikely to be noticeable (i.e., the AUC ratio would be smaller than 1.1, assuming $[I]/K_i = 1$).

Considering the validity of K_i and $[I]$ (83,84), for practical reasons a new drug candidate having a K_i value of 1 μmol/L could be viewed as a potent inhibitor, but a clinically relevant DDI would not be expected to occur if the max $[I]$ in plasma was expected to be less than 0.2 μmol/L. Plasma protein binding may also have to be taken into consideration. If a potent inhibitor ($K_i = 1$ μmol/L) binds extensively to plasma proteins (more than 99%), a significant DDI would be less likely to occur, even when the max $[I]$ reaches 10 μmol/L.

If a drug has a low K_m value, it implies that the drug strongly binds to the enzyme and cannot readily be inhibited by other inhibitors. Therefore, the ratio of the K_m of a substrate to the K_i of an inhibitor can be used as an important criterion for the assessment of the susceptibility of the substrate to the inhibitor.

Under conditions of reversible inhibition and linear substrate kinetics, the *in vivo* inhibition constant, $K_{i,i.v.}$, can be calculated when the formation of a metabolite is mediated by one enzyme. Tests of linearity and intercept for this equation require measurements of multiple formation clearances and simultaneous measurements of $[I]$. The $K_{i,i.v.}$ approach has been applied to several drug-interactions studies, such as carbamazepine/stiripentol (89), fluconazole/warfarin (90), and ritonavir-saquinavir (91). $K_{i,i.v.}$ has several features: (i) the difference in K_i values between *in vitro* and *in vivo* reflects the difference in $[I]$ around the enzyme in these two systems, assuming that the inhibitor binding affinity to the enzyme is the same and the same inhibition mechanism operates in both systems; (ii) because $K_{i,i.v.}$ is determined from the formation clearance of a metabolite, interindividual or intraindividual variations in absorption of the substrate do not affect its calculations; and (iii) $K_{i,i.v.}$ is a constant that is independent of concentrations of enzyme, substrate, and inhibitor, at least for one substrate/inhibitor binding site enzymes. Therefore, $K_{i,i.v.}$ should allow predictions of interactions with different doses of an inhibitor or interactions of the same inhibitor with different substrates of the enzyme.

There are several limitations that need to be considered when the clinical relevance of preclinical signals for a pharmacokinetic DDI is discussed.

Inhibition of intestinal metabolism of CYP3A4 substrates complicates *in vitro* predictions. However, particularly for CYP3A4 and Pgp substrates, the tremendous influence of intestinal activity on the oral bioavailability has been proven. Therefore, when the enzyme in question is expressed in the gut, a formal *in vivo* DDI study should be considered prior to phase 2 or 3 trials, even if an *in vitro* signal for a DDI is weak.

Concurrent induction of P450s with inhibition is another area of concern. While the HIV protease inhibitor ritonavir is a well-known and potent CYP3A inhibitor, DDI studies evaluating the clinical relevance of a ritonavir–CYP3A substrate interaction should dose ritonavir for several days in order to cover its CYP3A-inducing properties. Ritonavir's inhibiting effects are a direct interaction with the CYP3A enzyme and will most likely be immediately apparent, whereas the inducing effects require transcription and translation and need some days to be established.

The existence of multiple-drug transport pathways in addition to metabolic pathways complicates the prediction of *in vitro* data to the *in vivo* situation. As outlined for paclitaxel, this combination may be particularly apparent at the intestinal site after oral administration of drugs under consideration. To date, the most widely accepted human cell–based model for intestinal permeability is the human colon carcinoma cell line (Caco-2) cell system (92,93).

Other complexities in the prediction of inhibitor-based metabolic drug interactions can come from additional inhibition of non-CYP enzymes such as FMO, NAT, glucuronosyl transferases, and epoxide hydrolase, food–drug interactions, and interactions between herbal medicines and drugs.

Interindividual variability in the extent of DDI always complicates predictions. It has been emphasized that interpretations of interaction studies should consider not only the mean interaction effect but also the theoretically conceivable extreme effects in individual subjects (94). Differences in $f_{m,E}$ in the population contribute to the variability in extent of drug interactions *in vivo*, especially at high inhibitor doses.

SUMMARY

Because pharmaceutical DDIs are independent of host-bound determinants, they can be explored *in vitro* and should be avoidable in clinical practice. The increased understanding of the causes of pharmacokinetic DDIs has provided additional tools to assess a new drug's interaction potential during preclinical development. Even though extrapolation from *in vitro* data to the *in vivo* situation in humans is limited, these tools can semiquantitatively estimate the risk of clinical relevance of a DDI *in vivo*. Several considerations facilitating such a risk and prioritization assessment have been discussed in this chapter. It is understood that the elaboration of such principles overlaps with the traditional classification of pharmacokinetic DDI into ADME-related interactions. Therefore, the recognition of such principles changes the way in which DDIs are evaluated and assessed.

Cellular and animal models are used to estimate pharmacodynamic DDIs in humans. These preclinical studies should, whenever possible, be combined with pharmacokinetic/pharmacodynamic modeling and, thus, contribute to the design and interpretation of exploratory DDI in humans during the early stages of clinical drug development. Clearly, an understanding of the underlying principles of pharmaceutical and pharmacokinetic DDIs serves to better explore and manage pharmacodynamic DDI.

The goal of DDI studies during early clinical development of a new drug are to reassure the subjects' safety in subsequent clinical trials and to better design such studies in terms of efficacy assessment. The number of available methods to detect preclinical signals of DDIs has increased during recent years, and DDI studies in early development will achieve their goals only when their design appropriately addresses these preclinical signals. Then however, their impact on patient safety and on further decision making during the drug development process (i.e., their impact on both ethical and cost-saving considerations in clinical drug development) will be significant.

The authors thank H. Delesen, MSc (Department of Pharmacometry and Biometry, Bayer AG, Wuppertal) for providing expert review of the biostatistical aspects.

REFERENCES

1. Lazaron J, Pomeranz BH, Corey PN. Incidence of adverse drug reactions in hospitalized patients. *JAMA* 1998;279:1200–1205.

2. Borda IT, Slone D, Jick H. Assessment of adverse reactions within a drug surveillance program. *JAMA* 1968; 205:645–717.

3. Köhler GI, Bode-Böger SM, Busse R, et al. Drug-drug interactions in medical patients: effects on in-hospital treatment and relation to multiple drug use. *Int J Clin Pharmacol Ther* 2000;38:504–513.

4. Kuhlmann J, Mueck W. Clinical pharmacological strategies to assess drug interaction potential during drug development. *Drug Safety* 2001;24:715–725.

5. McDonnell PJ, Jacobs MR. Hospital admissions resulting from preventable adverse drug reactions. *Ann Pharmacother* 2002;36:1331–1336.

6. Morris JS, Stockley IH. Fundamentals of drug interactions. In: Sirtori C, Kuhlmann J, Telement JP, Vrhovac B, eds. *Clinical pharmacology*. New York: McGraw-Hill International, 2000:51–69.

7. Kuhlmann J. General aspects of drug interaction studies. In: Kuhlmann J, ed. *Drug interaction studies during drug development*. W. Zuckschwerdt Verlag, 1994.

8. Lamy P. The elderly and drug interactions. *J Am Geriatr Soc* 1986;34:586–592.

9. European Agency for the Evaluation of Medicinal Products. General considerations for clinical trials. Step 4: Consensus guideline. London: EMEA, 1997.

10. McLeod HL, Evans WE. Pharmcogenomics: Unlocking the human genome for better drug therapy. *Ann Rev Pharmacol Toxicol* 2001;41:101–121.

11. Phillips KA, Veenstra DL, Oren E, et al. Potential role of phamacogenomics in reducing adverse drug reactions: a systematic review. *JAMA* 2001;286:2270–2279.

12. Vesell ES. Advances in pharmacogenetics and pharmacogenomics. *J Clin Pharmacol* 2000;40:930–938.

13. Zuehlsdorf MT. Relevance of pheno- and genotyping in clinical drug development. *Int J Clin Pharmacol Ther* 1998;36:607–612.

14. Li RC, Lo KNM, Lam JS, et al. Effects of order of magnesium exposure on the postantibiotic effect and bactericidal activity of ciprofloxacin. *J Chemother* 1999;11:243–247.

15. Teng RL, Dogolo LC, Willavize SA, et al. Effect of Maalox and omeprazole on the bioavailability of trovafloxacin. *J Antimicrob Chemother* 1997;39[Suppl B]:93–97.

16. Bardelmeijer HA, Ouwehand M, Malingre MM, et al. Entrapment by Cremophor EL decreases the absorption of paclitaxel from the gut. *Cancer Chemother Pharmacol* 2002;49:119–125.

17. Malingre MM, Schellens JHM, van Tellingen O, et al. The co-solvent Cremophor EL limits absorption of orally administered paclitaxel in cancer patients. *Br J Cancer* 2001;85:1472–1477.

18. Malingre MM, Beijnen JH, Rosing H, et al. The effect of different doses of cyclosporine A on the systemic exposure of orally administered paclitaxel. *Anticancer Drugs* 2001;12:351–358.

19. van Tellingen O, Huiznig MT, Panday VR, et al. Cremophor EL causes (pseudo-)nonlinear pharmacokinetics of paclitaxel in patients. *Br J Cancer* 1999;81:330–335.

20. Kuhlmann J. Wechselwirkungen bei der Resorption von Arzneimitteln. *Med Klin* 1980;75:802–812.

21. Baumhaekel M, Kasel D, Rao-Schymanski RA, et al. Screening for inhibitory effects of antineoplastic agents on CYP3A4 in human liver microsomes. *Int J Clin Pharmacol Ther* 2001;39:517–528.

22. Kivistoe KT, Kroemer HK, Eichelbaum M. The role of human cytochrome P450 enzymes in the metabolism of anticancer agents: Implications for drug interactions. *Br J Clin Pharmacol* 1995;40:523–530.

23. Bohnenstengel F, Hofmann U, Eichelbaum M, et al. Characterization of the cytochrome P450 involved in side-chain oxidation of cyclophosphamide in humans. *Eur J Clin Pharmacol* 1996;51:297–301.

24. Chang TKH, Weber GF, Crespi CL, et al. Differential activation of cyclophosphamide and ifosphamide by cytochromes P-450 2B and 3A in human liver microsomes. *Cancer Res* 1993;53:5629–5637.

25. Walker D, Flinois J-P, Monkman SC, et al. Identification of the major human hepatic cytochrome P450 involved in activation and N-dechloroethylation of ifosfamide. *Biochem Pharmacol* 1994;47:1157–1163.

26. Monsarrat B, Chatelut E, Royer I, et al. Modification of paclitaxel metabolism in a cancer patient by induction of cytochrome P4503A4. *Drug Metab Dispos* 1998;26:229–233.

27. Kolars JC, Schmiedlin-Ren P, Schuetz JD, et al. Identification of rifampin-inducible P450IIIA4 (CYP3A4) in human small bowel enterocytes. *J Clin Invest* 1992;90:1871–1878.

28. Kolars JC, Lown KS, Schmiedlin-Ren P, et al. CYP3A expression in human gut epithelium. *Pharmacogenetics* 1994;4:247–259.

29. Gorski JC, Jones DR, Haehner-Daniels BD, et al. The relationship of intestinal and hepatic CYP3A to the interaction between midazolam and clarithromycin. *Clin Pharmacol Ther* 1998;64:133–143.

30. Paine MF, Shen DD, Kunze KL, et al. First-pass metabolism of midazolam by the human tissue. *Clin Pharmacol Ther* 1996;60:14–24.

31. Wandel C, Witte JS, Hall JM, et al. CYP3A activity in African American and European American men. Population differences and functional effect of the CYP3A4*1B 5'-promotor region polymorphism. *Clin Pharmacol Ther* 2000;68:82–91.

32. Relling MV, Pui CH, Sandlund JT, et al. Adverse effects of anticonvulsants on efficacy of chemotherapy for acute lymphoblastic leukaemia. *Lancet* 2000;356: 285–290.

33. Farabos C, Haaz MC, Gires P, et al. Hepatic extraction, metabolism, and biliary excretion of irinotecan in the isolated perfused rat liver. *J Pharm Sci* 2001;90:722–731.

34. Santos A, Zanetta S, Cresteil T, et al. Metabolism of irinotecan (CPT-11) by CYP3A4 and CYP3A5 in humans. *Clin Cancer Res* 2000;6:2012–2020.

35. Rodriguez-Galindo C, Radomski K, et al. Clinical use of topoisomerase I inhibitors in anticancer treatment. *Med Pediatr Oncol* 2000;35:385–402.

36. Okuda H, Nishiyama T, Ogura Y, et al. Lethal drug interactions of sorivudine, a new antiviral drug, with oral 5-fluorouracil prodrugs. *Drug Metab Dispos* 1997;25:270–273.

37. Schinkel AH, Smit JJM, van Tellingen O, et al. Disruption of the mouse mdr1a P-glycoprotein gene leads to a deficiency in the blood-brain barrier and to increased sensitivity to drugs. *Cell* 1994;77:491–502.

38. Schinkel AH, Wagenaar E, Mol CAAM, et al. P-glycoprotein in the blood-brain barrier of mice influences the brain penetration and pharmacological activity of many drugs. *J Clin Invest* 1996;97:2517–2524.

39. Sparreboom A, van Asperen J, Mayer U, et al. Limited oral bioavailability and active epithelial excretion of paclitaxel (Taxol) caused by P-glycoprotein in the intestine. *Proc Natl Acad Sci U S A* 1997;94:2031–2035.

40. Bartlett N, Lum BL, Fisher GA, et al. Phase I trial of doxorubicin with cyclosporine as a modulator of multidrug resistance. *J Clin Oncol* 1994;12:835–842.

41. Erlichman C, Moore J, Thiessen J, et al. A phase I trial of doxorubicin (D) and PSC833, a modulator of multidrug resistance (MDR). *Proc Am Soc Clin Oncol* 1993;13:134.

42. Malingre MM, Beijnen JH, Rosing H, et al. Co-administration of GF120918 significantly increases the systemic exposure to oral paclitaxel in cancer patients. *Br J Cancer* 2001;84:42–47.

43. Fisher GA, Sikic BI. Clinical studies with modulators of multidrug resistance. *Drug Resist Clin Oncol Haematol* 1995;9:363–382.

44. Boote DJ, Dennis IF, Twentyman PR, et al. Phase I study of etoposide with SDZ PSC833 as a modulator of multidrug resistance in patients with cancer. *J Clin Oncol* 1996;14:610–618.

45. Bates S, Kang M, Meadows B, et al. A phase I study with infusional vinblastine in combination with the P-glycoprotein antagonist PSC833 (valspodar). *Cancer* 2001;92:1577–1590.

46. Gianni L, Munzone E, Capri G, et al. Paclitaxel by 3-hour infusion in combination with bolus doxorubicin in women with untreated metastatic breast cancer. High antitumor efficacy and cardiac effects in a dose-finding and sequence-finding study. *J Clin Oncol* 1995;13:2688–2699.

47. Ryberg M, Nielsen D, Skovsgaard T, et al. Epirubicin cardiotoxicity: An analysis of 469 patients with metastatic breast cancer. *J Clin Oncol* 1998;16: 3502–3508.

48. Gianni L, Vigano L, Locatelli A, et al. Human pharmacokinetic characterization and in vitro study of the interaction between doxorubicin and paclitaxel in patients with breast cancer. *J Clin Oncol* 1997;15:1906–1915.

49. Graselli G, Vigano L, Capri G, et al. Clinical and pharmacologic study of the epirubicin and paclitaxel combination in women with metastatic breast cancer. *J Clin Oncol* 2001;19:2222–2231.

50. Wacher VJ, Wu CY, Benet LZ. Overlapping substrate specificities and tissue distribution of cytochrome P4503A and P-glycoprotein: Implications for drug delivery and activity in cancer chemotherapy. *Mol Carcinogen* 1995;13:129–134.

51. Wandel C, Kim RB, Kajiji S, et al. P-glycoprotein and cytochrome P-450 3A inhibition: Dissociation of inhibitory potencies. *Cancer Res* 1999;59:3944–3948.

52. Britten CD, Baker SD, Denis CJ, et al. Oral paclitaxel and concurrent cyclosporin A: Targeting clinically relevant systemic exposure to paclitaxel. *Clinical Cancer Res* 2000;6:3459–3468.

53. Desai PB, Duan JZ, Zhu YW, et al. Human liver microsomal metabolism of paclitaxel and drug interactions. *Eur J Drug Metab Phamacokinet* 1998;23:417–424.

54. Meerum-Terwogt JM, Malingre MM, Beijnen JH, et al. Coadministration of oral cyclosporin A enables oral therapy with paclitaxel. *Clin Cancer Res* 1999;5: 3379–3384.

55. Geick A, Eichelbaum M, Burk O. Nuclear receptor response elements mediate induction of intestinal MDR1 by rifampin. *J Biol Chem* 2001;276:14581–14587.

56. Greiner B, Eichelbaum M, Fritz P, et al. The role of intestinal P-glycoprotein in the interaction of digoxin and rifampin. *J Clin Invest* 1999;104:147–153.

57. Liddle C, Goodwin B. Regulation of hepatic drug metabolism: role of the nuclear receptors PXR and CAR. *Semin Liver Dis* 2002;22:115–122.

58. Synold TW, Dussault I, Forman BM: The orphan nuclear receptor SXR coordinately regulates drug metabolism and efflux. *Nat Med* 2001;7:584–590.

59. LeCluyse EL. Pregnane X receptor molecular basis for species differences in CYP3A induction by xenobiotics. *Chem Biol Interact* 2001;134:283–289.

60. Lehmann JM, McKee DD, Watson MA, et al. The human orphan nuclear receptor PXR is activated by compounds that regulate CYP3A4 gene expression and cause drug interactions. *J Clin Invest* 1998;102: 1016–1023.

61. Salphati L, Benet LZ. Modulation of P-glycoprotein expression by cytochrome P450 3A inducers in male and female rat livers. *Biochem Pharmacol* 1998;55:387–395.

62. Lehne G, de Angelis P, den Boer M, et al. Growth inhibition, cytokinesis failure and apoptosis of multidrug-resistant leukemia cells after treatment with P-glycoprotein inhibitory agents. *Leukemia* 1999;13:768–778.

63. Cabot MC, Giuliano AE, Han TY, et al. SDZ PSC833, the cyclosporine A analogue and multidrug resistance modulator, activates ceramide synthesis and increases vinblastine sensitivity in drug-sensitive and drug-resistant cancer cells. *Cancer Res* 1999;59:880–885.

64. Johnstone RW, Ruefli AA, Smyth MJ. Multiple physiological functions for multidrug transporter P-glycoprotein? *Trends Biochem Sci* 2000;25:1–6.

65. Chu XY, Kato Y, Sugiyama Y. Multiplicity of biliary excretion mechanisms for irinotecan, CPT-11, and its metabolites. *Cancer Res* 1997;57:1934–1938.

66. Fricker G, Miller D. Relevance of multidrug resistance proteins for intestinal drug absorption in vitro and in vivo. *Pharmacol Toxicol* 2002;90:5–13.

67. Schellens JHM, Malingre MM, Kruijtzer CMF, et al. Modulation of oral bioavailability of anticancer drugs: from mouse to man. *Eur J Pharm Sci* 2000;12:103–110.

68. Wijnholds J, Evers R, van Leusden MR, et al. Increased sensitivity to anticancer drugs and decreased inflammatory response in mice lacking the multidrug resistance-associated protein. *Nat Med* 1997;3:1275–1279.

69. Fromm MF, Kauffmann HM, Fritz P, et al. The effect of rifampin treatment on intestinal expression of human mrp transporters. *Am J Pathol* 2000;157:1575–1589.

70. Cvetkovic M, Leake B, Fromm MF, et al. OATP and P-glycoprotein transporters mediate the cellular uptake and excretion of fexofenadine. *Drug Metab Dispos* 1999;27:866–871.

71. Dresser GK, Bailey DG, Leake BF, et al. Fruit juices inhibit organic anion transporting polypeptide-mediated drug uptake to decrease the oral availability of fexofenadine. *Clin Pharmacol Ther* 2002;71:11–20.

72. Ahmed AAK, Kumagai M, Otake T, et al. Sevoflurane exposure time and the neuromuscular blocking effect of vecuronium. *Can J Anaesth* 1999;46(5Part1):429–432.

73. Jellish WS, Brody M, Sawicki K, et al. Recovery from neuromuscular blockade after either bolus and prolonged infusions of cisatracurium or recuronium using either isoflurane or propofol-based anesthetics. *Anesth Analg* 2000;91:1250–1255.

74. Evans M, Rees A. The myotoxicity of statins. *Curr Opin Lipidol* 2002;13:415–420.

75. Rosso R, Angiolini C. Basis for anti-tumoral therapy and rationale for multi-modality therapy. In: Sirtori C, Kuhlmann J, Telement JP, Vrhovac B, eds. *Clinical pharmacology*. New York: McGraw-Hill International, 2000: 547–553.

76. McInnes GT, Brodie MJ. Drug interactions that matter: a critical reappraisal. *Drugs* 1988; 36:83–110.

77. US Food and Drug Administration, Center for Drug Evaluation and Research, Center for Biologics Evaluation and Research. Guidance for industry: in vivo drug metabolism / drug interaction studies. Study design, data analysis, and recommendations for dosing and labeling. Rockville MD: US Dept. of Health and Human Services, 1999.

78. US Food and Drug Administration, Center for Drug Evaluation and Research, Center for Biologics Evaluation and Research. Guidance for industry: population pharmacokinetics. Rockville MD: US Dept. of Health and Human Services, 1999.

79. Kuhlmann J. Drug interaction studies during drug development: which, when, how. *Int J Clin Pharm Ther* 1994; 32:305–311.

80. Steinijans VW, Hartmann M, Huber R, et al. Lack of pharmacokinetic interaction as an equivalence problem. *Int J Clin Pharmacol Ther* 1991;29:323–328.

81. European Agency for the Evaluation of Medicinal Products, Committee for Proprietary Medicinal Products. Note for guidance on the investigation of drug interactions. London: EMEA, 1998.

82. Balis F. Pharmacokinetic drug interactions of commonly used anticancer drugs. *Clin Pharmacokinet* 1986;11:223–235.

83. Tucker GT, Houston JB, Huang S-M. Optimizing drug development: strategies to assess drug metabolism / transporter interaction potential–towards a consensus. *Br J Clin Pharmacol* 2001;52:107–117.

84. Lin JH. Sense and nonsense in the prediction of drug-drug interactions. *Curr Drug Metab* 2000;1:305–331.

85. Yao C, Levy R. Inhibition-based metabolic drug-drug interactions: Predictions from in vitro data. *J Pharm Sci* 2002;91:1923–1935.

86. Wilkinson GR. Clearance approaches in pharmacology. *Pharmacol Rev* 1987;39:1–47.

87. Levy RH, Trager WF. From in vitro to in vivo: an academic perspective. In: Levy RH, Thummel KE, Trager WF, Hansten PD, Eichelbaum M, eds. *Metabolic drug interactions*. Philadelphia: Lippincott-Raven Publishers, 2000:21–27.

88. Rowland M, Matin SB. Kinetics of drug-drug interactions. *J Pharmacokinet Biopharm* 1973;1:553–567.

89. Tran A, Rey E, Pons G, Rousseau M, et al. Influence of stiripentol on cytochrome P–450 mediated metabolic pathways in humans: In vitro and in vivo comparison and calculation of in vivo inhibition constants. *Clin Pharmacol Ther* 1997;62:490–504.

90. Kunze KL, Trager WF. Warfarin-fluconazole III. A rational approach to management of a metabolically based drug interaction. *Drug Metab Dispos* 1996;24:429–435.

91. Hsu A, Granneman GR, Cao G, et al. Pharmacokinetic interactions between two human immunodeficiency virus protease inhibitors, ritonavir and saquinavir. *Clin Pharmacol Ther* 1998;63:453–464.

92. Hidalgo IJ, Raub TJ, Borchardt RT. Characterization of the human colon carcinoma cell line (Caco-2) as a model system for intestinal epithelial permeability. *Gastroenterology* 1989;96:736–749.

93. Li AP. Screening for human ADME/Tox drug properties in drug discovery. *Drug Discov Today* 2001;6: 357–366.

94. Krayenbuhl JC, Vozeh S, Kondo-Oestreicher M, et al. Drug-drug interactions of new active substances: mibefradil example. *Eur J Clin Pharmacol* 1999;55: 559– 565.

12

Gene-Targeted Mice in Anticancer Drug Development

Thomas M. Donnelly

The Warren Institute, Ossining, New York 10562

The laboratory mouse has emerged as the primary mammalian system for genomics research and the preeminent surrogate model system for human disease and normative biology. Approximately 90% of human genes share homology with genes within the mouse genome. A rapidly evolving and increasingly sophisticated technology has developed for creating mouse models. The aim of this chapter is to:

- Review the conditional mouse models of cancer and examine the different techniques that allow experimental "switches" to turn genes on or off, where and when the researcher desires
- Highlight the diversity of the laboratory mouse's genetic background and alert researchers to the endogenous genetic and exogenous variables that contribute to mismanagement of transgenic lines
- Describe the mouse imaging systems that now enable noninvasive monitoring of tumor development, an area especially useful for preclinical testing of therapeutic intervention or chemoprevention strategies, and
- Provide a list of Web-based resources on mouse cancer models that can aid in the derivation and characterization of mouse models, and generate resources, information, and innovative approaches to their application in cancer research.

WHY USE GENE-TARGETED MICE FOR ANTICANCER DRUG DEVELOPMENT?

Preclinical animal models perform an essential role in evaluating drug efficacy and selecting lead compounds. Investigational New Drug applications require extensive preclinical studies to show efficacy and determine drug pharmacokinetics and dynamics. Transplantable rodent or human tumor grafts have traditionally been used for preclinical testing of anti-

neoplastic agents (see Chapter 10). Unfortunately not all drugs found to be chemotherapeutic in rodents are efficacious in humans (1,2). Drug companies often do not establish this failure of novel chemopreventive agents until phase 2 or 3 clinical trials, after they have made costly investments of time and money.

Improving the quality of targets and compounds is a priority for drug companies, which aim to reduce the time and money they have to spend on Investigational New Drug applications. Without a dependable animal model, cancer drug discovery has traditionally focused on targeting DNA synthesis and cell division (3). Although traditional cancer drugs showed efficacy (all chemotherapeutic agents that are efficacious in humans are also effective in rodents), their lack of selectivity for tumor cells over normal cells resulted in unwanted high toxicity. The discovery of cancer-causing genes, later called oncogenes, in 1978 suggested a logical, targeted approach to cancer drug discovery (Fig. 12.1). The development of imatinib (Gleevec, formerly known as Glivec) and other active protein-kinase inhibitors illustrates this process.

Chronic myeloid leukemia results from the action of BCR-ABL tyrosine kinase. Rowley (4) first characterized a reciprocal translocation between chromosomes 9 and 22 in human chronic myelogenous leukemia (CML). The shortened version of chromosome 22 (known as the Philadelphia chromosome) presented the first evidence of a genetic change associated with human cancer (5). Transpositioning chromosome 22 creates the *bcr-abl* oncogene that transcribes a protein with elevated tyrosine-kinase activity (6). In 1990, Daley et al. (7) demonstrated that introduction of the *bcr-abl* oncogene could induce CML in mice. As the tyrosine-kinase activity of Bcr-Abl is essential for its transforming activity, the enzymatic activity of Bcr-Abl was realized to be a drug target to treat Bcr-Abl–positive leukemias (8).

163

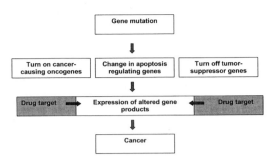

FIG. 12.1. Targeted drug therapy. The aim of rational drug design is to identify a drug target (e.g., an oncogene) that differs in its activity between neoplastic and normal cells.

For the first time, a drug target was identified that differed in its activity between leukemic and normal cells.

Our knowledge of gene variation in cancer, obtained by comparing the patterns of genes expressed in cancer patients and normal individuals, has distinguished transcriptional changes in thousands of genes as normal cells undergo transformation into cancer cells (9,10). We have learned to use *in vitro* techniques such as antisense oligonucleotides, ribozymes, and peptides to inhibit gene expression and study gene function. However, the most important method to study gene function in cancer is gene targeting in mice[1], i.e., introducing specific mutations into endogenous mouse genes that are subsequently transmitted through the mouse germ line. The first experiments occurred in 1984 when mouse eggs were microinjected with oncogenes. Brinster et al. (11) found that copies of the simian virus 40 (SV40) T antigen caused choroid plexus tumors, and Stewart et al. (12) found that the mouse mammary tumor virus *myc* gene caused mammary adenocarcinoma. A crucial advantage of gene-targeting approaches over

microinjection techniques is that homologous recombination in embryonic stem (ES) cells clearly defines the site of integration and allows for precise design of the introduced genetic change. With the use of conventional gene-targeting strategies, hundreds of alleles have been successfully engineered and the corresponding phenotypes analyzed (13,14).

We can investigate the function of genes with known sequences in two ways using mice. The first is through loss-of-function (i.e., knock-out), whereas the other is through gain-of-function (ie knock-in). Since the mid-1980s, research groups using different gene-targeting strategies such as defined mutations, including null mutations (elimination of a gene and loss-of-function of its activity by substituting another gene) or point mutations (substitution of one nucleotide for another resulting in a change in a single base pair), complex chromosomal rearrangements encompassing large deletions, and translocations (fragmentation of a chromosome and transfer of the broken-off portion to another chromosome, often of a different pair) or inversions (deletion and reinsertion of a chromosome segment in the same place but turned 180 degrees from its original orientation, so that the gene sequence for the segment is reversed with respect to that of the rest of the chromosome), have introduced mutant alleles into known mouse cancer genes (15–19). These oncogene-bearing transgenic mice (knock-ins) or tumor-suppressor gene knockout mice have generated numerous cancer-prone mouse strains.

Unfortunately, early gene-targeting work did not achieve the promise of useful cancer drug discovery information. Many genes have several roles, and when mutated in the germ line or overexpressed in developing organs, the result is an embryonic-lethal phenotype that makes the study of the effects of gene mutations in adult mice impossible (17,20–23). Consequently, transgenic and knockout mice have not become the optimal models once anticipated for drug testing. Instead, the pharmaceutical industry, the National Cancer Institute (NCI), and the US Food and Drug Administration (FDA) have relegated their use to efficacy and target-identification studies.

Since 1999, cancer-prone mice that have conditional knockouts (24–26) and carry regulatable oncogenes started to supersede "first-generation" mouse tumor models (27–32). In these mice, we can induce somatic mutations in specific tissues and at precise times, which more reliably models sporadic tumor formation. These second-generation models present opportunities to gain insight into the role of genes in the initiation, progression, and treatment of cancer.

---

[1] Genetically modified mice can be generated either by direct pronuclear injection of exogenous DNA into fertilized zygotes or by injection of genetically modified mouse ES cells into a blastocyst. Pronuclear microinjection results in random integration of the injected DNA in the genome and relies on the overexpression of the transgene to produce a phenotype. In contrast, homologous recombination occurs in the ES cells before we inject them into the blastocyst. In homologous recombination, a fragment of introduced genomic DNA finds and recombines with the endogenous homologous sequence, resulting in a genetic modification. This process is known as "gene targeting." In common usage, the term *transgenic* now refers to random (microinjected) integration.

MOUSE CANCER MODELS THAT USE CONDITIONAL GENE MUTATION

Sporadic cancer arises because individual cells sustain a series of sequential mutations that result in tumor growth. However, malignancy emerges from a tumor–host microenvironment in which the host is an active participant throughout the entire process of cancer etiology, progression, and metastasis (33). Indeed, the local microenvironment is the driving force in stimulating or suppressing the invasive and malignant behavior of cancer cells (34). Conventional transgenic mice mimic hereditary forms of cancer because the initiating gene mutation is present in all cells of the body, including those that make up the tumor microenvironment (35). Consequently, the effects of stromal cells in inhibition (e.g., immune response) or stimulation (e.g., angiogenesis) of tumor growth can be diminished (Fig. 12.2). The introduced gene mutation can also activate compensatory factors or pathways during embryonic development, resulting in embryonic death. Conventional transgenic mice are not good models of sporadic cancer because most human tumors are monoclonal in origin.

In contrast, conditional gene mutation allows researchers to examine neoplastic transformation in a normal, nonmutated microenvironment. Researchers can focus on a particular tissue and/or at a specific time. Furthermore, transgenic mice with a single controlled gene mutation can be crossbred to introduce multiple conditional alleles in one mouse. Crossbreeding allows researchers to evaluate the role of individual mutations to the tumor phenotype. For example, this could be a controllable *APC*, *BRCA*, *VHL*, or *trp53* tumor-suppressor gene knockout in a controllable *ras*, *myc*, or *abl* oncogene-activated, oncogene-expressing mouse. A real example is the conditional mouse model that Bex et al. reported (36). These mice permit study of time-controlled mutations of bladder-cancer–related tumor-suppressor genes when they are crossbred to other mice carrying floxed alleles for *Rb*, *trp53*, and *p16INK4a* either alone or in combination.

What is the ideal conditional mouse model? Lewandoski (27) described it as one in which investigators can turn on or off a transgene where and when they choose. Scientists have achieved conditional gene expression through a double-transgenic approach. Two components interact to control gene expression. Typically, the product of an effector transgene acts upon a "target" transgene. We can divide the double-transgenic systems into two categories. In one, the effector transgene transactivates transcription of the target transgene, which is usually an oncogene. In the other, the effector transgene is a tissue or site-specific DNA recombinase that rearranges the target gene, usually a tumor-suppressor gene, and inactivates it.

Theoretically, the ideal conditional transgenic mouse meets the following criteria:

- By itself, the effector transgene does not affect the expression of endogenous genes (this has been accomplished by using partial effector transgene sequences derived from bacteria or viruses)
- Control of the target transgene is fully conditional on the presence of the effector transgene (this has been realized by restricting expression of the target transgene only in the presence of an exogenously added inducer, such as tetracycline, which allows appropriate effector–gene product–target gene interaction)
- The effector transgene should be reversible so that defined periods or critical stages in disease can be appropriately monitored
- Induction kinetics should be fast and expression levels sufficiently high to produce a rapid and detectable effect.

There are exceptions and variations to these criteria, and for more detail the reader is referred to recent reviews on this subject (27–32,37). To illustrate the dramatic explosion in conditional gene targeting, between 2000 and 2002 approximately 1,000 articles were published on conditional mouse models of cancer. In the next section, I will review the genetic strategies used in these articles, citing specific experiments, and consider their advantages and limitations.

Inducible Transgenes

The most common conditional gene expression systems use tetracycline (tet)-inducible promoters (38). In these systems, the effector is a tissue-specific promoter that induces protein fusion between the herpes simplex virus VP16 transactivation domain and the *Escherichia coli* transposon Tn10 tetracycline repressor (TetR). This fusion protein, known as tTA, specifically binds both tetracycline and the Tet operon (*tetO*) in the target transgene. In the presence of doxycycline, a form of tetracycline, the tTA protein, binds the *tetO* sequences and represses target gene expression. A reverse tTA (rtTA) has also been created in which doxycycline activates target gene expression.

These inducible systems have been applied to the study of tumorigenesis primarily by investigating tissue-specific and time-controlled oncogenesis (Table 12.1). Adding doxycycline to food or water is the usual method to control transgene induction. Removal of the doxycycline turns off gene expression. This technique

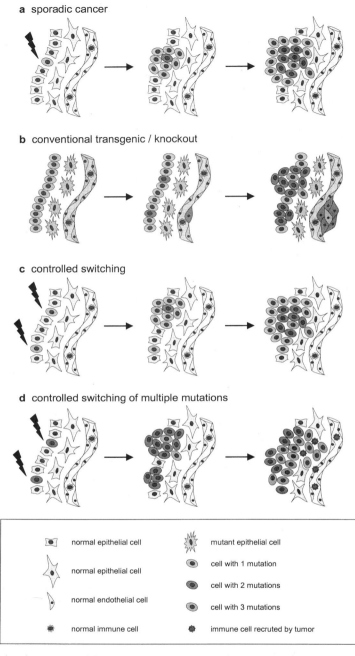

a sporadic cancer

b conventional transgenic / knockout

c controlled switching

d controlled switching of multiple mutations

normal epithelial cell	mutant epithelial cell
normal epithelial cell	cell with 1 mutation
normal endothelial cell	cell with 2 mutations
normal immune cell	cell with 3 mutations
	immune cell recruited by tumor

FIG. 12.2. Conventional versus conditional mouse tumor models. Cancer arises through the sequential accumulation of genetic and epigenetic changes that drive the conversion of normal cells into highly malignant derivatives. **A:** In sporadic cancer, the initiating mutation affects a single cell in an otherwise normal microenvironment. **B:** Conventional tumor-suppressor gene knockouts or oncogene-bearing transgenic mice do not mimic sporadic tumor development because the initiating mutation is present throughout the body or a particular tissue. Consequently, the functions of the microenvironment in stimulating or inhibiting tumor growth can be impaired. Other unwanted side effects include tumorigenesis outside the tissue of interest, or the induction of mechanisms that balance the effects of the mutation. **C:** Conditional gene-mutation strategies allow the induction of somatic mutations in a tissue-restricted and time-specific manner, and so can faithfully mimic sporadic tumor onset and progression under well-controlled conditions. **D:** Simultaneous induction of multiple mutations will result in the development of specific tumors with high penetrance and short latency. Reprinted from Jonkers J, Berns A. Conditional mouse models of sporadic cancer. *Nat Rev Cancer* 2002;2:251–265, with permission.

TABLE 12.1. *Tumor models that investigate inducible oncogenes*

Tissue	Tumor	Transactivator	Target oncogene	Reference
Hematopoietic cells	B-cell leukemia	rtTA	*bcr-abl1*	46
Hematopoietic cells	T-cell lymphoma and myelogenous leukemia	tTA	*myc*	47
Melanocytes	Melanoma	tTA	H-*ras*	40
Salivary gland	Hyperplastic ducts	rtTA	*SV40 Tag*	39
Suprabasal epidermis	Papilloma	ER/tamoxifen	c-*myc*	42

bcr-abl1, breakpoint-cluster-region Abelson murine leukemia virus; c-*myc*, avian myelocytomatosis viral oncogene homologue; H-*ras*, Harvey rat sarcoma viral oncogene; *myc*, avian myelocytomatosis viral oncogene; *SV40 Tag*, simian virus 40 large T antigen.

allows the researcher to turn on and off gene expression. Ewald et al. (39) used this method to investigate the SV40 T antigen (TAg) oncoprotein in maintaining cellular transformation. Expression of TAg in the submandibular gland of transgenic mice from birth to 4 months of age induced epithelial transformation and extensive ductal hyperplasia. The hyperplasia was reversed when they silenced TAg expression for 3 weeks. However, when they silenced TAg expression after 7 months, the hyperplasia persisted although TAg was absent. Chin et al. (40) used the TetR system to activate an inserted H-*ras* oncogene allele, and showed that its expression induces melanomas in an *INK4a*-null tumor-suppressor gene mouse.

Instead of a tetracycline-inducible promoter, some studies have used protein fusions between the target transgene and the tamoxifen-responsive hormone-binding domain of the estrogen receptor. This system induces gene expression by treatment with the antiestrogen tamoxifen or its derivative, 4-hydroxytamoxifen (41). An example of this method is the study by Pelangris et al. (42), who induced epidermal papillomas by activating c-*myc*.

The tumor-induction studies suggest prolonged expression of certain oncogenes cause genetic changes that eventually become independent of that oncogene's expression. Most important, they provide data that may lead to the production of oncogene-specific anticancer drugs (43).

The benefits of the TetR system are (a) the ability to reverse expression of the transactivator and target gene; (b) the sensitivity of transgene activation levels to inducer concentration, making gene expression "titration" possible; and (c) the ability to control the expression of more than one target transgene. Consequently, the TetR system is appropriate for gain-of-function experiments such as oncogene activation, in which phenotypes are generated by transgene overexpression.

The limitations of the TetR systems are leakiness (unwanted expression in the absence of the inducer) and poor inducibility (insufficient expression in the presence of the inducer). Leakiness is associated with *cis*-acting regulatory elements and regions of heterochromatin, a compacted silent form of DNA, near the insertions influencing gene expression (44,45). Poor inducibility is associated with the kinetics of doxycycline clearance and induction can take up to 7 days, and repeated switching on and off results eventually in unresponsiveness to further stimulation (45). Although the TetR system offers excellent temporal control of gene expression, tissue-specific or spatial control is limited; therefore, the mouse models are inappropriate for mimicking sporadic cancer (28).

Conditional Gene Inactivation with *Cre* Recombinase

The Cre recombinase protein encoded by the *E. coli* bacteriophage P1 promotes recombination of DNA at a specific site, called lox (*loxP*), and does not require any other protein factors (48). Using *Cre* site-specific DNA recombinase allows researchers to make precise DNA rearrangements and genetic switches when combined with inducible systems for controlling *Cre* expression and function (49). When the mouse genome is engineered to have *loxP* sites, using defined promoters to drive *Cre* can control DNA recombination in a spatial and temporal pattern. In such mouse tumor models, recombinase recognition sites flank the target gene, and because *loxP* sites flank the exons, we call it a "floxed" allele. In the presence of the recombinase, the intervening DNA segment is deleted, converting a functional allele to a null allele (Fig. 12.3). The *Cre/loxP* recombinase system is currently the most widely used method in mice to disrupt gene expression conditionally, and a *Cre* transgenic database exists

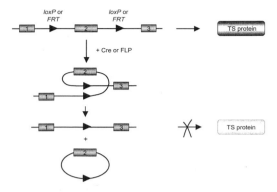

FIG. 12.3. Tumor model using *Cre/lox* recombination-mediated tumor-suppressor gene inactivation. *Cre/loxP* recombination-mediated tumor-suppressor gene inactivation can be achieved by inserting the 34-base pair *loxP* recombinase recognition sites into intron sequences in a direct orientation. Expression of the *Cre*-recombinase enzyme will catalyze the conservative recombination between the recognition sites, resulting in juxtaposition of exons 1 and 3, and excision of the intervening sequence that includes exon 2. The recombination event results in gene inactivation if this exon is essential for proper gene function. Reprinted from Jonkers J, Berns A. Conditional mouse models of sporadic cancer. *Nat Rev Cancer* 2002;2:251–265, with permission.

(50–52). Examples of *Cre/loxP* mouse tumor models are presented in Table 12.2. Cre recombinase can be introduced by viral delivery or by crossbreeding the floxed allele mice with transgenic mice in which *Cre* is expressed in a tissue-specific manner. Although the resulting compound mutant mice may have several conditional tumor-suppressor gene alleles, they can be bred without compromising viability.

Cre-mediated excision of genes has been used to avoid embryonic lethality associated with null alleles of some tumor suppression genes. For example, homozygous *Nf2*, *APC*, *BRAC1*, and *Rb* knockout mice die during embryogenesis. To avoid embryonic lethality, Xu et al. (53) used *Cre* expression to induce tissue-specific deletion of a conditional *BRCA1* allele in adult mammary-gland epithelium cells. *BRCA1* inactivation resulted in mammary tumors after a long latent period. However, tumor formation occurred faster when the investigators performed the same experiment in heterozygous null-*trp53* mice. In addition, the mammary tumors showed genetic instability. Jonkers et al. (54) observed similar synergistic effects between *BRCA2* and *trp53*.

In experiments for which tumor-suppressor gene inactivation does not cause embryonic death, *Cre*-mediated two-gene inactivation offers a technique to prevent unwanted tumorigenesis (55). Marino et al. (56) generated a mouse model of medulloblastoma in a *Cre*-mediated double knockout of *Rb* and *trp53* tumor-suppressor genes in glial cells. This gene-targeting strategy allowed the investigators to study the effect of *Rb* inactivation in glial cells, without the unwanted development of lymphomas that we commonly see in homozygous *trp53* knockouts (55).

The *Cre/loxP* recombinase system can also be used to investigate tissue-specific activation of oncogenes. Researchers use a transcriptional terminator (e.g., a green fluorescent protein reporter gene or *Stop* sequence, the DNA sequence occurring at the end of the gene causing RNA polymerase to stop transcription) flanked by recombinase target sites (*loxP*) to split a tissue-specific promoter from an oncogene (Fig. 12.4). Two different techniques for conditional expression of the activated oncoprotein K-Ras illustrate this strategy. In one technique, Jackson et al. (57) used a knock-in approach to achieve *Cre*-mediated K-*ras* expression. In the second technique, Meuwissen et al. (58) used transgenic mice in which *Cre* expression

TABLE 12.2. *Tumor models that investigate conditional gene inactivation with Cre recombinase*

Tissue	Tumor	Tissue-specific promoter	Floxed target gene	Reference(s)
Mammary gland epithelium	Mammary adenocarcinoma	MMTV-LTR	*BRCA1*^{loxP} + *trp53* +/–	53
Mammary gland epithelium	Mammary adenocarcinoma	K14	*BRCA2*^{loxP} + *trp53*^{loxP}	54
Cerebellar external granular layer	Medulloblastoma	GFAP	*Rb*^{loxP} + *trp53*^{loxP}	56
Pulmonary epithelium	Pulmonary adenocarcinoma	Adenovirus-Cre	*Stop*^{loxP} + K-*ras*	57,58

BRCA1, breast cancer gene 1; *BRCA2*, breast cancer gene 2; K-*ras*, Kirsten rat sarcoma virus oncogene; *Rb*, retinoblastoma gene; *trp53*, mouse tumor-suppressor gene 53; *Stop*, DNA sequence at the end of gene causing RNA polymerase to stop transcription.

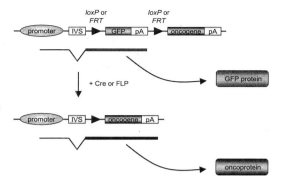

FIG. 12.4. Tumor model using *Cre/lox* recombination-mediated oncogene activation. *Cre/loxP* recombination-mediated oncogene activation can be achieved by using a floxed transcriptional terminator [e.g., a green fluorescent protein (GFP) reporter gene] to insulate the oncogene from a promoter. In the absence of the recombinase enzyme, GFP is expressed and the oncogene behind the polyadenylation (pA) signal remains silent. After recombinase-mediated excision of the GFP gene, the oncogene is placed under direct control of the promoter. IVS-intervening sequence. Reprinted from Jonkers J, Berns A. Conditional mouse models of sporadic cancer. *Nat Rev Cancer* 2002;2: 251–265, with permission.

caused recombination of activated K-*ras* to an active actin promoter. Both models used recombinant adenoviruses expressing *Cre* recombinase to activate K-*ras* in the lungs of mice, resulting in pulmonary adenocarcinomas. A major limitation of many mouse lung cancer models is the inability to control tumor numbers, resulting in mice dying early from respiratory failure due to an overwhelming number of early-stage tumors. The early mortality limits tumor progression. Furthermore, the inability to synchronize tumor development complicates analysis of tumor initiation and progression. These two studies overcame the limitations of the TetR system by still allowing control of tumor-initiation timing, but also by allowing control of tumor location and numbers. The resulting pulmonary adenocarcinomas closely mimic a human non–small cell carcinoma.

The *Cre/loxP* system is uniquely suited for tissue-specific and time-controlled gene activation and inactivation. When used in combination with established ES cell techniques, the *Cre/loxP* recombination system is the benchmark for transgenic mouse loss-of-function studies (52). The limitations of this system have only become apparent as the number of tissue-specific *Cre* mice grows. There is difficulty in properly regulating *Cre* expression. Vooijs et al. (59) showed that recombination efficiency is locus depen-

dent, which has important consequences when the study design needs simultaneous switching of multiple alleles within the same cell. Researchers have also found prolonged low levels of *Cre* activity (independent of *loxP*) permit recombination with accompanying genomic toxicity such as chromosomal aberrations and an increased number of sister chromatid exchanges (60,61). The difficulties in controlling *Cre* expression and its genomic toxicity at chronic low levels highlight the need for *Cre* techniques with controllable or self-inactivating recombinase activity.

Retroviral Gene Delivery

Cell-specific gene delivery based on avian retroviral–mediated gene delivery to cells expressing the avian retroviral receptor, tv-a, has developed in the laboratory of Harold Varmus (62,63). Mice do not express the tv-a receptor, which avian retroviruses require for cellular entry. Scientists in the Varmus laboratory have produced conventional transgenic mice to express tv-a under the control of cell-specific and tissue-specific promoters. These tissues are then susceptible to gene delivery with an avian pseudo-typed retrovirus that recognizes the tv-a receptor. The gene of interest (e.g., an oncogene) is cloned into a replication-competent avian proviral vector (RCAS) derived from avian Rous sarcoma virus. The retroviral vector is transfected into chicken fibroblasts to produce high-titer stocks of infectious pseudotyped viral particles containing avian leukosis virus coat protein that recognizes the tv-a receptor. The researchers then inject the virus into mice either as virus-producing cells or as viral particles.

This technique has been used extensively by Holland et al. (64,65) to model gliomagenesis in mice. The investigators designed an experiment to find out if signal transduction pathways involving Ras or Akt induce glioblastoma formation. Genes encoding activated forms of Ras and Akt were transferred by direct injection of cells producing RCAS vectors into the brains of newborn mice. They found that although activated Ras or Akt alone is insufficient to induce glioblastoma formation, the combination of activated Ras and Akt induces glioblastomas.

Mouse tumor models using retroviral gene delivery are suitable for drug-efficacy studies. The advantage of the system is that several genes (e.g., *ras, akt*) can be transferred simultaneously or sequentially into the same cells, making it ideal for investigating oncogene cooperation in tumorigenesis. Retroviral gene transfer can also be used to mimic human sporadic cancer development. For example, transfer of RCAS vectors with single or multiple genes leads to the production of a heterogenous population of cells that express different quantities and mixtures of the transferred gene products. This situation is similar to human cancer, in which a number of different genetic lesions occur in the same mass. In addition, retroviral gene transfer using a known viral titer can be used to infect a single cell that gives rise to a single tumor.

The limitations of retroviral gene transfer are the production of an immune response at the site of virus injection and the restricted use of small complimentary DNAs because the insert cannot be larger than 2.5 kilobases.

Sporadic Activation of Spontaneous Recombination

Using a novel gene-targeting technique, Johnson et al. (66) constructed mouse tumor models involving K-*ras*. The mice carry oncogenic alleles of K-*ras* that can be activated only when spontaneous recombination (i.e., shuffling of DNA segments) occurs either within or between chromosomes during cell division. An active wild-type K-*ras* or mutant K-*ras2* gene is generated in random tissues mimicking the sporadic occurrence of K-*ras* mutations that occur in many human tumors, such as adenocarcinoma of the pancreas (70%–90% prevalence), colon (50%), and lung (25%–50%) (67,68). The mice carrying the low but significant number of K-*ras* mutations are predisposed to a range of tumors (e.g., thymic lymphoma, skin papilloma), but predominantly develop an early-onset pulmonary adenocarcinoma.

Sporadic activation of a recombination system in mice allows researchers to introduce several genetic alterations at a defined time point in a subset of cells, increasing the ability to duplicate a wide range of human tumors (69). As the Ras pathway is considered an attractive target for chemotherapeutic intervention, these mice may be useful in evaluating the efficacy of Ras pathway–directed therapies (70). A limitation of this strategy is the lack of control that researchers have over gene expression.

EFFECT OF GENETIC VARIATION ON CONDITIONAL MOUSE MODELS

Besides allowing the induction of well-defined sporadic tumors with high penetrance and within a narrow time window, conditional mouse models of cancer should allow assessment of the contributions of individual mutations to the tumor phenotype. Ideally, measuring the effect of a single variable in an otherwise stable genetic background that contains a

fixed number of defined complementing mutations should be possible. In reality, it becomes crucial for the interpretation of any knockout and transgenic genotype to decide whether the targeted mutation causes the observed phenotypic difference or is the result of background genetic variation[2].

The Three Major Inbred Strains in Transgenic Research

Although more than 450 inbred strains of mice are described for biomedical research, three strains are the mainstays of genetically modified mouse models: the 129, C57BL/6 (B6), and FVB/N; however, none of these strains was originally developed for modern biomedical research (72)[3]. Clarence Little (also a founder and first director of the Jackson Laboratory) developed the C57BL strain in 1921 as a low-tumor, long-lived strain. Fortunately, because this strain is used in toxicology and aging research, a large amount of information on its background pathology is available (74,75). Transgenic technologies have increased the use of 129 and FVB strains. Only limited background pathology information is available on the129 strain (76).

Most transgenic mice are created from hybrid and outbred mice, especially Swiss[4] mice, because they have large pronuclei for injection. However, hybrid and outbred mice created in this way have limited value as research models because of their genetic heterozygosity. Consequently, we require backcrossing such mice onto a standard genetic background. Alternatively, inbred Swiss FVB mice have been heavily used because they offer the advantages of Swiss mice but are inbred (78). FVB mice originated from outbred NIH Swiss mice that were inbred for pertussis research and are characterized by vigorous reproductive performance and large litters. Fertilized FVB eggs contain prominent pronuclei and zygotes

---

[2] For several years, behavioral neuroscientists have been aware of the influence of genetic background on phenotype interpretation in genetically engineered mice. Consequently, the 1997 Banbury Conference on Genetic Background in Mice recommended that researchers maintain knockout mutations as standard inbred congenic lines so they are used as such in experiments, or as F1 hybrids between strains of two different backgrounds (71).

[3] For more detail on the origins and relationships of inbred mouse strains, refer to the review by Beck et al. (73).

[4] Swiss mice can be inbred or outbred strains. Their outbred character is only relative as they were derived from two male and seven female mice imported from a closed colony in 1926. For more information, refer to the paper by Clara Lynch (77).

survive well after DNA microinjection (78). Barthold (79) observed that FVB mice are likely to develop prolactin-secreting pituitary adenomas and hyperplasia. Because mammary gland involution does not occur after lactation, a significant amount of research using mice as human models of breast cancer has been with FVB transgenics.

Targeted mutagenesis (knock-ins and knock-outs) using ES cells makes extensive use of 129 mouse substrains (37). The targeted mutations are developed by homologous recombination of genes inserted into 129 ES cell lines, and selected ES cells are injected into the inner mass of blastocysts of a recipient (usually B6) mouse embryo to create a chimeric mouse. If the mutated gene is incorporated into germ cells, then backcrossing the chimeric mouse onto a B6 mouse strain can transmit the allele to successive generations.

The 129 strain was bred for its tendency to develop testicular teratomas, and the derivation of ES cells came from the initial work on teratocarcinoma stem cells (80). Simpson et al. (81) documented that outcrossing of 129 substrains has lead to extensive genetic variability between substrains and the ES cells derived from them. By using simple sequence length polymorphisms, Threadgill et al. (82) showed that the numerous substrains of 129 have demonstrable physiologic differences ie phenotype variation. They found that the 129/SvJ strain is significantly different from other 129 substrains. This mixed genetic background can complicate gene-targeting experiments by reducing homologous recombination efficiency when researchers do not derive their constructs and ES cells from the same 129 substrain. In addition, discrepancies due to different genetic backgrounds may arise when comparing phenotypes of genes targeted in different 129-derived ES cell lines.

The B6 embryos are highly compatible hosts for 129 ES cells, and facilitate chimerism. As a result, B6 mice are becoming the benchmark background genotype for most targeted mutations. Although they are more difficult to develop, there is a growing tendency for the creation of ES cell lines, including but not limited to B6 and BALB/c cell lines (83,84). Albino B6 mice or albino B6 ES cell lines offer solutions to select likely germ-line chimeras by coat color.

Transgene expression is often inconsistent because genetic and epigenetic processes control it (85,86). In theory, once integrated into the murine genome, the injected DNA can manifest its function. However, as the insertion occurs at random, positional variegation effects may occur. The insertion of the transgene may affect the function of the endogenous genes (insertional effects), and surrounding elements may compromise the expression of the transgene itself (variegation effects). Evidence for strain-specific major modifier locus effects has been found, suggesting that variegating gene expression in transgenic and gene-targeted mice is influenced by their genetic background (86–88).

Transgenic mice carry multiple alleles that either enhance or reduce the likelihood and phenotypic expression of developing specific types of tumors. For example, Donehower et al. (89) monitored p53-deficient mice of two different genetic backgrounds (129/Sv and mixed C57BL/6 × 129/Sv). Accelerated tumorigenesis occurred in p53+/− and p53−/− 129/Sv mice compared with the p53-deficient mixed C57BL/6 × 129/Sv mice. Although the range of tumors was similar in the two strains, half the 129/Sv p53−/− males developed malignant teratomas, whereas these tumors rarely arose in the C57BL/6 × 129/Sv mice and did not occur in the 129/Sv p53+/− males. Cory et al. (90) found that inserting an *Eμ-myc* allele causes lymphoma onset earlier on an SJL or BALB/c background than on a C57BL/6 background. Similarly, with plasmacytoma induction by an *Eμ-v-abl* transgene, the incidence in BALB/c mice was 80% within 7 months, but less than 20% at 12 months on a C57BL/6 background (91). Age can also influence expression of the transgene (92). Fortunately, the degree of gene silencing, variegation, or expression tends to be stable within a transgenic mouse (93).

In *Cre/loxP* mice, the potential for unwanted genetic variation is greater than other gene-targeted mice. These mice "start" as selected 129 ES cells with floxed target genes. The 129 ES cells are placed in recipient blastocysts (usually B6) to create chimeric mice. The chimeras expressing the target gene in germ cells are then backcrossed onto B6 mice. The resulting mice, often only partially backcrossed, are then crossed with *Cre*-recombinase transgenic mice (usually FVB or inbred strain hybrids) to create the *Cre/loxP* mouse. Consequently, there is the potential for four (or more) background genomes to influence the gene alteration.

Mouse Retroviruses

The mouse genome contains exogenous and endogenous murine leukemia viruses, mammary tumor viruses, replication-incompetent tumor viruses, and retrovirus-like elements (79). Thousands of copies of these viruses and viral-like elements are distributed throughout the mouse genome (79). The retroviruses can act as endogenous transgenes, recombining into different regions of the genome and resulting in null mutations and chromosomal rearrangements that contribute to strain characteristics, subline divergence, and new phenotypes. Through active recombination and transposition, retroviruses cause genetic subline divergence (94). Crossbreeding inbred strains enhances the opportunity for recombination and expression of endogenous retroviruses (95). The small size of mutant mouse colonies makes them highly vulnerable to subline divergence. Sublines of the same strain can have substantial genetic differences due to gene targeting, retrovirus integrations and excisions, residual heterozygosity and genetic contamination from a wild or escaped mouse. For example different sublines of inbred FVB mice vary in their prevalence of pituitary adenomas and hyperplasia, and differ in post lactational mammary gland involution (79).

X and Y Chromosomes

Nearly all commonly used ES cell lines have XY genotype (i.e., male) mice. However, when we insert XY ES cells into female recipient embryos, fertile male neonates are often produced. Although female ES cell lines are created as easily as XY lines, geneticists claim that their XX line is unstable because it can result in an XO sterile genotype, and are consequently less efficient for selecting for germ-line transmission. Besides effects of the X chromosome, maternal cells readily populate fetal bone marrow during gestation. Thus, the neonates are fetal-maternal chimeras to some degree. Although the maternal cells do not contribute to the germ-line, it is unknown if such fetal-maternal chimerisms are transmitted beyond the first generation through maternal lineages. Maternally derived chimeric cells can potentially express endogenous retroviruses that could insert as a replicant-competent virus in successive generations. Genetically, this means A ♂ × B ♀ F1 mice are not genetically the same as B ♂ × A ♀ F1 mice (96). Furthermore, Barthold (79) points out that when we backcross mice onto a specific background strain, mutant males are selected for breeding to females. However, unless we mate a mutant female to a male, the Y chromosome of the background strain will not be incorporated into the new transgenic mouse line.

Congenic Knockout Strains

An alternative to exclude genetic background effects is to perform all planned experiments with the same individual mouse before and after the induction of the reversible phenotype (97). Significantly, reversible gene-targeting strategies may demonstrate that the induced phenotype is clearly associated with the mutated gene, because reversion back to a functional gene should reverse the observed effect. However, the most common practice used to minimize genetic background effects is the time-consuming generation of congenic knockout strains (71). Complete backcrossing requires 10 generations to make a line congenic at the locus of interest. Congenic animals are genetically identical except for a single region containing the introduced change. Usually, this takes 2 or 3 years of backcrosses to a defined strain before the resulting genetic backgrounds are greater than 99% identical. The influence of each background genome, with a random mix of gene segregation still ongoing, renders the reproducibility of the phenotype in partially backcrossed mice questionable. The Jackson Laboratory offers a possible shortcut in this time-consuming backcrossing by carrying out genetic marker–assisted (microsatellites or single-nucleotide polymorphisms) selection of mice. This technique can reduce the time needed to generate a defined genetic background on backcrossed mice from 10 generations to five generations, shortening the time required by half. However, this process can underestimate achievement of congenic status by up to two generations (98).

Nongenetic Factors Affecting Phenotype

Besides genetic background variation, infectious disease can affect phenotype expression. Laboratory mice are a host to more than 60 infectious pathogens including viruses, bacteria, protozoa, fungi, helminths, and arthropods (99). The unregulated distribution of genetically altered mice between investigators and institutions has resulted in widespread infectious disease reemergence and spread. For example a report on *Demodex musculi* infestation in a specific-pathogen–free transgenic colony in 1999 illustrates this trend, because biologists had not seen Demodex in laboratory mice since 1917 (100). Biological products derived from mice such as cell lines, tissues and serum are also a source of infection. ES cells present a particularly high risk because they are of murine origin, involve the use of mouse feeder cells, and the medium contains mouse products (101). Lipman et al. (102) reported an outbreak of mousepox, of which the United States is free, in a major US medical school due to ectromelia virus–contaminated, imported mouse serum that was used to feed a murine spindle cell tumor line. Being aware of intercurrent infectious disease, even subclinical infections, is critical because it introduces unwanted variables.

Infectious disease can cause a variety of effects including immunomodulation, modified tumor kinetics, multiple actions on cell and tissue function and response, and altered patterns of the expression of strain-specific background pathology (79). Many effects are unpredictable and unknown as they depend on within experiment variables; experimental assay; infectious agent and its virulence and tropism; the mouse's strain, age and immune competence; epizootiology; and genomic manipulation.

IMAGING SYSTEMS FOR NONINVASIVE MONITORING IN MICE

Over the past several years specific small animal (SA) imaging technologies and devices, including magnetic resonance imaging (MRI), high-resolution x-ray computed tomography (micro-CT), positron emission tomography (PET), high-resolution single-photon emission tomography (SPECT), and bioluminescence imaging (BLI), have been developed. When coupled with mouse models of cancer, noninvasive imaging technologies are significant new tools for *in vivo* studies (103). Researchers can perform repetitive observations of the biological processes underlying cancer growth and development. They can test anticancer drugs on pathways affected by conditional-tumor–initiating mutations in the same mouse over time. The resolution with some SA-imaging modalities is the size of single cells, and imaging specific molecules and targets (i.e., molecular imaging) is now possible. Scientists can administer novel drugs to genetically engineered mice and follow the drug distribution and target binding, or they can image the target and look at receptor expression and downstream target modulation (104).

The NCI has funded substantial portions of the technology development for SA imaging by assisting institutions develop SA-imaging centers and making these resources available to cancer researchers (105). Three NCI biomedical imaging programs–Small Animal Imaging Resource Programs (SAIRPs), *In Vivo* Molecular and Cellular Imaging Centers (ICMICs), and Development of Clinical Imaging Drugs and Enhancers (DCIDE), are designed to improve SA-imaging technologies by improving the imaging devices as well as developing probes and ligands (106–108). Additional details on these programs are listed in Web Resources.

Different imaging techniques are complimentary rather than competitive. Detection and characterization of neoplasia by anatomical features are especially suitable to MRI and CT, while PET and SPECT offer the sensitivity to characterize neoplasia by its biological behavior and to monitor drug distribution, pharmacodynamics and pharmacokinetics. This section will focus on the primary uses of each imaging modality and their advantages and disadvantages. For information on the principles and mechanistic aspects of current imaging modalities in mouse models of cancer, Paulus and Weissleder provide excellent reviews (104,109,110).

Magnetic Resonance Imaging

MRI is important for *in vivo* anatomic studies of soft tissue structure. SA-imaging scanners generally have magnets with fields at 2, 4.7, 7, and 9.4 Tesla (T) compared with clinical scanner magnets that have fields between 0.5 and 1.5 T. Consequently, clinical scanners provide image resolutions about 3 to 5 mm, whereas SA-imaging systems give image resolutions less than 50 μm. Johnson et al. have obtained 20-μm resolution[5] images of isolated fixed mouse organs at 9.4 T for morphologic phenotyping of knockout mice (111,112). Song et al. (113) used diffusion-weighted MRI to detect tumors less than 1 mm in diameter in live transgenic mice (CR2-TAg) that have conditional prostate SV40 T antigen expression.

MRI analysis permits *in vivo* measurement of tumor angiogenesis parameters such as vascular volume, capillary permeability, and blood flow by replacing terminal histological procedures involving meticulous analysis of microvessel density (114,115). Weissleder et al. (116) used MRI to detect tumor-specific markers that allow noninvasive monitoring over time and can show when a gene is activated (Fig. 12.5). In mouse cancer models, MRI has been used to assess therapeutic efficacy of anticancer drugs by noninvasive quantitation of cell death, detect a therapeutic response before tumor volume change occurs, detect spatial heterogeneity of the tumor response, and quantitate transgene expression (117).

The advantage of MRI is the excellent high-resolution anatomical images, especially in soft tissue, where hydrogen atoms are abundant. SA-MRIs can also provide functional imaging capabilities when used with appropriate contrast-enhancing agents. The disadvantage of SA-MRI is the cost. One scanner can cost more than $1 million, and its operation frequently requires a trained magnetic resonance physicist.

---

[5] MRI resolution is often expressed as volumetric resolution. An image resolution of 3 to 5 mm, refers to a volumetric resolution of 3 to 5 mm^3; a 50 μm resolution describes a resolution of 50 $\times$ 50 $\times$ 50 μm. This volumetric resolution represents an increase of 25,000 times over clinical imaging; the work of Johnson et al. (111,112) represents an increase of 625,000 times over clinical magnetic resonance imaging.

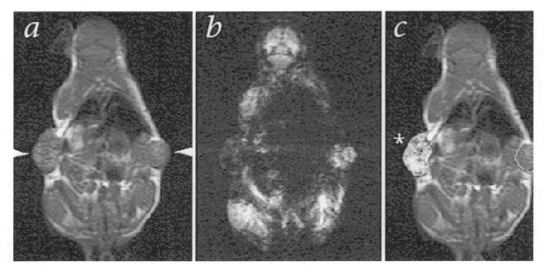

FIG. 12.5. *In vivo* magnetic resonance imaging (MRI) of a single mouse with orthoptic flank tumors containing engineered transferrin receptors (ETR+, left arrowhead) and no receptors (ETR-, right arrowhead). **A:** T1-weighted coronal spin-echo image (imaging time, 3.5 minutes; voxel resolution, 300 × 300 × 3,000 m). ETR- and ETR+ tumors have similar signal intensities. **B:** T2-weighted gradient-echo image corresponding to the image in **A**, showing substantial differences between ETR- and ETR+ tumors (imaging time, 8 minutes; voxel resolution, 300 × 300 × 3,000 m). As expected, ETR-mediated cellular accumulation of the superparamagnetic probe decreases signal intensity. These differences in MR signal intensity were most pronounced using T2- and T2*-weighted imaging pulse sequences, consistent with the increased transverse relaxation rate (R2) after cellular internalization. **C:** Composite image of a T1-weighted spin-echo image obtained for anatomical detail with superimposed R2 changes after administration of the receptor-targeted MR reporter Tf-MION. The reporter consists of a 3-nm monocrystalline iron oxide particle (MION), sterically protected by a layer of low-molecular-weight dextran to which human holo-transferrin (TF) is covalently conjugated. Asterisk indicates difference in R2 changes between the ETR+ and ETR - tumors. Reprinted from Weissleder R, Moore A, Mahmood U, et al. In vivo magnetic resonance imaging of transgene expression. *Nat Med* 2000;6:351–355, with permission.

High-Resolution X-ray Computed Tomography

Micro-CT has been used primarily for bone imaging studies due to the high contrast between calcified and soft tissue, and of thoracic imaging because the air-filled lung provides natural contrast between the vascular and bronchial structure of the lung. Micro-CT is also effective for soft-tissue imaging when iodinated contrast agents are employed. In mice, micro-CT has been used primarily to detect prostate, lung, and bone tumors (118,119). Micro-CT produces lung images that radiologists can evaluate from anesthetized mice, in contrast to high-resolution MRI images that can be obtained only after euthanasia when lungs are not moving (120).

The advantage of micro-CT is the relatively low cost of X-ray imaging hardware, making it among the least expensive SA-imaging modalities. Typical micro-CT systems cost about $200,000, are simple to operate, and readily achieve image resolutions comparable to MRI (approximately 50 μm). Data-acquisition times can be short, ranging from 5 to 30 minutes, depending on the required spatial and contrast resolution (109,118). The disadvantage of micro-CT is the need to couple the technique with other imaging modalities to evaluate cancer therapies. Using micro-CT, Kennel at al. (120) could identify lung tumors as small as 100 μm in diameter, but they could not evaluate radioimmunotherapy-induced regression of the tumors using micro-CT analyses alone.

Positron Emission Tomography

Unlike MRI and CT, which primarily image the anatomy of the subject, PET (and SPECT) image the anatomical distribution of radiolabeled compounds that reflect the presence of biological processes in the subject. Clinical PET scanners have intrinsic resolutions of about 6 mm in all spatial directions. In contrast, SA-PET systems have smaller bores and use smaller detectors to provide spatial resolutions of 1 or 2 mm. The higher resolution of dedicated SA-PET scanners allows the repetitive acquisition of quantitative kinetic data in mouse models so that each animal serves as its own control in experiments designed to evaluate the effects of a particular interventional strategy (121).

PET is of value in gene-expression studies because it can be used to monitor efficacy of gene-therapy vectors. Work from the laboratory of Ronald Blasberg has used the herpes simplex virus-1 thymidine kinase gene (*HSV1-tk*) and the radiolabeled nucleoside probe 5-iodo-2′-fluoro-2′deoxy-1-b-D-arabino-furanosyl-uracil (FIAU) to image and measure transgene expression (122–124). The *HSV1-tk* "marker/reporter" gene encodes for the HSV1-tk enzyme. The natural function of HSV1-tk is to phosphorylate thymidine; however, because HSV1-tk has relaxed substrate specificity, it also phosphorylates other nucleosides (e.g., uracil) or nucleoside analogs (e.g., ganciclovir or penciclovir) and traps them in a given cell. Cells that do not express HSV1-tk do not significantly trap radiolabeled reporter probes, such as FIAU; therefore, a very low level of background signal is present. Blasberg's group has shown that FIAU accumulation in cells is highly correlated with independent measures of *HSV1-tk* expression. In gene-therapy strategies, PET and a γ camera can evaluate gene-delivery efficiency by determining the distribution and magnitude of transgene expression in target tumor cells over time. A specific example is the viral infection kinetics study of rat 9L gliosarcoma cells by the replication-conditional HSV1 vector, hrR3, using *HSV1-tk* as a "marker gene" and FIAU as a "marker substrate" for the HSV1-tk enzyme (125,126).

The advantages of SA-PET systems are their high resolution, the ability to use a wide range of radiolabeled tracer compounds, and their high sensitivity to the tracer compounds (~200 cps/ μCi). However, PET scanners are expensive ($500,000–$750,000 per scanner) and must be located near a cyclotron producing the short-lived positron-emitting isotopes.

Single-Photon Emission Tomography

SPECT is a second nuclear imaging modality used for SA imaging (127). Like PET, SPECT uses position-sensitive γ cameras to image the distribution of radiolabeled tracers in the subject (128). SPECT isotopes include technetium-99m, indium-111, iodine-131, and iodine-123. Unlike PET isotopes, which are positron-emitting isotopes of elements found naturally in biological tissue such as carbon, nitrogen, oxygen, and fluorine, SPECT isotopes are attached chemically to biologically interesting molecules using chelators.

SA-SPECT scanners, like SA-PET scanners, can produce images with 1-mm or 2-mm resolution. The principal advantage of SPECT over PET is the wide commercial availability of isotopes, some of which can be produced in any laboratory using inexpensive generators. For longer-lived isotopes, researchers can purchase ready-to-use tracer compounds. SA-SPECT scanners are typically less expensive than SA-PET systems (approximately $300,000). The principal disadvantage of SPECT over PET is the greatly reduced sensitivity of the detector system caused by the mechanical collimation. Reported sensitivities of SA-SPECT scanners typically range from 1 to 10 cps/μCi (109).

A review by Michael Phelps at the University of California at Los Angeles, who together with Simon Cherry helped pioneer the development of high-resolution PET technology for small animals, emphasizes the potential of PET and SPECT imaging in drug discovery (129). Reporter gene assays are used to trace the location and temporal level of expression of therapeutic and endogenous genes. PET probes and drugs are being developed together, in small amounts, as molecular imaging probes (diagnostic radiopharmaceuticals) to image the function of targets without disturbing them, and in mass amounts to modify the target's function as a drug. In both instances, the compounds are the same or analogs of each other. PET can be used to titrate drugs to their sites of action within organ systems *in vivo* and to assay biological outcomes of the processes being modified in the mouse or the patient.

Bioluminescence Imaging

BLI is a recent development in SA imaging. Several groups have explored the use of bioluminescent compounds, such as luciferase, as tracers. These tracers emit visible light that can be detected using cooled charged-coupled-device cameras (Fig. 12.6). Generating transgenic mice with pituitary-specific expression of both *Cre* and luciferase, Vooijis et al. (130) has exploited luciferase-based BLI in a conditional mouse model of retinoblastoma-dependent (Rb) sporadic pituitary cancer. Mice homozygous for a conditional allele of *Rb* develop pituitary tumors with full penetrance over a short time. Injection of these mice with luciferin allows quantitative measurement of pituitary tumor growth as well as detection of tumor-free mice by luciferase expression in the pituitary glands. The authors measured the tumor-suppressive effects of doxorubicin treatment to demonstrate how effectively this model system can be used to test cancer prevention and treatment strategies.

One principal advantage of BLI is that because it is oxygen and adenosine triphosphate dependent, only live cells are detected. Therefore, compared with other techniques that measure total tumor volume, BLI is ideal for quantitating tumor-specific cell death, including necrotic areas. Another advantage of BLI is its use of nonnuclear tracer compounds and the relatively low cost of the imaging hardware (approximately $100,000). Recently, Ntziachristos et al. (131) overcame two disadvantages of BLI: namely, difficulty in imaging deep tissue tumor-bearing regions and inability to obtain tomographic images. Using near-infrared

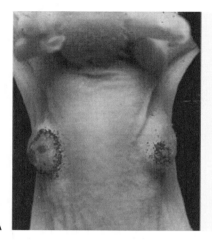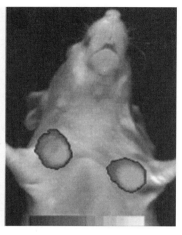

A   **B**

FIG. 12.6. Bioluminescent and fluorescent imaging in mice. **A:** Bilateral chest tumors expressing transgenic luciferase and imaged with a photon-counting camera after intraperitoneal injection of luciferin. The tumor on the
left expresses higher levels of luciferase than the tumor on the right. **B:** Near-infrared (NIR) fluorescence imaging
(700–900 nm) can be used to image deeper tumors than can be observed with fluorescence imaging in the visible light range. This example shows matrix metalloproteinase 2 (MMP-2) enzyme levels in bilaterally implanted
breast tumors using an NIR fluorescence probe coupled to an MMP-2 substrate. Reprinted from Weissleder R.
Scaling down imaging: molecular mapping of cancer in mice. *Nat Rev Cancer* 2002;2:11–18, with permission.

fluorescent molecular beacons and inversion techniques, they obtained three-dimensional *in vivo* images of a protease in orthotopic gliomas in nude mice.

IMPLICATIONS OF GENE TARGETING
IN MICE FOR ANTICANCER
DRUG DEVELOPMENT

Mouse cancer models using conditional gene expression allow us to generate tissue-restricted and time-
specific somatic mutations. Under controlled experimental conditions, these mutations more faithfully
copy sporadic tumor onset and progression that we see
in human cancer. With the rapidly evolving and highly
sensitive SA-imaging modalities, these mice are valuable models to evaluate experimental therapies that
use conventional and/or novel pharmacologic treatments, combination radiologic and drug therapies, and
pharmacologic prevention strategies.

Although science writers often describe imatinib
(Gleevec) as the prime example of a targeted anticancer drug, researchers established the relationship
between CML and the BCR-ABL tyrosine kinase in
parallel with the development of Gleevec. The development of erlotinib (Tarceva), and ZD1839 (Iressa),
inhibitors of the epidermal growth factor receptor
(EGFR) tyrosine kinase, illustrates a similar progression. The interactions between EGFR and the transformation of normal cells to neoplastic cells were
gradually established, in parallel with the develop-

ment of anti-EGFR drugs. With our greater knowledge of the molecular pathways of cancer, the success
of Gleevec, Tarceva, and Iressa highlight the enormous potential of rational cancer drug design and target validation in conditional mouse cancer models.

The genetic strategies for conditional gene expression permit modulation of the target not only over
time, but also in quantitative levels that may more accurately reflect the clinical picture of human cancer
progression rather than a static picture at one point in
the disease course. This allows evaluation of combination therapies (conventional and novel drugs) during different phases of the disease, and selection of
optimal combinations.

The gene-expression examples that I have described in this chapter emphasize single pathways. In
reality, individual gene pathways interact with each
other in transcriptional regulatory networks to cause
changes in living organisms. Lee et al. (132) recently
used an algorithm that combines genome-wide location analysis with gene-expression data to map transcriptional regulatory networks in the budding yeast
Saccharomyces cerevisiae. Astonishingly, the automated algorithm required no previous biological
knowledge, yet assigned all regulators to the correct
cell-cycle stages. An important observation arising
from this work is that control of cellular processes involves transcriptional regulation of other regulators
(Fig. 12.7). This has significant consequences for mutation analysis—gene-expression profiling is as likely

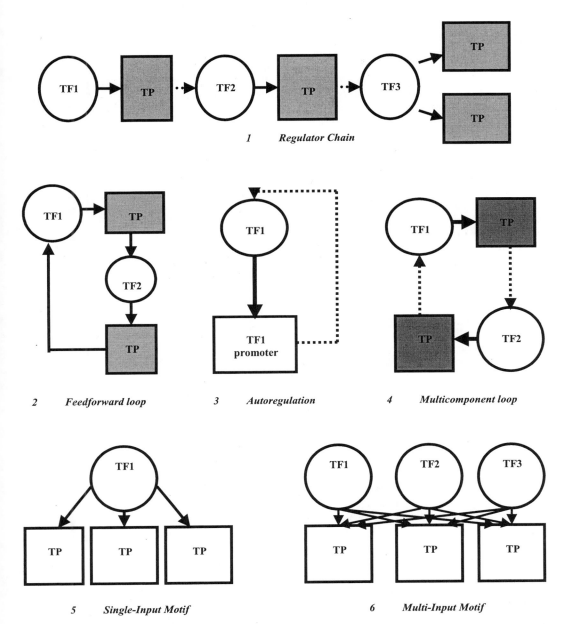

FIG. 12.7. Types of transcriptional regulatory networks. The control of cellular processes involves not only individual transcriptional pathways, but also how they interact to bring about changes in the living organism. The control of cellular processes involves transcriptional regulation of other regulators and appears to fall into six basic regulatory motifs that are the building blocks of larger regulatory networks. TF indicates transcription factor; TP, target promoter. Modified from Lee TI, Rinaldi NJ, Robert F, et al. Transcriptional regulatory networks in Saccharomyces cerevisiae. *Science* 2002;298:799–804, with permission. Copyright 2003 American Association for Advancement of Science.

to reveal direct targets of a mutated regulation as it is to reveal the effects of network disruption.

Work from the laboratory of Allan Balmain has increased our understanding of the multistage nature of *in vivo* tumor progression by providing a new view of two genes, *ras* and *Smad,* cooperating to promote tumor development in a regulatory network (133). They showed that H-*ras* induces nuclear accumulation of phosphorylated *Smad2* and consequent upregulation of *Smad2*-mediated transcription. Balmain's group previously proposed that sequential increases in H-*ras* levels during tumor progression may be required to activate different effector pathways to provide the necessary survival signals at later stages of tumorigenesis (134). Taken together, the changes in gene-expression patterns suggest that both mechanisms—cooperativity of H-*ras* and *Smad2* on certain promoters and antagonism on others—are functional during H-*ras*- and transforming growth factor (TGF)-driven tumor progression. They see the coordinate upregulation of both Ras and TGF as a mechanism that allows the tumor cell to adopt the cell-fate change and invasive properties required for progression without dying because of increased levels of proapoptotic signals. This pathway will provide important targets for drug discovery.

How is this relevant for using conditional mouse models of cancer? We know that some human tumors express several oncogenes, drug-resistance proteins, and repair mechanisms. The *Cre*-expression system allows us to generate compound mutant mice that may have several conditional alleles mimicking these human tumors. Thus, not only may it be possible to study the effect of the drug on the mutated gene, but we can also look at the effect of the mutated gene on the drug. Using Balmain's work as an example, we know that upregulation of *Smad2* requires a sequential increase of H-*ras* expression. H-*ras* upregulates TGF-β, and *Smad2* is a downstream target of TGF-β signaling. What happens to a drug directed against TGF-β? Although the TGF-β–targeted drug may stop *Smad2* upregulation, does the increased H-Ras affect any other network that could inhibit or enhance the targeted TGF-β drug? The researchers who have developed and studied conditional mouse cancer models have focused more on the biological behavior of neoplasia than on the pharmacologic treatment of cancer. Drug discovery programs now have an opportunity not only to look at ways to enhance current drug regimens, but to continue the development of novel targeted anticancer drugs by modifying their structure to optimize their mode of action in different tumor environments. In addition, just as conditional mouse models have provided a forward approach to understanding gene function, they too can allow a forward approach to pharmacogenetics. We do not have to rely on finding a person who has a negative reaction to discover what specific genetic defect caused the reaction.

Elimination of the physiologic differences between humans and mice limiting the predictive value of mouse models for human tumor response to drugs is an important challenge in the future. Two important areas are differences in signaling pathways associated with malignant transformation and xenobiotic metabolizing enzymes. Hahn and Weinberg (135) review the signaling pathways that function differently in humans and mouse models. For example, human cells must avoid replicative senescence, or M1, and apoptotic cellular crisis, or M2, to achieve immortalization, an essential prerequisite for malignant transformation. Telomere shortening and the RB, p53, H-Ras, and ST-PP2A pathways have prominent roles in limiting human cell lifespan. Removing the ARF-p53 pathway is enough to immortalize murine cells, whereas telomere shortening does not seem to limit the lifespan of murine cells. Gonzalez and Kimura (136) review the human and murine species differences in expression and catalytic activities of the xenobiotic metabolizing enzymes of the cytochrome P-450 enzyme system that may cause mice to respond to drug therapy differently than humans. Genetically engineered mice with a humanized drug and carcinogen metabolism might provide more accurate information on the therapeutic effects of anticancer drugs.

WEB RESOURCES

Conditional Mouse Models Databases

Tet Mouse Base

Laboratory of Ernesto Bockamp Web site with a comprehensive list of currently available general and tissue-specific tet-on/tet-off effector and reporter strains of mice.

URL: http://www.zmg.uni-mainz.de/tetmouse/

Cre *Transgenic Database*

Laboratory of Andras Nagy Web site with a wide-ranging list of *Cre*- and *Flp*-based conditional mouse strains.

URL: http://www.mshri.on.ca/nagy/default.htm

Transgenic and Knockout Databases

Transgenic/Targeted Mutation Database (TBASE)

TBASE organizes information on transgenic animals and targeted mutations generated and analyzed worldwide.

URL: http://tbase.jax.org/

The German Genetrap Consortium (GGTC)

A reference library of gene-trap sequence tags from insertional mutations generated in mouse ES cells.
URL: http://tikus.gsf.de/

Mouse Knockout and Mutation Database (MKMD)

Elsevier's commercial database of phenotypic information related to knockouts and classical mutations in mice.
URL: http://research.bmn.com/mkmd

Omnibank

A commercial library of Lexicon Genetics with more than 200,000 knockout mouse ES cell clones corresponding to more than 50% of mammalian genes.
URL: http://www.lexgen.com

Mouse Strain Repositories

Mutant Mouse Regional Resource Centers (MMRRC) Program

The MMRRC network comprises an Informatics Coordinating Center and four regional mutant mouse distribution facilities capable of husbandry, cryopreservation, storing and reconstructing embryos, phenotypic characterization (structural and behavioral), genetic quality control, maintenance of a mouse resource database, and distribution of genetically modified mice.
URL: http://www.mmrrc.org

The Jackson Laboratory (JAX)

Three important centers within JAX are (1) the Induced Mutant Resource, which selects, imports, cryopreserves, maintains, and distributes congenic targeted mutant mice; (2) the Mouse Mutant Gene Resource, which develops and maintains strains of mice with specific mutant genes, and (3) the Cryopreservation of Murine Germplasm repository, which contains frozen eight-cell mouse embryos and sperm from more than 2,300 inbred and mutant strains of laboratory mice.
URL: http://www.jax.org

Mouse Models of Human Cancers Consortium (MMHCC)

MMHCC is an NCI-funded repository for mouse cancer models and associated strains.
URL: http://web.ncifcrf.gov/researchresources/mmhcc/default.asp

European Mouse Mutant Archive (EMMA)

EMMA collects, archives (via cryopreservation), and distributes mutant mouse strains. It is a partnership of European laboratories and institutions.
URL: http://www.emma.rm.cnr.it/

Mouse Pathology

Mouse Tumor Biology (MTB) Database

MTB Database provides access to descriptions of mouse tumors (organized by strain and organ of origin), tumor frequency and latency data, and tumor pathology reports and images.
URL: http://tumor.informatics.jax.org/FMPro?-db=TumorInstance&-format=mtdp.html&-view

Pathbase

Pathbase is a European program providing a searchable database of histopathology images from experiments on genetically manipulated mice and a reference covering mouse pathology. It has 100 links to other resources.
URL: http://eulep.anat.cam.ac.uk/What_is_Pathbase/index.php

HistoBank

HistoBank is an interactive histology atlas that allows retrieval of annotated, high-resolution mammary gland histology images. It also provides a forum for veterinary and human pathologists to exchange opinions on the classification of mammary lesions in gene-targeted mice.
URL: http://histology.nih.gov/

Mouse Genetics and Genomics

NCI Cancer Genome Anatomy Project (CGAP)

CGAP provides genomic data for mouse and human, and informatics tools to determine the gene-expression profiles of normal, precancer, and cancer cells. The site includes a slide tour and education resource that explains the science behind GCAP, and is an excellent resource for those who are not familiar with genomics. For the first-time user, there are clear instructions for use of the informatics tools.
URL: http://cgap.nci.nih.gov/

NCBI Mouse Genome Resources (MGR)

MGR is a gateway to mouse genomic resources.
URL: http://www.ncbi.nlm.nih.gov/genome/guide/mouse/

JAX Mouse Genome Informatics (MGI) Database

MGI provides integrated access to data on the genetics, genomics, and biology of the laboratory mouse
URL: http://www.informatics.jax.org/

Mammalian Gene Collection (MGC)

MGC provides full-length (open reading frame) sequences and complimentary DNA clones of expressed genes for human and mouse.
URL: http://mgc.nci.nih.gov/

RIKEN Institute

Full-length complimentary DNA encyclopedia of the mouse.
URL: http://genome.rtc.riken.go.jp/

Edinburgh Mouse Atlas Project (EMAP) and Gene Expression (EMAGE)

EMAP is a digital atlas and database of mouse development for spatially mapped data such as *in situ* gene expression and cell lineage; EMAGE is a spatial database of gene-expression patterns in the developing mouse embryo.
URL: http://genex.hgu.mrc.ac.uk/intro.html

Harwell Mammalian Genetics Resource (MGR)

MGR is an integrated campus for mouse genetics research with facilities for molecular genetics, genomics, mutagenesis, transgenesis, and informatics.
URL: http://www.mgu.har.mrc.ac.uk/

Ensembl

Mouse sequencing genome consortium's mouse genome server containing more than 95% of the mouse genome.
URL: http://www.ensembl.org/Mus_musculus/

Human Cancer Gene Databases

Sanger Cancer Genome Project (CGP)

CGP identifies somatically acquired sequence variants/mutations in the development of human cancers.
URL: http://www.sanger.ac.uk/CGP/

GeneCards

A database of human genes, their products, and their involvement in diseases.
URL: http://nciarray.nci.nih.gov/cards/

Comprehensive Mouse Links

Mouse Models of Human Cancers Consortium (MMHCC)

NCI's MMHCC Web site provides information, resources, and innovative approaches to the application of mouse models in cancer research.
URL: http://emice.nci.nih.gov/emice/

Mouse Genome

Nature's complete initial sequence and analysis of the mouse genome with all content from the mouse genome special issue.
URL:http://www.nature.com/nature/mouse-genome/

Trans-NIH Mouse Initiative

A central information resource on funding opportunities for mouse genomics and genetics resources, funded grants, mouse genomics and genetics resources, and courses and scientific meetings related to the mouse.
URL: http://www.nih.gov/science/models/mouse/

International Mammalian Genome Society

A society that fosters and stimulates research in mammalian genetics. Links are organized by individual countries' research and organisms studied.
URL: http://imgs.org

Small Animal Imaging

Small Animal Imaging Resource Program (SAIRP)

NCI's Biomedical Imaging Program-funded resource that supports shared imaging research resources to be used by cancer investigators, and research related to small animal imaging technology. The site lists the ten current SAIRP institutions and principal investigators.
URL: http://www3.cancer.gov/bip/sairp.htm

In Vivo *Cellular and Molecular Imaging Centers (ICMICs)*

NCI's Biomedical Imaging Program-funded resource designed to facilitate interactions among scientists who conduct multidisciplinary research on cellular and molecular imaging related to cancer. The site lists the 16 current planning grants for establishing an institutional ICMIC.
URL: http://www3.cancer.gov/bip/ICMICs.htm

Development of Clinical Imaging Drugs and Enhancers (DCIDE)

NCI-funded program for the development and use of labeled therapeutic agents as compounds for imaging studies, and imaging agents that will be used as metabolic markers of response to newly developed therapeutic agents. Most of the preclinical evaluations of the new drugs will use SA imaging.

URL: http://www3.cancer.gov/bip/DCID_des.htm

REFERENCES

1. Kerbel RS. What is the optimal rodent model for antitumor drug testing? *Cancer Metastasis Rev* 1998; 17:301–304.
2. Bibby MC. Making the most of rodent tumour systems in cancer drug discovery. *Br J Cancer* 1999;79: 1633–1640.
3. Steele VE, Boone CW, Lubet RA, et al. Preclinical drug development paradigms for chemopreventives. *Hematol Oncol Clin North Am* 1998;12:943–961, v–vi.
4. Rowley JD. Chromosomal patterns in myelocytic leukemia. *N Engl J Med* 1973;289:220–221.
5. Nowell PC, Hungerford DA. The etiology of leukemia: some comments on current studies. *Semin Hematol* 1966;3:114–121.
6. Online Mendelian inheritance in man OT. MIM Number 151410. Breakpoint Cluster Region; BCR (NCB1 Literature Database). Available at: http://www.ncbi. nlm.nih.gov/entrez/dispomim.cgi?id=151410. Last update April 13, 2003.
7. Daley GQ, Van Etten RA, Baltimore D. Induction of chronic myelogenous leukemia in mice by the P210bcr/abl gene of the Philadelphia chromosome. *Science* 1990;247:824–830.
8. Lugo TG, Pendergast AM, Muller AJ, et al. Tyrosine kinase activity and transformation potency of bcr-abl oncogene products. *Science* 1990;247:1079–1082.
9. Ramaswamy S, Tamayo P, Rifkin R, et al. Multiclass cancer diagnosis using tumor gene expression signatures. *Proc Natl Acad Sci U S A* 2001;98:15149–15154.
10. Golub TR, Slonim DK, Tamayo P, et al. Molecular classification of cancer: class discovery and class prediction by gene expression monitoring. *Science* 1999; 286:531–537.
11. Brinster RL, Chen HY, Messing A, et al. Transgenic mice harboring SV40 T-antigen genes develop characteristic brain tumors. *Cell* 1984;37:367–379.
12. Stewart TA, Pattengale PK, Leder P. Spontaneous mammary adenocarcinomas in transgenic mice that carry and express MTV/myc fusion genes. *Cell* 1984; 38:627–637.
13. Jackson Laboratory. The transgenic/targeted mutation database [online database]. Available at: http://tbase. jax.org. Accessed November 30, 2002.
14. BioMedNet. Mouse knockout and mutation database [online database]. Available at: http://research.bmn. com/mkmd. Accessed November 30, 2002.
15. Andres AC, Bchini O, Schubaur B, et al. H-ras induced transformation of mammary epithelium is favoured by increased oncogene expression or by inhibition of mammary regression. *Oncogene* 1991;6:771–779.
16. Lavigueur A, Bernstein A. p53 transgenic mice: accelerated erythroleukemia induction by Friend virus. *Oncogene* 1991;6:2197–2201.
17. Johnson RS, van Lingen B, Papaioannou VE, et al. A null mutation at the c-jun locus causes embryonic lethality and retarded cell growth in culture. *Genes Dev* 1993;7:1309–1317.
18. Corral J, Lavenir I, Impey H, et al. An Mll-AF9 fusion gene made by homologous recombination causes acute leukemia in chimeric mice: a method to create fusion oncogenes. *Cell* 1996;85:853–861.
19. Liao MJ, Zhang XX, Hill R, et al. No requirement for V(D)J recombination in p53-deficient thymic lymphoma. *Mol Cell Biol* 1998;18:3495–3501.
20. van Deursen J, Boer J, Kasper L, et al. G2 arrest and impaired nucleocytoplasmic transport in mouse embryos lacking the proto-oncogene CAN/Nup214. *EMBO J* 1996;15:5574–5583.
21. Jones SN, Roe AE, Donehower LA, et al. Rescue of embryonic lethality in Mdm2-deficient mice by absence of p53. *Nature* 1995;378:206–208.
22. Tutois S, Salaun J, Mattei MG, et al. Tg (9 HSA-MYC), a homozygous lethal insertion in the mouse. *Mamm Genome* 1991;1:184–190.
23. McMahon AP, Bradley A. The Wnt-1 (int-1) proto-oncogene is required for development of a large region of the mouse brain. *Cell* 1990;62:1073–1085.
24. Capecchi MR. The new mouse genetics: altering the genome by gene targeting. *Trends Genet* 1989;5: 70–76.
25. Capecchi MR. Altering the genome by homologous recombination. *Science* 1989;244:1288–1292.
26. Rajewsky K, Gu H, Kuhn R, et al. Conditional gene targeting. *J Clin Invest* 1996;98:600–603.
27. Lewandoski M. Conditional control of gene expression in the mouse. *Nat Rev Genet* 2001;2:743–755.
28. Jonkers J, Berns A. Conditional mouse models of sporadic cancer. *Nat Rev Cancer* 2002;2:251–265.
29. Jackson-Grusby L. Modeling cancer in mice. *Oncogene* 2002;21:5504–5514.
30. Tuveson DA, Jacks T. Technologically advanced cancer modeling in mice. *Curr Opin Genet Dev* 2002;12: 105–110.
31. Van Dyke T, Jacks T. Cancer modeling in the modern era: progress and challenges. *Cell* 2002;108:135–144.
32. Herzig M, Christofori G. Recent advances in cancer research: mouse models of tumorigenesis. *Biochim Biophys Acta* 2002;1602:97–113.
33. Liotta LA, Kohn EC. The microenvironment of the tumour-host interface. *Nature* 2001;411:375–379.
34. Huang S, Van Arsdall M, Tedjarati S, et al. Contributions of stromal metalloproteinase-9 to angiogenesis and growth of human ovarian carcinoma in mice. *J Natl Cancer Inst* 2002;94:1134–1142.
35. Hanahan D, Weinberg RA. The hallmarks of cancer. *Cell* 2000;100:57–70.
36. Bex A, Vooijs M, Horenblas S, et al. Controlling gene expression in the urothelium using transgenic mice with inducible bladder specific Cre-lox recombination. *J Urol* 2002;168:2641–2644.

37. Bockamp E, Maringer M, Spangenberg C, et al. Of mice and models: improved animal models for biomedical research. *Physiol Genomics* 2002;11: 115–132.

38. Baron U, Bujard H. Tet repressor-based system for regulated gene expression in eukaryotic cells: principles and advances. *Methods Enzymol* 2000;327:401–421.

39. Ewald D, Li M, Efrat S, et al. Time-sensitive reversal of hyperplasia in transgenic mice expressing SV40 T antigen. *Science* 1996;273:1384–1386.

40. Chin L, Tam A, Pomerantz J, et al. Essential role for oncogenic Ras in tumour maintenance. *Nature* 1999; 400:468–472.

41. Eilers M, Picard D, Yamamoto KR, et al. Chimaeras of myc oncoprotein and steroid receptors cause hormone-dependent transformation of cells. *Nature* 1989;340: 66–68.

42. Pelengaris S, Littlewood T, Khan M, et al. Reversible activation of c-Myc in skin: induction of a complex neoplastic phenotype by a single oncogenic lesion. *Mol Cell* 1999;3:565–577.

43. Berns A. Turning on tumors to study cancer progression. *Nat Genet* 1999;5:989–990.

44. Chin L, DePinho RA. Flipping the oncogene switch: illumination of tumor maintenance and regression. *Trends Genet* 2000;16:147–150.

45. Kistner A, Gossen M, Zimmermann F, et al. Doxycycline-mediated quantitative and tissue-specific control of gene expression in transgenic mice. *Proc Natl Acad Sci U S A* 1996;93:10933–10938.

46. Huettner CS, Zhang P, Van Etten RA, et al. Reversibility of acute B-cell leukaemia induced by BCR–ABL1. *Nat Genet* 2000;24:57–60.

47. Felsher DW, Bishop JM. Reversible tumorigenesis by MYC in hematopoietic lineages. *Mol Cell* 1999;4: 199–207.

48. Sauer B, Henderson N. Site-specific DNA recombination in mammalian cells by the Cre recombinase of bacteriophage P1. *Proc Natl Acad Sci U S A* 1988;85: 5166–5170.

49. Sauer B. Inducible gene targeting in mice using the Cre/lox system. *Methods* 1998;14:381–392.

50. Nagy A. Cre recombinase: the universal reagent for genome tailoring. *Genesis* 2000;26:99–109.

51. Nagy A. Published Cre transgenic lines [online database]. Available at: http://www.mshri.on.ca/nagy/Cre-pub.html. Accessed November 30, 2002.

52. Kaartinen V, Nagy A. Removal of the floxed neo gene from a conditional knockout allele by the adenoviral Cre recombinase in vivo. *Genesis* 2001;31:126–129.

53. Xu X, Wagner KU, Larson D, et al. Conditional mutation of Brca1 in mammary epithelial cells results in blunted ductal morphogenesis and tumour formation. *Nat Genet* 1999;22:37–43.

54. Jonkers J, Meuwissen R, van der Gulden H, et al. Synergistic tumor suppressor activity of BRCA2 and p53 in a conditional mouse model for breast cancer. *Nat Genet* 2001;29:418–425.

55. Donehower LA, Harvey M, Slagle BL, et al. Mice deficient for p53 are developmentally normal but susceptible to spontaneous tumours. *Nature* 1992;356: 215–221.

56. Marino S, Vooijs M, et al. Induction of medulloblastomas in p53-null mutant mice by somatic inactivation of Rb in the external granular layer cells of the cerebellum. *Genes Dev* 2000;14:994–1004.

57. Jackson EL, Willis N, Mercer K, et al. Analysis of lung tumor initiation and progression using conditional expression of oncogenic K-ras. *Genes Dev* 2001;15: 3243–3248.

58. Meuwissen R, Linn SC, van der Valk M, et al. Mouse model for lung tumorigenesis through Cre/lox controlled sporadic activation of the K-Ras oncogene. *Oncogene* 2001;20:6551–6558.

59. Vooijs M, Jonkers J, Berns A. A highly efficient ligand-regulated Cre recombinase mouse line shows that LoxP recombination is position dependent. *EMBO Rep* 2001;2:292–297.

60. Schmidt EE, Taylor DS, Prigge JR, et al. Illegitimate Cre-dependent chromosome rearrangements in transgenic mouse spermatids. *Proc Natl Acad Sci U S A* 2000;97:13702–13707.

61. Loonstra A, Vooijs M, Beverloo HB, et al. Growth inhibition and DNA damage induced by Cre recombinase in mammalian cells. *Proc Natl Acad Sci U S A* 2001;98:9209–9214.

62. Federspiel MJ, Bates P, Young JA, et al. A system for tissue-specific gene targeting: transgenic mice susceptible to subgroup A avian leukosis virus–based retroviral vectors. *Proc Natl Acad Sci U S A* 1994;91:11241–11245.

63. Fisher GH, Orsulic S, Holland EC, et al. Development of a flexible and specific gene delivery system for production of murine tumor models. *Oncogene* 1999;18: 5253–5260.

64. Holland EC. Gliomagenesis: genetic alterations and mouse models. *Nat Rev Genet* 2001;2:120–129.

65. Holland EC, Celestino J, Dai C, et al. Combined activation of Ras and Akt in neural progenitors induces glioblastoma formation in mice. *Nat Genet* 2000;25: 55–57.

66. Johnson L, Mercer K, Greenbaum D, et al. Somatic activation of the K-ras oncogene causes early onset lung cancer in mice. *Nature* 2001;410:1111–1116.

67. Bos JL. ras oncogenes in human cancer: a review. *Cancer Res* 1989;49:4682–4689.

68. Cho KR, Vogelstein B. Genetic alterations in the adenoma—carcinoma sequence. *Cancer* 1992;70: 1727–1731.

69. Berns A. Cancer. Improved mouse models. *Nature* 2001;410:1043–1044.

70. Lerner EC, Hamilton AD, Sebti SM. Inhibition of Ras prenylation: a signaling target for novel anti-cancer drug design. *Anticancer Drug Des* 1997;12:229–238.

71. Banbury Conference on genetic background in mice. Mutant mice and neuroscience: recommendations concerning genetic background. *Neuron* 1997;19: 755–759.

72. Morse 3rd HC. The laboratory mouse - a historical perspective. In: Foster HL, Small JD, Fox JG, eds. *The mouse in biomedical research.* New York: Academic Press, 1981:1–16.

73. Beck JA, Lloyd S, Hafezparast M, et al. Genealogies of mouse inbred strains. *Nat Genet* 2000;24:23–25.

74. Turusov VS, Mohr U, eds. *Tumours of the mouse.* Lyon, France: International Agency for Research on Cancer, 1994.

75. Mohr U, Dungworth DL, Capen CC, et al., eds. *Pathobiology of the aging mouse.* Washington, D.C.: International Life Sciences Institute, 1996.

76. Haines DC, Chattopadhyay SK, Ward JM. Pathology of aging B6;129 mice. *Toxicol Pathol* 2001;29: 653–661.

77. Lynch CJ. The so-called Swiss mouse. *Lab Anim Care* 1969;19:214–220.

78. Taketo M, Schroeder AC, Mobraaten LE, et al. FVB/N: an inbred mouse strain preferable for transgenic analyses. *Proc Natl Acad Sci U S A* 1991;88: 2065–2069.

79. Barthold SW. "Muromics": genomics from the perspective of the laboratory mouse. *Comp Med* 2002;52:206–223.

80. Silver LM, Martin GR, Strickland S. *Teratocarcinoma stem cells.* Cold Spring Harbor: Cold Spring Harbor Laboratory, 1983.

81. Simpson EM, Linder CC, Sargent EE, et al. Genetic variation among 129 substrains and its importance for targeted mutagenesis in mice. *Nat Genet* 1997;16: 19–27.

82. Threadgill DW, Yee D, Matin A, et al. Genealogy of the 129 inbred strains: 129/SvJ is a contaminated inbred strain. *Mamm Genome* 1997;8:390–393.

83. Noben-Trauth N, Kohler G, Burki K, et al. Efficient targeting of the IL-4 gene in a BALB/c embryonic stem cell line. *Transgenic Res* 1996;5:487–491.

84. Ledermann B, Burki K. Establishment of a germ-line competent C57BL/6 embryonic stem cell line. *Exp Cell Res* 1991;197:254–258.

85. Whitelaw E, Martin DI. Retrotransposons as epigenetic mediators of phenotypic variation in mammals. *Nature Genetics* 2001;27:361–365.

86. Martin DI, Whitelaw E. The vagaries of variegating transgenes. *Bioessays* 1996;18:919–923.

87. Dobie K, Mehtali M, McClenaghan M, et al. Variegated gene expression in mice. *Trends Genet* 1997;13:127–130.

88. Opsahl ML, McClenaghan M, Springbett A, et al. Multiple effects of genetic background on variegated transgene expression in mice. *Genetics* 2002;160: 1107–1112.

89. Donehower LA, Harvey M, Vogel H, et al. Effects of genetic background on tumorigenesis in p53-deficient mice. *Mol Carcinogen* 1995;14:16–22.

90. Cory S, Vaux DL, Strasser A, et al. Insights from Bcl-2 and Myc: malignancy involves abrogation of apoptosis as well as sustained proliferation. *Cancer Res* 1999;59:1685s–1692s.

91. Harris AW, Strasser A, Bath ML, et al. Lymphomas and plasmacytomas in transgenic mice involving bcl2, myc and v-abl. *Curr Top Microbiol Immunol* 1997; 224:221–230.

92. Robertson G, Garrick D, Wilson M, et al. Age-dependent silencing of globin transgenes in the mouse. *Nucleic Acids Res* 1996;24:1465–1471.

93. Robertson G, Garrick D, Wu W, et al. Position-dependent variegation of globin transgene expression in mice. *Proc Natl Acad Sci U S A* 1995;92:5371–5375.

94. Coffin JM, Hughes SH, Varmus HE. Interactions of retroviruses and their hosts. In: Coffin JM, Hughes SH, Varmus HE, eds. *Retroviruses.* Plainview: Cold Spring Harbor Laboratory Press, 1997.

95. Jenkins NA, Copeland NG. High frequency germline acquisition of ecotropic MuLV proviruses in SWR/J-RF/J hybrid mice. *Cell* 1985;43:811–819.

96. Brownstein DG. Genetically engineered mice: the holes in the sum of the parts. *Lab Anim Sci* 1998; 48:121–122.

97. Lee P, Morley G, Huang Q, et al. Conditional lineage ablation to model human diseases. *Proc Natl Acad Sci U S A* 1998;95:11371–11376.

98. Wakeland E, Morel L, Achey K, et al. Speed congenics: a classic technique in the fast lane (relatively speaking). *Immunol Today* 1997;18:472–477.

99. Percy DH, Barthold SW. *Pathology of laboratory rodents and rabbits,* 2nd ed. Ames: Iowa State University Press, 2001.

100. Hill LR, Kille PS, Weiss DA, et al. *Demodex musculi* in the skin of transgenic mice. *Contemp Top Lab Anim Sci* 1999;38:13–18.

101. Nicklas W, Weiss J. Survey of embryonic stem cells for murine infective agents. *Comp Med* 2000;50: 410–411.

102. Lipman NS, Perkins S, Nguyen H, et al. Mousepox resulting from use of ectromelia virus-contaminated, imported mouse serum. *Comp Med* 2000;50:426–435.

103. Luker GD. Special conference of the American Association for Cancer Research on molecular imaging in cancer: linking biology, function, and clinical applications in vivo. *Cancer Res* 2002;62:2195–2198.

104. Rudin M, Weissleder R. Molecular imaging in drug discovery and development. *Nat Rev Drug Discov* 2003;2:123–131.

105. Hoffman JM, Croft BY. Future directions in small animal imaging. *Lab Anim (NY)* 2001;30:32–35.

106. Cancer Imaging NCI. Development of clinical imaging drugs and enhancers. Available at: http://www3.cancer.gov/bip/DCID_des.htm. Accessed August 30, 2002.

107. Biomedical Imaging Program Funded Projects and Resources, National Cancer Institute. In vivo cellular and molecular imaging centers. Available at: http://www3. cancer.gov/bip/ICMICs.htm. Accessed November 30, 2002.

108. Biomedical Imaging Program, National Cancer Institute. Small animal imaging resource program (SAIRP). Available at: http://www3.cancer.gov/bip/sairp.htm. Accessed November 30, 2002.

109. Paulus MJ, Gleason SS, Easterly ME, et al. A review of high-resolution x-ray computed tomography and other imaging modalities for small animal research. *Lab Anim (NY)* 2001;30:36–45.

110. Weissleder R. Scaling down imaging: molecular mapping of cancer in mice. *Nat Rev Cancer* 2002;2:11–18.

111. Johnson GA, Cofer GP, Fubara B, et al. Magnetic resonance histology for morphologic phenotyping. *J Magn Reson Imaging* 2002;16:423–429.

112. Johnson GA, Cofer GP, Gewalt SL, et al. Morphologic phenotyping with MR microscopy: the visible mouse. *Radiology* 2002;222:789–793.

113. Song SK, Qu Z, Garabedian EM, et al. Improved magnetic resonance imaging detection of prostate cancer in a transgenic mouse model. *Cancer Res* 2002;62: 1555–1558.

114. Lewin M, Bredow S, Sergeyev N, et al. In vivo assessment of vascular endothelial growth factor-induced angiogenesis. *Int J Cancer* 1999;83:798–802.

115. Weissleder R, Cheng HC, Marecos E, et al. Non-invasive in vivo mapping of tumour vascular and interstitial volume fractions. *Eur J Cancer* 1998;34:1448–1454.

116. Weissleder R, Moore A, Mahmood U, et al. In vivo magnetic resonance imaging of transgene expression. *Nat Med* 2000;6:351–355.

117. Ross BD, Chenevert TL, Rehemtulla A. Magnetic resonance imaging in cancer research. *Eur J Cancer* 2002;38:2147–2156.

118. Paulus MJ, Gleason SS, Kennel SJ, et al. High resolution x-ray computed tomography: an emerging tool for small animal cancer research. *Neoplasia* 2000;2: 62–70.
119. Borah B, Gross GJ, Dufresne TE, et al. Three-dimensional microimaging (MRmicroI and microCT), finite element modeling, and rapid prototyping provide unique insights into bone architecture in osteoporosis. *Anat Rec* 2001;265:101–110.
120. Kennel SJ, Davis IA, Branning J, et al. High resolution computed tomography and MRI for monitoring lung tumor growth in mice undergoing radioimmunotherapy: correlation with histology. *Med Phys* 2000;27: 1101–1107.
121. Cherry SR, Gambhir SS. Use of positron emission tomography in animal research. *ILAR J* 2001;42: 219–232.
122. Tjuvajev JG, Finn R, Watanabe K, et al. Noninvasive imaging of herpes virus thymidine kinase gene transfer and expression: a potential method for monitoring clinical gene therapy. *Cancer Res* 1996;56:4087–4095.
123. Tjuvajev JG, Chen SH, Joshi A, et al. Imaging adenoviral-mediated herpes virus thymidine kinase gene transfer and expression in vivo. *Cancer Res* 1999;59: 5186–5193.
124. Blasberg RG, Tjuvajev JG. Herpes simplex virus thymidine kinase as a marker/reporter gene for PET imaging of gene therapy. *Q J Nucl Med* 1999;43: 163–169.
125. Bennett JJ, Tjuvajev J, Johnson P, et al. Positron emission tomography imaging for herpes virus infection: Implications for oncolytic viral treatments of cancer. *Nat Med* 2001;7:859–863.
126. Jacobs A, Tjuvajev JG, Dubrovin M, et al. Positron emission tomography-based imaging of transgene expression mediated by replication-conditional, oncolytic herpes simplex virus type 1 mutant vectors in vivo. *Cancer Res* 2001;61:2983–2995.
127. Weber DA, Ivanovic M. Ultra-high-resolution imaging of small animals: implications for preclinical and research studies. *J Nucl Cardiol* 1999;6:332–344.
128. Groch MW, Erwin WD. Single-photon emission computed tomography in the year 2001: instrumentation and quality control. *J Nucl Med Technol* 2001;29: 12–18.
129. Phelps ME. PET: the merging of biology and imaging into molecular imaging. *J Nucl Med* 2000;41:661–681.
130. Vooijs M, Jonkers J, Lyons S, et al. Noninvasive imaging of spontaneous retinoblastoma pathway-dependent tumors in mice. *Cancer Res* 2002;62:1862–1867.
131. Ntziachristos V, Tung CH, Bremer C, et al. Fluorescence molecular tomography resolves protease activity in vivo. *Nat Med* 2002;8:757–760.
132. Lee TI, Rinaldi NJ, Robert F, et al. Transcriptional regulatory networks in Saccharomyces cerevisiae. *Science* 2002;298:799–804.
133. Oft M, Akhurst RJ, Balmain A. Metastasis is driven by sequential elevation of H-ras and Smad2 levels. *Nat Cell Biol* 2002;4:487–494.
134. Frame S, Balmain A. Integration of positive and negative growth signals during ras pathway activation in vivo. *Curr Opin Genet Dev* 2000;10:106–113.
135. Hahn WC, Weinberg RA. Modelling the molecular circuitry of cancer. *Nat Rev Cancer* 2002;2:331–341.
136. Gonzalez FJ, Kimura S. Role of gene knockout mice in understanding the mechanisms of chemical toxicity and carcinogenesis. *Cancer Lett* 1999;143:199–204.

PART 4

Analytical Laboratory Techniques

13

Modern and Practical Guide for Bioanalysis

Surendra K. Bansal and Zhenmin Liang

Hoffmann-La Roche, Inc., Nutley, New Jersey 07110

Bioanalysis determines concentrations of drugs and metabolites in biofluids and, therefore, provides building blocks for pharmacokinetic determinations in clinical and toxicological studies. The pharmacokinetic data can be only as good and reliable as the underlying bioanalytical data. With today's advanced tools and techniques, the bioanalysts determine these concentrations accurately, precisely, and rapidly. These tools and techniques, which were only dreams in the past, are results of a continuous search for higher sensitivity, specificity, and speed for bioanalysis. The tool that has had the greatest impact on the bioanalytical field is a triple quadrupole mass spectrometer coupled to a high-pressure liquid chromatography (HPLC), commonly known as LC/MS/MS. The bioanalysts are now using LC/MS/MS almost exclusively, because of its speed and high sensitivity and selectivity. Very few cases exist where classical HPLC or gas chromatography (GC) methods are still in use. The standard HPLC method is used for older bioanalytical methods or for analyzing compounds that cannot be ionized efficiently for mass spectral analysis, whereas GC or GC/MS is used for some volatile compounds that are difficult to ionize for LC/MS/MS. Overall, LC/MS/MS appears to be the instrument of choice for bioanalytical work.

This chapter will provide an overview of the current instrumentation, techniques, principles, logistics, and regulatory guidance for bioanalysis. Because LC/MS/MS is now the predominant method used for bioanalysis, emphasis is placed on this technology. However, the general principles of bioanalysis provided in this chapter are applicable for any technology. This chapter is intended to educate the users of bioanalytical data, but can also serve as a summary for bioanalysts in the field.

ORIGIN OF SAMPLES AND THEIR BIOANALYSIS

Biological samples, such as plasma, serum, whole blood, and urine, are obtained from many types of studies. The most common studies that generate samples for bioanalysis are discovery pharmacokinetics or pharmacology, including cassette pharmacokinetic (N-in-1 dosing), non-GLP (Good Laboratory Practice) toxicokinetic, GLP toxicokinetic, and clinical studies.

Bioanalytical methods (assays) for new compounds are generally developed at about the same time as the discovery studies are performed. Historically, the methods used at this stage were highly insensitive and the sensitivity was improved as experience was gained in analysis. With the use of LC/MS/MS, this situation has changed and more sensitive methods are being developed at early discovery stages. Although these early methods are not fully optimized, they are quite adequate to support the analysis of samples from discovery and non-GLP toxicokinetic studies. As the compound moves forward in a drug development program, the bioanalytical methods are optimized. During optimization, stable-isotope–labeled internal standards (IS) are also added to increase precision and accuracy. After proper optimization, the assays are validated and used for analysis of samples from GLP toxicokinetic or clinical studies.

ADVANTAGES OF LC/MS/MS ANALYSIS IN EARLY PHASES OF DRUG DISCOVERY

One of the most important contributions of LC/MS/MS in the bioanalytical field is the shortening of time required for method development. This has tremendously benefited sample analysis at the discovery stage. These samples could not have been analyzed in a timely fashion and with the needed sensitivity and specificity before the development of LC/MS/MS. These samples are now being analyzed rapidly with highly sensitive and selective methods. The ability to analyze samples from cassette pharmacokinetics is another important advantage of LC/MS/MS at the discovery stage (1,2). Cassette pharmacokinetics has become a popular technique for conducting high-throughput pharmacokinetic screening in early drug discovery research. In a cassette-pharmacokinetic study, a dosing formulation containing a mixture of several compounds (up to six typically) is administered to an animal. Plasma samples are collected and analyzed to obtain the pharmacokinetic profiles for all compounds. With this approach, one can accomplish pharmacokinetic screens at a high speed and with a fraction of the resources compared with conventional single-compound pharmacokinetics. A disadvantage of cassette pharmacokinetics is that there is a potential for drug–drug interaction, causing the pharmacokinetic results to be unreliable. To overcome this drawback, multiple compounds have been dosed in parallel, but singly, in animal studies. The blood samples at a given time point are pooled from several animals dosed with different compounds. Pooled samples containing multiple compounds are analyzed by LC/MS/MS (3). This approach avoids the drug–drug interaction potential, but does dilute the samples for any given compound. The dilution of samples may not be a problem because

of high sensitivity of LC/MS/MS. If needed, one can avoid the dilution of samples by creating calibration standards and quality controls (QCs) with multiple compounds, and analyzing the samples without pooling. All of these variants of cassette-pharmacokinetic analysis have been possible only because of the high specificity and sensitivity of LC/MS/MS.

INSTRUMENTS AND TECHNIQUES

LC/MS/MS Instrumentation

LC/MS/MS consists of two major components: front-end HPLC and back-end mass spectrometer (MS). The HPLC separates the analytes of interest from potential interfering compounds in biological matrices prior to their introduction to the MS. Many types of mass spectrometers can be coupled to an HPLC for LC/MS analysis. One type, the triple quadrupole MS, stands out as the best in sensitivity, precision, accuracy, and specificity when operated under the MS/MS (tandem MS) mode. The triple quadrupole MS consists of the following five major sections (Fig. 13.1): ion source, first mass analyzer (first quadrupole, MS1), collision chamber (second quadrupole or multipole), second mass analyzer (third quadrupole, MS2), and detector.

The ion sources widely used for LC/MS are electrospray and atmospheric pressure chemical ionization. Both of the these ionization sources operate under atmospheric pressure, in contrast to mass analyzers which operate under high vacuum. During a

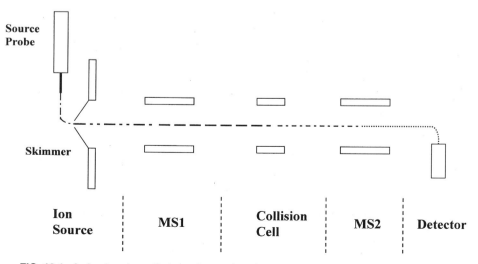

FIG. 13.1. A simple schematic for major sections in a triple quadrupole mass spectrometer.

typical quantitative LC/MS/MS analysis, the eluents from an HPLC column are introduced into the ion source, where ions are formed in the gas phase. The ions are directed to the first mass analyzer (MS1) by electrical potentials. The MS1 selectively passes an ion beam with a preset mass (more accurately, mass-to-charge ratio) corresponding to the target analyte into the collision chamber. The ions in the collision chamber collide with a collision gas (an inert gas, such as argon) and undergo fragmentation to form product ions. The product ions exit the collision chamber and move toward the second mass analyzer (MS2), which is set to pass a specific ion beam with a preset mass-to-charge ratio corresponding to a characteristic product ion from the analyte. The product ion beam travels further to be detected by a detector mounted after MS2.

A simpler instrument that does not have the collision chamber and MS2 is called a single-stage quadrupole MS. Only one mass analyzer is utilized to detect target analytes in single-stage LC/MS analysis, making LC/MS less specific for analysis than LC/MS/MS. Although LC/MS is also used for bioanalysis, LC/MS/MS is more prevalent.

In summary, LC/MS/MS provides several dimensions of separation and selection: namely, the HPLC separation, selection of precursor ions in MS1, formation of unique product ions, and selection and detection of unique product ions. These multiple dimensions of separation and selection make the assays based on LC/MS/MS highly selective and specific for an analyte. High specificity coupled with the instrument's high sensitivity makes LC/MS/MS the instrument of choice for bioanalytical work.

Sample-preparation Techniques

Biological samples in most cases are processed or prepared for injection into an HPLC column for LC/MS/MS analysis. During sample preparation, some components that could interfere with the quantitation of the analytes are removed from samples. Because the LC/MS/MS provides many dimensions of selection beyond HPLC separation, a relatively simple sample preparation is sufficient, making the LC/MS/MS method development easy. Minimal sample preparation for LC/MS/MS is in contrast to an extensive sample preparation needed for classical HPLC analysis using ultraviolet-light detection. Extensive sample preparation and low specificity of the ultraviolet detectors make these types of HPLC assays difficult to develop. Although LC/MS/MS methods need simple sample processing, a proper sample preparation is essential for a rugged and reliable assay. Some

of the most common techniques used for sample preparation prior to LC/MS/MS analysis are described below.

Protein Precipitation

Protein precipitation is the simplest procedure used for preparation of biological samples for LC/MS/MS analysis. In this technique, an organic solvent is added to an aliquot of sample to precipitate most of the proteins. Commonly used precipitating solvents are acetonitrile, methanol, or ethanol, with acetonitrile being the most used. After a thorough mixing and centrifugation, the supernatant is analyzed by LC/MS/MS. This technique is simple and provides a quick and universal cleanup procedure for plasma and urine samples. It produces acceptable-quality data, which are most suited for drug discovery and early drug development. A disadvantage of this technique is that the sample cleanup is less effective than other sample preparation techniques, making the overall analytical method less rugged.

Liquid–Liquid Extraction

Liquid–liquid extraction was employed in the past as the most frequently used sample cleanup technique. It utilizes the solubility difference between the analytes and the matrix components to extract the analytes preferentially into one liquid phase while leaving interfering components in the other liquid phase. A properly optimized method can give a very clean sample with this technique. Liquid–liquid extraction is the least generic of the sample-processing techniques, requiring specific method development efforts.

Solid-phase Extraction

Solid-phase extraction (SPE) is another popular sample cleanup technique. The principle of SPE is similar to chromatographic separation, which utilizes an interaction of the analyte between solvent and the stationary phases. The extracts produced by this method are quite clean. This technique is more generic than liquid–liquid extraction. SPE can be performed using several available formats of extraction cartridges of various adsorbent types. Selection of the SPE cartridge is based on the type of analyte, sample volume, and the type of automation instrument used. A frequently used extraction cartridge is C18 silica in a 96-well-plate format. An alternative to this offline SPE is online extraction, which is described in the next section.

Online Extraction

Online extraction is performed by coupling extraction onto the HPLC flow path. Several instruments and cartridges are available to perform online extraction. A simple, effective, and popular technique is the use of extraction column or cartridge with column switching. A raw or pretreated plasma sample is injected to an extraction column in this technique. The analytes bind to the stationary phase of the extraction column. Solvent is passed through the extraction column to wash out some matrix components. The solvent composition is then changed to elute the analytes off the extraction column to another column (the analytical column). The LC/MS/MS analysis continues as usual on the analytical column. This method provides clean and consistent extraction like the SPE method, with minimum manual involvement.

Automation

Many steps are being automated to improve efficiency and precision of the method. Most attention is being given to automate the sample-preparation step. All of the previously described sample-preparation procedures can be automated to varying degrees. A popular format for automating sample preparation is the 96-well microtiter plate. Samples are loaded to the microtiter plate using an automated liquid handler with four or eight pipettes. Once the samples are in a 96-well format, they are more amenable to other types of automation, because instruments are available with 96 pipettes for liquid addition or removal and for performing SPE. Autosamplers are also available for injection of samples directly from the 96-well-format plates. Automation provides better reproducibility and allows the analyst to perform other useful tasks, such as reviewing the data, managing projects, and writing reports.

BIOANALYTICAL METHOD DEVELOPMENT, VALIDATION, AND USE FOR ANALYSIS

Method Development

The first step in bioanalysis of a drug is to develop a suitable method. There are three steps to method development for an LC/MS/MS assay. Sample preparation is the first step. Any of the previously described techniques can be used for sample preparation. At the early discovery phase, a quick and generic method is needed. Therefore, the protein-precipitation technique is a preferred choice for early method development. As the method matures and goes for validation,

some other technique may be required to make the method more rugged. The second step in assay development is the optimization of MS settings, which is usually performed by infusing the compound to the mass spectrometer and optimizing the MS response manually or through some automated optimization feature of the instrument. The third step is the development of an HPLC method. Most pharmaceutical compounds can be analyzed on a C-18 HPLC column with simple mobile phases consisting of solvents such as, water, acetonitrile, or methanol. Some pH modifiers (volatile acids or bases) or volatile buffers may also be added to the mobile phase to facilitate ionization of the analytes and improve chromatography. The processed samples are then applied to the HPLC and eluents are measured by MS.

Method Validation

Bioanalytical methods used for analysis of biological samples from bioavailability, bioequivalence, and pharmacokinetic studies in humans and animals must be validated prior to their use. A brief description of validation is provided here and the details can be found in widely accepted guidance publications (4,5).

Method validation is performed using a blank biological matrix, the same as in the intended test samples. The blank matrix is spiked with known amounts of analyte(s) to prepare calibration standards and QC samples. These samples are used to obtain the following validation parameters. The fundamental parameters required according to the guidance document (4) and the conference report (5) are given in italics. Fundamental parameters must be determined for all assays, and the other parameters should be determined as applicable for a specific assay:

- *Accuracy*
- *Precision*
- *Selectivity*
- *Sensitivity*
- *Reproducibility*
- *Stability*
- Calibration range and concentration–response function (linear or nonlinear)
- Extraction efficiency
- Positional differences within the run
- Dilution integrity for analyzing samples above the limit of quantitation

Multipoint (six to eight points) calibration curves are used in bioanalytical methods to quantify the unknown samples. QC samples at three concentrations (within the range of the method) are generally added to assess the method's quality. The accuracy and precision is determined by analyzing five QC samples at each concentration. Interday precision and accuracy is determined for a minimum of 3 independent days of analysis. The accuracy is determined by the difference between the observed mean concentration of the QC sample and its nominal value. The accuracy should be within 15% of the nominal concentration of the QC samples, except for the QC prepared at the lower limit of quantitation (LLOQ), in which case the accuracy can be within 20% of its nominal concentration. The precision is determined by the coefficient of variation (CV) obtained at each QC concentration. The CV should not exceed 15% at each concentration, except 20% if the QC concentration is at the LLOQ level. The lowest standard on the calibration curve is accepted as the limit of quantitation and should meet the 20% rule (allowed inaccuracy and CV of 20%). Several types of stability for the analyte are determined during validation–stock solution, freeze-thaw, short-term room temperature, processed sample, and long-term storage stability. Determination of the long-term storage stability continues after the initial validation is complete. All other needed validation parameters are determined, and a final report that includes information regarding the bioanalytical methods used is written.

Analysis of Test Samples

Calibration standards and QC samples (minimum of duplicates at three concentrations), prepared in the same biological matrix as the intended samples, are included with each batch of sample analysis. The analytical batch is accepted if the calibration standards and QC samples meet the following criteria. The backcalculated concentration for a minimum of 75% of the standards should fall within 15% of their nominal concentration or within 20% for the LLOQ standard. The observed concentration of the QC samples should not differ from the nominal concentration by more than 15% at all concentrations, except 20% if the QC is made at the LLOQ level. At least four of the six QC samples should meet these criteria, and the two not meeting the criteria must not be from the same concentration. The number of QC samples within a batch should be at least 5% of the total unknown samples. Concentrations of test samples from clinical or GLP toxicology studies are reported only when these acceptance criteria are met. Similar acceptance criteria may be difficult to achieve for early discovery studies because the methods are not optimized or validated. In such cases, the acceptance criteria may be relaxed by 5% to 10%, but it is recommended that the QC samples be used for discovery studies also.

Certain samples need to be reanalyzed because of analytical problems or if concentrations do not seem to fit the pharmacokinetic profile. Standard procedures must be set *a priori* for handling the repeat analysis. A table for the repeat analytical results should be provided, giving the initial, repeat, and final results. The reasons for repeating and accepting results should also be provided. Repeat-analysis criteria vary among laboratories and can be complex, but in brief, the samples for analytical anomalies are reanalyzed singly and the repeat-analytical results are reported. When the analytical results are suspect without obvious analytical reasons, the samples are analyzed in duplicate and the median value from the original and reanalysis results is reported.

Documentation of Bioanalytical Work

The guidance document (4) provides some specific requirements for documentation of bioanalytical work. An attempt is made here to simplify the documentation of bioanalytical work required by this document. Laboratories working under GLP should have a set of standard operating procedures for conducting the bioanalytical work. When methods are validated, formal validation reports must be written. When samples are analyzed, a bioanalytical report must be written for each study. The bioanalysis usually generates a large amount of raw data and information that must be documented and archived. Table 13.1 summarizes the types of information generated during the analysis of samples (column 1). The information should be readily available for audit by the regulatory agencies and should be kept with the raw data or provided in the bioanalytical report. Table 13.1 provides a suggested location for documenting and archiving the information under columns 2 and 3. A check mark indicates that the available information should be documented under the section specified in the column, whereas a blank space indicates that the information is not kept in that section. Also included in the table are specific details about what information for the item is kept in the indicated section.

COMMON BIOANALYTICAL ISSUES AND POSSIBLE SOLUTIONS

Sample Stability

The stability of the analyte(s) in biological matrix is unknown at the beginning. A preliminary assessment of the stability of the analyte in biological matrix should be made during method development. Knowledge of the stability will provide confidence that the observed

TABLE 13.1. *Documentation for bioanalytical work*

Documentation item	Store with raw data	Provide in report
Evidence of identity and purity (COA) for standards	Certificate of analysis	Purity information
Sample identification	✓	✓
Collection dates	✓	
Shipping information	✓	
Storage condition prior to shipping	✓	
Sample condition	✓	Abnormal sample condition that could affect sample results
Storage condition prior to analysis	✓	✓
Analytical run identification	✓	✓
Date and time of analysis	✓	Dates for analytical runs
Assay method	✓	Method description, identification, or validation report number containing the method
Names of analysts	✓	✓
Analysis start and stop times	✓	
Significant equipment and material changes	✓	Changes affecting the analysis
Any potential issue or deviation from validated method	✓	✓
Equation for back calculation of results	✓	✓
Tables for calibration data and quality control results	✓	✓
Samples results including assay run identification, raw data and back-calculated results, integration, and/or other reporting codes	✓ (Full information kept)	Calculated results for samples in tabular format
Complete chromatograms from 5%–20% of subjects with standards and quality controls	✓ Choose subjects prior to analysis of clinical samples for printing of chromatograms for submission; provide chromatograms from 5% subjects for all studies and 20% subjects from bioequivalence studies	Print chromatograms to paper or a computer (.pdf) file without printing them to paper; if the bioanalytical report is provided electronically, attach the .pdf file to the bioanalytical report; provide the chromatograms from the full run containing the preidentified subjects
Reasons for missing samples	✓	Identify missing samples
Documentation for repeat analysis of samples	✓ Repeat samples according to a standard operating procedure; record name of requestor for repeat analysis and supervisory approval for repeat analysis	Repeat-analysis results table containing initial, repeat, and finally reported results, reasons for repeating and accepting results
Documentation for reintegrated data	✓ Initial and repeat integration results, reason for reintegration and supervisory approval	
Deviations with justifications	✓	List deviations
Abbreviations and codes used in the bioanalytical report	✓	Provide descriptions of the abbreviations and codes used in the report
References	Keep referenced material	Reference to the referenced material
Standard operating procedures	Kept in department records	Make references as necessary

concentrations are actual concentrations of the analyte. The stability should be determined at ambient and/or elevated temperature (e.g., 37°C). It is desirable to obtain a stability profile over a few time points for a period up to overnight. Extrapolation and trend analysis of these data can provide information on how the samples should be stored. Long-term stability at the actual storage temperature should be determined during and after the validation of the bioanalytical method.

Matrix Interference

Because LC/MS/MS is highly selective, one does not see many interfering peaks in the LC/MS/MS chromatogram. It is true that LC/MS/MS is almost free from the types of interference that ultraviolet HPLC methods exhibit because of low specificity of the ultraviolet detector. However, LC/MS/MS methods can be affected by components coeluting with the analyte, even though these components are transparent in MS/MS detection. This interference by matrix is called *matrix effect on ionization* (6). Matrix interference is a major issue confronting bioanalysis by LC/MS/MS. Matrix interference arises from the fact that the ionization efficiency for an analyte in the two types of ion sources (electrospray and atmospheric pressure chemical ionization) used in LC/MS/MS are influenced by other components present in the eluent stream. Most frequently, the presence of matrix components suppresses the ionization of an analyte, thereby artificially reducing the response of the analyte. On rare occasions, matrix components can also enhance the ionization of an analyte, artificially increasing the response of the analyte. The degree of ionization suppression or enhancement varies with the quality and quantity of matrix components. There is no universal accepted quantitative measure for matrix interference. The term *matrix factor* (MF) was recently introduced to quantify the matrix interference (7), and is defined as a ratio of the analyte peak response (peak area, height, or a ratio with added internal standard) in presence of matrix components to the analyte peak response in absence of matrix components:

$$MF = \frac{Peak\ response\ in\ presence\ of\ matrix}{Peak\ response\ in\ absence\ of\ matrix}$$

Matrix interference can be compensated for by use of suitable internal standards. When an IS is subject to matrix interference similar to that of the analyte, the ratio of the responses tends to compensate for the matrix interference. The most appropriate IS for the LC/MS analyses are stable-isotope–labeled compounds. Such compounds have the same chemical properties and have almost the same retention times as the analytes. Therefore, stable-isotope–labeled IS are

subject to a similar interference as the analyte, and provide excellent compensation for matrix interference. If an IS is used in the analysis, the matrix factor should be determined for both analyte and the IS. A ratio of MF for the analyte and IS would provide "IS-adjusted MF," which can also be obtained when the response used in the equation for MF is peak area ratio or peak height ratio. An MF value of one indicates no matrix interference, an MF value of less than one suggests ionization suppression, and an MF value greater than one may be due to ionization enhancement or to analyte sticking in the absence of matrix during LC/MS/MS analysis.

Matrix Interference from Intravenously Administered Formulations

When intravenous formulations containing surfactants are given to test subjects, the plasma samples may exhibit abnormally high matrix interference (8). This interference is due to the intravenous formulation excipients, specifically the surfactants, mixing with the blood and causing matrix interference. The excipients must be extracted from the samples prior to LC/MS/MS analysis to avoid experimental anomalies (9). Such a precaution is specially needed for discovery-samples analysis, because IS is generally not available at this early stage. Without the proper IS, the matrix interference in intravenously administered samples is enhanced and may lead to erroneous results. Enhanced ion suppression in intravenously administered samples would yield low concentrations in intravenous plasma samples compared to the samples obtained after the drug is orally administered, producing erroneously higher oral bioavailability data.

Simultaneous Assay of Metabolites

With LC/MS/MS methods, it is easy to analyze metabolites simultaneously with the drug molecule. However, a decision to analyze metabolite(s) should be made judiciously, and not just because the analysis of metabolites is easy. If the metabolites are minor, their concentrations compared to the drug molecule could also be too small to measure them together. One may need to analyze a diluted sample to measure the drug concentration and another undiluted sample to measure the metabolite. The usefulness of concentration data for minor metabolites may also be in question (10).

Bioanalytical Data Transfer

Bioanalytical data for clinical and GLP regulated studies need to go through several checks before they can be finalized. If needed, preliminary data can be released prior to the release of final data. But, it should be understood that the preliminary data could change after a thorough review, and therefore should be used only for a preliminary pharmacokinetic evaluation. Preliminary data are checked by the analysts and/or their supervisors, and are audited by the quality assurance unit before they become final. The final quality-assurance–reviewed data are provided in the bioanalytical reports.

Concentration Dependent Clinical Trials

When escalation of dosing is dependent on the concentrations of the biological samples from the previous dose, the clinicians would want to know the pharmacokinetic parameters or bioanalytical concentrations prior to the next dosing. Because the bioanalytical laboratory is usually not at the same site as the clinic, the samples need to be transferred from the clinic to a bioanalytical laboratory. These samples are analyzed in the laboratory and the data transferred to a pharmacokinetist. The logistics for sample and data transfer are equally important to bioanalysis of samples in such cases, to achieve a minimal overall turnaround time.

Proactive Solutions for Bioanalytical Problems

As stated previously, bioanalysis is required for samples from many types of studies from early discovery to late-stage development of a compound. Although the analytical process is similar for analysis of samples from any stage of drug discovery or development, the handling of the samples and data, expectation for timing of analysis, review and release of data, and writing of bioanalytical reports are much different at different stages. Requirements of each stage must be understood and addressed proactively to provide the best bioanalytical support. As the modern tools and techniques for bioanalysis advance, these methods must be used very carefully to take full advantage of their capabilities and avoid any pitfalls.

The US Food and Drug Administration's guidance document (4) provides generally accepted principles for validation of bioanalytical methods, criteria for acceptance of bioanalytical runs, and documentation requirements. These guidelines are very similar to those presented in the position papers developed by the bioanalysts at the workshops and conferences held in Arlington, VA (5,11). Bioanalysis is an important process for any drug discovery or development program, and requires careful attention by both the users and providers of bioanalytical data. An early partnership between the users and providers will ensure the quality of the bioanalytical data and, in turn, the quality of the pharmacokinetic results.

The authors thank Stan Kolis and Corinne Martinelli of Hoffmann-La Roche, Inc., for proofreading and providing valuable suggestions.

REFERENCES

1. Berman J, Halm K, Adkinson K, et al. Simultaneous pharmacokinetic screening of a mixture of compounds in the dog using API LC/MS/MS analysis for increased throughput. *J Med Chem* 1997;40:827–829.
2. Bayliss MK, Frick LW. High-throughput pharmacokinetics: cassette dosing. *Curr Opin Drug Discov Dev* 1999;2:20–25.
3. Kou BS, Van Noord T, Feng MR, et al. Sample pooling to expedite bioanalysis and pharmacokinetic research. *J Pharm Biomed Anal.* 1998;16:837–846.
4. US Food and Drug Administration. Guidance for industry: bioanalytical method validation, US Department of Health and Human Services, May 2001.
5. Shah VP, Midha KM, Findlay JWA, et al. Bioanalytical method validation: a revisit with a decade of progress. *Pharm Res* 2000;17:1551–1557.
6. Tang L, Kebarle P. Dependence of ion intensity in electrospray mass spectrometry on the concentration of the analytes in the electrosprayed solution. *Anal Chem* 1993;55:3654–3668.
7. Bansal SK, Liang Z. Matrix factor and extraction uniformity: novel quantitative tools for assessing matrix effects in LC/MS/MS during assay validations. Presented at the 50th annual conference of the American Society of Mass Spectrometry; June 2002; Orlando, FL.
8. Liang, Z, Weigl, P, Nieuwenhuis, T, et al. Issues Covering Rapid Bioanalytical Method Development and Sample Analysis. Presented at the 46th annual conference of the American Society of Mass Spectrometry; May 1998; Orlando, FL.
9. Weigl, P, Liang, Z, Mallalieu, N, et al. Removal of ionization suppression in LC/MS/MS methods due to additives in IV formulation. Presented at the annual meeting and exposition of the American Association of Pharmaceutical Scientists; November 2002; Toronto, Canada.
10. Bailie TA, Cayen MN, Fouda H, et al. Contemporary issues in toxicology: drug metabolites in safety testing. *Toxicol Appl Pharmacol* 2002;198:188–196.
11. Shah VP, Midha KM, Dighe S. Analytical methods validation: bioavailability, bioequivalence, and pharmacokinetic studies. *J Pharm Sci* 1992;81:309–312.

14

Good Laboratory Practice and the Development of Anticancer Agents

Jinee D. Rizzo

Institute for Drug Development, Cancer Therapy and Research Center, San Antonio, Texas 78229

HISTORY

An ancient Japanese proverb states, "Nature makes no mistakes." However, people are not so infallible, and we often do make mistakes. In 1976, in response to mistakes and other discrepancies found in laboratory studies submitted as part of a New Drug Application (NDA) by a major pharmaceutical company, the US Food and Drug Administration (FDA) established the Bioresearch Monitoring Program to develop a strategy to handle the problem of data validity in the areas of safety studies and clinical testing. As a result, the FDA published a first draft of the Good Laboratory Practice regulations, or GLPs as they are often referred. Final regulations were published in 1978 with revisions issued in 1980, 1987, 1989, and 1991. These regulations are found in the Code of Federal Regulations (21CFR Part 58) and continue to evolve based on improvements and advances in laboratory science and instrumentation.

The original intent of the regulations was to outline standards for the conduct of *nonclinical* laboratory studies designed to establish the safety of products regulated by the FDA. Scientific judgment in the design and conduct of the studies was not to be restricted. The ideal outcome of following GLP guidelines is that studies would be well designed, properly conducted, closely monitored, accurately reported, and fully reconstructible. These studies included all manner of toxicity studies, from *in vitro* mutagenicity studies to acute, subchronic, and long-term toxicity and/or carcinogenicity. The regulations did not include basic research, studies utilizing human subjects, or clinical trials.

Analytical laboratories performing quantitative analysis of drugs and metabolites from biological fluids, including plasma and urine, obtained during the conductance of phase 1, 2, and 3 clinical trials are not specifically addressed in the GLPs. In the past, at least in phase 1 oncology trials, adhering to strict GLP guidelines was not required. Indeed, proving that a laboratory followed "good laboratory science" was enough. In addition, since many phase 1 oncology trials are conducted at academic institutions, GLP is not required. However, in today's highly regulated, global environment, most pharmaceutical companies now require that GLP guidelines be followed in the performance of any analytical study used to obtain data from a clinical trial.

BECOMING GLP COMPLIANT

Laboratories that adhere to GLP are referred to as "GLP compliant." The process of attaining GLP compliance may take anywhere from 1 to 3 years, depending on the size of the laboratory, and is not a task for the faint-hearted. In general terms, the primary things that must be accomplished include: (a) writing standard operating procedures (SOPs), (b) creating a system for study sample as well as test and control article accountability, (c) validating all analytical instrumentation, (d) maintaining costly service agreements and maintenance records with instrument manufacturers of all major equipment, (e) creating calibration/maintenance logs for balances and other appropriate equipment, and (f) developing/implementing a computer compliance plan to include software validation, data accountability in terms of audit trail capabilities, as well as data and system security procedures. Maintaining compliance in the laboratory is an ongoing process that continually evolves to meet new regulatory requirements and/or changes. The most recent addition to the GLPs includes 21CFR Part 11, addressing computer systems security and validation as well as electronic signatures and electronic FDA submissions.

As well as a significant investment of time, the costs involved in setting up and maintaining a fully GLP-compliant laboratory can be substantial. Some of these costs include instrument service/maintenance agreements, 24-hour on-call refrigerator/freezer monitoring systems, computer hardware and software validation, and the ongoing continuing education of skilled employees. Depending on the size of the laboratory, a quality assurance unit (QAU) or individual must be available to perform routine laboratory inspections, audit data, and review final reports.

Similar to most other classes of therapeutic agents, the development of new and promising oncology agents requires that safety and toxicity studies be carried out in at least two animal species, most commonly the dog and rat. As mentioned previously, these preclinical or "' nonclinical' laboratory studies" were the original focus of the FDA when drafting the GLP guidelines. Subsequently, over the past decade, the importance of a complete data audit trail and evidence of consistent laboratory procedure have been recognized as significant in the generation of pharmacokinetic data from clinical trials intended as part of an NDA. Because the accurate and precise quantitation of analyte levels are the foundation of pharmacokinetic results, it has become industry standard that bioanalytical laboratories adopt and function under GLP guidelines.

FDA-GLP REGULATIONS

The Code of Federal Regulations outlines the GLP regulations (21CFR Part 58), dividing these guidelines into nine subparts (A–K). An outline of these subparts and their divisions is given in Table 14.1. A discussion of these subparts and sections will be presented in this chapter, although it is not intended to be an exhaustive review of the regulations. The Internet contains not only the actual GLP guidance documents (1), but also Web sites dedicated to discussion regarding these regulations (2). In addition, *Good Laboratory Practice Regulations*, a reference source edited by Sandy Weinberg (3), is a valuable tool for any laboratory implementing GLP compliance.

Subpart A: General Provisions

58.1 Scope

Scope describes *all* of the conditions that must be met before a study will be regulated by GLP, including:

- Study of a product regulated by the FDA (except cosmetics)
- *In vivo* or *in vitro* study

- Study in which the FDA-regulated product is administered to nonhuman animals (toxicology), plants, microorganisms, or subparts of any of these listed
- Study results submitted or intended to be submitted to the FDA in support of the approval of an application for research or marketing permit (NDA)
- Study results that may be used to predict adverse events and/or to establish safe use characteristics for the product

Examples of oncology studies that can be GLP regulated include median lethal dose (LD_{50}), any specific toxicity study such as phototoxicity or dermal toxicity, target animal absorption, distribution, metabolism and excretion (ADME), subchronic or chronic multiple-dosing studies, and general toxicological safety studies. These studies are all preclinical in nature. Examples of studies that would not be regulated include, pharmacology experiments, dose-range finding, studies to develop new experimental techniques (i.e., analytical method development), and human efficacy studies. Clinical trials involving phase 1, 2, or 3 studies are monitored under a separate set of guidelines, similarly named Good Clinical Practice (GCP).

58.3 Definitions

In order to interpret the GLPs, an understanding of the terminology used is essential. As mentioned previously, the regulations were originally written to cover nonclinical laboratory studies. According to the GLPs, a nonclinical laboratory study means an "*in vivo* or *in vitro* experiment in which test articles are studied in test systems under laboratory conditions to determine their safety." The term does not include studies involving human subjects or clinical studies. The term *test article* refers to any food or color additive, biological product, medical device for human use, or any other article subject to regulation under the Federal Food, Drug and Cosmetic Act. Along with test article, the term *control article* is also used frequently and refers to any food or color additive, biological product, medical device for human use, or any article other than a test article, food, or water that is administered to the test system in the course of a nonclinical study for the purpose of establishing a basis for comparison with the test article. For example, a vehicle, solvent, or other drug carrier material when given to control animal groups as part of a safety study is referred to as the control article. The control article is also called the *positive control*.

In regard to the bioanalytical laboratory, the control article is usually referred to as the *reference standard*.

TABLE 14.1. *Major subparts and sections for Good Laboratory Practice guidelines*

Subpart A. General provisions
    58.1   Scope
    58.3   Definitions
    58.15   Inspection of a testing facility
Subpart B. Organization and personnel
    58.29   Personnel
    58.31   Testing facility management
    58.33   Study director
    58.35   Quality assurance unit
Subpart C. Facilities
    58.41   General
    58.43   Animal care facilities
    58.45   Animal supply facilities
    58.47   Facilities for handling test and control articles
    58.49   Laboratory operation areas
    58.51   Specimen and data-storage facilities
Subpart D. Equipment
    58.61   Equipment design
    58.63   Maintenance and calibration of equipment
Subpart E. Testing facilities operation
    58.81   Standard operating procedures
    58.83   Reagents and solutions
    58.90   Animal care
Subpart F. Test and control article
    58.105 Test and control article characterization
    58.107 Test and control article handling
    58.113 Mixtures of articles and carriers
Subpart G. Protocol for and conduct of a nonclinical laboratory study
    58.120 Protocol
    58.130 Conduct of a nonclinical laboratory study
Subparts H–I. (Reserved)
Subpart J. Records and reports
    58.185 Reporting of nonclinical laboratory study results
    58.190 Storage and retrieval of records and data
    58.195 Retention of records
Subpart K. Disqualification of testing facilities
    58.200 Purpose
    58.202 Grounds for disqualification
    58.204 Notice and opportunity for hearing on proposed disqualification
    58.206 Final order on disqualification
    58.210 Actions upon disqualification
    58.213 Public domain of information regarding disqualification
    58.215 Alternative or additional actions to disqualification
    58.217 Suspension or termination of a testing facility by a sponsor
    58.219 Reinstatement of a disqualified testing facility

The reference standard is the cornerstone that quantitative analytical assays are built on. Proper handling and storage of standards are essential to the integrity of the data generated from the assay. FDA compliance requires that each separate batch of reference standard or control article be appropriately characterized in terms of identity, purity, expiration date, and other significant characteristics such as light or temperature sensitivity. The stability and appropriate storage conditions should be determined by the testing facility or the study sponsor. Quite often, the long-term stability of a control article will not have been established prior to study initiation. Therefore, it is necessary that periodic reanalysis or recertification be performed to document continued batch stability. The reanalysis must be carried out using an analytical method that is "stability indicating." That is, the assay is capable of quantitating the control article and any degradation products of the control article to the extent required by the FDA. Documentation proving characterization and batch recertification must be maintained. GLP regulations require that reference standards kept in the *same* storage container throughout the duration of the study. The container must be labeled by name, batch number, expiration date, if established, and appropriate storage conditions. The FDA requires that the receipt and distribution of each batch of reference standard or control article are documented. Accountability of standards is maintained with detailed records indicating the amount and date initially received as well as a system for documenting the date and quantity removed for each use over the course of the study.

A few other useful definitions include "sponsor" (i.e., the organization that bears ultimate responsibility for the study), "study director" (the individual responsible for the overall scientific conduct of the study and serves as the single point of study control), "study initiation date" (the date the study is signed by the study director), "study completion date" (the date the final report is signed by the study director), "raw data" (any laboratory worksheets, records, notes, or exact copies that are the result of original observations and activities of the nonclinical study and that are necessary for the preparations and evaluation of the final report), and "quality assurance unit" (any person or persons, except the study director, designated by management to perform duties relating to quality assurance of the study).

58.15 Inspection of a Testing Facility

The FDA is allowed to inspect any facility conducting GLP studies during normal business hours and they are *not* required to give prior notice as to when an inspection will take place. Auditing of a facility usually includes inspection of the laboratory and any appropriate instrumentation as well as inspection and collection of any specimens required to be maintained during or after the course of the study. The photocopying of any records pertinent to the study is also allowed. One important exception to the inspection of study records are quality assurance inspection and audit findings as well as any corrective actions recommended and subsequently carried out. If a facility refuses to allow an FDA inspector to audit a study, the data generated from the facility will *not* be considered in support of an NDA application.

Subpart B: Organization and Personnel

58.29 Personnel

Fully trained personnel are essential for proper study conduct and the production of a final report appropriate for regulatory decision making. Almost one third of GLP regulations are directed at describing relevant personnel behavior. The FDA requires that each individual involved in any aspect of study conduct must have the appropriate level of education, training, and experience to perform his or her assigned functions. It is the responsibility of laboratory management to assure employees are qualified and to maintain detailed documentation that supports their qualifications. This documentation should include an education history, an employment history relevant to the current job position, and a description of any on-the-job training, such as workshops or seminars provided to the employee. Part 58.29 also states that there should be a sufficient number of personnel for timely and proper study conduct. If a laboratory takes on more work than it can handle, the quality of the data will be compromised and there may be a temptation to create fraudulent data. QAU and personnel involved in GLP studies include primarily the study director, the study analyst(s), the quality assurance unit, and management. The GLPs designate responsibilities for each position.

58.31 Testing Facility Management

Responsibilities of management are more administrative than scientific. One of the primary responsibilities of management is to designate the study director prior to study initiation.

58.33 Study Director

The study director has overall responsibility for the scientific conduct of the study. She/he is responsible for ascertaining the protocol has been approved by study sponsor management and that all GLP regulations are followed. Interpretation, analysis, documentation, and reporting of results are also the responsibility of the study director.

58.35 Quality Assurance Unit

The QAU has many responsibilities throughout the conduct of a GLP study. The QAU interfaces with sponsor management to affirm the study is conducted with the proper equipment, personnel, methods, documentation, and controls. At least once while a study is in progress, the QAU must observe and report to the study director and management on compliance with study protocol, laboratory SOPs, and GLP regulations. Data generated during the study as well as any final written reports are audited by the QAU for accuracy and completeness before being signed by the study director. A statement is prepared by the QAU and included in the final study report specifying the dates inspections and/or audits were performed and any findings reported to the appropriate personnel. Finally, the QAU must keep a copy of all protocols, and a copy of the detailed master schedule describing all laboratory studies including study initiation date (date protocol is signed by study director), current status, study director, test article, and study sponsor. QA usually oversees the long-term data storage archives and determines when and who will be allowed to remove study records. A laboratory should take the necessary precautions to protect both the health and safety of employees by requiring them to wear lab coats and change them frequently. Likewise, the test and control articles should be protected from contamination. The FDA requires that a laboratory have a generic policy for the safe handling of chemicals and special policies for the handling of hazardous materials.

Subpart C: Facilities

58.41 General

This section of the GLPs are primarily concerned with assuring the FDA that a facility has the required space and is constructed in a manner appropriate to performing nonclinical studies.

Animal Care Facilities

Animal care facilities must be adequate for the housing, treatment, and isolation of animals as needed.

Animal Supply Facilities

Animal supply facilities must include storage areas for feed, bedding, supplies, and equipment. Feed and bedding must not be stored where animals are housed and must be protected against infestation and vermin.

Facilities for Handling Test and Control Articles

Separate areas are necessary to prevent contamination or mix-ups between the test and control articles as well as between the test and/or control article and the test systems. One of the primary goals of 58.47 is to ensure the test and control article are not mixed-up or cross-contaminated. In a bioanalytical laboratory only a control article is used to prepare stock solutions, so a mix-up is not usually possible.

Test and control articles are stored under lock and key with the laboratory director maintaining records as to who has been issued keys to the storage areas or containers. In addition, the test/control article must be stored under proper conditions to maintain its chemical stability throughout the term of the study. If the article is stored in a refrigerator or freezer, the entire unit must be locked or the articles stored within a lock box within the unit.

58.49 Laboratory Operation Areas

This regulation states that a laboratory must provide adequate separate space for the performance of routine procedures such as surgery, cleaning of equipment, preparation of reagents, and handling of biohazardous materials.

58.51 Specimen and Data Storage Facilities

If a laboratory conducts GLP studies, a separate area (i.e., archive) must be provided for safe, lockable storage and retrieval of raw data as well as all specimens generated during the study. Access to the archive is defined in an SOP and is usually controlled by the QA unit. Material transfer to archive is expected within a "reasonable" period of time after the study director has signed the final report.

Subpart D: Equipment

Equipment Design

Equipment used to generate or assess study data or to monitor facility environmental control must be of appropriate design to function adequately according to the protocol. This equipment, be it for freezer monitoring, chromatography (high-pressure liquid chromatography, liquid chromatography/mass spectrometry, gas chromatography), blood analysis, analytical balances or computers, should undergo a validation procedure to ensure it can consistently function as intended. For analytical equipment, this process is usually broken down into three areas: installation qualification, performance qualification, and operational qualification. Installation qualification is performed by the instrument manufacturer to ensure the equipment is set up correctly after purchase. Performance qualification is designed to ensure the equipment performs within the design specifications (e.g., injection precision of an autosampler), whereas operational qualification ensures the equipment operates correctly with a specific method used within the laboratory. System suitability samples are often used to validate operational qualification prior to each analytical run.

Maintenance and Calibration of Equipment

In addition to validation, equipment used to generate or assess data must also be calibrated and maintained on a consistent basis. The specialized analytical instrumentation mentioned previously, such as chromatographs and balances, are usually calibrated annually by the manufacturer. Other instruments or laboratory equipment, such as pH meters, precision pipettes, and centrifuges, can be calibrated by a qualified laboratory individual. All calibration and maintenance procedures must be meticulously recorded in instrument diaries or notebooks. All laboratory procedures for calibration, maintenance, cleaning, and testing of equipment must be clearly outlined by the laboratory SOPs.

Subpart E: Testing Facilities Operation

58.81 Standard Operating Procedures

All laboratories must have standard operating procedures that outline study methods and ensure the laboratory adheres to GLP regulations. The SOPs provide guidance to study personnel on the accepted conduct for routine study procedures. Any deviation from SOPs must be approved by the study director. A historical file of SOPs must be retained so that it is possible to see which SOPs were in effect at any time during a laboratory's history.

58.83 Reagents and Solutions

All reagents and solutions must be labeled to provide identity, concentration, storage condition, and expiration date. Outdated reagents must not be used.

58.90 Animal Care

Prior to use in a laboratory study, animals must be quarantined until their health status can be evaluated. More in-depth information about animal care and supply facilities may be found in the regulations posted on the FDA Web site (1).

Subpart F: Test and Control Article

58.105 Test and Control Article Characterization

The GLP regulations specify that the identity, strength, purity, and composition of the test and control (reference standard) article must be defined and documented for each batch. A storage container is assigned to the test or control article batch for the duration of a study. However, aliquots of test or control article may be placed in "working" containers that are properly labeled. The label must include the name, chemical abstract number or code number, batch number, expiration date, and storage conditions

required to maintain stability. Standard solutions are prepared from weighings removed from the "working" container.

58.107 Test and Control Article Handling

The accountability of the test or control must be maintained throughout its period of use. Laboratory records must be kept indicating the receipt date, amount received, who received it, and whom it was received from. A method for documenting the date, amount used and by whom for each use of test or control article should also be developed.

58.113 Mixtures of Articles and Carriers

For more detailed information on the regulations involving of subpart F, 58.113, please visit the FDA Web site (1) or refer to the work of Weinberg (3).

Subpart G: Protocol For and Conduct of a Nonclinical Laboratory Study

58.120 Protocol

Every GLP study must have a written protocol approved by the study director that outlines the objectives and general methods of the study. The purpose of this requirement is to be certain that all study personnel have a clear understanding of the purpose of the study and what needs to be done to carry out the goal(s) intended. Any changes to the protocol must be documented, dated, and signed by the study director. Changes are usually issued as "protocol amendments."

58.130 Conduct of a Nonclinical Laboratory Study

Simply stated, the study shall be performed in accordance with the protocol and the test system(s) or methodology used to carry out the study will be monitored as required to assure conformity to the protocol.

A very important aspect of study performance, particularly bioanalytical work, involves the handling of biological specimens. The proper handling of plasma and/or urine samples is critical to the integrity of the data generated from them. Section 58.130 addresses this issue and states that specimens should be identified minimally with study name, nature, and date/time of collection. This information must be on the sample or accompany it in such a way as to prevent any errors in recording or storage of data. In addition, "chain of custody" documentation is important to ensure the sample was not mishandled. Sample log-in sheets are often used to confirm which samples were received, by whom, the condition of the sample on arrival in the laboratory (frozen/thawed), and storage site for the similar samples. Data must be recorded in ink throughout all aspects of a GLP study. Errors are corrected by drawing a *single* line through the mistake. The person correcting the error must sign, date, and provide a reason for the change. Study samples must be stored in refrigerators or freezers that are monitored on a daily basis for temperature control either by laboratory personnel or by electronic monitoring systems. A log of temperatures must be maintained throughout any study and eventually archived with study data.

Subparts H through I (Reserved)

No GLP regulations are outlined in these sections.

Subpart J: Records and Reports

58.185 Reporting of Nonclinical Laboratory Study Results

A final report is required for each nonclinical study, and the FDA is specific as to the minimum of what should be included. The requirements are numerous and can be reviewed on the FDA Web site (1). One of the most important requirements, however, is a statement prepared by the QAU designating dates the study was audited as well as the date of review of final report. A report is "final" once signed by the study director. Any subsequent changes must be in the form of an amendment.

58.190 Storage and Retrieval of Records and Data

Archives must be created to retain study data, protocols, specimens, and final reports in an environment that will minimize deterioration of records. A single person, usually quality assurance personnel, is responsible for the archive. Material removed from the archive can be signed out for a limited period of time and must be returned in a timely manner. A record is maintained as to who removed and returned materials to the archive and when.

58.195 Retention of Records

Specific time periods that original or photocopies of original records must be retained are outlined in this section of the GLPs. The length of time records must be kept usually depends on the original purpose of the study (1).

Subpart K: Disqualification of Testing Facilities

58.200 Purpose

The obvious purpose of this subpart of the GLPS is to outline the consequences once the FDA has determined that during the conduct of a study, a laboratory has failed to comply with the GLP guidelines. Subsequently, the study submitted for review may not be scientifically sound or may consist of primarily poor documentation and quality assurance. Subpart K further describes the legal and administrative procedures that control aspects of the disqualification process.

58.202 Grounds for Disqualification

The FDA must find *all three* of the following conditions before it can disqualify a laboratory: (a) the testing facility failed to comply with one or more of the regulations outlined in the GLPs; (b) the noncompliance adversely affected the validity of the laboratory studies; and (c) other less stringent regulatory actions (e.g., warnings) have not been, nor will most likely be, adequate to achieve compliance with the GLPs. See Table 14.1 for additional section headings of Subpart K. A further discussion of this subpart can also be found on the FDA Web site (1).

21 CFR PART 11

The latest section of the guidelines under CFR 21 was developed to deal with the ubiquitous involvement of computers in the today's scientific laboratory. This section is referred to as Part 11 and is divided into three subparts: general provisions, electronic records, and electronic signatures. These regulations outline the criteria under which the FDA considers electronic records, electronic signatures, and handwritten signatures executed to electronic records to be trustworthy, reliable, and generally equivalent to paper records and handwritten signatures executed on paper. Validation of computer hardware and software must be performed to demonstrate the hardware and software of a computer are consistently doing what they are designed to do and that any invalid or altered data can be recognized. The use of time-stamped audit trails is important for maintaining the integrity and security of data generated and stored on computers. The proper level of security and authority checks should be in place to determine that only authorized personnel can use a system to alter data or electronically sign a record. It is certain that as technology changes, Part 11 will also continue to evolve.

SUMMARY

This chapter is intended to provide a general overview of the subparts and sections of the Code of Federal Registry that comprise the Good Laboratory Practice guidelines. A brief discussion on regulations and guidelines particularly pertinent to the analysis of drugs and their metabolites, pharmacodynamic markers (e.g., vascular endothelial growth factor), and other analytes quantitated from plasma or urine recovered during oncology phase 1, 2, or 3 trials is presented. Although strict adherence to the GLP guidelines does not guarantee a scientifically sound study design or methodology, it does ensure that there will exist a trail of documentation that, if sufficiently created, should provide clues to confirm or deny the validity of the study. In the increasingly complex and global world of drug development, the GLPs, similar to the Good Manufacturing Practices, bring a commonality of design to nonclinical studies such as toxicological and/or efficacy studies performed in various laboratories around the world. Although GLP guidelines have been adhered to for quite some time in other types of pharmaceutical studies, such as bioequivalence and/or bioavailability studies, only recently have they become standard practice in bioanalytical/pharmacokinetic studies designed to support phase 1 oncology clinical trials. It is relatively safe to say that if an analytical laboratory is not GLP compliant, they will not be participating in many industry-sponsored studies for investigational new drugs or NDA-oriented studies. Becoming GLP compliant is a long, expensive, arduous process, but as yet another ancient Japanese proverb tells us, "As water carves through stone, those that persevere will win."

REFERENCES

1. Available at: www.accessdata.fda.gov/scripts/cdrh/cfdocs/cfcfr/CFRSearch.cfm.
2. Available at: www.fda.gov/ora/compliance_ref/bimo/GLP/qna.htm.
3. Weinberg S, ed. *Good laboratory practice regulations,* 2nd ed. New York: Marcel Dekker Inc, 1995.

PART 5

Delivery Systems

15

Pharmaceutical Formulation of Novel Anticancer Agents

Bastiaan Nuijen

Department of Pharmacy and Pharmacology, Slotervaart Hospital/The Netherlands Cancer Institute, Louwesweg 16 1066 EC, Amsterdam, The Netherlands

After its identification as a potential anticancer agent, several hurdles have to be overcome before a drug candidate can enter the clinic. Among these is the development of a clinical feasible pharmaceutical formulation, which is a prerequisite for the assessment of toxicity, kinetics, and efficacy in humans. Only in rare instances is an active pharmaceutical ingredient (API) administered to the patient as a pure compound. Instead, the API is almost always transformed or formulated into a well-defined pharmaceutical product containing a specified quantity of the drug suitable for its intended use (1). Pharmaceutical formulations are often mixtures containing the API together with excipients like bulking agents, stabilizers, buffering agents, and solubilizers.

Anticancer drugs at the early stage of development are generally administered as an intravenous bolus injection or infusion in order to obtain absolute bioavailibility, circumvent possible disturbance of or degradation in the gastrointestinal tract, and to be able to adjust or stop administration of the drug in case of acute toxicity. Consequently, the development of a pharmaceutical formulation of a novel anticancer agent is generally focused on issues associated with the design of sterile and stable injectable products.

The successful development of a pharmaceutical formulation requires a broad knowledge of analytical techniques, pharmaceutical sciences, regulatory guidelines (e.g., Good Manufacturing Practices), and clinical practice. Table 15.1 summarizes the pharmaceutical formulation development route of an investigational anticancer agent. In this chapter, this route will be discussed and illustrated by highlighting aspects of the pharmaceutical development of representative compounds. Although biotechnology products will become increasingly important in anticancer therapy and many of the issues discussed here are also

applicable to these products, this chapter will focus on the pharmaceutical development of small molecules. For more information on the pharmaceutical formulation of biotechnology compounds, the reader is referred to some excellent reviews (2,3). Guidelines for the formulation of investigational cytotoxic agents have been established by the Joint Formulation Working Party of the Cancer Research Campaign, European Organization for Research and Treatment of Cancer, and National Cancer Institute (4). Furthermore, guidelines for development pharmaceutics have been issued by the regulatory authorities (18,19).

ANALYTICAL CHARACTERIZATION AND METHOD DEVELOPMENT

Before the initiation of the pharmaceutical formulation development of an investigational anticancer agent, it is pivotal to confirm its molecular structure and to analytically characterize the compound in order to define a reference standard for each batch submitted for further research. Structural characterization is carried out by using techniques like nuclear magnetic resonance (NMR) spectroscopy, mass spectroscopy, and infrared spectroscopy.

Analytical characterization is performed using methods such as ultraviolet/visible spectrophotometry, liquid, gas, or size-exclusion chromatographic methods coupled to various detection techniques (e.g., ultraviolet light, fluorescence, mass spectroscopy, refractive index). These methods are used as well for purity determinations to determine the levels of related substances, degradation products, and intermediates or impurities from synthesis or purification pathways. Additionally, methods for quantification of residual water (e.g., thermogravimetric analysis, Karl-Fischer titration) and residual solvents (gas

TABLE 15.1. *The pharmaceutical formulation development route*

Analytical characterization and method development
Pharmaceutical formulation
  Preformulation studies (solubility, stability)
  Lyophilization
  Solubilization approaches
Manufacture
Stability studies
  Stability testing of pharmaceutical product
  Stability in and compatibility with administration sets
Biocompatibility studies

chromatography) are used. In order to establish the physical state of the investigational drug substance, which is of importance with respect to its solubility, hygroscopicity, and stability properties, techniques like differential scanning calorimetry (DSC), x-ray diffraction analysis, NMR, and infrared spectroscopy are applied. Table 15.2 gives the tests and specifications for AP5280 drug substance, a novel N-(2-hydroxypropyl)methacrylamide (HPMA) polymer-conjugated platinum compound designed for tumor targeting. As can be seen, a broad spectrum of analyt-

ical techniques is used to characterize AP5280, which combination provides a meaningful picture of structure, size, and integrity of this complex molecule (7).

During formulation development of an investigational anticancer drug, at least some methods have to be in place in order to be able to evaluate solubility and stability of the compound. Crucial in this respect is the development of a stability-indicating assay that can discriminate between the parent compound and degradation products. The method should also be capable of separating the parent compound from impurities and excipients used in the pharmaceutical product. The most commonly applied method in the case of investigational substances is high-performance liquid chromatography (HPLC) coupled to ultraviolet detection, a highly specific and sensitive method if the drug of interest contains an exploitable chromophore. The development of a stability-indicating assay can result in serious challenges. This is illustrated by the development of a stability-indicating ultraviolet HPLC assay of aplidine, a marine-derived anticancer agent belonging to the didemnin-family (8). The development of this method was complicated by the existence of multiple conformations of aplidine, which was confirmed by NMR analysis. The initial assays, both normal-

TABLE 15.2. *Overview of the tests and specifications of AP5280 drug substance*

Test method/item	Specification
Appearance	Light brown, flaky substance, with no visible signs of contamination
^{195}Pt NMR spectroscopy	
Identity	A single peak at $\delta = -2,048 \pm 10$ ppm
Purity	Absence of other signals than at $\delta = -2048 \pm 10$ ppm
^{1}H NMR spectroscopy	
Identity	Peaks are present at 0.8–1.0, 1.1, 1.6, 1.7–2.0, 3.0–3.3, 3.9, 4.4, 7.3, 7.4, 7.5, and 7.7 ppm
Purity	No other accompanying signals are present
F-AAS	
Free platinum	2.0 ± 0.1 mg/mL AP5280 in WfI contains ≤ 1.0% free Pt (with respect to the total Pt content) at room temperature (20°–25°C).
Release of small platinum species	2.0 ± 0.1 mg/mL AP5280 in PBS at 37°C releases ≤1.5% small Pt species after 3 h and ≤3.5% free Pt after 24 h (with respect to the total Pt content)
GF-AAS	8.0 ± 0.5% (w/w)
Total platinum content	
Size-exclusion chromatography	
M_w	A. $M_w = 24 \pm 3$ kd
M_n	B. $M_n = 14.5 \pm 3$ kd
Polydispersity index	C. PI = 1.2–2.3
Shape of the peak	D. Monomodal
IR spectroscopy	AP5280 exhibits major absorption bands at approximately 3,700–3,100, 2,970, 2,920, 1,630, 1,520, 1,380, 1,290–1,230, 1,190, 1,140–1,050, and 960–900 cm^{-1}

Pt, platinum; NMR, nuclear magnetic resonance; F-AAS, flame atomic absorption spectrometry; PBS, phosphate-buffered saline; GF-AAS, graphite-furnace atomic absorption spectrometry; w/w, weight-to-weight ratio; IR, infrared; WfI, water for injection; Mw, weight-average molecular weight; Mn, number-average molecular weight.

phase, isocratic, and gradient HPLC methods, showed two peaks in the chromatograms referring to the equilibrium between *cis* and *trans* isomers of the pyruvoyl–proline amide bond present in the molecule. Although quantification of aplidine concentrations on the total area of both isomer peaks was satisfactory in terms of linearity, accuracy, and reproducibility, the stability-indicating capacity of the assay was not. It was shown that during stress testing, degradation peaks coeluted with the aplidine-isomer complex. Finally, by adjusting the analytical column temperature, a stability-indicating assay for aplidine was obtained, with a good selectivity for impurities and degradation products (Fig. 15.1).

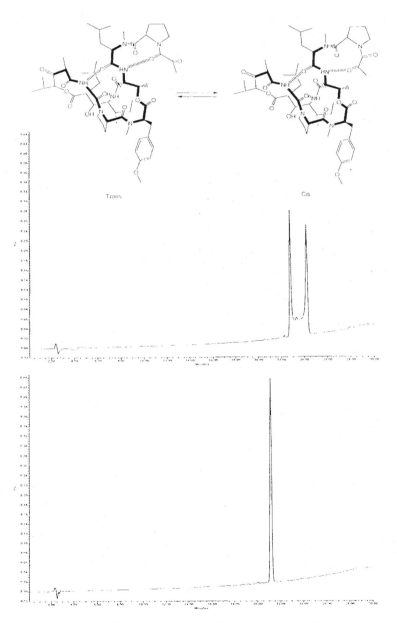

FIG. 15.1. *Cis-trans* isomerism of aplidine at the peptide binding between the proline and pyruvoyl moieties. This results in two peaks in the chromatogram at a column temperature of 25°C. For analysis, a column temperature of 80°C was selected, resulting in one aplidine peak with good selectivity for impurities and degradation products.

TABLE 15.3. *General quality control test items for active pharmaceutical ingredient (API) and final intravenous products*

Test Items	
API	Final pharmaceutical product
Appearance	Appearance
Identity	Identity
Potency	Reconstitution time*
Purity	Content
Residual solvents	Content uniformity
Water content	Purity
Bacterial endotoxins	pH (after reconstitution*)
Bioburden	Particulates
	Sterility
	Bacterial endotoxins
	Residual solvents*
	Water content*

*In case of a lyophilized product.

In parallel with the pharmaceutical formulation study, a full set of validated analytical techniques has to evolve to enable quality control of the API and the final product (9–13). Table 15.3 summarizes the general test items for the active drug substance and the final pharmaceutical product for intravenous use. Preliminary specifications are generally accepted by the regulatory authorities at the time of the investigational new drug (IND) application, with the exception of critical items like sterility and bacterial endotoxin testing (14,15). The robustness of a product in terms of formulation, manufacture, and analytical methodology will grow in the course of the development program, allowing the setting of final, often tighter specifications at the time of filing of the New Drug Application (NDA) (16).

Excipients used in the pharmaceutical development and final product need to comply and to be tested according to pharmacopeial standards (e.g., European Pharmacopeia, United States Pharmacopeia/National Formulary).

PHARMACEUTICAL FORMULATION

Basically, two types of pharmaceutical formulations can be discerned. The first type offers the API a pharmaceutically optimal vehicle in terms of solubility and stability, but is not intended to interfere with its mode of action after administration. The second type of pharmaceutical formulation is specifically designed to optimize the activity or reduce toxicity of the API by altering its pharmacokinetic or pharmacologic characteristics (e.g., prolongation of residence time, targeting to the tumor site).

To reduce the lag time between discovery and clinical evaluation, novel promising anticancer agents are pharmaceutically formulated using the most straightforward methods available. Experience with currently marketed formulations is often used, thereby minimizing concerns on part of the regulatory authorities (17–19). Only after well-proven activity in clinical practice and additional pharmacokinetic and pharmacological data, second-generation formulations, such as long-circulating PEGylated liposomes are developed (e.g., doxorubicin, Doxil).

From a pharmaceutical point of view, the most straightforward formulation is a stable, sterile, low-in-endotoxin, isotonic, and isohydric aqueous solution of the compound of interest. An example of such a formulation is the antimetabolite cladribine (Leustatin), which is formulated as a solution for intravenous infusion in normal saline at pH 5.5 to 8. However, due to the low aqueous solubility and stability displayed by many investigational anticancer agents, this often cannot be realized. Usually, various solubilization and stabilization techniques have to be applied to succesfully formulate a compound. In this respect, the parenteral drug development of an anticancer agent does not differ from other therapeutic agents, although more "heroic" formulation approaches are allowed considering the life-threatening nature of the disease. For example, the taxane paclitaxel (Taxol) is formulated using the nonionic surfactant Cremophor EL, which is dosed up to 40 mL and administered intravenously per course of treatment. In order to prevent anaphylactic reactions due to this excipient, antihistaminic premedication is required (20).

PREFORMULATION STUDIES

Solubility

The intravenous administration route requires solubilization of the investigational anticancer agent in a pharmaceutically acceptable administration vehicle (1,17,18). The necessary solubility for the investigational drug formulation depends on the starting dose in the clinical phase 1 dose-finding study and the estimated human maximal tolerated dose (MTD_{human}). The human starting dose is calculated from the dose lethal for 10% of the test animal population (LD10, mice or rats) found in preclinical studies using a surface area conversion formula (21):

Human dose$_{start}$ (mg/m^2)

$$= 1/10 \times [3 \times LD10_{mouse} \text{ (mg/kg)], or}$$

Human dose$_{start}$ (mg/m^2)

$$= 1/10 \times [6 \times LD10_{rat} \text{ (mg/kg)]}$$

TABLE 15.4. *Solubilization approaches*

pH adjustment
Cosolvent and surfactant systems
Emulsions
Colloidal systems
Complexation

Taking the MTD_{human} at 10 times the starting dose, this calculation provides a rough estimate of the human dosing range during early clinical studies.

A number of solubilization approaches, which will be discussed in more detail later in this section, is available for parenteral dosage form development (Table 15.4). The feasibility of an approach is, besides the stability of the drug in the pharmaceutical vehicle, dependent on the amount of the investigational drug to be administered, the solubility of the drug in the vehicle, and the intrinsic toxicity of the vehicle on intravenous administration. This accounts in particular for cosolvent and surfactant systems, which are often applied in the formulation of investigational anticancer drugs and which all display vehicle-related side effects to a higher or lesser degree. From the maximal amount of the potential pharmaceutical vehicle or excipient and available literature (19,22–25), it can be determined if its application would be in correspondence with current clinical practice and if formulation-related toxicity can be expected.

During preformulation studies, the solubility of an investigational anticancer agent is screened in vehicles representing various formulation approaches (e.g., water, buffer solutions, cosolvents, surfactant-solutions, cyclodextrin-solutions, oils) both qualitatively as well as quantitatively. The standard method used to determine solubility is the shake-flask or equilibrium method. The concentration at saturation is determined after adding an excess of drug to a medium, stirring the suspension during a defined period of time, filtering or centrifuging the suspension, and measuring the amount dissolved.

Before applying various solubilization techniques, it is usefull to consider the possibility of water-soluble salt formation of the investigational substance (18). Counter ions applied in salt formation include sodium, meglumine, potassium, tromethamine (cations) and hydrochloride, sulfate, mesylate, and acetate (anions) (22).

Also, the formation of water-soluble prodrugs may be a valuable approach. Prodrugs are therapeutically inactive derivatives of the therapeutically active parent compound. Within the body, the prodrug is trans-formed by spontaneous hydrolysis or enzymatic degradation to its active form. For successful derivatization, the presence of a functional group that offers a handle for prodrug synthesis is a prerequisite. Disadvantages of the use of prodrugs are that derivatization is, in general, a costly and difficult process, and the pharmacokinetic and pharmacodynamic properties may be altered undesirably (1). However, drug carriers may offer the possibility of targeted drug delivery. Examples are prodrugs in which the active compound is conjugated to polyethylene glycols (PEG), albumin, or hydroxypropylmethacrylamide (HPMA) (26–28). All are highly water-soluble macromolecules that are well distributed in the organism and expected to be concentrated in tumor tissues because of enhanced vascular permeability and lack of lymphatic drainage (enhanced permeation and retention [EPR] effect). Marketed antineoplastic prodrugs are the phosphate esters etoposide phosphate (Etopophos) and fludarabine phosphate. Another example is irinotecan hydrochloride (Camptosar), which is converted to the active SN-38 by carboxylesterase-mediated carbamate hydrolysis (29).

Furthermore, as mentioned previously, the physical state (amorphous, crystalline, polymorph) of the raw drug substance is of importance with respect to its solubility. The amorphous form of a drug provides the highest solubility because it represents, in theory, the most energetic state of a material. If multiple crystalline forms of a drug exist (polymorphism), these can display different solubilities due to their different thermodynamic properties (30). A notorious example of this phenomenon is ritonavir, an antiviral agent used in the treatment of AIDS, and formulated as a semisolid capsule for oral use (Norvir, Abbott Laboratories). In 1998, several lots of the ethanol/water filled capsules failed the dissolution requirement because of the appearance of a polymorph with a significant lower solubility. It became clear that the hydroalcoholic solution of ritonavir was 400% supersaturated with respect to this polymorph, making this formulation unmanufacturable. At the time, this event seriously threatened the supply of Norvir and necessitated immediate reformulation (31). This example stresses the importance of physical characterization studies of an investigational anticancer agent as a part of the pharmaceutical formulation process. Moreover, changes in the production method of a raw drug substance, not uncommon during the development phase, can alter the physical properties of the compound. On the other hand, solid-state manipulation can be used to obtain the most favorable physical form of a drug in terms of solubility.

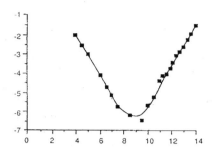

FIG. 15.2. The pH-rate profile of EO9 at 25°C. x-axis, pH; y-axis, log k_{obs} (sec^{-1}).

Stability

Systematic chemical stability studies are performed during preformulation studies to provide information on the degradation kinetics of the investigational substance as a function of pH, buffer composition, ionic strength, temperature, and additives. Together with solubility data, these stability data are used for selection of the most optimal pharmaceutical formulation. Besides low aqueous solubility, a common characteristic of many anticancer agents is the limited chemical stability in solution. Figure 15.2 shows the pH-rate profile of the investigational aziridinylquinone EO9 (32). Although most stable at pH 8 to 9, an aqueous solution does not offer sufficient shelf life as pharmaceutical formulation. In this case, lyophilization of the EO9 solution at pH 9 was applied as stabilizing technique (33).

Design of Experiments

A helpful tool in formulation studies is the application of Design of Experiments (DoE). DoE allows to study the effect of multiple parameters on a selected determinant. Influence of independent variables as well as interactions are evaluated by multivariate analysis. By setting up an experiment, parameters, ranges, outcomes, and type of design must be selected with care. Advantage of DoE is that the number of experiments to be conducted in order to optimize a system are minimized, thereby reducing time and the amount of test material required. DoE may not only be applied in formulation studies assessing the effect of various parameters on, for example, solubility or stability, but also in validation (e.g., analytical method robustness studies) or production process optimization (34–36).

Lyophilization

Currently, 45% of the cytotoxic agents marketed in the United States are formulated as lyophilized prod-

ucts (22). Lyophilization or freeze-drying is a stabilizing technique that is widely used to increase the shelf life of chemically unstable compounds. In this processing method, water or solvent is extracted from a frozen formulation solution containing the unstable compound by sublimation, resulting in a dry powder or cake. The final composition of the freeze-dried product, its appearance, stability, and lyophilization cycle parameters are defined by the constituents of the formulation solution. Inherent to the instability of the formulation, lyophilization is generally part of an aseptic manufacturing procedure (4).

A freeze-dryer consists of three major parts (Fig. 15.3). The freeze-drying chamber contains shelves on which the solution to be lyophilized is placed. The shelves can be cooled and heated while the drying chamber can be evacuated to a desired vacuum. The condensor is connected to the drying chamber and held at a low temperature (approximately −65°C). Its purpose is to remove the condensable solvent vapor from the gases that pass from the drying chamber. Together with the condensor, the vacuum pumping system provides the necessary low pressures for conducting the lyophilization process.

The freeze-drying process can be subdivided into three subsequent steps: freezing, primary drying, and secondary drying (Fig. 15.4). In order to rationally de-

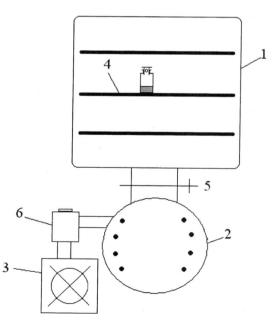

FIG. 15.3. Schematic depiction of a freeze-dryer drying chamber (1), condensor (2), vacuum pump (3), shelf with product vial (4), valve (5), and cold trap (6, optional).

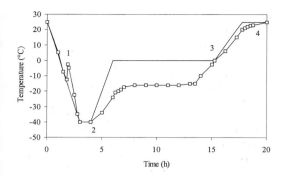

FIG. 15.4. Example of a lyophilization cycle. Solid line indicates T_{shelf}; □, $T_{product}$; 1, freezing stage with supercooling event of formulation solution; 2, initiation of primary drying (T_{shelf} to 0°C, P_c to 0.2 mbar); 3, initiation of secondary drying phase (T_{shelf} to +25°C, P_c to 0.02 mbar); 4, end of cycle.

velop an optimal lyophilization cycle, thermal properties of the formulation solution like the eutectic temperature (T_e), glass transition temperature (T_g'), metastable states, degree of crystallization, and the ice melting temperature must be established beforehand. These data can be obtained by thermal analysis methods like differential thermal analysis (DTA) and DSC (37).

After dispensing into the primary containers and semistoppering, freezing of the formulation solution is performed on the shelves of the freeze-dryer. Other freezing techniques are snap freezing (induced in an evacuation chamber) or immersion freezing (e.g., using liquid nitrogen), but these are not widely applied. The principal function of the freezing process is to separate the solvent(s) and solutes, and provide a matrix structure with minimal impedence to the vapor flow during drying. The temperature of the formulation solution is reduced from ambient to a temperature below the T_e or below the T_g' if an amorphous phase is present. Upon freezing, water will separate as ice crystals, ideally forming channels throughout the matrix allowing vapor flow from the matrix during drying. Noncrystalline, unfreezable water together with excipients form interstitial, glassy regions in the matrix. The degree of crystallization is defined as the ratio of ice formed during the freezing process to the total amount of freezable water in the formulation. Optimal drying rates are obtained with degrees of crystallization approaching 1. Below 0.5, most of the water is present in the interstitial, amorphous phase, which will greatly reduce the sublimation rate. The size of the ice crystals formed is determined by the freezing rate. Rapid cooling, resulting in small ice crystals, is associated with fast sublimation rates (38). If a system does not (fully) crystallize but forms

an amorphous mass, the solution should be frozen below its T_g'. Around T_g', the viscosity of the system changes dramatically with a "rubbery," mobile state above and a glassy state with a viscosity near zero below T_g'. The T_g' is dependent on the water content of the system and will increase during the drying process. In order to obtain a completely frozen, immobile system before initiation of the primary drying phase, freezing to −40°C is generally sufficient. In case of the presence of a metastable state within the frozen matrix, thermal treatment (i.e., heating above the metastable onset temperature followed by refreezing) can induce full crystallization of the system. In order to fully freeze the system, the fill height of the formulation solution in the container should be taken into account in the total freezing time.

The second step involves the primary drying process, in which the unbound solvent is sublimed by establishing a vacuum over the frozen product. During the primary drying process, the temperature of the product ($T_{product}$) should be below T_e or T_g' with a safety margin of approximately 5°C in order to prevent collapse. Collapse of the product results in a poor cake formation as well as a strongly reduced drying rate. The $T_{product}$ is governed by the chamber pressure (P_c), which induces the sublimation process, and the shelf temperature (T_{shelf}), which keeps the product at $T_{product}$. Both should be adjusted and controlled in such a way that an optimal drying rate is obtained at a $T_{product}$ without jeopardizing the quality of the final product throughout the cycle. Several models have been developed to describe the sublimation process and take into consideration the various factors influencing this complex process (e.g., vial shape, stopper resistence, heat transfer routes, P_c, resistence of cake) (37). Finalization of the primary drying phase can be taken as the time $T_{product} = T_{shelf}$ and when P_c no longer rises above a predetermined level when isolating the condensor from the drying chamber (pressure rise test).

Depending on temperature and composition of the product, a 5% to 10% weight-to-weight ratio of water can be absorbed onto the surface of the cake after the primary drying stage. During the final step of the freeze-drying process, the secondary drying phase, this so-called bound water is removed to the level of residual moisture ensuring the desired stability of the final product. This desorption process is usually performed at a higher T_{shelf} compared to that during primary drying and a further reduced P_c. Again, $T_{product}$ is kept below T_g. As for the primary drying phase, a pressure rise test can be used to determine completion of the secondary drying phase. Alternatively, the successful use of a one-step lyophilization cycle combining the primary and secondary drying steps has been reported (39).

Excipients used in freeze-drying are solvents, bulking agents, buffering agents, lyoprotectants, and cryoprotectants. Preferably, the drug of interest is lyophilized from water as solvent. However, in case of insufficient aqueous solubility, organic solvents or mixtures of water and organic solvents may be applied. Examples of suitable organic solvents are tertiary butanol and dimethyl sulfoxide (40). In particular, tertiary butanol has favorable freeze-drying characteristics. It is completely miscible with water, has a high melting point (25.3°C), and has a vapor pressure higher than water even at low temperatures (36). Furthermore, tertiary butanol has been reported to enhance freeze-drying efficiency by modifying the crystal habit of ice, forming large needle-shaped ice crystals resulting in a more porous and thus less resistent cake (41,42). With respect to stability, the addition of an organic solvent may reduce the chemical degradation rate of a drug. Various agents, among which the investigational anticancer agents bryostatin 1, rhizoxin, and aplidine have been successfully lyophilized from tertiary butanol/water mixtures (43–46). In case of a low drug concentration, a bulking agent is required to prevent product blowout during sublimation and to provide a visually attractive solid cake. Probably the most commonly applied is polyol mannitol. When frozen slowly or after thermal treatment, mannitol is completely crystallized and provides an excellent supporting matrix. Disadvantage of mannitol is the extensive vial breakage that can occur as a result of large fill heights and volumes, high concentrations of solute, and rapid freezing rates (47–49). Examples of amorphous bulking agents are polyvinyl pyrrolidone or disaccharides like sucrose and trehalose. The bulking agent should be selected carefully in order to obtain a stable product. For instance, the polypeptide anticancer agent kahalalide F appeared more stable in an amorphous sucrose matrix compared to a crystalline mannitol matrix (35). Other bulking agents used are glycine, lactose, dextran, sodium chloride, sodium bicarbonate, PEG3400, and sorbitol (2,3,37,50,51). Buffering agents have to be selected with care because they can induce drastic pH changes during freezing. For example, with sodium phosphate the dibasic form will readily crystallize, resulting in a frozen sample in which the pH in the remaining amorphous phase can be reduced to 4 or lower. Similarly, crystallization of the dihydrogen salt of potassium phosphate results in a pH near 9. It is clear that these pH shifts can be detrimental to the stability of the active component. The best approach is to avoid sodium or potassium phosphate buffers and to use buffers with minimal pH change upon freezing like citric acid, histidine, and Tris (3). Cryoprotectants

and lyoprotectants are mainly used in protein formulations to prevent protection of the active component during freezing and drying. However, cryoprotectants are also applied in the freeze-drying of liposomes to stabilize the phospholipid bilayer (52). Disaccharides have been shown effective in this respect. The final composition of the lyophilized product (active substance, excipients and their weight ratios, residual moisture or solvent content) determines its chemical and physical stability. In case of an amorphous phase, product should be stored below its T_g.

Dissolution or reconstitution of the lyophilized product is necessary before administration to the patient. Lyophilization may increase the aqueous solubility of an active substance because of the fine dispersion in the product, a changed physical state (e.g., from crystalline to amorphous), or the hygroscopicity of the freeze-dried cake. However, when the product cannot be dissolved in an aqueous solution, a suitable reconstitution vehicle must be developed. For example, freeze-dried melphalan (Alkeran) is reconstituted with a diluent composed of propylene glycol and ethanol before further dilution in infusion fluid. Similarly, the experimental agents kahalalide F, aplidine, and rhizoxin have to be reconstituted with vehicles composed of Cremophor EL/ethanol/water or propylene glycol/ethanol/water, respectively (35,43,44).

Formulation Approaches

pH Adjustment

Adjustment of pH is the first approach of choice for improving the aqueous solubility of a novel drug substance. It is intended to bring the drug of interest in its ionized form that has higher aqueous solubility compared to the neutral species. To what extend a compound is ionized is determined by its pKa(s) and the pH of the solution according to the Henderson-Hasselbalch equation. Normally, weak acids are formulated at pH greater than 5 and weak bases at pH less than 7. Zwitterionic molecules are characterized by more than one ionizable group, and the preferred ionic state with respect to solubility has to be determined. The optimal pH can be obtained from a pH-solubility profile, in which the maximum solubility of the drug is assessed as a function of pH using buffering agents. To maintain a constant pH, buffers are generally added to the formulation solution. Examples include citric acid/citrate (pH range application, 2.2–6.2), acetic acid/acetate (4.0–6.5), and trometamol (7.2–9.0). With respect to biocompatibility, however, the buffer capacity should be minimal (see also the Biocompatibility section). Intravenous pharmaceuticals in the pH range of 2 to 12 are applied in clinical practice [e.g., doxycycline hyclate (Vibramycin), pH 1.8–3.3; phenytoin sodium (Dilantin), pH 10–12.3].

Cosolvent and Surfactant Systems

The use of cosolvents and/or surfactants is probably the most widely employed formulation approach to increase drug solubility. Cosolvents are miscible with water, thereby forming homogeneous binary, ternary, or quartenary solvent systems with polarities between that of pure water and the pure cosolvent. The use of appropriate cosolvents can increase the aqueous solubility of a drug by several orders of magnitude and is primarely dependent on the polarity of the drug with respect to the system (53). The major drawback of cosolvent formulations, however, is the possible precipitation of the solubilized drug during cooling or dilution in infusion fluids. Therefore, cosolvents are often used in combination with surface-active agents. Surfactant molecules are composed of polar and nonpolar regions that orient themselves to form micelles when added to an aqueous solution in concentrations above their critical micelle concentration. Because the interior of the micelles is much less polar than water, nonpolar drug molecules can be kept dissolved, thus preventing drug precipitation during dilution. Table 15.5 lists examples of cosolvents and surfactants used in parenteral drug formulation. Besides solubility increase, the use of cosolvents and surfactants allows the exclusion of water for compounds susceptible to hydrolysis, thus increasing drug stability (1). As mentioned previously, another drawback to cosolvents and surfactants is their potential toxicity, which is exemplified by the ongoing search for an alternative formulation of paclitaxel devoid of Cremophor EL (54). Of the antineoplastic agents currently licensed in the United States, approximately 25% is formulated using a cosolvent and/or surfactant system [e.g., docetaxel solubilized in polysorbate 80 (Taxotere), paclitaxel solubilized in Cremophor EL/ethanol (Taxol), busulfan solubilized in dimethylacetamide/PEG 400 (Busulfex), etoposide solubilized in PEG 300/ethanol/Tween 80 (VePesid), teniposide solubilized in Cremophor EL/ethanol/dimethylacetamide (Vumon)] (29). Furthermore, the cosolvency/surfactant solubilization approach is often followed in the pharmaceutical development of investigational anticancer agents (35,43,44,55–59). Although several (predictive) cosolvency models as well as models describing the combined use of cosolvency, surfactant, complexation, and pH-solubilization approaches have been developed, the formulation scientist still has to rely on empirical observations (53,61–64). This can, however, be systemized using experimental design approaches.

Emulsion Systems

Parenteral emulsions consist of an oleaginous (o) phase dispersed in a continuous aqueous phase (w), generally stabilized by an emulsifier as third component resulting in an oil-in-water (o/w) mixture. Typical emulsions contain triglyceridic vegetable oils and lecithin and may contain nonionic surfactants as emulsifying agents (18). Formulation of a drug using emulsion systems can be applied only when the drug of interest has sufficient lipid solubility. Formulation challenges are to obtain an efficient and stable incorporation of the drug into the dispersed phase, and to develop a consistent manufacturing method (1). Emulsions may be prepared *de novo* or by extemporeneous addition to a commercially available fat emulsion (e.g., Intralipid). The latter method, however, often results in insufficient capture of the drug in the lipid droplets causing unstable systems in which phase separation and precipitation readily occurs. Several emulsion compositions have been reported as promising vehicles for investigational anticancer agents (65–70). For example, a lipid emulsion consisting of triolein as oil core, dipalmitoyl phosphatidylcholine (DPPC) as principal emulsifier, and polysorbate 80 and polyethylene glycol-dipalmitoyl phosphatidylethanolamine (PEG-DPPE) as stabilizers was used in the development of an alternative paclitaxel formulation. The obtained submicron emulsion (droplet size of approximately 40 nm) was stable for several months at 4°C. Furthermore, lyophilization from 5% dextrose resulted in a stable product that

---

TABLE 15.5. *Examples of cosolvents and surfactants used in parenteral drug formulations.*

Cosolvents
  Propylene glycol
  Dimethylacetamide
  Dimethyl sulfoxide
  Ethanol
  Polyethylene glycols (PEGs)
  Sorbitol
  Glycerin
  N-methyl-2-pyrrolidone
Surfactants
  Polysorbates (Tweens)
  Pluronics
  Cremophor EL

---

could readily be reconstituted with distilled water (71). Thus far, no emulsion formulations of anticancer agents have been marketed.

Colloidal Systems

Over the past few years, the development of colloidal systems (liposomes, nanoparticles) as an alternative to cosolvent systems for the intravenous delivery of water insoluble drugs have gained a lot of attention. Liposomes are microparticulate lipid vesicles consisting of one or more phospholipid bilayers (lamellae) surrounding discrete aqueous compartments. Phospholipids are amphiphilic and self-assemble to spherical bilayers in aqueous media. Depending on the method of preparation and lipids used, the characteristics of liposomes vary in terms of the number of bilayers and size (e.g., multilameller vesicles, 0.1–5.0 μm; small unilamellar vesicles, 20–50 nm; large unilamellar vesicles, from 60 nm), morphology, bilayer fluidity, and surface characteristics such as charge and hydrophilicity. Liposomes can encapsulate drugs with various lipophilicities by entrapment of lipophilic drugs in the lipid bilayer and water soluble drugs within the aqueous vesicle compartment. Liposomes can be prepared either by hydration of lipids followed by high-intensity agitation or by the emulsion method, which involves the dissolution of lipids in an organic solvent, in addition to an aqueous medium under vigorous agitation, and the subsequent removal of the organic solvent under reduced pressure. The resulting dispersions are sized by filtration or extrusion. Drug substances can be incorporated by encapsulation (hydration of a lipid with an aqueous solution of the drug), partitioning (codissolution of a low-aqueous soluble drug with lipids in organic solvent followed by emulsification resulting in intrabilayer entrapment), or reverse loading (entrapment by charging the drug after passive loading by adjusting the internal liposome pH) (72). Advantages of liposomal formulations may be the circumvention of toxic solubilizing agents and, by altering the pharmacokinetic properties, decreasing systemic toxicity or (passive) targeting the drug to the site of action. For example, a Stealth liposome formulation of cisplatin, SPI-77, was developed to increase the total dose of cisplatin that can be administered without an increase in systemic toxicity (73). Because they are small (approximately 110 nm), and because of their long circulation time and reduced interaction with blood components, sterically stabilized (methoxypolyethylene glycol–coated, Stealth) liposomes are expected to accumulate in tumours, also as a result of the EPR effect mentioned previously. Indeed, significantly altered phar-

macokinetic characteristics (which appeared to be mainly governed by its liposomal properties) and toxicity profile of SPI-77 compared to "free" cisplatin were found in phase 1 clinical studies (73). Currently, several liposomal formulations of anticancer agents have been marketed [e.g., doxorubicin, Doxil (PEGylated Stealth liposome), Myocet; daunorubicin, DaunoXome; cytarabine, DepoCyte], all second-generation formulations intended to reduce toxicity or activity by improving residence time of the active compound (74–76).

Microencapsulation involves the application of a thin film composed of synthetic (e.g., polyesters, polyanhydrides, polyphosphazenes) or natural (e.g., albumin, dextran, collagen) polymers around a micronized solid or liquid, resulting in nanocapsules or microspheres. An investigational lipid (dioleoyl-phosphatidylserine, PS-dioleoyl-phosphatidylcholine, PC) coated, nanocapsule formulation of cisplatin was developed using a freeze-thaw technique (77). It is believed that using this technique, small cisplatin aggregates are formed during freezing, covered by positively charged aquo-species of cisplatin. These aggregates subsequently interact with the negatively charged lipid vesicles, resulting in the formation of nanocapsules with unprecedented encapsulation efficiency (drug-to-lipid ratio of approximately 3.3 mg cisplatin per μmol phospholipid). The entrapment efficiency (in relation to the expected dosing range) and stability greatly determine the applicability of a colloidal formulation for an investigational drug substance. Furthermore, challenges as sterilization of the formulation, reproducibility of (large-scale) manufacture, and long-term storage stability apply. For more information, the reader is referred to dedicated handbooks (78,79).

Complexation

Cyclodextrins are cyclic oligosaccharides consisting of covalently (α-1,4)-linked α-D-glucopyranose rings containing a relatively hydrophobic central cavity and hydrophilic outer surface (80–82). Cyclodextrins are able to form noncovalent complexes by incorporating a lipophilic guest molecule or lipophilic moieties of the guest molecule within its inner core. Naturally occurring cyclodextrins are α-, β-, and γ-cyclodextrin, which consist of six, seven, and eight glucopyranose rings, respectively. A number of chemically modified cyclodextrins have been developed to overcome the low aqueous solubility and toxicity (in particular renal) associated with natural cyclodextrins and increase their usefulness. Among these are hydroxypropyl-β-cyclodextrin (HPβCD) and the anionic

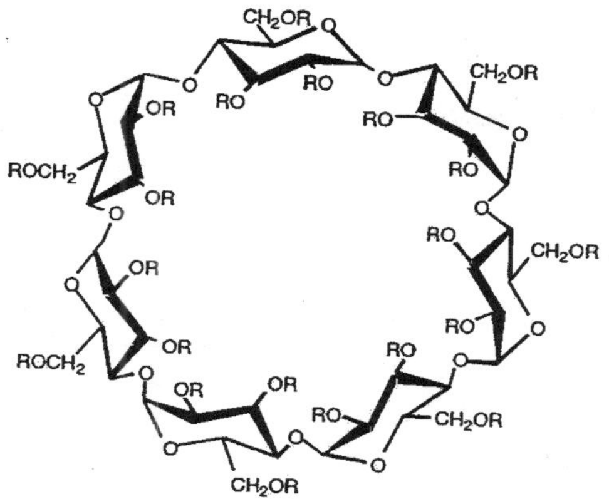

FIG. 15.5. Structural formula of HPβCD (R = $CH_2CHOHCH_3$) and SBEβCD (R = $-(CH_2)_4SO_3Na$ or $-H$).

sulfobutylether-β-cyclodextrin (SBEβCD), both of which are of particular interest because of their suitability in parenteral formulations (Fig. 15.5). Complexation of a guest molecule with cyclodextrin leads to a change in its physicochemical properties, which can result in increased solubility, stability, and tolerability. Formation of a drug–cyclodextrin complex can be induced by several methods including coprecipitation, lyophilization, and solubilization. Phase-solubility diagrams (plots of drug versus cyclodextrin concentration) are generally used to examine complex formation. Linear diagrams (A_L-type) indicate formation of 1:1 drug–cyclodextrin complexes (slope less than one), or higher-order complexation (e.g., 2:1 drug/cyclodextrin, slope value greater than one). Slope values greater than unity, however, may also indicate aditional solubilization due to aggregate formation of, for example, drug–cyclodextrin complexes (83). For a 1:1 drug–cyclodextrin complex, the complexation efficiency is defined by the slope of the phase-solubility diagram divided by (1 − slope). A positive deviation from linearity (A_P-type phase-solubility diagrams) suggests formation of a higher-order complex with respect to cyclodextrin (e.g., 1:2, 1:3 drug/cyclodextrin). Complexation is further analytically characterized using techniques like NMR, DSC, Fourier transform (FT)-infrared, and x-ray diffraction analysis. Addition of polymers such as polyvinyl pyrrolidone as well as cosolvents or surfactants may affect the solubility of the drug of interest (62,80,82,84). Besides their solubilizing and stabilizing capabilities, cyclodextrins are easy to process and have a high chemical stability, which makes them suitable for both solid (lyophilized) and liquid formu-

lations. Complexation using cyclodextrins is an attractive formulation approach for investigational anticancer agents, and reformulation studies of mitomycin C, paclitaxel, camptothecin, melphalan, and carmustine have been reported (85–89). Furthermore, cyclodextrins have been selected as a first-choice formulation approach for several experimental agents (e.g., flavopiridol, aphidicolin, all-*trans* retinoic acid, NSC-639829, bropirimine) (62,90–93). Cyclodextrin formulations for the intravenously administered antifungal agents itraconazole (Sporanox, HPβCD) and voriconazole (Vfend, SBEβCD), and the antipsychotic agent ziprasidone mesylate (Geodon, SBEβCD), have gained market approval.

MANUFACTURE

After definition of the pharmaceutical formulation prototype of the investigational anticancer agent, a manufacturing process must be established and validated (5,94,95). This process should be capable of the consistent manufacture of product of the required quality. Furthermore, it should be flexible with respect to product content and batch size during early clinical trials, and upscalable at the time of further development.

In general, a manufacturing process consists of weighing of API and excipients, compounding, sterilization, filling, and if necessary freeze-drying or additional formulation-specific processing steps (e.g., liposome sizing by extrusion) (74). The method of sterilization is determined by the stability of the investigational anticancer agent and/or formulation. For instance, heat lability precludes the use of terminal sterilization of the product by moist heat, the sterilization method of first choice (96,97). Sterile filtration in combination with aseptic processing generally offers a solution for heat-labile formulations. Figure 15.6 depicts the flow chart of an aseptically manufactured, lyophilized product.

Pharmaceutical manufacture of investigational anticancer drugs to be used in clinical trials, although generally performed on a small scale, has to comply with the principles of Good Manufacturing Practices (6). This requires that an organizational structure be in place in which responsiblities for production, quality control, and quality assurance are separate. Release of the final product is reserved to a responsible person. Obviously, all personnel should be trained for their tasks. Furthermore, the facilities and equipment used in the manufacturing process must be fully validated (design, installation, operational, performance qualification) for their purpose. For example, an aseptic processing method requires high standard environ-

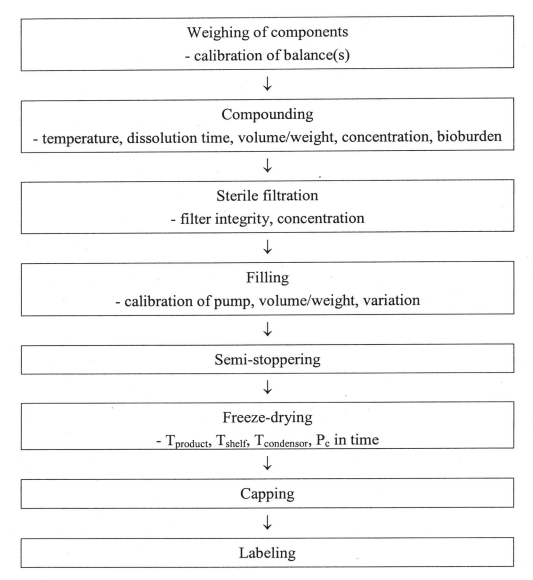

FIG. 15.6. Flow chart of the aseptic manufacture of a lyophilized product with critical parameters. Throughout the process, recovery of product is assessed and monitoring (particulates, microorganisms) of production facilities and personnel is performed.

mental conditions of the production facilities with respect to particulate and microorganism levels, both at rest and at operating state (Table 15.6). Cleaning and disinfection procedures should be in place, as well as methods to determine product or cleaning agent residuals.

Excipients, primary packaging materials (e.g., vials, stoppers), and other materials (e.g., filters, tubing) used in the manufacture need to be compatible with the formulation, comply with pharmacopeial standards (e.g., European Pharmacopeia, United States Pharmacopeia/National Formulary), and must be obtained from reliable sources. Furthermore, the primary packaging material must offer absolute container-closure integrity to prevent ingress of microorganisms. Procedures should be in place for the pretreatment of production materials (e.g., washing and sterilization of primary packaging materials and com-

TABLE 15.6. *Environmental levels of particles and microbial contamination during aseptic processing*

Maximum permitted number of particles/m³ equal or above	At rest		In operation	
	A	B	A	B
0.5 μm	3,500	3,500	3,500	350,000
5.0 μm	0	0	0	2,000
Microbial contamination limits				
Air sample (cfu/m³)		n.s.	<1	10
Settle plates (cfu/4 h)		n.s.	<1	5
Contact plates (cfu/plate)		n.s.	<1	5
Glove print (five fingers, cfu/glove)		n.s.	<1	5

Grade A, zone for high-risk operations (e.g., filling, stoppering, open vials); grade B, background of grade A zone; cfu, colony-forming unit; n.s., no specification (6).

pounding vessels). Critical steps in the manufacture process must be defined and controlled by adequate in-process controls. Examples are filter integrity testing, monitoring of filling weight, and bioburden assessment of the formulation solution. Labeling of investigational products must be performed according to regulatory guidelines (6). Documentation should be provided with each lot manufactured appropriately describing the formulation procedures, quality-control methods, and product specifications and recording details from manufacture as well as quality control. This documentation is extremely important for regulatory control and retrieval of historical data in the event of questionable product problems, and is to be archived until at least 2 years after finalization of the clinical study (6). For the same reason, a sample of the lot enabling full quality control whenever necessary is archived. Finally, a recall procedure should be in place.

STABILITY STUDIES

Pharmaceutical stability refers to storage life or utility time (i.e. the period of time a raw drug substance, excipient, final product, reconstituted product, or infusion solution remains within its specification limits under certain environmental conditions such as temperature, humidity, and light). Stability can be subdivided in chemical (i.e., incessant, irreversible degradation of the parent molecule), physical (e.g., precipitation, collapse of lyophilized product), and microbial stability.

Stability Testing of Pharmaceutical Product

The aim of the pharmaceutical development of an investigational anticancer agent is constitution of a product that has a sufficient shelf life (longer than 1 year) at a practically convenient storage condition [room temperature, $25°C \pm 2°C/60\% \pm 5\%$ relative humidity (RH)] or refrigerated condition, $5°C \pm 3°C$). During the investigational status of a new compound, other storage conditions can be accepted, but not with large-scale, commercial distribution. Real-time stability testing of the pharmaceutical product at the designated long-term storage condition is required, but can be performed in parallel with clinical evaluation of the investigational anticancer drug. Also, to anticipate fluctuations that can occur (e.g., during shipment of product), stability testing of the final product at defined intermediate and/or accelerated storage conditions must be carried out (e.g., $40°C \pm 2°C/75\% \pm 5\%$ RH) (98). Furthermore, photostability testing is required (99,100). Items to be monitored during the stability study must be selected, and generally include appearance, content, and purity. Also, sterility of the product throughout its shelf life must be assured. The information obtained will allow for future adjustments to the label storage recommendations and provide necessary information for assignment of retest dates or expiration dates. For further details, the reader is referred to regulatory guidelines (98,99).

Stability in and Compatibility with Administration Sets

Before administration of the investigational anticancer agent, infusions or injections have to be prepared from the pharmaceutical dosage form for the individual patient. This involves reconstitution of the lyophilized pharmaceutical product (if applicable), dilution of the product with infusion solution, and transfer into the final administration container or syringe. If necessary, the administration set is completed with an infusion line and/or in-line filter.

Therefore, chemical and physical stability of the investigational anticancer agent in commonly applied infusion solutions (e.g., 0.9% weight/volume sodium chloride, normal saline; 5% weight/volume dextrose, D5W) as well as compatibility testing with administration sets over the concentration range and under the conditions (e.g., temperature, light) intended in the clinical setting must be assessed prior to the start of the study. Stability from a microbial point of view depends on the preparation conditions, composition of the infusion solution (e.g., presence of preservative), and storage condition.

Figure 15.7 shows the stability profile of AP5280 in normal saline and D5W, depicted as the release of platinum from the HPMA-polymer backbone in time. Based on these data, which show an ongoing, apparently chloride-driven release of platinum species, AP5280 was administered during clinical studies using D5W as infusion solution (101). Besides stability of the infusion solution during the actual administration period, additional time required for preparation and logistics (timespan of transport from the hospital pharmacy to installation at the bedside) should be taken into consideration. This sometimes requires that subsequent activities are optimally geared up. For example, the final infusion solution of the experimental ruthenium compound NAMI-A is chemically stable for just 4 hours after preparation (7). Taken into consideration a 1-hour infusion duration, short lines between hospital pharmacy and clinic are pivotal for succesful treatment. Sometimes the limited stability of a pharmaceutical formulation forces the use of laborious administration methods. To administer the physically instable pharmaceutical formulation of the phenylbenzoylurea derivative clanfenur to the patient, a two-pump infusion system with in-line filter was

TABLE 15.7. *Recovery of the investigational anticancer agent aplidine from different infusion sets*

Aplidine infusion concentration	PVC administration set	PVC-free administration set
5.9 μg/mL	48.3%	78.3%
28.8 μg/mL	77.4%	93.1%
84.7 μg/mL	83.6%	97.8%

PVC, polyvinyl chloride.

applied. This system prevented the almost immediate precipitation of the drug from its Cremophor EL/ethanol vehicle on dilution (102). Because this may not be attractive during later stages of development, adaptation of the formulation is generally indicated.

Stability of infusion solutions is generally studied in various infusion container materials [e.g., polyvinyl chloride (PVC), low-density polyethylene, glass] at 25°C ± 2°C and 5°C ± 3°C in light and dark conditions. *In vitro* real-time infusion simulations can give insight into the percentage of the intended dose, which will eventually be administered to the patient using a specific administration set, infusion concentration, and infusion duration (103,104). This is of particular interest when dealing with hydrophobic, low-dosed compounds, which are prone to adsorb to administration set surfaces. Table 15.7 shows the results of infusion simulations with aplidine, intended to be administered down to concentrations of approximately 6 μg/mL in the phase 1 clinical study. These data show a significant loss of drug at these low concentrations, in particular in the PVC administration set. Therefore, aplidine should be administered in infusion concentrations equal to or above 28.8 μg/mL using a PVC-free administration set (103).

If the pharmaceutical formulation contains cosolvents or surfactants, compatibility with intravenous administration devices is often limited due to leaching of components from the material under influence of these excipients. The nonionic surfactants Cremophor EL and polysorbate 80 are notorious for leaching of the plasticizer diethylhexyl phthalate (DEHP) from PVC administration sets (103–108). Furthermore, compound-specific incompatibilities can occur. For instance, the platinum compounds cisplatin and carboplatin are known to interact with aluminium-containing devices, resulting in a black precipitate (109).

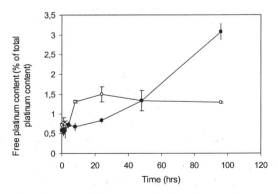

FIG. 15.7. Free platinum content of AP5280 solutions in normal saline and 5% dextrose (■ indicates normal saline; ○, 5% dextrose).

BIOCOMPATIBILITY STUDIES

Biocompatibility studies are performed to assess the local and systemic toxicity associated with precipitation, hemolysis, or altered pH after intravenous administration of a novel pharmaceutical formulation. In this way, formulation and administration-related adverse effects can be anticipated prior to clinical use. To minimize patient discomfort, the pharmaceutical formulation may be modified (e.g., the addition of tonicifiers) and the optimal injection or infusion parameters (e.g., concentration, speed, duration, peripheral or central vein) are selected (103,110,111).

Precipitation during injection may lead to phlebitis or tissue necrosis, embolus formation, or altered drug pharmacokinetics. Precipitation can occur as a consequence of dilution of a drug from a dosage form containing solubilizing agents (e.g., cosolvents or surfactants), changes in the ionization state of the drug due to differences in pH between the dosage form and blood or infusion medium, or salting-out of the drug by various mechanisms (112). Several *in vitro* precipitation test models have been developed (113). An *in vitro* dynamic flow model, using spectrophotometric detection of precipitate after injection of the formulation into a running "blood" flow (usually isotonic Sorensen's phosphate buffer), simulates the *in vivo* situation (Fig. 15.8) (114,115). Furthermore, static models using dog or human blood plasma have been described (112,116).

Hemolysis or the destruction of red blood cells caused by intravenous administration of pharmaceutical vehicles results in the release of hemoglobin into the plasma, which is associated with vascular irritation, phlebitis and even anemia, jaundice, kernicterus,

and acute renal failure. For example, hemolysis can be induced by cosolvents or surfactants (117,118). However, vehicles like SBEβCD or lipid emulsions can have a protective effect on red blood cells (119,120). As for precipitation, hemolysis can be studied *in vitro* using both static and dynamic flow models. The dynamic model is believed to give a more reliable description of the *in vivo* situation (Fig. 15.8) (121). The degree of hemolysis is expressed as the hemoglobin concentration in the test solution related to this in a 100% lysed sample, commonly induced by water. Hemolytic potentials of several pharmaceutical excipients have been reported (122).

Bolus injections at pH ranging from 2 to 11 do not induce phlebitis, as determined *in vivo* in a rat ear model (123). Vascular irritation is related to the time vein tissue is exposed to a nonphysiologic-pH environment. This is of particular importance in case of an intravenous infusion, which takes place over a longer period. Therefore, the capacity of blood to maintain the physiological pH (7.40 ± 0.05) on injection or infusion of a pharmaceutical formulation solution outside this range is of interest. This can be expressed as the FB ratio (i.e., the ratio of formulation solution volume and volume of blood simulator necessary to make up a pH of 7.40 ± 0.05) (110). Comparison with currently marketed pharmaceuticals can be helpful in assessing applicability (111). For more information the reader is referred to dedicated handbooks (122).

CONCLUSIONS

Solubility and stability issues are often the major hurdles to be overcome during the pharmaceutical development of an investigational anticancer drug. Classical solubilization approaches (e.g., pH adjustment, cosolvent/surfactant systems) are the most straightforward and generally result in clinically feasible, injectable pharmaceutical formulations. A disadvantage, however, may be the formulation-related toxicity of excipients contributing to the overall toxicity of the drug. After well-proven activity in humans and additional pharmacokinetic and pharmacological data, second-generation formulations (e.g., colloidal systems such as liposomes) become of interest because they may offer more specific drug delivery and reduced toxicity. Complexation of an investigational anticancer drug with cyclodextrins seems to be an attractive formulation approach, because this may increase both aqueous solubility and stability with limited additional vehicle-related toxicity. Lyophilization is the stabilizing technique of choice used to provide sufficient shelf life in investigational products with

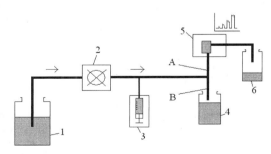

FIG. 15.8. *In vitro* dynamic precipitation **(A)** and hemolysis **(B)** test model. 1, blood or blood simulator (ISPB at pH 7.4 and 37°C, ± albumin); 2, pump; 3, syringe pump with formulation solution; 4, vessel for quenching hemolytic reaction (normal saline) before hemoglobin analysis; 5, ultraviolet/visible spectrophotometer with flow-through cell and example of opacity recordings due to precipitation; 6, waste vessel. For both methods, the ratio formulation:blood is determined by the infusion rate:flow rate; contact time is determined by the flow rate, the diameter of the tubing and the distance from the injection point to 4 or 5.

limited chemical stability. Besides solubility and stability issues, analytical method development, manufacturing, and (bio)compatibility testing are important aspects in the formulation of a novel anticancer agent.

In conclusion, the development of a pharmaceutical formulation of an investigational anticancer drug enables clinical assessment of the compound and is a prerequisite for its further development.

REFERENCES

1. Jonkman-de Vries JD, Flora KP, Bult A, et al. Pharmaceutical development of investigational anticancer agents for parenteral use. *Drug Dev Ind Pharm* 1996; 22:475.
2. Crommelin DJA. Formulation of biotech products, including biopharmaceutical considerations. In: Crommelin DJA, Sindelar RD, eds. *Pharmaceutical biotechnology: an introduction for pharmacists and pharmaceutical scientists.* Amsterdam: Harwood Academic Publishers, 1997:71–99.
3. Carpenter JF, Pikal MJ, Chang BS, et al. Rational design of stable lyophilized protein formulations: some practical advice. *Pharm Res* 1997;14:969–975.
4. Davignon JP, Slack JA, Beijnen JH, et al. EORTC/CRC/NCI guidelines for the formulation of investigational cytotoxic drugs. *Eur J Clin Oncol* 1988;24:1535–1538.
5. CPMP/QWP/155/96. Note for guidance on development pharmaceutics. Available at: http://www.emea.eu.int/index/indexh1.htm.
6. European Commission. Pharmaceutical Legislation volume 4: medicinal products for human and veterinary use: Good Manufacturing Practices. Available at: http://pharmacos.eudra.org/F2/eudralex/vol-4/home.htm
7. Bouma M. *Pharmaceutical development of the novel metal-based anticancer agents NAMI-A and AP5280* [thesis]. University of Utrecht, 2002.
8. Nuijen B, Rodrigues-Campos IM, Noain CP, et al. HPLC-UV method development and impurity profiling of the marine anticancer agent aplidine in raw drug substance and pharmaceutical dosage form. *J Liq Chromatogr* 2001;24:3119–3139.
9. International Conference on Harmonization. Guideline Q2A: text on validations of analytical procedures. Available at: http://www.ich.org/ich5q.html.
10. International Conference on Harmonization. Guideline Q2B: validation of analytical procedures: methodology. Available at: http://www.ich.org/ich5q.html.
11. International Conference on Harmonization. Guideline Q3A (R): impurities in new drug substances. Available at: http://www.ich.org/ich5q.html.
12. International Conference on Harmonization. Guideline Q3B: impurities in new drug products. Available at: http://www.ich.org/ich5q.html.
13. International Conference on Harmonization. Guideline Q3C. Impurities: residual solvents. Available at: http://www.ich.org/ich5q.html.
14. International Conference on Harmonization. Guideline Q6A. Specifications: test procedures and acceptance criteria for new drug substances and new drug products. Chemical substances. Available at: http://www.ich.org/ich5q.html.
15. Geigert J. Appropriate specifications at the IND stage. *PDA J Pharm Sci Technol* 1997;51:78–80.
16. Stafford J. Calculating the risk of batch failure in the manufacture of drug products. *Drug Dev Ind Pharm* 1999;25:1083–1091.
17. Nuijen B, Bouma M, Manada C, et al. Pharmaceutical development of anticancer agents derived from marine sources. *Anticancer Drugs* 2000;11:793–811.
18. Sweetana S, Akers MJ. Solubility principles and practices for parenteral drug dosage form development. *PDA J Pharm Sci Technol* 1996;50:330–342.
19. Akers MJ: Excipient-drug interactions in parenteral formulations. *J Pharm Sci* 2002;91:2283–2300.
20. Nannan Panday VR, Huizing MT, ten Bokkel Huinink WW, et al. Hypersensitivity reactions to the taxanes paclitaxel and docetaxel. *Clin Drug Invest* 1997;14:418–427.
21. European Organization for Research and Treatment of Cancer New Drug Development Committee. EORTC guidelines for phase I clinical trials with single agents in adults. *Eur J Clin Oncol* 1985;21:1005–1007.
22. Strickley RG. Parenteral formulations of small molecules therapeutics marketed in the United States (1999) Part II, III. *PDA J Pharm Sci Technol* 2000;54:69–96,152–169.
23. Nema S, Washkuhn RJ, Brendel RJ. Excipients and their use in injectable products. *PDA J Pharm Sci Technol* 1997;51:166–171.
24. Wade A, Weller P, eds. *Handbook of pharmaceutical excipients,* 2nd ed. London: The Pharmaceutical Press, 1994.
25. Powell MF, Nguyen T, Baloian L. Compendium of excipients for parenteral formulations. *PDA J Pharm Sci Technol* 1998;52:239–311.
26. Greenwald RB. PEG drugs: an overview. *J Control Rel* 2001;74:159–171.
27. Dosio F, Brusa P, Crosasso P, et al. Preparation and characterization and properties *in vitro* and *in vivo* of a paclitaxel-albumin conjugate. *J Control Rel* 1997;47:293–304.
28. Duncan R: Drug-polymer conjugates: potential for improved chemotherapy. *Anticancer Drugs* 1992;3:175–210.
29. Hatefi A, Amsden B. Camptothecin delivery methods. *Pharm Res* 2002;19:1389–1399.
30. Hancock BC, Parks M: What is the true advantage for amorphous pharmaceuticals? *Pharm Res* 2000;17:397–404.
31. Bauer J, Spanton S, Henry R, et al. Ritonavir: an extraordinary example of conformational polymorphism. *Pharm Res* 2001;18:859–866.
32. Jonkman-de Vries JD, Kettenes-van den Bosch JJ, Henrar REC, et al. A systematic study on the chemical stability of the novel indoloquinone antitumor agent EO9. *Int J Pharm* 1993;100:181–188.
33. Jonkman-de Vries JD, Talsma H, Henrar REC, et al. Pharmaceutical development of a parenteral lyophilized formulation of the novel indoloquinone antitumor agent EO9. *Cancer Chemother Pharmacol* 1994;34:416–422.
34. Box GEP, Hunter WG, Hunter JS, eds. *Statistics for experimenters: an introduction to design, data analysis,*

and model building. New York: Wiley, 1978.

35. Nuijen B, Bouma M, Talsma H, et al. Development of a lyophilized, parenteral pharmaceutical formulation of the investigational polypeptide marine anticancer agent kahalalide F. *Drug Dev Ind Pharm* 2001;27: 767–780.

36. Baldi G, Gasco MR, Pattinaro F. Statistical procedures for optimizing the freeze-drying of a model drug in ter-butyl alcohol:water mixtures. *Eur J Pharm Biopharm* 1994;40:138–141.

37. Jennings TA. *Lyophilization: introduction and basic principles.* Englewood, CO: Interpharm Press, 1999.

38. Pikal MJ. Freeze-drying of proteins. Part I: process design. *Biopharm Drug Dispos* 1990;3:18–27.

39. Chang BS, Fischer NL. Development of an efficient single-step drying cycle for protein formulations. *Pharm Res* 1995;12:831–837.

40. Teagarden DL, Baker DS. Practical aspects of lyophilization using non-aqueous co-solvent systems. *Eur J Pharm Sci* 2002;15:115–133.

41. Kasraian K, DeLuca PP. Thermal analysis of the tertiary butyl alcohol-water system and its implications on freeze-drying. *Pharm Res* 1995;12:484–490.

42. Wittaya-Areekul S, Nail SL. Freeze-drying of *tert*-butyl alcohol/water cosolvent systems: effects of formulation and process variables on residual solvents. *J Pharm Sci* 1998;87:491.

43. Nuijen B, Bouma M, Henrar REC, et al. Pharmaceutical development of a parenteral lyophilized formulation of the novel antitumor agent aplidine. *PDA J Pharm Sci Technol* 2000;54:193–208.

44. Stella VJ, Umprayn K, Waugh WN. Development of parenteral formulations of experimental cytotoxic agents. I. Rhizoxin (NSC-332598). *Int J Pharm* 1988; 43:191–199.

45. Ni N, Tesconi M, Tabibi SE, et al. Use of pure *t*-butanol as a solvent for freeze-drying: a case study. *Int J Pharm* 2001;226:39–46.

46. Wittaya-Areekul S, Needham GF, Milton N, et al. Freeze-drying of *tert*-butanol/water cosolvent systems: a case report on formation of a friable freeze-dried powder of tobramycin sulfate. *J Pharm Sci* 2002;91: 1147–1155.

47. Williams NA, Lee Y, Polli GP, et al. The effects of cooling rate on solid phase transitions and associated vial breakage occurring in frozen mannitol solutions. *J Parent Sci Technol* 1986;40:135–141.

48. Williams NA, Dean T. Vial breakage by frozen mannitol solutions: correlation with thermal characteristics and effect of stereoisomerism, additives and vial configuration. *J Parent Sci Technol* 1991;45:94–100.

49. Williams NA, Guglielmo J. Thermal mechanical analysis of frozen solutions of mannitol and some related stereoisomers: evidence of expansion during warming and correlation with vial breakage during lyophilization. *J Parent Sci Technol* 1993;47:119–123.

50. Kovalcik TR, Guillory JK. The stability of cyclophosphamide in lyophilized cakes. Part I. Mannitol, lactose, and sodium bicarbonate as excipients. *J Parent Sci Technol* 1988;42:29–37.

51. Gibson M, Denham AJ, Taylor PM, et al. Development of a parenteral formulation of trimelamol, a synthetic S-triazine carbinolamine-containing cytotoxic agent. *J Parent Sci Technol* 1990;44:306–313.

52. Van Winden ECA. *Freeze-drying of liposomes* [thesis]. University of Utrecht, 1996.

53. Yalkowsky SH, ed. *Techniques of solubilization of drugs.* New York: Marcel Dekker, 1981.

54. Nuijen B, Bouma M, Schellens JHM, et al. Progress in the development of alternative pharmaceutical formulations of taxanes. *Invest New Drugs* 2001;19: 143–153.

55. Azmin MN, Setanoians A, Blackie RGG, et al. Formulation of 1,3,5–triglycidyl-S-triazinetrione (α-TGT) for intravenous injection. *Int J Pharm* 1982;10: 109–118.

56. Mojaverian P, Repta AJ. Development of an intravenous formulation for the unstable investigational cytotoxic nucleosides 5-azacytosine arabinoside (NSC 281272) and 5-azacytidine (NSC 102816). *J Pharm Pharmacol* 1984;36:728–733.

57. Krishna G, Mao J, Almassian B. Development of a parenteral formulation of an investigational anticancer drug, 3-aminopyridine-2-carboxaldehyde thiosemicarbazone. *Pharm Dev Technol* 1999;4:71–80.

58. Menon K, Teicher BA. Antitumor activity of cryptophycins: effect of infusion time and combination studies. *Proc Am Assoc Cancer Res* 1999;40:A1907.

59. Prendiville J, Crowther D, Thatcher N, et al. A phase I study of bryostatin 1 in patients with advanced cancer. *Br J Cancer* 1993;68:418–424.

60. Rubino T, Yalkowsky SH. Cosolvency and cosolvent polarity. *Pharm Res* 1987;4:220–230.

61. Li P, Tabibi E, Yalkowsky SH. Solubilization of ionized and un-ionized flavopiridol by ethanol and polysorbate 20. *J Pharm Sci* 1999;88:507–509.

62. Li P, Tabibi E, Yalkowsky SH. Solubilization of flavopiridol by pH control combined with cosolvents, surfactants, or complexants. *J Pharm Sci* 1999;88: 945–947.

63. Barzegar-Jalali M, Jouyban-Gharamaleki A. A general model from theoretical cosolvency models. *Int J Pharm* 1997;152:247–250.

64. Jouyban-Gharamaleki A, Valaee L, Barzegar-Jalali M, et al. Comparison of various cosolvency models for calculating solute solubility in water-cosolvent mixtures. *Int J Pharm* 1999;177:93–101.

65. Tarr BD, Sambandan TG, Yalkowsky SH. A new parenteral emulsion for the administration of Taxol. *Pharm Res* 1987;4:162–165.

66. Lundberg B. Preparation of drug-carrier emulsions stabilized with phosphatidylcholine-surfactant mixtures. *J Pharm Sci* 1994;83:72–75.

67. Lundberg B. The solubilization of lipophilic divatives of podophyllotoxins in sub-micron sized lipid emulsions and their cytotoxic activity against cancer cells in culture. *Int J Pharm* 1994;109:73–81.

68. Simamora P, Dannenfelser RM, Tabibi SE, et al. Emulsion formulations for intravenous administration of paclitaxel. *PDA J Pharm Sci Technol* 1998;52:170–172.

69. Kan P, Chen ZB, Lee CJ, et al. Development of nonionic surfactant/phospholipid o/w emulsion as a paclitaxel delivery system. *J Control Release* 1999;58: 271–278.

70. Fukushima S, Kishimoto S, Takeuchi Y, et al. Preparation and evaluation of o/w type emulsions containing antitumor prostaglandin. *Adv Drug Deliv Rev* 2000;45: 65–75.

71. Lundberg BB. A submicron lipid emulsion coated with amphipathic polyethylene glycol for parenteral administration of paclitaxel (Taxol). *J Pharm Pharmacol* 1997;49:16–21.

72. Chrai SS, Murari R, Ahmad I. Liposomes, Part I: Man-

ufacturing issues. Biopharm Europe, September 2002
73. Meerum Terwogt JM, Groenewegen G, Pluim D, et al. Phase I and pharmacokinetic study of SPI-77, a liposomal encapsulated dosage form of cisplatin. *Cancer Chemother Pharmacol* 2002;49:201–210.
74. Ceh B, Winterhalter M, Frederik PM, et al. Stealth® liposomes: from theory to product. *Adv Drug Deliv Rev* 1997;24:165–177.
75. Forssen EA. The design and development of DaunoXome® for solid tumor targeting in vivo. *Adv Drug Deliv Rev* 1997;24:133–150.
76. Waterhouse DN, Tardi PG, Mayer LD, et al. A comparison of liposomal formulations of doxorubicin with drug administered in free form. *Drug Saf* 2001;24:903–920.
77. Burger KHJ, Staffhorst RWHM, De Vijlder HC, et al. Nanocapsules: lipid-coated aggregates of cisplatin with high cytotoxicity. *Nat Med* 2002;8:81–84.
78. New RRC. *Liposomes: a practical approach.* Oxford: Oxford University Press, 1990.
79. Crommelin DJA, Schreier H. Liposomes. In: Kreuter J, ed. *Colloidal drug delivery systems.* New York: Marcel Dekker, 73–157.
80. Brewster ME, Simpkins JW, Singh Hora M, et al. The potential use of cyclodextrins in parenteral formulations. *J Parent Sci Technol* 1989;43:231–240.
81. Bekers O, Uijtendaal EV, Beijnen JH, et al. Cyclodextrins in the pharmaceutical field. *Drug Dev Ind Pharm* 1991;17:1503–1549.
82. Loftsson T, Brewster ME. Pharmaceutical applications of cyclodextrins. 1. Drug solubilization and stabilization. *J Pharm Sci* 1996;85:1017–1025.
83. Loftsson T, Magnúsdóttir A, Másson M, et al. Self-association and cyclodextrin solubilization of drugs. *J Pharm Sci* 2002;91:2301–2316.
84. Mura P, Faucci MT, Bettinetti GP. The influence of polyvinylpyrrolidone on naproxen complexation with hydroxypropyl-β-cyclodextrin. *Eur J Pharm Sci* 2001;13:187–194.
85. Bhardwaj R, Dorr RT, Blanchard J. Approaches to reducing toxicity of parenteral anticancer drug formulations using cyclodextrins. *PDA J Pharm Sci Technol* 2000;54:233–239.
86. Sharma US, Balasubramanian SV, Straubinger RM. Pharmaceutical and physical properties of paclitaxel (Taxol) complexes with cyclodextrins. *J Pharm Sci* 1995;84:1223–1230.
87. Ma DQ, Rajewski RA, Vander Velde D, et al. Comparative effects of $(SBE)_{7m}$-β-CD and HP-β-CD on the stability of two anti-neoplastic agents, melphalan and carmustine. *J Pharm Sci* 2000;89:275–287.
88. Ma DQ, Rajewski RA, Stella VJ. New injectable melphalan formulations utilizing $(SBE)_{7m}$-β-CD or HP-β-CD. *Int J Pharm* 1999;189:227–234.
89. Kang J, Kumar V, Yang D, et al. Cyclodextrin complexation: influence on the solubility, stability, and cytotoxicity of camptothecin, an antineoplastic agent. *Eur J Pharm Sci* 2002;15:163–170.
90. Michaelis M, Cinati J, Vogel JU, et al. Treatment of drug-resistant human neuroblastoma cells with cyclodextrin inclusion complexes of aphidicolin. *Anticancer Drugs* 2001;12:467–473.
91. Lin HS, Chean CS, Ng YY, et al. 2-Hydroxypropyl-beta-cyclodextrin increases aqueous solubility and photostability of all-trans-retinoic acid. *J Clin Pharm Ther* 2000;25:265–269.
92. Jain N, Yang G, Tabibi SE, et al. Solubilization of

NSC-639829. *Int J Pharm* 2001;225:41–47.
93. Echezaretta-López M, Torres-Labandeira JJ, Castiñeiras-Seijo L, et al. Complexation of the interferon inducer, bropirimine, with hydroxypropyl-β-cyclodextrin. *Eur J Pharm Sci* 2000;9:381–386.
94. CPMP/QWP/848/96. Note for guidance on process validation. Available at: http://www.emea.eu.int/index/indexh1.htm.
95. CPMP/QWP/486/95. Note for guidance on manufacture of the finished dosage form. Available at: http://www.emea.eu.int/index/indexh1.htm.
96. Morris JM. Sterilization decision trees development and implementation. *PDA J Pharm Sci Technol* 2000; 54:64–68.
97. CPMP/QWP/054/98. Decision trees for the selection of sterilization methods: annex to note for guidance on development pharmaceutics. Available at: http://www. emea.eu.int/index/indexh1.htm.
98. International Conference on Harmonization. Guideline Q1A (R): stability testing of new drugs and products. Available at: http://www.ich.org/ich5q.html.
99. International Conference on Harmonization. Guideline Q1B: photostability testing. Available at: http://www. ich.org/ich5q.html.
100. Bouma M, Nuijen B, Jansen MT, et al. Photostability profiles of the experimental antimetastatic ruthenium complex NAMI-A. *J Pharm Biomed Anal* 2002;30: 1287–1296.
101. Bouma M, Nuijen B, Stewart DR, et al. Stability and compatibility of the investigational polymer-conjugated platinum anticancer agent AP 5280 in infusion solution and its hemolytic potential. *Anticancer Drugs* 2002;13:915–924.
102. Jonkman-de Vries JD, Van den Bemt BJ, ten Bokkel-Huinink WW, et al. Pharmaceutical development of a parenteral formulation of the investigational anticancer drug clanfenur. *PDA J Pharm Sci Technol* 1997;51: 89–95.
103. Nuijen B, Bouma M, Henrar REC, et al. Compatibility and stability of aplidine, a novel marine-derived depsipeptide antitumor agent, in infusion devices, and its hemolytic and precipitation potential upon i.v. administration. *Anticancer Drugs* 1999;10:879–887.
104. Nuijen B, Bouma M, Manada C, et al. Compatibility and stability of the investigational polypeptide marine anticancer agent kahalalide F in infusion devices. *Invest New Drugs* 2001;19:273–281.
105. Faouzi ME, Dine T, Luyckx M. Stability, compatibility and plasticizer extraction of miconazole injection added to infusion solutions and stored in PVC containers. *J Pharm Biomed Anal* 1995;13:1363–1372.
106. Maas B, Huber C, Krämer I. Plasticizer extraction of Taxol®-infusion solution from various infusion devices. *Pharm World Sci* 1996;18:78–82.
107. Mazzo DJ, Nguyen-Huu JJ, Pagniez S, et al. Compatibility of docetaxel and paclitaxel in intravenous solutions with polyvinyl chloride infusion materials. *Am J Health Syst Pharm* 1997;54:566–569.
108. Hanawa T, Muramatsu E, Asakawa K, et al. Investigation of the release behaviour of diethylhexyl phthalate from the polyvinyl-chloride tubing for intravenous administration. *Int J Pharm* 2000;210:109–115.
109. Trissel LA. *Handbook on injectable drugs*, 11th ed. Bethesda: American Society of Health-Sytem Pharmacists, Inc, 2001.
110. Nuijen B, Bouma M, Henrar REC, et al. In Vitro bio-

compatibility studies with the experimental anticancer agent BIBX1382BS. *Int J Pharm* 2000;194: 261–267.

111. Nuijen B, Bouma M, Manada C, et al. In vitro biocompatibility studies with the novel marine anticancer agent kahalalide F and its reconstitution vehicle Cremophor EL/ethanol. *PDA J Pharm Sci Technol* 2001; 55:223–229.

112. Rubino JT, Nellore R, Parmar B. Dynamic compatibility testing of DMP 840, an experimental antitumor agent. *PDA J Pharm Sci Technol* 1997;51:130–136.

113. Li P, Vishnuvajjala R, Tabibi SE, et al. Evaluation of in vitro precipitation methods. *J Pharm Sci* 1998;87: 196–199.

114. Yalkowsky SH, Valvani SC, Johnson BW. *In vitro* method for detecting precipitation of parenteral formulations after injection. *J Pharm Sci* 1983;72: 1014–1017.

115. Davio SR, McShane MM, Kakuk TJ, et al. Precipiatation of the renin inhibitor ditekiren upon iv infusion: *in vitro* studies and their relationship to the *in vivo* precipitation in the cynomolgus monkey. *Pharm Res* 1991;8:80–83.

116. Gupta SL, Patel JP, Jones DL, et al. Parenteral formulation development of renin inhibitor Abott-72517. *J Pharm Sci Technol* 1994;48:86–91.

117. Krzyzaniak JF, Raymond DM, Yalkowsky SH. Lysis of human red blood cells 2: effect of contact time on cosolvent induced hemolysis. *Int J Pharm* 1997;152: 193–200.

118. Krzyzaniak JF, Yalkowsky SH. Lysis of human red blood cells 3: effect of contact time on surfactant-induced hemolysis. *PDA J Pharm Sci Technol* 1998;52: 66–69.

119. Jumaa M, Müller BW. Lipid emulsions as a novel system to reduce the hemolytic activity of lytic agents: mechanism of the protective effect. *Eur J Pharm Sci* 2000;9:285–290.

120. Nagase Y, Hirata M, Arima H, et al. Protective effect of sulfobutyl ether β-cyclodextrin on DY-9760-induced hemolysis *in vitro*. *J Pharm Sci* 2002;91: 2382–2389.

121. Krzyzaniak JF, Alvarez Núñez FA, Raymond DM, et al. Lysis of human red blood cells 4: comparison of *in vitro* and *in vivo* hemolysis data. *J Pharm Sci* 1997;86: 1215–1217.

122. Gupta PK, Brazeau GA, eds. *Injectable drug development: techniques to reduce pain and irritation*. Englewood, CO: Interpharm Press, 1999.

123. Simamora P, Pinsuwan S, Alvarez JM, et al. Effect of pH on injection phlebitis. *J Pharm Sci* 1995;84: 520–522.

16

Liposomal Drug Carriers for Cancer Diagnosis and Therapy

Martin Brandl

*Department of Pharmaceutics and Biopharmaceutics, Institute of Pharmacy,
University of Tromsø, Tromsø N-9037, Norway*

WHAT ROLE CAN LIPOSOME CARRIERS PLAY IN CANCER DIAGNOSIS AND DRUG THERAPY?

The potential benefit that can be gained from using liposomal carriers depends on the physicochemical characteristics of the drug, the desired pharmacological intervention, and both the sites of application and action. Principally, it can be assigned to one or more of the six mechanisms outlined in Table 16.1. This chapter will not discuss the details of the various anticancer liposomal agents described in the literature; rather, we will survey the common underlying technologies and try to identify the major challenges to be addressed when developing liposomal anticancer drugs for use in humans.

LIPOSOME TECHNOLOGY

Lipids

The primary lipid used in liposomal drug carriers is phosphatidylcholine. This lipid has a hydrophilic head group consisting of the quaternary ammonium moiety choline, which is linked to the glycerol backbone by a phosphoric ester (Fig. 16.1). Because the phosphate is negatively charged at physiologic pH levels, phosphatidylcholine is zwitterionic and liposomes made of it have no overall net charge. The remaining two hydroxyl groups of the glycerol backbone are esterified with fatty acids of varying chain lengths and degrees of saturation (number of double bonds). The preferred state of self-organization of hydrated phosphatidylcholine is in the form bilayer leaflets, where the hydrophilic head groups of the lipid molecules are oriented towards the water phase whereas the alkyl chains of the two monolayers are oriented towards the middle of the membrane (Fig.

16.1). The chain length and degree of saturation of the acyl chains mainly determines at which temperature (i.e., the main transition temperature) the membrane "melts," or goes over from a rigid, well-oriented "gel state" to a liquid crystalline, less-ordered "fluid state" (Fig. 16.1). Both states are truly lamellar, but the fluid state is more flexible and permeable (i.e., susceptible to the formation of transient water channels, which allow flux of hydrophilic molecules across the bilayer). Furthermore, membrane flexibility and lateral mobility determine to which degree guest molecules, such as lipophilic drugs (see the Incorporation and Association sections or plasma proteins (see the Behavior *In Vivo* section) may be incorporated into or adsorbed onto the membrane. A surface charge is introduced by partly replacing phosphatidylcholine with charged phospholipids, such as phosphatidylglycerol, which induces electrostatic repulsion of the liposomes and thus stabilization. A hydrophilic coat on the liposome surface is achieved by implementing approximately 5 mol% polyoxyethylene-phosphatidylethanolamine (PEG-PE) (1,2). This results in an improved thermodynamic stability of the lipid assembly (3).

Preparation of Liposomal Drug Carriers for Anticancer Drugs

In general, the process comprises hydration of the lipids resulting in the formation of liposomes, adaptation of liposome size, and loading of the active ingredient into the liposomes. These three steps of liposome preparation may be carried out one after another or take place simultaneously. In general, bigger liposomes are also more heterogeneous in size and lamellarity (number of lamellae). The formation of liposomes is a self-accomplishing process. It can be

TABLE 16.1. *Potential benefits of liposomal carriers for anticancer drugs and diagnostics*

Action	Mechanism	Consequences for cancer therapy and diagnosis
Solubilization	Incorporation/association of poorly soluble drugs with a vesicle membrane	Stable aqueous formulations for IV injection or infusion
Entrapment, controlled release	Liposome membranes provide an effective penetration barrier for entrapped drug, resulting in release at programmed rates	Altered drug pharmacokinetics; e.g. prevent premature metabolic inactivation or excretion allowing for extended drug exposure, avoiding toxic peak plasma levels and thus acute toxic effects
Altered biodistribution	Due to particulate character: after IV application, restrict extravasation into normal tissues and promote accumulation in MPS organs and solid tumors (passive targeting); after local administration, retain the drug within the compartment (locoregional therapy)	Reduce drug levels in healthy organs, thus reducing toxic side effects; accumulate drug in tumors with enhanced vascular permeability and thus increase therapeutic effect; Improve therapeutic index
Directed delivery	Liposomes with moieties on their surface that aim for specific interaction with structures of the target site may cause accumulation of the drug at the target site (active targeting)	Accumulate drug in tumors with overexpression of the L antigen and thus increase therapeutic effect
Overcoming biological barriers	Through receptor-mediated uptake guide the active entity through cell membranes; deliver it to specific compartments (e.g., nucleus) of cells	Increase level of therapeutic agent within target cells, thereby improving the therapeutic effect; circumvent efflux mechanisms, thus overcoming multidrug resistance; gene therapy
Enhancing immune response	Liposomes may present the active entity in a preferred conformation/orientation or copresent it together with other immune response-enhancing structures	Immune modulation; vaccination

IV, intravenous, MPS, mononuclear phagocytic system.

supported by mechanical agitation or transient use of organic solvent (4) or detergents (5).

Large-vesicular Carriers

After swelling of phospholipid in water, multilamellar large vesicles (MLVs) are formed. This type of liposome has not found widespread use due to its poor reproducibility and heterogeneity, both in size and lamellarity, except as an intermediate for further treatment by high-pressure homogenization or filter extrusion. A schematic drawing comparing small and large unilamellar and multilamellar vesicles is given in Figure 16.1.

Vesicular phospholipid gels (VPGs) are semisolid phospholipid pastes or gels of high lipid content. VPGs consist of vesicular structures and are obtained

by high-pressure homogenization. Under appropriate production conditions, pastes with a small-unilamellar-vesicular morphology, very much like densely packed small unilamellar vesicles (SUVs), are obtained (6), and appear to be suitable as depot formulations for controlled release of drugs (7).

Multivesicular lipid-based particles (DepoFoam) are particles in the micrometer size range with an aqueous interior and, like liposomes, are surrounded by a phospholipid-bilayer membrane, but with a multivesicular interior characterized by a foamlike chamber (8). Neighbored chambers share one membrane. The manufacturing process is a two-step emulsification process (9). First, the drug-containing water phase is emulsified under high input of mechanical energy within an organic solvent containing the lipids. This emulsion is then emulsified within a drug-

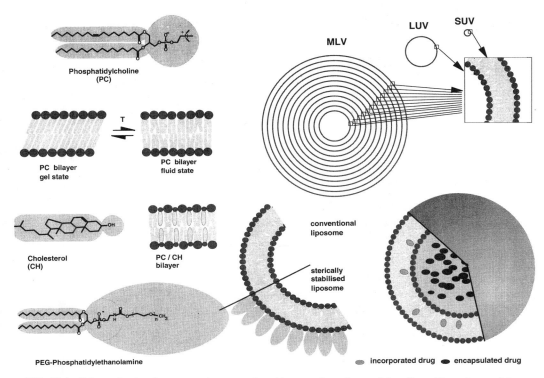

FIG. 16.1. Schematic drawing comparing a small and large unilamellar vesicle with multilamellar vesicles.

free water phase using less energetic mechanical agitation such that a water-in-oil-in-water (w/o/w) double emulsion is formed. The organic solvent is removed by purging with nitrogen such that the lipids take on a closely packed polyhedral structure. Several water-soluble molecules (e.g., cytarabine, amikacin, and morphine) have been entrapped in multivesicular lipid-based particles (9).

These large-vesicular structures are better suited for intramuscular or subcutaneous injection or instillation into body cavities (intrathecal, epidural, intraperitoneal) than for intravenous administration. The particles are retained at the injection site and control the release of the drug (sustained release).

Smaller Unilamellar Vesicles

Small to large unilamellar vesicles are a first choice for intravenous injection.

Conversion of Lipid Solutions to Liposomes

To convert lipid solutions to large unilamellar vesicles (LUVs), the lipid precipitates when an ethanolic solution of lipid(s) is mixed with an aqueous medium and forms large, mostly unilamellar vesicles. For improved homogeneity and reproducibility of liposome size, the ethanol injection technique may be combined with in-line high-shear homogenization or filter extrusion (10). Techniques for in-line removal of the organic solvent have been described elsewhere (10).

Conversion of Mixed Micelles to Liposomes

Phospholipids are solubilized by tensides like octyl-glucoside or cholate to form mixed micelles, and convert to liposomes when the tenside concentration in the preparation is lowered (detergent removal technique) (5). Liposome size can be adopted within certain limits (approximately 50–200 nm) with good size homogeneity and lamellarity close to one. Various attempts have been made to improve efficiency and scalability of this laboratory technique (11), which is suited for incorporation of membrane-associated moieties within liposomes and is being applied to the manufacture of virosomes (12). However, because of poor entrapment efficiency, this technique is not suitable for water-soluble drugs.

Conversion of Vesicular Phospholipid Gels
to Liposomes

Vesicular phospholipid gels, when blended with excess aqueous medium, are readily transferred into "classical" SUV dispersions (13).

Preparation of Small Unilamellar Vesicles by
High-Pressure Homogenization

Various high-pressure homogenization techniques (14–16) can reduce liposome size and lamellarity. High-pressure homogenization, regardless of the type of homogenizer used or the operating conditions employed, results in SUVs (less than 100 nm) with quite narrow size distribution. The liposome size can be manipulated to some extent only by higher homogenization pressures and repeated recycling. Bypassing the formation and hydration of a lipid film may be achieved by the so-called one-step liposome preparation technique, which yields homogeneous vesicles in just one step (14,17). Insufficient hydration may affect this result (18). In case of binary lipid blends, such as phosphatidylcholine and cholesterol, the dissolution of the lipids in organic solvent and removal of organic solvent appear inevitable to ensure homogeneous distribution of the lipids over the bilayer (17,19). Liposome production using high-pressure homogenization is being used within industrial processes because it can easily be scaled up and carried out under Good Manufacturing Practice (GMP) conditions.

Preparation of Large Unilamellar Vesicles
by Filter Extrusion

To manufacture vesicles of defined sizes in the range of approximately 50 to 200 nm, the filter extrusion technique is a suitable tool (20). Raw liposome dispersions (MLVs) are passed through polycarbonate membrane filters with straight pores of defined size. Usually, sequential extrusion through filters of decreasing pore sizes (from 100 to 30 nm) is performed, resulting in liposome diameters slightly above the pore size of the final membrane (21,22). Attempts have been made to scale up the process (23,24). With higher lipid concentrations and long-chain saturated lipids (below their phase transition temperature), however, clogging of the membrane is a common problem (25). This problem can be avoided by using high-pressure filter extrusion at pressures of up to 10 MPa (26). Industrial production is feasible; e.g., sequential high-pressure extrusion down to a final pore size of 0.2 μm and using lipid concentrations of up to 200 mg/g (27).

Loading with Drug

The choice of the most suitable technology for loading liposomes with a specific drug primarily depends on the physicochemical characteristics of the drug. Drug substances can be divided into two main categories according to their ability to interact with the liposome membrane:

1. *Water-soluble* substances. After loading into liposomes, these substances are truly entrapped or encapsulated within the aqueous core of the vesicles and/or aqueous spaces between the lamellae. The techniques that may be used to entrap hydrophilic drugs include (a) passive entrapment in the course of the liposome preparation and (b) remote loading via a pH or ion gradient or passive loading of vesicular phospholipid gels.
2. *Amphiphilic* or *lipophilic* substances. After loading into liposomes, these substances are somehow associated with the bilayer(s). Terms such as "entrapped" or "encapsulated" are often used to describe lipophilic substances; however, a more appropriate term is "incorporated" or "associated." A schematic diagram of drug-containing liposomes is shown in Figure 16.1. For some drugs one has a choice, they may be truly entrapped or alternatively associated with liposomes depending on acid dissociation constant (pKa) and lipid composition, especially in the case of charged phospholipids (28).

Incorporation and Association

Drugs that are loaded into or onto liposomes via incorporation are often virtually insoluble in water but soluble in nonpolar solvents (e.g., oil). These lipophilic compounds are treated as lipid compounds, in that they are transferred into a molecular mixture with the lipid components before hydration (e.g., by dissolving the drug and lipid in organic solvent and removing the latter to form a thin film). The amount of hydrophobic drug that can be incorporated in a liposome is dependent on packing restrictions within the bilayer. It is thus vital to choose an appropriate lipid formulation (see section "Lipids"). As long as the drug concentration does not exceed maximum incorporation capacity, the majority of drug will remain within the liposomes. The association of amphiphilic drugs with liposomes is often less stable than that of lipophilic compounds (29).

Passive Entrapment

Passive entrapment is taking place if the formation (and sizing) of the liposomes is carried in a drug-containing aqueous medium. Together with a certain portion of the aqueous medium, a certain portion of the drug ends up encapsulated within the liposomes. The encapsulation efficiency, the percentage of drug encapsulated as compared to the total amount of drug present, depends on liposome size, lamellarity, and total lipid content of the preparation. For classical MLVs, solute entrapment is low because of tight packing of the concentric lamellae and the little aqueous space in between them. For other big, oligolamellar to multilamellar vesicles, such as freeze/thaw multilamellar vesicles, reverse-phase evaporation vesicles (30), or dehydration/rehydration vesicles (31), this figure is much higher and may reach magnitudes of 40% or 50%. For SUVs, this figure typically is in the magnitude 1% to 10%.

Remote Loading

There are in principle two techniques described to load preformed vesicles with drug: pH- or ion-gradient–induced active loading and passive loading of VPGs.

The technique of *active loading* can be applied to drugs of the type amphiphilic weak base or weak acid, which show a pH-dependent difference in bilayer-membrane permeability (32). Anthracyclines for example readily permeate through the liposome bilayer in the base form, whereas they are relatively membrane impermeable when protonated. Thus, pH gradients can be employed for active loading (i.e., filling of preformed "empty" liposomes with such drugs) (33). The principle is as follows. Outside the liposomes a high pH value causes a shift of the dissociation equilibrium of the drug towards the unprotonated base. The base diffuses through the bilayer following the concentration gradient. Inside the liposomes, at a low pH value, the arriving base is protonated, which holds the concentration of the unprotonated form inside the liposomes constantly low, and thus maintains the concentration gradient over the bilayer. It has been shown that this loading process may continue until virtually all drug is carried over to the interior of the liposomes. A 100-fold accumulation inside the vesicles is achievable under certain circumstances. The same is, in principle, achieved by ammonium-sulfate gradients (34).

Doxorubicin accumulated within the liposomes beyond the limit of solubility forms *gel-like precipitates* (35). Both, citrate- and sulphate-induced precipitation of doxorubicin results in fibrous bundles comprised of stacked doxorubicin molecules electrostatically bridged by the multianions. This prevents osmotic-stress–induced vesicle rupture (36). In the case of ammonium-sulphate gradients, the sulphate ions stabilize the retention of the trapped drug in the long-term because they have a very low membrane permeability. Doxorubicin–metal complexes may also form precipitates (37). With this type of loading, removal of unentrapped drug is unnecessary.

The process of *passive loading* of VPGs (38,39) takes advantage of two facts: (i) bilayer-membrane permeability towards most drugs is greatly enhanced when the liposomes are warmed close to their thermotropic phase transition temperature; (ii) within vesicular phospholipid gels, the ratio of aqueous medium inside and outside liposomes is relatively high. Drug added to preformed "empty" vesicular phospholipid gels permeates at elevated temperatures through the leaky bilayer into the vesicles until equilibrium between the interior of the vesicles and the surrounding medium is reached (usually within 30–240 minutes). After recooling and subsequent dilution of the VPG into SUV dispersions, encapsulation efficiencies beyond 40% may be reached. Removal of unentrapped drug can in most cases be omitted.

Both previously discussed remote-loading techniques have several common advantages. No active ingredient is present during the preparation of the liposomes, which may greatly reduce the extent of safety precautions that have to be taken when toxic drugs are handled. The composition of the dispersion medium of the liposomes and of the drug preparation may be chosen independently and thus be optimized with respect to increased shelf life (e.g., pH 6.5 for liposomes and pH 4 for doxorubicin) (40) or freeze-dried state for highly sensitive drugs. These techniques allow loading of the liposomes at the bedside. In this case, drug and liposomes do not come in contact with each other until shortly before application, and interactions that induce degradation can be avoided (41).

Removal of Unentrapped Drug

With substances that do associate with the bilayer, it usually is not necessary to remove extraliposomal drug because the majority of the drug is liposome bound. However, for water-soluble, truly entrapped compounds, the bilayer membrane usually represents a diffusion barrier (i.e., after removal of extraliposomal drug the liposome will maintain a concentration gradient, at least for a certain period). Whether it is necessary to remove unentrapped drug primarily depends on the loading efficiency of the liposome-loading technique and on the efficacy and toxicity profile of free compared to liposomal drug. Several techniques are well established on a laboratory scale for removal of unentrapped drug from liposomes, such as gel chromatography (size-exclusion chromatography), ion-exchange chromatography, ultracentrifugation, and techniques employing semipermeable membranes. None of them is easy to scale up and perform under aseptic precautions. Therefore, this step is difficult to accomplish in the course of industrial production and should be avoided.

Sterilization

Two principally different approaches are used to ensure sterility of a parenteral product: terminal sterilization of the finished product in its final container, preferably by steam sterilization, and aseptical manufacturing. Terminal sterilization is generally preferred over aseptical manufacturing due to the higher sterility assurance level achieved and the lower validation and in-process control effort needed. Unfortunately, terminal sterilization does not seem possible with many liposomal drug carrier formulations. Aseptic production regimens for liposomal drug carriers may involve steps to reduce microbiological burden of the raw materials, intermediates, or final drug preparation, such as γ-irradiation (42), microbial retentive filtration (sterile filtration) (43), or heat treatment. Passing a liposome preparation through microbe-retentive filters may cause loss of bigger liposomes due to geometrical constraints or loss of certain species of lipids due to specific adsorption to the filter surface (18,43). Because lipid loss is difficult to predict, quantitative determination of lipid content after filtration appears mandatory.

CHALLENGES IN THE DESIGN AND MANUFACTURE OF LIPOSOMAL ANTICANCER DRUGS

Liposome Characteristics

The manufacturing process for a liposomal drug preparation should be suited to reproducibly achieve defined product characteristics in terms of lipid composition, liposome size and lamellarity, drug load (lipid-to-drug ratio), state of dispersion (aggregation), and sterility in a manner that can easily be accomplished under settings typical for industrial production of parenteral products for human use. The main challenge here is to achieve an efficient loading of the drug into vesicles of mostly small size and to retain the drug payload within the liposomes during storage time. From a technical standpoint, liposome size is directly correlated with the volume of the aqueous core. The volume of the aqueous core in turn determines the capacity to carry a hydrophilic drug, at least if the drug is truly entrapped (see the Loading with Drug section).

Storage Stability

Shelf life of liposomal drug carriers may be limited by insufficient chemical stability of both the active ingredient and the lipids or by insufficient physical stability of the liposomes.

In terms of *chemical stability* of phospholipids in aqueous dispersion, there are two major degradation reactions: hydrolysis and oxidation. Hydrolysis comprises cleavage of the ester bond, which results first in a free fatty acid and 1-acyl lysophospholipid, because cleaving off of the second fatty acid is slower as lysophospholipids accumulate. This hydrolysis is a pseudo–first-order reaction, which is catalyzed by acids and bases. The hydrolytic stability is thus pH dependent and is optimal around pH 6.5 (44,45). Cholesterol has no effect, and negatively charged phosphatidylglycerol shifts the surface charge density, which increases hydrolysis rate in acidic medium (46). Certain drug substances promote liposomal phospholipid hydrolysis (41). It is not clearly established yet to which degree the formation of lysophospholipid in liposomal drug carriers is acceptable.

Lysophospholipids have tenside character and affect bilayer stability, but changes in liposome size and phase separation occur only when hydrolysis reaches degrees of 60% (47). Lysophospholipids in liposomes, however, evoke lethal toxic reactions and decrease the phagocytic activity of macrophages, at least under certain conditions (48,49). Oxidation of the unsaturated fatty acids contained in certain phospholipids as well as of cholesterol is characterized by a change in color and smell. However, it is difficult to establish hard quantitative data because of the poor sensitivity of the established analytical methods.

Physical stability of liposome dispersions may affect particle size and drug content of the liposomes (leakage). A growth in primary particle size is due to fusion of vesicles and represents an irreversible process whereas a growth in secondary particle size is due to aggregation or flocculation of vesicles and in many cases reversible. A dispersion of hydrogenated soy phosphatidylcholine and cholesterol treated by a high-pressure homogenizer immediately after homogenization may cause fusion of vesicles with diameters of 20 nm, exhibiting extreme curvatures (17). If sedimentation or flotation in a liposome preparation occurs during shelf life, this often indicates aggregation. Vesicles bearing a net charge on their surface are less susceptible to aggregation because of electrostatic repulsion. Precipitation of cationic dimethyl-aminoethyl-carbamoyl (DC)-cholesterol/dioleylphos-phatidylethanolamine liposomes with increase of apparent particle size was observed (18). *Leakage* occurs, when entrapped drugs start to diffuse through the liposome membrane. This happens as soon as a concentration gradient over the membrane occurs (e.g., during active loading or when the nonentrapped drug is removed from the preparation). The rate and extent of leakage depend on both type of drug and lipid formulation. If the drug has a high tendency to leak out of liposomes, the preparation may be stabilized by using a lipid formula, which results in tighter membranes such as long-chain saturated phospholipids in combination with cholesterol or steric stabilization. Drugs that have been accumulated in liposomes via a pH or ion gradient are retained, at least as long as the gradient persists.

Behavior *In Vivo*

The desired route of administration (e.g., intravenous, intramuscular, or topical) and the desired type of action (local or systemic) is of key importance for the design of a drug carrier. The challenges described in this chapter refer to those associated with intravenous injection, the most common route. For a good therapeutic effect, the liposomal drug should be unavailable to nontarget cells/tissue while traveling in the blood stream, but available to target cells/tissue once the agent has arrived at the target site. This is influenced by:

- Pharmacokinetics and biodistribution of liposomal drugs
- Retention of liposomal drug within the central compartment
    minimal loss of the drug from the liposomal carrier
    minimal phagocytic elimination of the liposomes
       by the mononuclear phagocytic system (MPS)
- Accumulation of liposomal drugs in tumors
    extravasation of the liposomal drug at the
       tumor site
    internalization of the drug carrier into tumor
       cells
    release of drug from the liposomes near the
       tumor cells for uptake via diffusion

Retention of Liposomal Drug within the Central Compartment

After intravenous injection, a liposomal drug is designed to circulate in the blood stream and reach the desired target organ or tissue (if this is not the blood pool itself). Under ideal circumstances, the fate of the liposomal drug (i.e., the tissue or organ in which it ends up), is no longer dependent on the drug itself, but controlled by the characteristics of the liposomal carrier. This of course is only true as long as the drug remains associated with the carrier. The biodistribution and pharmacokinetics of the carrier primarily depend on the size and surface characteristics of the liposome. The retention of drug is determined by the physicochemical characteristics of the drug and by the lipid composition of the vesicle. In general, liposomes and their associated drug are largely confined to the central compartment. Uptake of drug into regular tissues is therefore decreased, leading to decreased toxicities in certain sensitive tissues; e.g., dermis in the case of vincristine (50) or heart muscle in the case of doxorubicin (51–53).

The Role of Membrane Composition and Liposome Surface Characteristics

The choice of lipids with regard to membrane fluidity and surface characteristics of the liposomes is of importance for clearance. A key role for the biopharmaceutical fate of liposomes is the adsorption of plasma proteins (opsonins) onto the surface (54). Up to lipid doses of 20 to 50 mg/kg body weight, interaction with high-density lipoprotein or its apolipoprotein may lead to solubilization of pure phosphatidylcholine liposomes. At lower doses, phosphatidylcholine liposomes acquire some apolipoproteins from HDL and lose some phosphatidylcholine, which induces leakiness of the liposomes (premature loss of drug load) (55). Furthermore, opsonization causes priming for recognition by the MPS and removal from circulation. This can be circumvented by (i) stiffening the membrane, (ii) shielding the surface, or (iii) increasing the lipid dose (or predose with empty liposomes) (56). Therefore, phosphatidylcholine is hardly ever used alone in liposomal lipid formulations. Blends of phosphatidylcholine with other lipids are used primarily to improve both *in vitro* and *in vivo* stability of the liposomes. Cholesterol is added to induce a tighter packing (stiffening) of the membrane, which above levels of 30 mol% results in reduced leakiness (55) and adsorption of membrane proteins (opsonins). In general, uncharged liposomes with a tightly packed membrane can escape opsonization to some degree. PEG-PE forms a steric stabilizing shield that inhibits protein binding and cellular recognition (2,57). Application of higher liposome doses saturates the phagocytic system, and the use of a polymer coat does not result in prolonged circulation times as compared with conventional lipid formulations (58).

The Role of Type of Drug Association with the Liposome

Actively loaded liposomes that exhibit a pH gradient retain their drug *in vivo*. In fact, even the loading works *in vivo*. A study found that liposomes exhibiting a transmembrane pH gradient, if injected intravenously, accumulated subsequently injected doxorubicin while circulating in the bloodstream (59). Another means to improve drug retention within liposomes is the previously described precipitation of doxorubicin. Membrane-associated drugs tend to rapidly redistribute *in vivo* to lipophilic biogenous sinks such as HDL. In the case of adriamycin, a burst of leakage of bilayer-incorporated drug shortly after injection was seen (60).

The Role of Liposome Size

It is a well-established fact that big liposomes (i.e., greater than 200 nm in diameter) made of phospholipids are rapidly taken up by macrophages and disappear from the circulation within short periods (61). These liposomes primarily end up in spleen (62). Therefore, bigger liposomes are not appropriate for applications in which a distant solid tumor is to be reached (60), except if the target is the MPS. However, liposomes of intermediate size (i.e., 70–200 nm in diameter) have a better chance of escaping the MPS and thus circulate long enough (e.g., blood-pool imaging by liposomal-contrast agents) or reach targets within or close to the vascular bed. Small liposomes (i.e., less than 70 nm in diameter) show shorter circulation, again because of extravasation through the fenestrated capillary walls in the liver.

In summary, sufficient circulation lifetimes of liposomal carriers can be achieved when relatively small (100-nm) neutral liposomes containing at least 30 mol% cholesterol are used at doses of 10 mg/kg or above (63) or alternatively by steric stabilization, independent of the dose administered (64).

Extravasation of the Liposomal Drug at the Site of Action

Only small liposomes may reach targets outside the vasculature. Within sites of inflammation and solid tumors, the architecture of the vascular blood supply is extraordinary. The lining of the vascular bed is less perfect with more and bigger gaps, which allow more extravasation. In tumors, the system of lymph vessels is less well established and the lymphatic drainage is reduced. This allows small liposomes to escape vasculature preferentially within tumors and accumulate there (65–67), a phenomenon called *enhanced perme-ability and retention*. In consequence, small liposomes are ideally suited to reach solid tumors and accumulate there via passive targeting effects (see section regarding the role of liposome size). Selective tumor localization of doxorubicin from sterically stabilized liposomes *in vivo* was proven (68). Whether sterically stabilized liposomes improve tumor localization compared with conventional liposomes is controversial (66,69,70).

For injections other than into the veins and for all other applications (e.g., topical administration), different rules apply in terms of desired liposome size and surface characteristics. In most of these applications, the primary role of liposomes is to retain and localize the drug in the form of a reservoir at the site of administration. A high drug-carrying capacity and prolonged retention is best achieved with large multilamellar or multivesicular liposomes (see sections regarding MLVs and multivesicular lipid-based particles).

Release of Drug from the Liposomes Near the Tumor

Once it has arrived at the target site, the liposome, if not taken up as a whole, should release the drug so that it can reach the cancer cells via diffusion. In principle, the same previously outlined rules apply for the design of liposome membranes in terms of permeability of drugs. This means that lipid membranes, which are tight during transit, will result in slow release rates of the drug at the target site as well. Too-slow release rates may impair the therapeutic effect. Metastable liposomes with a steric coat of a defined half-life have been described; PEG-PEs redistribute from the bilayer of the liposome drug carrier to other bilayers with exchange rates that are closely related to their chain lengths (71,72). A novel approach to induce remote release of doxorubicin from liposomes is the use of temperature-sensitive liposomes, which release drug in hyperthermic conditions (73).

Uptake of the Liposomal Carrier by Tumor Cells

There is certain evidence that liposomes are internalized by tumor cells, primarily for so-called immunoliposomes (74). *Immunoliposomes* with ligands (mostly antibodies) on their surface were designed to specifically interact with receptors or antigens being overexpressed by tumor cells (75–77). Although specific interaction of various types of immunoliposomes with tumor cells *in vitro* was found (78), their passage through the blood compartment appears to

TABLE 16.2. *Approved liposome-based anticancer drugs*

Trade name(s)	Drug	Lipid formula, vesicle type Drug to lipid ratio	Application; indication	Pharmaceutical company	Characteristics
Doxil (United States) Caelyx (European Union)	Doxorubicin	HSPC/CH/PEG-PE, LUV (80–110 nm) 1:8	IV; Kaposi's sarcoma, refractory ovarian cancer	Alza Corp. (Sequus)	Remote loaded and precipitated by ammonium sulfate gradient; sterically stabilized by PEG coat; prolonged retention in the central compartment; passive targeting due to EPR effect
Myocet	Doxorubicin	EPC/CH LUV (150 nm) 1:4	IV; metastatic breast cancer	Elan Corp. (Liposome Co.)	Remote loaded and precipitated by citrate gradient; prolonged retention in the central compartment; passive targeting due to EPR
DaunoXome	Daunorubicin	DSPC/CH SUV (35–65 nm) 1:19	IV; Kaposi's sarcoma	Gilead Sciences (NeXstar)	Delivered as liquid liposome suspension containing a citrate salt solution of the drug; passive targeting due to EPR; endocytosis-mediated uptake
DepoCyte	Cytarabine	DepoFoam lipid particles (micrometer range)	Intrathecal; lymphomatous meningitis	Chiron Corp. Elan Corp. Nippon Shinyaku (Skye Pharma)	Local retention and sustained release
Visudyne	Verteporfin	EPG, DMPC	IV; age-related macular degeneration	CIBA Vision (QLT PhotoTherapeutics, Inc.)	Drug incorporated in membrane; local activation by laser beam; photodynamic therapy

HSPC, hydrogenated soy phosphatidylcholine; CH, cholesterol; PEG, phosphatidylcholine; PE, polyoxyethylene; LUV, large unilamellar vesicle; IV, intravenous; EPR, enhanced permeability and retention; EPC, egg phosphatidylcholine; DSPC, di-stearoyl-phosphatidylcholine; SUV, small unilamellar vesicle; DMPC, di-myristoyl-phosphatidylcholine.

be compromised by the surface modification to an extent, making clinical application impossible. *pH-sensitive liposomes* undergo destabilization when encountering an intracellular acidic stimulus within the endosomal compartment (79). Metastable pH-sensitive liposomes are expected to be stable during transit, but become pH sensitive after the PEG coat is cleaved (80)

Multidrug Resistance

Cross-resistance of certain tumors to various cyto-toxic agents such as anthracyclines, vinca alkaloids, or taxanes due to an overexpression of permeability glycoprotein, an efflux pump, may be overcome by liposomal entrapment of these agents. Although the exact mechanism is unknown, possibilities include a blockade of the transporter by liposomal lipid or a protection of the drug after endosomal uptake of the whole carrier (81–86).

CONCLUDING REMARKS

Liposomal Drugs in Clinical Use

When the first reports of liposomal anticancer drug carriers were published (87), expectations were flying high. Liposomes were even compared with the "magic bullets" postulated by Paul Ehrlich. However, in terms of liposomal drug products approved for clinical use today, only a small number of liposomal or liposomelike dosage forms have been approved for parenteral use in humans. Table 16.2 summarizes the clinical applications of some of these preparations (88).

An impressing therapeutic benefit in terms of improved activity and reduced side effects could be demonstrated for a number of intravenously administered liposomal cytostatics formulations. Despite enormous research and development efforts, the commercialization of the first liposomal drugs occurred only recently. The main challenge represented a sufficient stabilization of the loaded carrier by an optimized lipid formula and preparation and loading technique (e.g., ion-gradient–induced loading and precipitation and steric stabilization). Many of these approaches, however, are specific for a certain type of drug (e.g., anthracyclines) and cannot be applied, at least not without major adaptation to other types of drugs. Many of the challenges thus persist, including efficient loading with *all* types of drugs and sufficient stability both *in vitro* (during storage and terminal sterilization) and *in vivo* (i.e., retention in the central compartment and accumulation within the tumor). The breakthrough for active targeting concepts has not been achieved, and further intense efforts in liposome research are required.

The authors thank M. Skar for assistance during literature research, A.M. Sætern for drawing the formula, and J. Zirkel, A. Dhanikula, and U. Massing for helpful discussions.

REFERENCES

1. Lasic DD, Martin FJ, Gabizon A, et al. Sterically stabilized liposomes: a hypothesis on the molecular origin of the extended circulation times. *Biochim Biophys Acta* 1991;1070:187–192.
2. Torchilin VP, Omelyanenko VG, Papisov MI, et al. Polyethylene glycol on the liposome surface: on the mechanism of polymer-coated liposome longevity. *Biochim Biophys Acta* 1994;1195:11–20.
3. Tirosh O, Barenholz Y, Katzhendler J, et al. Hydration of polyethylene glycol-grafted liposomes. *Biophys J* 1998;74:1371–1379.
4. Perrett S, Golding M, Williams WP. A simple method for the preparation of liposomes for pharmaceutical applications: characterization of the liposomes. *J Pharm Pharmacol* 1991;43:154–161.
5. Milsmann MHW, Schwendener RA, Weder HG. The preparation of large single bilayer liposomes by a fast and controlled dialysis. *Biochim Biophys Acta* 1978; 512:147–155.
6. Brandl M, Drechsler M, Bachmann D, et al. Morphology of semisolid aqueous phosphatidylcholine dispersions, a freeze fracture electron microscopy study. *Chem Phys Lipids* 1997;87:65–72.
7. Tardi C, Brandl M, Schubert R. Erosion and controlled release properties of semisolid vesicular phospholipid dispersions. *J Control Release* 1998;55:261–270.
8. Spector MS, Zasadzinski JA, Sankaram MB. Topology of multivesicular liposomes, a model biliquid foam. *Langmuir* 1996;12:4704–4708.
9. Mantripragada S. A lipid based depot (DepoFoam® technology) for sustained release drug delivery. *Prog Lipid Res* 2002;41:392–406.
10. Martin FJ. Pharmaceutical manufacturing of liposomes. *Drugs Pharm Sci* 1990;41:267–316.
11. Asanger M, Weder HG. Development of liposome production technique by counter-current-flow-dialysis (CCFD). *Acta Pharm Technol* 1985;31:215–223.
12. Hunziker IP, Zurbriggen R, Glueck R, et al. Perspectives: towards a peptide-based vaccine against hepatitis C virus. *Mol Immunol* 2001;38:475–484.
13. Brandl M, Drechsler M, Bachmann D, et al. Preparation and characterization of semi-solid phospholipid dispersions and dilutions thereof. *Int J Pharm* 1998;170: 187–199.
14. Brandl M, Bachmann D, Drechsler M, et al. Liposome preparation by a new high pressure homogenizer Gaulin Micron LAB 40. *Drug Dev Ind Pharm* 1990;16: 2167–2191.
15. Bachmann D, Brandl M, Gregoriadis G. Preparation of

liposomes using a Mini-Lab 8.30 H high-pressure homogenizer. *Int J Pharm* 1993;91:69–74.

16. Talsma H, Ozer AY, Van Bloois L, et al. The size reduction of liposomes with a high pressure homogenizer (Microfluidizer). Characterization of prepared dispersions and comparison with conventional methods. *Drug Dev Ind Pharm* 1989;15:197–207.

17. Brandl MM, Bachmann D, Drechsler M, et al. Liposome preparation using high-pressure homogenizers. In: Gregoriadis G., ed. *Liposome technology,* 2nd ed. Boca Raton: CRC, 1993:49–65.

18. Sorgi FL, Huang L. Large scale production of DC-Chol cationic liposomes by microfluidization. *Int J Pharm* 1996;144:131–139.

19. Brandl M. High-pressure homogenization techniques for the production of liposome dispersions: potential and limitations. In: Müller RH, Benita S, Böhm N, eds. *Emulsions and nanosuspensions for the formulation of poorly soluble drugs.* Stuttgart: Medpharm Scientific Publishers, 1998:266–294.

20. Olson F, Hunt CA, Szoka FC, et al. Preparation of liposomes of defined size distribution by extrusion through polycarbonate membranes. *Biochim Biophys Acta* 1979; 557:9–23.

21. Mayer LD, Hope MJ, Cullis PR. Vesicles of variable sizes produced by a rapid extrusion procedure. *Biochim Biophys Acta* 1986;858:161–168.

22. Jousma H, Talsma H, Spies F, et al. Characterization of liposomes. The influence of extrusion of multilamellar vesicles through polycarbonate membranes on particle size, particle size distribution and number of bilayers. *Int J Pharm* 1987;35:263–274.

23. Amselem S, Gabizon A, Barenholz Y. Evaluation of a new extrusion device for the production of stable oligolamellar liposomes in a liter scale. *J Liposome Res* 1990;1:287–301.

24. Turanek J. Fast-protein liquid chromatography system as a tool for liposome preparation by the extrusion procedure. *Anal Biochem* 1994;218:352–357.

25. Nayar R, Hope MJ, Cullis PR. Generation of large unilamellar vesicles from long-chain saturated phosphatidylcholines by extrusion technique. *Biochim Biophys Acta* 1989;986:200–206.

26. Schneider T, Sachse A, Roessling G, et al. Large-scale production of liposomes of defined size by a new continuous high pressure extrusion device. *Drug Dev Ind Pharm* 1994;20:2787–2807.

27. Schneider T, Sachse A, Roessling G, et al. Generation of contrast-carrying liposomes of defined size with a new continuous high pressure extrusion method. *Int J Pharm* 1995;117:1–12.

28. Nicolay K, Van der Neut R, Fok JJ, et al. Effects of adriamycin on lipid polymorphism in cardiolipin-containing model and mitochondrial membranes. *Biochim Biophys Acta* 1985;819:55–65.

29. Mayer LD, Bally MB, Hope MJ, et al. Techniques for encapsulating bioactive agents into liposomes. *Chem Phys Lipids* 1986;40:333–345.

30. Szoka F, Jr., Papahadjopoulos D. Procedure for preparation of liposomes with large internal aqueous space and high capture by reverse-phase evaporation. *Proc Natl Acad Sci U S A* 1978;75:4194–4198.

31. Kirby C, Gregoriadis G. Dehydration-rehydration vesicles: a simple method for high yield drug entrapment in liposomes. *Biotechnology* 1984;2:979–984.

32. Deamer DW, Prince RC, Crofts AR. Response of fluorescent amines to pH gradients across liposome membranes. *Biochim Biophys Acta* 1972;274:323–335.

33. Madden TD, Harrigan PR, Tai LCL, et al. The accumulation of drugs within large unilamellar vesicles exhibiting a proton gradient: a survey. *Chem Phys Lipids* 1990; 53:37–46.

34. Haran G, Cohen R, Bar LK, et al. Transmembrane ammonium sulfate gradients in liposomes produce efficient and stable entrapment of amphipathic weak bases. *Biochim Biophys Acta* 1993;1151:201–215.

35. Lasic DD, Frederik PM, Stuart MCA, et al. Gelation of liposome interior. A novel method for drug encapsulation. *FEBS Lett* 1992;312:255–258.

36. Li X, Hirsh DJ, Cabral-Lilly D, et al. Doxorubicin physical state in solution and inside liposomes loaded via a pH gradient. *Biochim Biophys Acta* 1998;1415:23–40.

37. Abraham S, Edwards K, Karlsson G, et al. Formation of transition metal-doxorubicin complexes inside liposomes. *Biochim Biophys Acta* 2002;1565:41.

38. Unger C, Massing U, Moog R. *Method for the production of liposomal substance formulations.* Ger. Offen., 1999.

39. Moog R, Burger AM, Brandl M, et al. Change in pharmacokinetic and pharmacodynamic behavior of gemcitabine in human tumor xenografts upon entrapment in vesicular phospholipid gels. *Cancer Chemother Pharmacol* 2002;49:356–366.

40. Beijnen JH, Van der Houwen OAGJ, Underberg WJM. Aspects of the degradation kinetics of doxorubicin in aqueous solution. *Int J Pharm* 1986;32:123–131.

41. Moog R, Brandl M, Schubert R, et al. Effect of nucleoside analogs and oligonucleotides on hydrolysis of liposomal phospholipids. *Int J Pharm* 2000;206:43–53.

42. Stensrud G, Redford K, Smistad G, et al. Effects of gamma irradiation on solid and lyophilized phospholipids. *Rad Phys Chem* 1999;56:611–622.

43. Goldbach P, Brochart H, Wehrle P, et al. Sterile filtration of liposomes: retention of encapsulated carboxyfluorescein. *Int J Pharm* 1995;117:225–230.

44. Grit M, Underberg WJM, Crommelin DJA. Hydrolysis of saturated soybean phosphatidylcholine in aqueous liposome dispersions. *J Pharm Sci* 1993;82:362–366.

45. Grit M, Zuidam NJ, Underberg WJM, et al. Hydrolysis of partially saturated egg phosphatidylcholine in aqueous liposome dispersions and the effect of cholesterol incorporation on hydrolysis kinetics. *J Pharm Pharmacol* 1993;45:490–495.

46. Grit M, Crommelin DJA. The effect of surface charge on the hydrolysis kinetics of partially hydrogenated egg phosphatidylcholine and egg phosphatidylglycerol in aqueous liposome dispersions. *Biochim Biophys Acta* 1993;1167:49–55.

47. Zhang J-aA, Pawelchak J. Effect of pH, ionic strength and oxygen burden on the chemical stability of EPC/cholesterol liposomes under accelerated conditions. Part 1: lipid hydrolysis. *Eur J Pharm Biopharm* 2000;50:357–364.

48. Lutz J, Augustin A, Jaeger L, et al. Acute toxicity and depression of phagocytosis in vivo by liposomes: influence of lysophosphatidylcholine. *Life Sci* 1994; 56:99–106.

49. Brandl M, Bachmann D, Augustin AJ, et al. Depression

of the phagocytic activity of the RES by liposomes: influence of lipids. *Pharm Pharmacol Lett* 1994;4:1–4.

50. Boman NL, Tron VA, Bally MB, et al. Vincristine-induced dermal toxicity is significantly reduced when the drug is given in liposomes. *Cancer Chemother Pharmacol* 1996;37:351–355.

51. Herman EH, Rahman A, Ferrans VJ, et al. Prevention of chronic doxorubicin cardiotoxicity in beagles by liposomal encapsulation. *Cancer Res* 1983;43:5427–5432.

52. Working PK, Newman MS, Sullivan T, et al. Reduction of the cardiotoxicity of doxorubicin in rabbits and dogs by encapsulation in long-circulating, PEGylated liposomes. *J Pharmacol Exp Ther* 1999;289:1128–1133.

53. Northfelt DW, Martin FJ, Working P, et al. Doxorubicin encapsulated in liposomes containing surface-bound polyethylene glycol: pharmacokinetics, tumor localization, and safety in patients with AIDS-related Kaposi's sarcoma. *J Clin Pharmacol* 1996;36:55–63.

54. Patel HM. Serum opsonins and liposomes: their interaction and opsonophagocytosis. *Crit Rev Ther Drug Carrier Syst* 1992;9:39–90.

55. Scherphof G, Van Leeuwen B, Wilschut J, et al. Exchange of phosphatidylcholine between small unilamellar liposomes and human plasma high-density lipoprotein involves exclusively the phospholipid in the outer monolayer of the liposomal membrane. *Biochim Biophys Acta* 1983;732:595–599.

56. Rodrigueza WV, Phillips MC, Williams KJ. Structural and metabolic consequences of liposome-lipoprotein interactions. *Adv Drug Deliv Rev* 1998;32:31–43.

57. Lasic DD. Sterically stabilized vesicles. *Angew Chem* 1994;106:1765–1779. See also *Angew Chem Int Ed Engl* 1994;1733(1717):1685–1790.

58. Sachse A, Leike JU, Schneider T, et al. Biodistribution and computed tomography blood-pool imaging properties of polyethylene glycol-coated iopromide-carrying liposomes. *Invest Radiol* 1997;32:44–50.

59. Mayer LD, Reamer J, Bally MB. Intravenous pretreatment with empty pH gradient liposomes alters the pharmacokinetics and toxicity of doxorubicin through in vivo active drug encapsulation. *J Pharm Sci* 1999;88:96–102.

60. Gabizon A, Chisin R, Amselem S, et al. Pharmacokinetic and imaging studies in patients receiving a formulation of liposome-associated adriamycin. *Br J Cancer* 1991;64:1125–1132.

61. Abra RM, Hunt CA. Liposome disposition in vivo. III. Dose and vesicle-size effects. *Biochim Biophys Acta* 1981;666:493–503.

62. Liu D, Mori A, Huang L. Role of liposome size and RES blockade in controlling biodistribution and tumor uptake of GM1-containing liposomes. *Biochim Biophys Acta* 1992;1104:95–101.

63. Senior J, Crawley JCW, Gregoriadis G. Tissue distribution of liposomes exhibiting long half-lives in the circulation after intravenous injection. *Biochim Biophys Acta* 1985;839:1–8.

64. Allen TM, Hansen CB, de Menezes DEL. Pharmacokinetics of long-circulating liposomes. *Adv Drug Deliv Rev* 1995;16:267–284.

65. Wu NZ, Da D, Rudoll TL, et al. Increased microvascular permeability contributes to preferential accumulation of Stealth liposomes in tumor tissue. *Cancer Res* 1993;53:3765–3770.

66. Yuan F, Leunig M, Huang SK, et al. Microvascular permeability and interstitial penetration of sterically stabilized (stealth) liposomes in a human tumor xenograft. *Cancer Res* 1994;54:3352–3356.

67. Yuan F, Dellian M, Fukumura D, et al. Vascular permeability in a human tumor xenograft: molecular size dependence and cutoff size. *Cancer Res* 1995;55:3752–3756.

68. Symon Z, Peyser A, Tzemach D, et al. Selective delivery of doxorubicin to patients with breast carcinoma metastases by stealth liposomes. *Cancer* 1999;86:72–78.

69. Unezaki S, Maruyama K, Ishida O, et al. Enhanced tumor targeting and improved antitumor activity of doxorubicin by long-circulating liposomes containing amphipathic poly(ethylene glycol). *Int J Pharm* 1995; 126:41–48.

70. Hong RL, Huang CJ, Tseng YL, et al. Direct comparison of liposomal doxorubicin with or without polyethylene glycol coating in C-26 tumor-bearing mice: is surface coating with polyethylene glycol beneficial? *Clin Cancer Res* 1999;5:3645–3652.

71. Li WM, Xue L, Mayer LD, et al. Intermembrane transfer of polyethylene glycol-modified phosphatidylethanolamine as a means to reveal surface-associated binding ligands on liposomes. *Biochim Biophys Acta* 2001;1513:193–206.

72. Adlakha-Hutcheon G, Bally MB, Shew CR, et al. Controlled destabilization of a liposomal drug delivery system enhances mitoxantrone antitumor activity. *Nat Biotechnol* 1999;17:775–779.

73. Needham D, Anyarambhatla G, Kong G, et al. A new temperature-sensitive liposome for use with mild hyperthermia: characterization and testing in a human tumor xenograft model. *Cancer Res* 2000;60:1197–1201.

74. Duzgunes N, Nir S. Mechanisms and kinetics of liposome-cell interactions. *Adv Drug Deliv Rev* 1999;40:3–18.

75. Huang A, Kennel SJ, Huang L. Interactions of immunoliposomes with target cells. *J Biol Chem* 1983;258:14034–14040.

76. Suzuki S, Inoue K, Hongoh A, et al. Modulation of doxorubicin resistance in a doxorubicin-resistant human leukemia cell by an immunoliposome targeting transferring receptor. *Br J Cancer* 1997;76:83–89.

77. Koning GA, Gorter A, Scherphof GL, et al. Antiproliferative effect of immunoliposomes containing 5-fluorodeoxyuridine dipalmitate on colon cancer cells. *Br J Cancer* 1999;80:1718–1725.

78. Maruyama K, Ishida O, Takizawa T, et al. Possibility of active targeting to tumor tissues with liposomes. *Adv Drug Deliv Rev* 1999;40:89–102.

79. Hafez IM, Cullis PR. Roles of lipid polymorphism in intracellular delivery. *Adv Drug Deliv Rev* 2001;47:139–148.

80. Kirpotin D, Hong K, Mullah N, et al. Liposomes with detachable polymer coating: destabilization and fusion of dioleoylphosphatidylethanolamine vesicles triggered by cleavage of surface-grafted poly(ethylene glycol). *FEBS Lett* 1996;388:115–118.

81. Michieli M, Damiani D, Ermacora A, et al. Liposome-encapsulated daunorubicin for PGP-related multidrug resistance. *Br J Haematol* 1999;106:92–99.

82. Michieli M, Damiani D, Ermacora A, et al. Liposome encapsulated daunorubicin doubles anthracycline toxicity in cell lines showing a non-PGP related multidrug resistance. *Haematologica* 1999;84:1151–1152.

83. Thierry AR, Jorgensen TJ, Forst D, et al. Multidrug resistance in Chinese hamster cells: effect of liposome-

encapsulated doxorubicin. *Cancer Commun* 1989;1: 311–316.

84. Rahman A, Husain SR, Siddiqui J, et al. Liposome-mediated modulation of multidrug resistance in human HL–60 leukemia cells. *J Natl Cancer Inst* 1992;84: 1909–1915.

85. Wang Y, Eksborg S, Lewensohn R, et al. In vitro cellular accumulation and cytotoxicity of liposomal and conventional formulations of daunorubicin and doxorubicin in resistant K562 cells. *Anticancer Drugs* 1999;10: 921–928.

86. Goren D, Horowitz AT, Tzemach D, et al. Nuclear delivery of doxorubicin via folate-targeted liposomes with bypass of multidrug-resistance efflux pump. *Clin Cancer Res* 2000;6:1949–1957.

87. Gregoriadis G, Neerunjun ED. Treatment of tumor bearing mice with liposome-entrapped actinomycin D prolongs their survival. *Res Commun Chem Pathol Pharmacol* 1975;10:351–362.

88. Harrington KJ. Liposomal cancer chemotherapy: current clinical applications and future prospects. *Expert Opin Invest Drugs* 2001;10:1045–1061.

17

Polymer-Drug Conjugates

Ruth Duncan

*Centre for Polymer Therapeutics, Welsh School of Pharmacy, Cardiff University,
Cardiff CF10 3XF, United Kingdom*

Over the last decade, 11 polymer–drug conjugates have entered phase I or II clinical trial as intravenous injectable anticancer agents. Their early clinical profile looks promising. These macromolecular prodrugs comprise a minimum of three components: a natural or synthetic water-soluble polymeric carrier (usually molecular weight 10–100 kd); a biodegradable polymer–drug linkage, and a bioactive antitumor agent. In certain cases, ligands for receptor-mediated targeting have also been incorporated, but with less success. Only one targeted polymer conjugate has so far reached clinical trial. With careful design of the polymer–drug linker, the toxicity of bound drug can be significantly reduced (a more than fivefold increase in the maximum tolerated dose has been reported clinically for a polymer–doxorubicin conjugate). Antitumor activity has been seen in chemotherapy-refractory patients with hints (preclinical and clinical) that polymer conjugation may bypass multidrug resistance. This new class of polymer therapeutic radically changes the pharmacokinetics of the bound drug. Conjugates with prolonged circulation times target tumors by the enhanced permeability and retention (EPR) effect. Once in the tumor interstitium, the polymer–drug can only enter cells by the endocytic route, leading to lysosomotropic drug delivery. Several conjugates have peptidyl polymer–drug linkers amenable to cleavage by lysosomal thiol-dependent proteases. In this case, prodrug activation occurs intracellularly. In contrast, other conjugates that contain an ester link between drug and polymer can release drug by chemical hydrolysis or esterase degradation extracellularly. This chapter will review those polymer–drug conjugates that have entered clinical development, summarize the rationale for design of preclinical lead compounds, and discuss the challenges facing effective and clinical development of these complex macromolecular prodrugs.

BACKGROUND

Helmut Ringsdorf first proposed the concept of polymer–anticancer conjugates in 1975 (1). These macromolecular prodrugs comprise a minimum of three components (shown schematically in Fig. 17.1): a natural or synthetic water-soluble polymeric carrier (molecular weight 10–100 kd), a biodegradable polymer–drug linkage, and a bioactive antitumor agent. Not surprisingly, the first conjugates synthesized incorporated the most important anticancer agents of that era, particularly anthracycline antibiotics (daunorubicin and doxorubicin), alkylating agents (cyclophosphamide and melphalan), and antimetabolites (methotrexate and fluorouracil). In the early 1990s, these first-generation conjugates entered clinical trial (2). More recently, an increasing number of conjugates containing more modern anticancer agents, particularly paclitaxel and camptothecin, are being transferred into the clinic (Table 17.1).

Normally, polymer–drug conjugates achieve tumor-specific targeting because of the EPR effect (3). Hyperpermeable angiogenic tumor vessels allow preferential extravasation of circulating macromolecules and liposomes, and once in the interstitium they are retained there because of lack of intratumoral lymphatic drainage. This leads to significant tumor targeting (more than 10-fold to 100-fold compared with free drug) and levels up to 20% dose/g have been reported, depending on tumor size. Smaller tumors exhibit the highest concentration of polymer–drug. Conjugates can also been synthesized to contain ligands to promote receptor-mediated targeting (antibodies, peptides, and saccharides). Although this is an attractive possibility, so far only one such conjugate has progressed into phase I trial.

Initially, people were slow to accept this concept. Polymer–drug conjugates were viewed as an impractical mix of polymer and organic chemistry resulting in compounds so complicated they would never be developed clinically. These conceptual difficulties

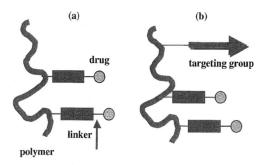

FIG. 17.1. Polymer–anticancer conjugates designed for **(A)** passive tumour targeting by the enhanced permeability and retention (EPR) effect and **(B)** receptor-mediated targeting.

were compounded by the fact that polymers used medically have many different forms, including implants, gels, and pharmaceutical excipients in the form of tablets and as solutions for injection. Oncologists have become increasingly familiar with biodegradable polymeric implants. Either used as a subcutaneous depot to slowly release luteinizing hormone-releasing hormone analogues (e.g., goserelin acetate, Zoladex; leuprolide acetate, Lupron Depot) (4) for treatment of prostate and other hormone-dependent cancers, or for implantation used after surgery to locally deliver chemotherapy for the treatment of patients with residual or recurrent disease (e.g., Gliadel) (5).

Our research [supported by the Cancer Research Campaign (CRC) and Farmitalia Carlo Erba (now Pharmacia) in collaboration with the Institute of Macromolecular Chemistry, Prague] designed the first two synthetic polymer–drug conjugates to enter clinical trial as intravenous injectable anticancer agents (6–12). Transfer of these N-(2-hydroxypropyl)methacrylamide (HPMA) copolymer–drug conjugates into good clinical practice (GCP) clinical trials in Europe, coupled with the commercialization

of polymer–protein conjugates (e.g., polyethylene glycol (PEG)-L-asparaginase, Oncaspar) in the United States (13), was the breakthrough that led to exponential growth of interest in polymer therapeutics.

Eleven polymer–drug conjugates have now entered phase I and II trials and further compounds are reported in preclinical development. In this chapter, these compounds are reviewed, lessons learned regarding design of polymer–drug conjugates are summarized, and the challenges for effective preclinical and clinical development are discussed. It should be emphasized that there are still few primary publications reporting verified clinical data, and the latest information has often been presented in abstract form or posted on company Web sites; furthermore, conjugate chemistry is often inadequately defined. Nonetheless, the emerging clinical results provide a great opportunity for the first time to compare and contrast preclinical and clinical data for each compound, and also to begin to understand how best to optimize the clinical dose and schedule for this exciting and completely novel class of antitumor agents.

POLYMER–DRUG CONJUGATES IN CLINICAL DEVELOPMENT

Conjugates that have entered phase I clinical trial are listed in Table 17.1. Early results have generally been promising, and antitumor activity has been seen in chemotherapy-refractory patients in many studies. These conjugates can be categorized into three groups as follows:

1. Conjugates that have progressed further to phase I and II trials, which include HPMA copolymer–doxorubicin (PK1), HPMA copolymer–doxorubicin-galactose (PK2), HPMA copolymer–platinate (AP5280), and poly(L-glutamic acid) (PG)-paclitaxel (CT-2103).

TABLE 17.1. *Polymer–drug conjugates in early clinical trials as anticancer agents*

Polymer–drug conjugate	Status	Reference(s)
Dextran–doxorubicin (AD-70, DOX-OXD).	Phase 1	14
HPMA copolymer–doxorubicin (PK1, FCE28068)	Phase 2	2,15
HPMA copolymer–doxorubicin-galactosamine (FCE28069)	Phase 1/2	16–18
HPMA copolymer–paclitaxel (PNU166945)	Phase 1	19
HPMA copolymer–camptothecin (MAG-CPT, PCNU166148)	Phase 1	20,21
HPMA copolymer–platinate (AP5280)	Phase 1	22–24
PG–paclitaxel (CT-2103)	Phase 1/2	25–27
PG–camptothecin (CT-2106)	Phase 1	28
PEG–camptothecin (PROTHECAN)	Phase 1	29
PEG–paclitaxel	Phase 1	30
Polysaccharide camptothecin (DE-310)	Phase 1	31,32

HPMA, N-(2-hydroxypropyl)methacrylamide; PG, poly(L-glutamic acid); PEG, polyethylene glycol.

2. Conjugates that have failed because of unacceptable toxicity of the conjugate, such as HPMA copolymer–paclitaxel (PNU166945), and HPMA copolymer–camptothecin (PNU166148), probably because the polymer–drug linkage is inadequate.

3. Conjugates that have failed, such as dextran–doxorubicin (AD-70, DOX-OXD), probably because of toxicity of the polymer carrier.

HPMA Copolymer Conjugates

The first synthetic polymer–drug conjugate to enter clinical evaluation was HPMA copolymer–doxorubicin (PK1, FCE28068) in 1994 (2). Since then, four other anticancer compounds and two γ-camera imaging agents derived from this polymer have been evaluated clinically. The homopolymer[1] poly-HPMA was originally developed in the Czech Republic as a plasma expander (33). It was nontoxic in preclinical tests at doses up to 30 g/kg, did not bind blood proteins, and was not immunogenic. Moreover, like PEG, grafting of HPMA copolymer chains to proteins reduces their immunogenicity (34).

To include the functionality needed for drug conjugation, HPMA copolymers[2] were prepared (35). Synthesis involves free-radical precipitation polymerization of HPMA and methacryloylated (MA)-peptidyl-nitrophenylester (ONp) as co-monomers. Normally, a monomer feed ratio of HPMA:MA-peptide-ONp of 95:5 is used, although this ratio has been varied. MA-tyrosinamide has also been included as a third comonomer (1 mol%[3]) to prepare analogues for radioiodination. These analogues have been used for pharmacokinetic (^{125}I labeling) (36,37) and γ-camera imaging studies (^{131}I or ^{123}I-labelling) (2,17,38,39). Depending on comonomer chemistry it is possible to synthesize an HPMA copolymer precursor of relatively narrow molecular weight distribution (Mw/Mn = 1.2–1.5)[4]. Early studies showed doxoru-

---

[1] A homopolymer consists of a single monomer that has been polymerized to give the polymer.

[2] A copolymer consists of two or more monomers that have been copolymerized to give the polymer.

[3] Mol% describes the fraction of monomers per 100 along the backbone of the polymer chain. Thus, 1 mol% indicates a ratio of 1 per 100 monomer units.

[4] Polymer molecular weight is defined in terms of the weight average molecular weight (Mw) and number average molecular weight (Mn). The distribution of molecular weights in any product is defined by the term polydispersity = Mw/Mn. A polymer preparation containing molecules of uniform chain length has a Mw/Mn = 1. Many natural polymers have a Mw/Mn > 2. Such a wide range of molecular weights in each batch of polymer is a major disadvantage for pharmaceutically active polymers. The different pharmacokinetics of polymer chains of significantly different size can lead to unacceptable variation in toxicity and efficacy.

bicin attachment to HPMA copolymers led to a more than 10-fold increase in solubility. This "solubilizing" property of hydrophilic polymers has subsequently been used to improve the formulation properties of other lipophilic drugs. The -C-C-HPMA copolymer main chain is not biodegradable, so all conjugates developed clinically have been limited to a molecular weight of less than 40,000 d to ensure eventual renal elimination.

HPMA Copolymer–Doxorubicin (PK1, FCE28068)

PK1 was the first lead compound arising from our research program supported by CRC and licensed to Farmitalia Carlo Erba. Both institutions supported clinical development via the CRC Phase I/II Clinical Trials Programme. FCE28068 was synthesized by aminolysis of an HPMA copolymer-Gly-(D,L)Phe-Leu-Gly-ONp precursor (HPMA:MA-peptide-ONp 95:5) with doxorubicin (Fig. 17.2) (40–42). The conjugate used in phase I clinical trial had a molecular weight of approximately 30,000 d, a doxorubicin content of approximately 8.5 wt%, and a free doxorubicin content of less than 2% of the total doxorubicin. The

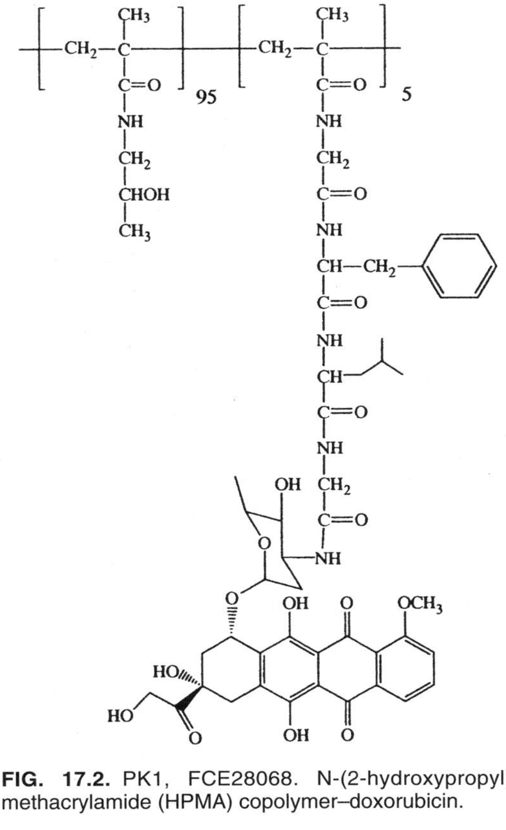

FIG. 17.2. PK1, FCE28068. N-(2-hydroxypropyl) methacrylamide (HPMA) copolymer–doxorubicin.

Gly-Phe-Leu-Gly linker was designed for cleavage by thiol-dependent proteases, particularly lysosomal cathepsin B (43). Racemization of -Phe- was an unfortunate artifact of the synthetic procedure first used to prepare the tetrapeptide linker (i.e., sequential addition of the dipeptides). However, comparison of (D,L)Phe-, (D)Phe- and (L)Phe-containing linkers confirmed that the racemization had no significant effect on drug release rate or antitumor activity *in vivo*. In aqueous solution, PK1 molecules form unimolecular micelles (44) that are approximately 6 nm in diameter. The Phe-Leu–containing peptidyl side chains and approximately four molecules of doxorubicin per polymer chain associate to form a more hydrophobic internal core, whereas the hydrophilic polymer orients to the exterior. It is noteworthy that early estimates of the Mw of HPMA copolymer–anthracycline conjugates were low (Mw = 20,000–25,000 d); however, these values were estimated using nonvalidated methods with inappropriate polymer calibration standards.

Preclinical studies showed remarkable antitumor activity of PK1 coupled with reduced toxicity, and these observations justified the move to clinical evaluation (7,15). During a phase I trial, FCE28068 was administered as a short infusion every 3 weeks (2). Conscious of the potential osmotic impact of a macromolecular prodrug, the infusion rate (4.16 mL/min) and concentration (2 mg/mL doxorubicin-equivalent) were kept the same during dose escalation, and thus infusion time was gradually extended. Dose escalation progressed cautiously as neither poly-HPMA nor any HPMA copolymers had previously been administered to humans. Standard phase I entry criteria were used for patient selection. However, because vascular permeability was considered not only an opportunity for EPR-mediated tumor targeting but also potentially toxic, patients with known brain metastases were excluded from this trial. A starting dose of 20 mg/m^2 (doxorubicin equivalent) was chosen [one tenth the dose estimated as lethal for 10% of the test animal population (LD$_{10}$) in mouse preclinical studies (45)] and escalation progressed to a maximum tolerated dose (MTD) of 320 mg/m^2 (doxorubicin equivalent) (2). An FCE28068 dose of 280 mg/m^2 was recommended as the phase II dose.

No polymer-related toxicity (or immunogenicity) was observed. The dose-limiting toxicity (DLT) was typical of the anthracyclines and included febrile neutropenia and mucositis. The time to nadir of neutrophil counts was typically 15 to 21 days. Interestingly, alopecia was not observed until dose escalation to 180 mg/m^2 or above, and nausea was mild without need for antiemetics up to doses of 240 mg/m^2. However, the usual anthracycline cardiotoxicity was ab-

sent, despite individual cumulative FCE28068 doses of up to 1,680 mg/m^2 (doxorubicin-equivalent). It should be noted that these cumulative doses represent more than 20 g/m^2 of HPMA copolymer. Lack of any HPMA copolymer-associated toxicity justified the subsequent clinical trails of the related conjugates based on this polymer.

FCE28068 administration produced two partial and two minor responses in the cohort of 36 patients enrolled. These were in patients with non–small cell lung cancer (NSCLC), colorectal cancer, and anthracycline-resistant breast cancer at 80 mg/m^2 (doxorubicin-equivalent) and anthracycline-naive breast cancer. Observation of antitumor activity in cancers considered resistant/refractory to conventional chemotherapy at lower doxorubicin doses (80–180 mg/m^2) was consistent with contribution of the EPR effect to tumor targeting and activity in an epirubicin-resistant patient.

Preclinical pharmacokinetics showed very little free doxorubicin in plasma after PK1 administration in mice (46). Compared to free drug (t$_{1/2}$ α = 4 min) the conjugate t$_{1/2}$ was considerably longer than 1 or 2 hours. Clinical pharmacokinetics were assessed by HPLC and also using a ^{131}I-labelled analogue for γ-camera imaging (2). The distribution profile in humans was similar to that seen in the preclinical studies: prolonged plasma circulation, absence of liver accumulation, and significant renal elimination (50%–75% over 24 h) over time. FCE28068 had a t$_{1/2}$ α = 1.8 hours and t$_{1/2}$ β = 93 hours. There was no evidence of dose dependency of pharmacokinetics. Imaging with a ^{131}I-labelled FCE28068 analogue generally showed poor resolution. Uptake was however seen in known tumor sites in 6 of the 21 patients studied, and radioactivity was particularly visible in a head-and-neck primary tumor. Here, the tumor levels of radioactivity were 2.2% dose at 2 or 3 hours, 1.3 % dose at 24 hours, and 0.5 % dose after 8 days. Although full publication of the phase II results are awaited, it has been reported that FCE28068 showed no activity in a colorectal cancer, but again activity has been seen in breast cancer and NSCLC (47).

HPMA Copolymer–Doxorubicin-galactosamine (PK2, FCE28069)

PK2, FCE28069 was the second compound emanating from our CRC-funded research program. It was also developed via the CRC Phase I/II Clinical Trials Programme in collaboration with Farmitalia Carlo Erba. FCE28069 (Fig. 17.3) contains doxorubicin bound to the polymer backbone via a Gly-(D,L)Phe-Leu-Gly linker and it also contains galactosamine,

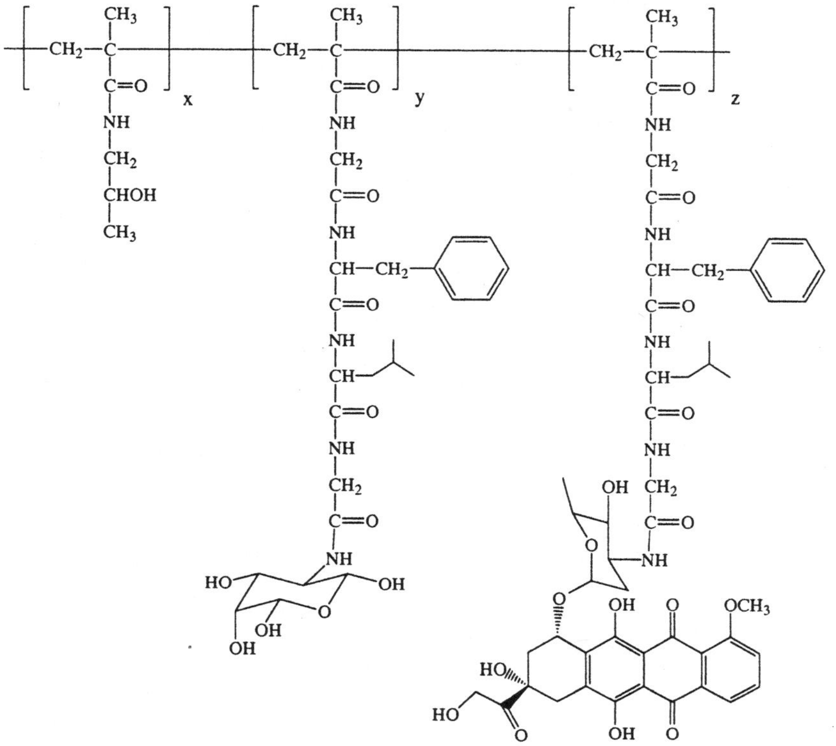

FIG. 17.3. PK2, FCE28069. N-(2-hydroxypropyl)methacrylamide (HPMA) copolymer–doxorubicin-galactosamine.

included to promote liver targeting. In this case, the polymer precursor is synthesized using a monomer feed ratio of HPMA:MA-peptide-ONp adjusted to 90:10 (40–42) to provide the additional side chains needed for conjugation of both doxorubicin and galactosamine. FCE28069 has a slightly lower molecular weight (Mw approximately 25,000 d) because of the changed polymerization conditions, a doxorubicin content of approximately 7.5 wt%, and a free doxorubicin content less than 2% total doxorubicin. The galactosamine content was 1.5 to 2.5 mol%. PK2 is less water soluble than PK1 because of the increased content of relatively hydrophobic Phe-Leu–containing side chains.

This galactosamine-containing conjugate was the first synthetic biomimetic (of an asialoglycoprotein) polymer. It is also the only "targeted" polymer–drug conjugate to enter a GCP clinical trial so far. Physiologically, loss of terminal sialic acid residues from ageing glycoproteins exposes galactose signaling plasma clearance. Endocytic uptake by hepatocytes after interaction with the asialoglycoprotein receptor (ASGR) leads to lysosomal trafficking and their sub-

sequent degradation (48). PK2 was designed with the aim of improving treatment of primary hepatocellular carcinoma and metastatic liver disease. The latter would only be feasible if released drug diffused into liver metastases and could act via to the "bystander effect." PK1 is not inherently hepatotropic, but preclinical studies confirmed that addition of galactosamine to HPMA copolymers promoted significant hepatocyte targeting after intravenous injection (approximately 80% of the dose) (16). The magnitude of targeting (percent dose) was markedly dose dependent because of ASGR receptor saturation (49).

Phase I evaluation of FCE28069 was conducted in 31 patients, 23 of whom had primary hepatoma (18). In this case, the objectives were establishment of both the MTD and pharmacokinetics using a ^{123}I-labelled FCE28069 γ-camera imaging analogue and HPLC analysis. FCE28069 was given intravenously every 3 weeks. The initial infusion rate was 4.16 mL/min (2 mg/mL doxorubicin-equivalent), but because of pain during infusion, this was reduced to 2 mL/min with a 1.0-mg/mL solution. Six patients were given FCE28069 by 24-hour infusion to see if this improved targeting efficiency. The starting dose was again 20 mg/m^2 (doxorubicin-equivalent) and the FCE28069 MTD was 160 mg/m^2. As for FCE28068, the DLTs were typical of anthracyclines, principally myelosuppression and mucositis. Interestingly the FCE28069 MTD was significantly lower than seen for FCE28068, and the authors speculated that this might be due to the presence of extrahepatic galactose receptors. Although this is possible, the pharmacokinetic data were not indicative of normal tissue targeting, other than the hint of lung localization at early times in the γ-camera images. It is more likely that the reduced solubility of FCE28069 contributed to this change in toxicity profile. The reactions seen on infusion would be consistent with this hypothesis, as would transient lung localization of polymer aggregates. The lower MTD of FCE28069 emphasizes the need to examine carefully the physico-chemical properties of each HPMA copolymer conjugate on its own merit. In this case FCE28069 does have a higher content of the relatively hydrophobic peptidyl side chains (10 mol%).

Of the 23 patients treated who had primary hepatocellular carcinoma, 2 had a measurable partial response, which at the time of report were lasting longer than 26 and 47 months, respectively (18). A third patient showed reduction in tumor volume and 11 had stable disease. Plasma levels of FCE28069 determined by HPLC were indistinguishable from those seen using radioactivity, and pharmacokinetics were linear with increasing dose. Less than 0.1% of the plasma levels of doxorubicin were free drug, and urinary excretion at 24 hours was 5%. Single-photon emission computed tomography γ-camera imaging showed FCE28069 liver levels of 15% to 20% dose at 24 hours. The majority of radioactivity was associated with normal liver (16.9% after 24 hours) with lower accumulations within hepatic tumor (3.2% dose). This was fivefold lower than levels seen in normal liver, but not surprising because hepatoma loses the ASGR receptor as disease progresses. Even so, it was estimated that this doxorubicin concentration in hepatoma would still be 12-fold to 50-fold higher than could be achieved with administration of free doxorubicin. Interestingly, a clavicular metastasis arising in a hepatoma patient showed clear FCE28069 localization using γ-camera imaging.

The extent of FCE28069 liver localization seen clinically was lower than observed in preclinical studies with PK2 (16), possibly because of a lower number of ASGR receptors present on human versus rat hepatocytes. However, it is noteworthy that the FCE28069 conjugates used in the clinic had lower galactose content (1.5–2.0 mol%) than suggested as optimal for liver targeting in preclinical studies (approximately 4 mol%) (16). It is well known that the asialoglycoprotein receptor requires a multivalent ligand, and so a high galactose density along the polymer chain is crucial if maximum liver targeting is to be achieved. Lack of increased liver uptake after a 24-hour infusion of FCE28069 was suggested as indicative of lack of receptor saturation. However, comparisons of liver levels were made at 24 hours, which may not be the best time point for comparative studies because hepatocyte targeting is usually rapid (approximately 5 min), and at longer time points, liver levels are complicated by elimination due to hepatobiliary transfer and excretion.

HPMA Copolymer–Paclitaxel (PNU166945)

The poor water solubility of paclitaxel combined with hypersensitivity reactions associated with the standard ethanol and Cremophor formulation made it a good candidate for polymer conjugation. Pharmacia developed an HPMA copolymer conjugate of paclitaxel, with the aim of improving drug solubility and subsequent "controlled release" of paclitaxel thereafter. First, a glycine derivative of paclitaxel was synthesized via the 2′ position of paclitaxel, and this was attached to an HPMA copolymer precursor containing -Gly-Phe-Leu- peptide side chains. In this case, drug is linked via the same tetrapeptide linkage used to create PK1 and PK2 with the addition of a terminal ester bond. The resulting conjugate (PNU166945) (Fig. 17.4) was more soluble than paclitaxel (more than 2 mg/mL conjugate compared to 0.0001 mg/mL paclitaxel) and had a drug content of approximately 5 wt%. (19). This loading is low considering the decreased potency of paclitaxel compared to doxorubicin. Theoretically, paclitaxel or peptidyl derivatives will be released from the polymer by hydrolytic or enzymatic (esterase) degradation of the ester bond, or by proteolytic cleavage of the peptidyl linker.

In the phase I study, PNU166945 was administered by a 1-hour infusion every 3 weeks (19). The starting dose of 80 mg/m^2 (paclitaxel-equivalent) was one third the MTD in dogs. The highest PNU166945 dose administered was 196 mg/m^2 (paclitaxel-equivalent), although no DLTs were seen at this level. The toxicity observed was consistent with commonly observed paclitaxel toxicities, including flulike symptoms, mild nausea and vomiting, mild hematologic toxicity, and neuropathy. Neurotoxicity (grade 2) occurred in two patients at a dose of 140 mg/m^2 (although these patients had preexisting grade 1 neurotoxicity on study entry) and one patient at 196 mg/m^2 had grade 3 neuropathy after the fourth cycle. Interestingly, alopecia

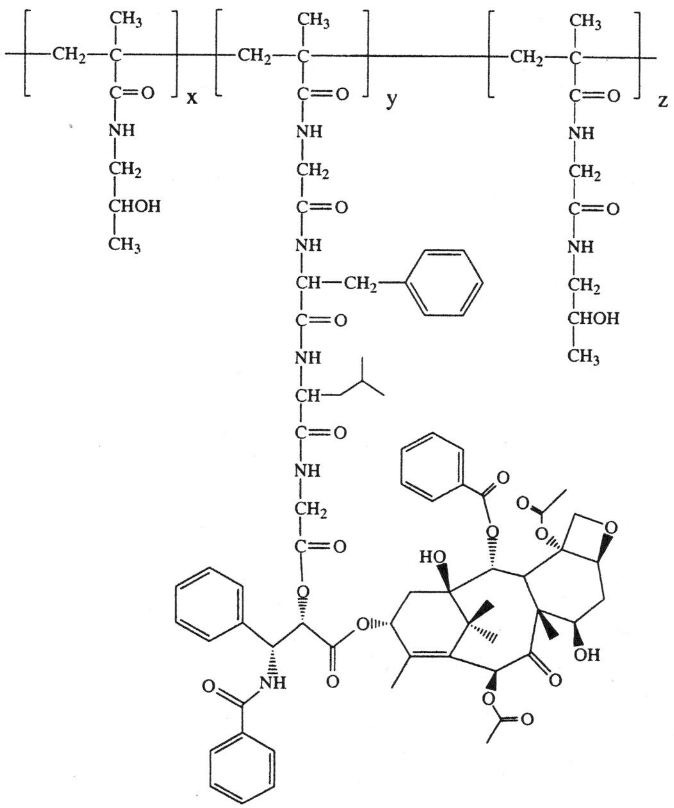

FIG. 17.4. N-(2-hydroxypropyl)methacrylamide (HPMA) copolymer–paclitaxel.

was absent throughout the study. Disappointingly, dose escalation was discontinued prematurely in this trial. Apparently, studies were curtailed because of concerns of potential clinical neurotoxicity following observations in preclinical animal studies (19) and fear that the risks might outweigh the benefits. Even so, in this small patient cohort antitumor activity was also observed. A patient with paclitaxel-refractory breast cancer showed remission of skin metastases after two courses at 100 mg/m^2 (paclitaxel equivalent). Two other patients had stable disease at a dose of 140 mg/m^2. Plasma pharmacokinetics were measured over 48 hours using HPLC and was linear with dose both for PNU166945 and the released paclitaxel. The conjugate had a t$_{1/2}$ approximately 6.5 hours and its volume of distribution indicated plasma circulation. Free paclitaxel released from the conjugate had a t$_{1/2}$ of approximately 1.2 hours and free drug levels were low, approximately1% of the paclitaxel present in plasma as conjugate. It is noteworthy that, as for FCE28068, antitumor activity was seen at a relatively low paclitaxel dose (100 mg/m^2). Conclusion of the phase I trial would have been interesting, as data regarding the phase II dose and possible schedule optimization would have been made available.

HPMA Copolymer–Camptothecin (MAG-CPT; PNU 166148)

Camptothecins have poor solubility and their nonspecific toxicity has also made them attractive candidates for polymer conjugation. Pharmacia also developed a series of HPMA copolymer–camptothecin conjugates (20,50). Again, the only option for drug conjugation was an ester linkage. The HPMA copolymer–camptothecin conjugates (so-called MAG-CPT derivatives) were synthesized from an HPMA copolymer precursor composed of HPMA: methacryloyl-glycine (MA-Gly)-ONp 95:5 or 90:10 (Fig. 17.5); hence, the MAG acronym used to describe this copolymer. This has caused some confusion and, to be clear, the MAG polymer is simply an HPMA copolymer synthesized

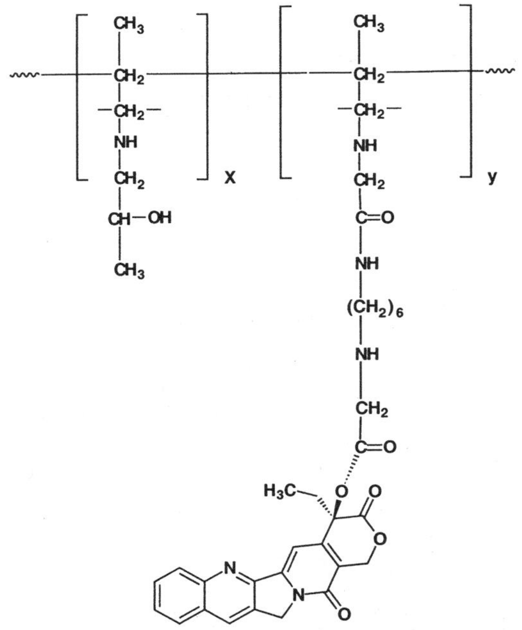

FIG. 17.5. N-(2-hydroxypropyl)methacrylamide (HPMA) copolymer–camptothecin.

via a different route. Camptothecin was first modified at the C-20 α-hydroxy group to give a peptidyl prodrug (e.g., Gly-camptothecin) and then bound to the polymer intermediate. The resultant conjugates had an Mw of 20,00 to 30,000 d depending on their side-chain content, and a camptothecin loading of 5 to 10 wt%. Although conjugates containing a library of different peptidyl linkers were examined preclinically, the conjugate PNU166148 (MAG-CPT) containing the Gly-C_6-Gly-linkage was selected for phase I clinical studies. Camptothecin is released from this conjugate either by chemical or by esterase-mediated hydrolysis.

Two dosing schedules were studied during phase I evaluation of MAG-CPT: an intravenous infusion over 30 minutes every 28 days (21), and as an alternative (three times) daily treatment repeated every 4 weeks (51). In the first study (21), 62 patients were entered starting at a dose of 30 mg/m^2 (camptothecin equivalent). Dose escalation progressed to an MTD of 240 mg/m^2 with 200 mg/m^2 as the recommended dose for further studies. At 240 mg/m^2, the DLTs included grade 4 neutropenia and thrombocytopenia and grade 3 diarrhea. Severe and unpredictable cystitis was also seen.

In the recently reported phase I study (51), MAG-CPT was administered as a 30-minute infusion on 3 consecutive days every 4 weeks. The starting dosage was 17 mg/m^2 per day and this was escalated to 130 mg/m^2 per day (i.e., total dose per cycle = 390 mg/m^2). Hematologic toxicity was rare, but cumulative bladder toxicity was dose limiting at doses of 68 mg/m^2 or greater. This could only be resolved by withdrawal of treatment. Of the 16 patients entered in this trial, 11 were evaluable for clinical responses after two courses. These two phase I studies were the first involving HPMA copolymer conjugates in which no objective clinical responses were seen. However, one patient with renal cell carcinoma had tumor shrinkage, and a patient with colon cancer had stable disease for 62 days.

Using HPLC analysis, no dose dependency of plasma clearance of either MAG-CPT or the released drug was seen (51,52). Plasma levels of free camptothecin were 100 times lower than conjugated drug, and there was no significant difference in terminal half-lives (approximately 8–10 days) of free and polymer bound drug. Camptothecin (measured as total drug) was still appearing in urine at 4 weeks with approximately 69% dose excreted in urine after 4 days. Patients with the most severe symptoms of renal toxicity had a relatively higher plasma area under the curve of MAG-CPT, which was attributed to impaired renal function.

Bladder toxicity of MAG-CPT had not been anticipated. However, early studies with camptothecins did highlight toxicities, including vomiting, diarrhea, and chemical or hemorrhagic cystitis. The acidic environment in bladder causes formation of the insoluble lactone form of camptothecin. Bladder toxicity of MAG-CPT has been attributed to variable conversion of the inactive open ring form to the active closed ring form of the drug. However, the biodistribution of the compound would also have contributed to this effect. HPMA copolymer molecular weight has been specifically optimized to ensure effective renal elimination. This has been clearly visualized by γ-camera imaging of other HPMA copolymer conjugates. There is always a likelihood of kidney or bladder toxicity if the polymer–drug linker degrades in urine to deliver high local doses of any cytotoxic agent. As urinary excretion of the MAG-CPT is very high (66% at 24 hours) and the conjugate was still detectable in urine after 4 weeks (51,52), bladder toxicity was perhaps not surprising.

HPMA Copolymer–Platinate (AP5280)

Although the HPMA copolymer–melphalan conjugates that we developed in the 1980s (53) did not proceed to clinical development, more recently a library of HPMA copolymer–platinates synthesized as "cis-platin" or "carboplatin" mimetics (22,23) (Fig. 17.6) have produced a clinical candidate. These conjugates were also prepared from HPMA copolymer precursors containing either -Gly-Gly-ONp or Gly-Phe-Leu-Gly-ONp side chains (5 or 10 mol%). The side chains were modified by hydrolysis (-COOH) or aminolysis with ethylenediamine (en), aminomalonate, or aminoaspartate to provide the terminal ligands for platination. An HPMA copolymer Gly-Phe-Leu-Gly-en-Pt required lysosomal activation to release active platinum species, and this was confirmed by the observation that conjugates containing the nondegradable linker -Gly-Gly-en-Pt were completely inactive *in vivo*. Whereas the -COO-Pt released platinum species much too rapidly for useful delivery (i.e., it would simply fall apart in plasma after injection), the malonate derivative showed a slower, more useful rate of hydrolysis (23). Access Pharmaceuticals selected this compound for preclini-

cal development. Using platinum nuclear magnetic resonance (NMR), it has been shown that the malonate ring rearranges with time to the more thermodynamically favorable structure (AP5280) shown in Figure 17.7. AP5280 has a Mw = 25,000 d and Mw/Mn = 1.7; the platinum content is approximately 7 wt%. Phase I studies were conducted in Europe and although the results have not yet been formally reported, Access Pharmaceuticals have stated that the initial AP5280 dose administered was 90 mg/m^2 (platinum-equivalent) with escalation to 1,440 mg/m^2 (platinum-equivalent) without observation of DLT. It is also stated that a phase II program is being planned. A second lead HPMA copolymer–platinate (AP5346) has been identified with a similar Gly-Phe-Leu-Gly-aminomalonate side chain, but in this case terminating in a 1,2-diaminocyclohexyl (DACH) platinate (Fig. 17.7) (54). The compound, AP5346, is currently under preclinical development with trials planned to commence at the end of 2002.

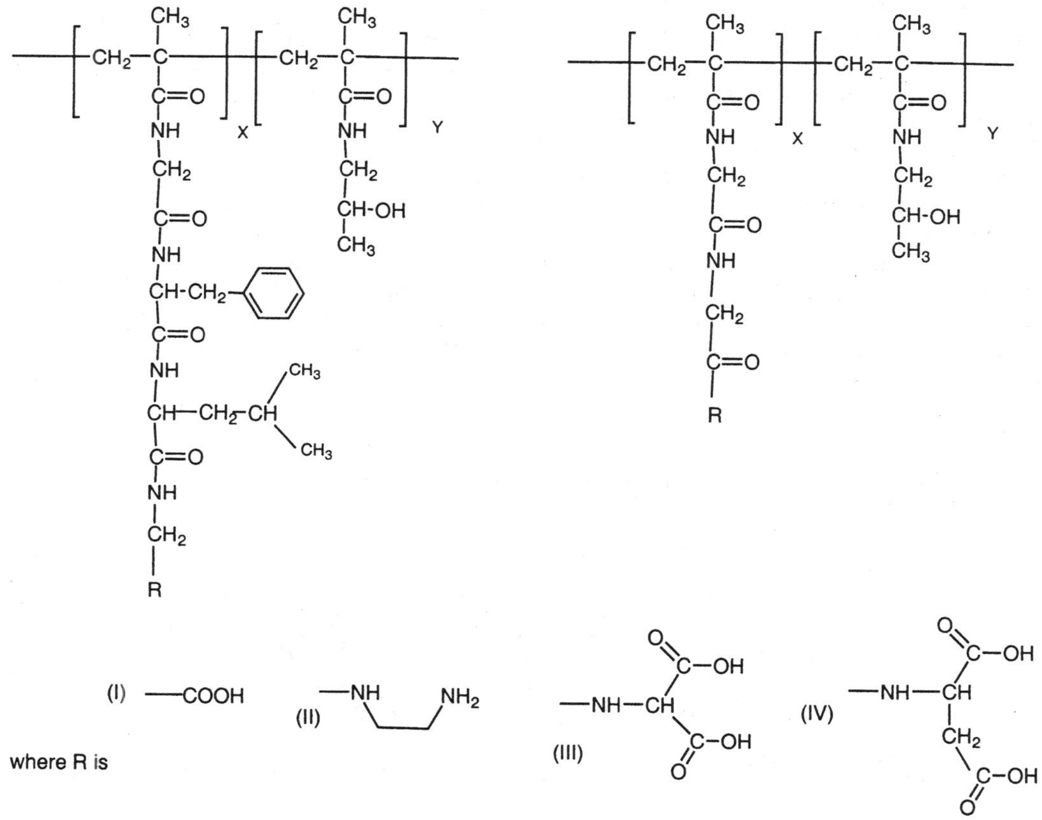

FIG. 17.6. First-generation N-(2-hydroxypropyl) methacrylamide (HPMA) copolymer–platinates where X:Y is 95:5 or 90:10.

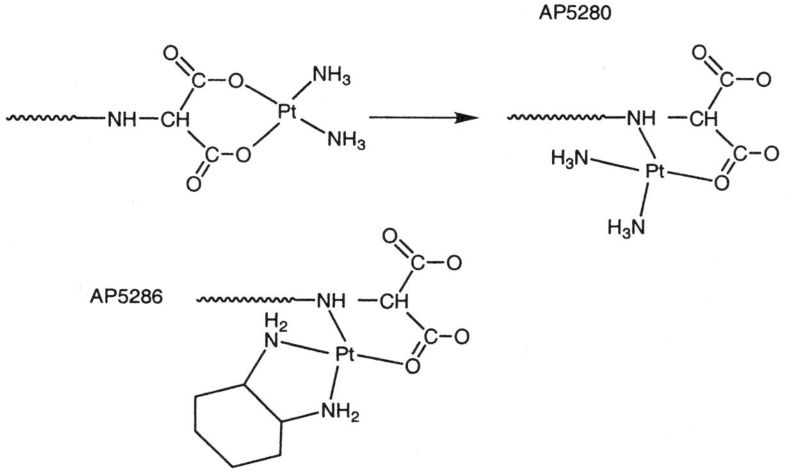

FIG. 17.7. New N-(2-hydroxypropyl)methacrylamide (HPMA) copolymer–platinates.

Poly(L-glutamic acid)—Paclitaxel (CT-2103, XYOTAX)

The use of poly(L-glutamic acid) (PG) as an anti-cancer carrier was first proposed in the 1980s, but the PG–doxorubicin conjugate synthesized at that time did not progress to clinic (55). Use of this carrier was successfully revisited in the 1990s by Wallace et al. (25), and a PG–paclitaxel conjugate (acquired by Cell Therapeutics, Inc.), CT-2103, has been advancing successfully and very rapidly through an early clinical development program.

In CT-2103, the paclitaxel is linked through the 2' position to the ester bond to the α-carboxylic acid of PG (Fig. 17.8). The conjugate has a molecular weight of approximately 40,000 d and contains 37 wt% paclitaxel. Moreover, it is 80,000 more soluble than paclitaxel. This conjugate has the advantage of a biodegradable PG polymer backbone, and it has been found that exposure to cathepsin B results in liberation of diglutamyl-paclitaxel (56). Remarkable antitumor activity was seen in a variety of *in vivo* tumor models that, together with evidence of tumor targeting by the EPR effect, paved the way for clinical testing (25,57,58). Interestingly, it has been shown in preclinical studies combining conjugate administration with radiation treatment that tumor targeting of PG–paclitaxel by the EPR effect is significantly increased, leading to enhanced antitumor activity (59). This has important implications for possible clinical development of this and other polymer–drug conjugates. Clinical studies combining CT-2103 and radiotherapy recently have received approval.

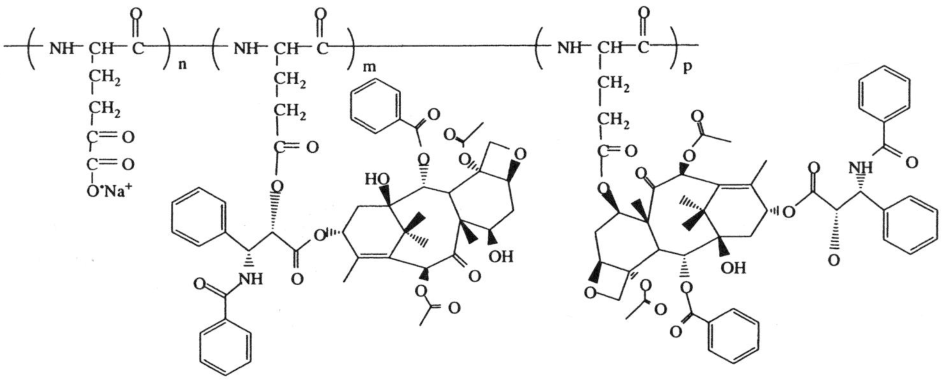

FIG. 17.8. Poly(L-glutamic acid) (PG)–paclitaxel.

CT-2103 is currently undergoing an extensive phase I/II program in Europe and the United States (26,60–66). In addition, recently announced is the initiation of a phase III trial in which CT-2103 will be given in combination with carboplatin to ovarian cancer patients. Preliminary results of the phase I and II trials have been presented in abstract form in recent months (60–66), and updated details are given on the Cell Therapeutics Web site. In one phase I study, CT-2103 was administered intravenously as a single agent for 30 minutes every 3 weeks. The starting dose was approximately 11 mg/m^2 (paclitaxel-equivalent) and dose escalation progressed to a MTD of 266 mg/m^2 (61). In another phase I study, a fixed dose of cisplatin (75 mg/m^2) or carboplatin was given with escalating doses of CT-2103 every 21 days. CT-2103 was administered first by a 10-minute intravenous infusion followed by platinate by intravenous infusion. In these studies, CT-2103 has shown manageable toxicity and a significant number of patients displayed partial responses or stable disease (mesothelioma, renal cell carcinoma, NSCLC, and paclitaxel-resistant ovarian cancer).

In the phase II program, CT-2103 is being evaluated against recurrent colorectal cancer, recurrent ovarian, fallopian tube, or peritoneal cancer, and NSCLC. Conjugate is administered at doses of 175 mg/m^2 or 210 mg/m^2 (platinum-equivalent) and in certain trials is given in combination with cisplatin or carboplatin. Early results show antitumor activity and minimal toxicity. Except for some hypersensitivity reactions, no serious drug-related events have been reported. The final outcome of this program is awaited with interest.

Poly(L-glutamic acid)–Camptothecin (CT-2106)

Cell Therapeutics Inc. is also developing a camptothecin conjugate using the same PG polymeric carrier (28). Conjugates containing different linkers including -Gly, -Glycolic acid, -α Glu and -β-Ala have been described. These were synthesized using polymers with a molecular weight of 33,000 to 74,000 d. The lead conjugate PG-Gly-CPT (CT-2106) containing 33 to 35 wt% camptothecin and with a molecular weight of 50,000 d entered phase I trials early in 2002 with plans to start other trials later in the year.

Polyethylene Glycol–Camptothecin (PROTHECAN)

Polyethylene glycol (PEG) is a widely used pharmaceutical excipient and in recent years has been brought to market in the form of PEG-protein conjugates. PEG-asparagase (Oncaspar) (13) is an anticancer conjugate used to treat acute lymphoblastic leukemia, and PEG-interferon α-2b (PEG-Intron) was commercialized as a treatment for hepatitis C. It is also under clinical development as an anticancer treatment. The safety profile of PEG is well documented, so its use as a potential drug carrier has been obvious for more than 20 years and many conjugates have been described in the literature (67–72).

Although the HPMA copolymer conjugates and PG conjugates that have been described thus far all contain multiple pendant functional groups for drug attachment, PEG contains only two terminal -OH groups suitable for conjugation. This severely limits drug carrying capacity to two drug molecules per PEG chain unless more sophisticated chemistry is used to amplify the number of terminal binding sites. This is disadvantageous, particularly for less potent drugs, but PEG does have an important advantage. The PEG polymer chain can be reproducibly synthesized to give molecules of uniform molecular weight (Mw/Mn approximately 1.0), which considerably improves the homogeneity of the product. A large number of PEG–anticancer conjugates and linking chemistries have been described using PEG chains of molecular weight 5,000 to 40,000 d.

Enzon, Inc. selected a PEG–camptothecin conjugate (PEG-CPT; PROTHECAN) for initial phase I pharmacokinetic and safety trials (29) (Fig. 17.9). In PEG-CPT, camptothecin is linked to PEG conjugate at the C-20-OH position, thus favoring the desired lactone ring configuration (Fig. 17.9). The ratio of PEG-CPT to active drug is reported as 60:1, suggesting a drug content of 1.7 wt%, which is very low. In the phase I study, PEG-CPT was administered every 3 weeks at doses of 600 to 4,800 mg/m^2 (conjugate) (estimated to represent approximately 10–82 mg/m^2 camptothecin equivalent using a drug content of 1.7 wt%). DLT included neutropenia and thrombocytopenia, both observed at the highest dose level. Preliminary pharmacokinetic studies suggested that PEG-CPT produced prolonged circulating levels of camptothecin ($t_{\frac{1}{2}} > 72$ hours). Enzon recently announced (July 2002) the initiation of a phase II trial in patients with small cell lung cancer. Interestingly, the MTD for PEG-CPT is lower than that reported for HPMA copolymer–camptothecin (MAG-CPT; PNU 166148), which had an MTD of 200 mg/m^2 (camptothecin equivalent). As pharmacokinetics and the drug-release rate are determined by the molecular weight of the polymer carrier used and conjugation chemistry, such differences are not surprising and do not necessarily reflect the potential therapeutic index of a particular compound.

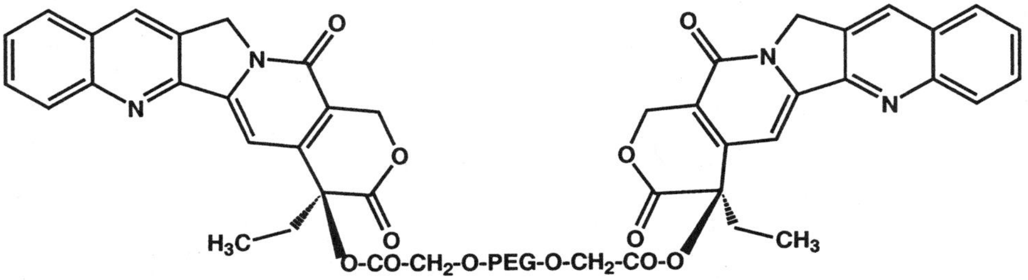

FIG. 17.9. Polyethylene glycol (PEG)–camptothecin.

Polyethylene Glycol–Paclitaxel

In May 2001, Enzon reported the start of a phase I clinical trial using a PEG–paclitaxel conjugate. The protocol has been designed to determine the safety, tolerability, and pharmacology of PEG–paclitaxel in patients with advanced solid tumors and lymphomas. Although PEG–paclitaxel conjugates have been reported in preclinical studies (69), no information is available regarding the chemistry of this particular conjugate or its clinical progress to date.

Dextran–Doxorubicin (AD-70, DOX-OXD)

Polysaccharides have long been a popular choice for synthesis of polymer–drug conjugates (10,73,74). Dextran (mainly $\alpha 1,6$ polyglucose, with some $\alpha 1,4$ branching) has been particularly popular owing to its clinical approval for use as a plasma expander. A dextran–doxorubicin conjugate (AD-70) was tested clinically. A dextran polymer with a molecular weight of approximately 70,000 d was used to prepare the conjugate, but no precise details synthesis or conjugate characteristics (bound and free doxorubicin, content) have been given. Drug conjugation seemed to be by Schiff base formation using oxidized dextran also modified with glycine as a pendant group for reaction with the anthracycline (14). The rationale of this conjugation approach was to utilize hypoxic conditions in the tumor to promote drug liberation. Alpha Therapeutic GmbH supplied the clinical formulation.

In a phase I trial involving 13 patients, AD-70 was administered every 21 to 28 days by a 30-minute infusion. A starting dose of 40 mg/m^2 (doxorubicin equivalent) was chosen as one tenth the mouse LD$_{10}$. However, unexpected toxicities occurred and the dose was reduced in the range 12.5 to 40 mg/m^2 (14). At the lowest level, there was minimal toxicity and 12.5 mg/m^2 was suggested as a phase II dose. The conjugate MTD was 40 mg/m^2 (doxorubicin-equivalent). Thrombocytopenia and severe hepatotoxicity were

the DLTs. Hepatotoxicity lasted for several weeks, suggesting liver localization of the conjugate with slow release of doxorubicin over time thereafter. Toxicity was attributed to uptake of the polysaccharide by the reticuloendothelial cells in the liver. This would result from use of dextran (polyglucose) as a carrier (there is a macrophage receptor for glucose) and/or the fact that doxorubicin was conjugated to oxidized dextran via a Schiff base—residual aldehydes would surely be present after drug conjugation. To better explain why this compound failed, it would be necessary to have more information on its chemistry, the formulation used, and the kinetics of doxorubicin release.

Other Compounds

A polysaccharide–camptothecin (DE-310) conjugate containing the new camptothecin analogue DX-8951f is currently in phase I trial. Drug is covalently bound to the carrier via a Gly-Gly-Phe-Gly peptide linker (31,32). A dextrin–doxorubicin (α-1,4 polyglucose) conjugate developed in our laboratory (75,76) is currently in preclinical development (ML Laboratories, Inc.).

PRECLINICAL DEVELOPMENT OF POLYMER–DRUG CONJUGATES

The unique features of polymer–drug conjugates (most closely related to protein conjugates and immunoconjugates) requires a paradigm shift in design, techniques used for preclinical screening and the drug development. Approximately 7 years lapsed from the "in principle" acceptance of PK1 as a clinical candidate by the CRC Phase I/II Committee in 1987 to recruitment of the first patient on study in 1994. Although slow, the meticulous preclinical program and considerable expertise in Farmitalia Carlo Erba/Pharmacia (especially in chemistry, pharmaceutical development and clinical), and manufacturing expertise of Polymer Laboratories, Inc. has laid the standards for subsequent projects. With an experienced team in the field, it is now possible to initiate a polymer–drug project, identify a lead compound, and progress to first clinical entry within 3 to 5 years. This timeframe has been achieved for our HPMA copolymer–platinate project (Access Pharmaceuticals) and the PG–paclitaxel conjugate of Cell Therapeutics, Inc. Moreover, such timelines are typical of any novel low-molecular-weight compound. Although the CRC/Pharmacia program laid the foundations for conjugate design and *in vitro* and *in vivo* preclinical screening methods paved the way for acceleration of conjugate transfer from laboratory to clinic, progress with the clinical development of HPMA copolymer conjugates has been disappointingly slow. FCE28068 and FCE28069 have still not been tested in a broad clinical development program, and their real potential remains undefined. In contrast, lessons can be learned from the early clinical development of CT-2103. This compound has progressed rapidly, and the strategic clinical development program will assess the compound's full potential with timely conclusion.

Polymer Therapeutics as New Chemical Entities

Polymer–drug conjugates are a subclass of the family of novel drugs and drug-delivery systems that have been defined as "polymer therapeutics" (9,10). Polymer therapeutics include polymeric drugs (polymeric molecules that are biologically active in their own right), polymer–drug conjugates as described here, polymer–protein conjugates, polymeric micelles to which the drug is covalently bound, and polymeric nonviral vectors for gene delivery. This term was coined to distinguish the above from pharmaceutical formulations developed to stabilize, solubilize, and/or control the release of a drug (polymer depot). Polymer therapeutics are more correctly viewed as "new chemical entities" with the polymer and drug (or protein) components as the two primary metabolites. A precise list of the requirements for regulatory approval of polymer–drug conjugates will only emerge with the market approval of first compounds. However, a useful reference is the activities undertaken to allow approval of polymeric drugs (e.g., Copaxone), polymer-protein conjugates (e.g., Oncaspar), and immunoconjugates (e.g., Mylotarg). It is clear that the development package will vary depending on whether the polymer used has already been accepted for routine human use (i.e., it is generally approved as safe, such as PEG), or is progressing for the first time through human studies (e.g., HPMA copolymers and PG).

General Terminology

There are still relatively few individuals with bridging expertise relating to polymer chemistry, organic and peptide chemistry, cell and molecular biology, pharmaceutical sciences, and the clinical development of polymer–drug conjugates. Even fewer have industrial development experience with such compounds. Successful (and safe) research and development in this field can only occur with consistent terminology. The current literature (including the many publications cited here) is peppered with inconsistencies and inaccuracies. For example:

- It is misleading to call a polymer–drug conjugate a "formulation." Like any other drug, a polymer–drug conjugate must be prepared as a stable formulation suitable for storage and clinical administration. It is a conjugate (like an immunoconjugate) or polymer–prodrug.

- It is misleading to use terminology that can be construed as either a homopolymer or a copolymer. These polymer molecules are chemically very different and would likely have a very different safety and efficacy profile. For example, it is incorrect to label the HPMA copolymer conjugates described here as "poly-HPMA." The latter suggests that drug is bound to an HPMA homopolymer. Standardized terminology (and abbreviations) should be adopted for all polymer chemistries.

- The chemical composition of a polymer–drug product can be markedly different depending on the scale of manufacture, route to synthesis, and purification procedures. Polymers are by definition heterogeneous. For example, the laboratory-scale PK1 product described in early publications is significantly different from the manufactured product FCE28068, which was manufactured to defined specification set to ensure batch-to-batch reproducibility. Thus, it is essential that compounds bear the designated reference code in all preclinical and clinical publications. For example, PK2 should be described as FCE28069 in all phase I or II reports. The compounds are different. This is also essential if preclinical studies purport to describe the mechanism of action of a compound in clinical development—it may not even be the same compound, and may have a different molecular weight and drug content.

- All publications (preclinical and clinical) should ensure adequate definition of polymer conjugate molecular weight and polydispersity, total drug content (wt%), and the free drug impurity (% total) as a minimum characterization. All these factors will have a major impact on the *in vitro*, *in vivo* and biological and clinical profile.

- It can be confusing to describe polymer–drug doses in terms of mg/kg (preclinical studies) or mg/m² (clinical trial) without clearly defining whether this is *drug content* or *conjugate dose*. It is essential that the dose specifies the amount of bioactive administered. Qualification with definition of the wt% drug in the conjugate allows also a clear appreciation of the amount of polymer administered to the patient.

It is noteworthy that some of the individual and cumulative polymer doses given clinically appear extremely high (more than 10 g/m²) (2). As such, this could have potential safety or osmotic implications. Of note is the fact that all intravenous injectable drugs are prepared either as lyophilized formulations for reconstitution with water or as ready-to-use solutions for injection. These pharmaceutical formulations typically contain very large amounts of lactose, surfactants, and polymeric excipients to aid drug solubility and/or stability. In the case of polymer–drug conjugates, the integral solubilizing and bulking agent properties of the polymeric carrier often replace the need for some of these ingredients. Perception of doses should take consideration of total formulation composition.

Chemistry: Designing a Lead Compound

History tells us that effective polymer–drug conjugates are the product of rational design. Synthesis of interesting chemical libraries without due attention to the now-known chemical and biological requirements for conjugate design leads to failure, as does use of polymers with inadequate biocompatibility or impracticality for scale-up manufacture (6–10). The main considerations for selection of the three principle components of a polymer–drug conjugate are:

The Polymer

- It must be water soluble and able to solubilize the drug payload even if the compound is extremely hydrophobic. Inadequate solubility can lead to precipitation on injection (toxicity) and/or creation of hydrophobic molecules that are rapidly cleared by the reticuloendothelial system.
- The chemistry must include sufficient functional groups along the polymer chain to allow drug conjugation.
- If the polymer mainchain is nondegradable, the molecular weight must be sufficiently low to allow renal elimination (less than 40,000 d for a random coiled water soluble polymer).

- Ideally, the polymer backbone should be biodegradable to aid eventual elimination after repeated administration and also to allow use of higher-molecular-weight polymers that can optimize EPR-mediated targeting.
- The polymer and its metabolites must be nontoxic and nonimmunogenic.
- Synthesis must be amenable to scale-up production (and costs should be commercially viable).

The Linker

- For perfect targeting, the linker should be completely stable in the circulation and release drug at the appropriate rate within the tumor. It has long been known that rapid drug liberation in the bloodstream after intravenous injection brings no therapeutic benefit compared to the parent compound (77).
- Stability of the linker during conjugate elimination (e.g., via hepatobiliary transfer or in urine) is important to avoid normal tissue damage (e.g., kidney or gastrointestinal tract).
- If the drug is linked via a hydrolytically unstable bond, it is not necessary to use an (expensive) peptidyl linker for conjugation.

The Drug

- Requires appropriate functionality for polymer conjugation.
- It is essential that the conjugate has adequate drug loading in relation to the potency of the compound. Typically for doxorubicin, camptothecin, and cisplatin, this would be a minimum of approximately 10 wt%. Even higher loading with preserved solubility and appropriate pharmacokinetics of the conjugate is advantageous.
- In conjugates designed for lysosomotropic delivery, it is essential that the drug has required stability at low pH (lysosomal pH can be as low as 2). Also, the drug must be resistant to lysosomal catabolism.
- If drug is liberated intralysosomally, it must be able to traverse the lysosomal membrane to access pharmacological targets in the cytosol or nucleus.

Pharmacokinetics and Pharmacology: Biological Rationale and Preclinical Screening

The fundamental aim of polymer–drug conjugation is to modify pharmacokinetics at the whole organism and cellular level, thus promoting increased tumor targeting while minimizing exposure of sensitive normal tissues (6,7) (Fig. 17.10). So far, preclinical pharmacokinetics (in mice and rats) have shown good correlation with the clinical measurements, thus validating animal studies as a useful model. An optimized con-

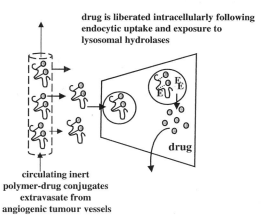

drug is liberated intracellularly following endocytic uptake and exposure to lysosomal hydrolases

drug

circulating inert polymer-drug conjugates extravasate from angiogenic tumour vessels

FIG. 17.10. Scheme showing the proposed mechanism of tumour-selective delivery.

jugate will have a longer $t_{1/2}$ plasma circulation (optimum seems to be 1–12 hours) compared to the free drug. This is essential to promote EPR-mediated targeting (78). It has been shown using ^{125}I-labelled HPMA copolymers that tumor targeting can be achieved over a wide range of polymer molecular weight up to 800,000 d (78). Conjugates that are not rapidly subject to glomerular filtration (i.e., have a molecular weight of more than 40,000 d) and thus circulate longest in plasma show greatest tumor accumulation. If the polymer–drug linker is stable in the circulation and if targeting is effective, no free drug should appear in the plasma (8). In phase I clinical studies, plasma free-drug levels were usually less than 100 times lower than the conjugated drug values, and this is consistent with the fact that the formulations administered typically contained 1% to 2% free drug.

The perfect conjugate will contain a linker that is stable in the circulation, thus the polymer prodrug will be inert during transit, but liberate drug intratumorally at a rate tailored to best suit the drug's mechanism of action (Fig. 17.10). For example, the HPMA copolymer conjugates PK1 and PK2 were designed for activation by the lysosomal thiol-dependent proteases, particularly cathepsin B (43), to liberate doxorubicin over a 24-hour to 48-hour period. It is now apparent that PG-paclitaxel is also degraded by this enzyme (56). To ensure cellular entry of lysosomotropic conjugates, the molecular weight of the polymer must be less than 100,000 d because higher-molecular-weight polymers are excluded from epithelial cells (79). Polymers of net neutral charge are preferable. Positively or negatively (and often hydrophobic) conjugates often

bind nonspecifically to the cell surface and have a tendency to localize in liver, lung, or endothelial cells after intravenous injection (up to 80% of dose-administered dose). This first-pass removal can jeopardize any chance of tumor delivery. Bearing in mind the above requirements, the following preclinical screening protocol has been developed in our laboratory to all rapid optimization of conjugate structure:

- Evaluation of polymer cytotoxicity, hematotoxicity, and immunogenicity (immunoglobulin G or M responses). The polymeric carrier must be biocompatible.
- Preliminary *in vivo* biodistribution studies are conducted to ensure that the *polymer itself* is not inherently hepatotropic (or targets other normal tissues).
- Conjugates containing a library of polymer–drug linkers are subjected to degradation studies *in vitro*. The plasma stability (and urine stability if this is an issue) and the rate of drug liberation are optimized. Typically, experiments are conducted at a variety of pH levels. (5.5–7.4) chosen to mimic the environments likely to be encountered *in vivo*. Linker degradation is also assessed in the presence of a mixture of isolated lysosomal enzymes if peptidyl side chains are involved.
- Preliminary *in vivo* biodistribution studies are carried out to ensure that the *polymer–drug conjugate* is not inherently hepatotropic (or targets other normal tissues). Then the whole-body distribution of the selected candidate(s) assessed in mice bearing a subcutaneous tumor to measure the extent of EPR-mediated targeting and also to identify any "potential" normal-tissue targeting that might have toxicological implications. *In vivo* biodistribution studies using a small library of conjugates is the primary screen which allows optimization of polymer conjugate design with respect to drug loading the molecular weight for best tumor targeting.
- Finally, antitumor activity of polymer–drug conjugates is evaluated using a panel murine and xenograft of tumor models. It is essential to have prior knowledge of the vascular permeability properties of the tumor models used and also changes that occur with respect to permeability with increasing tumor size (80). Only with this information can the model be standardized to allow reproducible comparisons between families of conjugates in subsequent experiments.

Use of this stepwise program allows rapid optimization to produce a lead candidate suitable for clinical evaluation. If the polymer or the conjugate fails at any stage, an alternative is sought.

It is important to note that conventional *in vitro* antitumor screening (e.g., the National Cancer Institute's Compare screen) is inappropriate for profiling polymer–drug conjugates because of their altered cellular pharmacokinetics. IC_{50} values (concentration required to destroy 50% of cells) seen *in vitro* are not predictive of therapeutic index *in vivo*. The IC_{50} values are strongly influenced by the free drug content of the conjugate and/or the rate of drug release into tissue-culture medium during the incubation. *In vitro* evaluation of HPMA copolymer–doxorubicin and HPMA copolymer–platinates is influenced by the free doxorubicin impurity (even if it is less than 0.1% total doxorubicin content) or the rapidly released platinum species in the case of the platinate conjugates (22). Investigations using *in vitro* cell-based models to study the molecular mechanisms of action of polymer conjugates are also affected by the previously mentioned limitations. Mechanistic studies using tumor samples taken after conjugate administration to animals or patients will prove more useful in terms of determining mechanisms of action.

It should also be noted that the protocols adopted to assess antitumor activity *in vivo* should use a dosing schedule that will reflect (in some way) the likely clinical protocol. Its not surprising that some of the dramatic antitumor responses seen *in vivo* have not been reproduced in the early clinical trials because many investigators use a repeated-conjugate dosing schedule (often daily for 3 days or an even more intensive daily administration) that has never been applied clinically.

Preclinical Toxicology

Once a promising clinical candidate emerges, the conjugate must then be subject to a conventional program of preclinical toxicology, as is the case for any other new drug. The program usually involves the following elements:

1. Single-dose and multiple-dose studies in two rodent species as a minimum. Depending on country, dog studies are frequently required as standard.
2. Studies designed to examine the potential immunogenicity of the macromolecular conjugate. For example, the potential immunogenicity of HPMA copolymer conjugates PK1 and PK2 was rigorously examined (81).
3. Additional studies may be requested, depending on the known toxicological profile of conjugated drug. For example, proof of reduced cardiotoxicity of HPMA copolymer–doxorubicin conjugates was

requested prior to acceptance for phase I entry (82,83).
4. At some stage it will be necessary to document the fate of the polymer carrier after administration. This is particularly important if a nondegradable polymer is used. The polymer and conjugates drug are considered two primary metabolites.

The only preclinical program reported so far describes FCE28068 toxicology (45). In preliminary studies, the LD_{50} of PK1 in MF1 mice after a single intravenous injection was found to be approximately 63 mg/kg (doxorubicin–equivalent). Subsequently, PK1 was administered to MF1 mice (22.5 or 45 mg/kg) in a single-dose study, and was administered to MF1 mice or Wistar rats weekly for 5 consecutive weeks at 12.0 or 22.5 mg/kg (mice) or 3 and 5 mg/kg (rats) in a multiple-dose study. PK1 induced hematologic changes in rats and mice shortly after treatment, and in the single-dose study alanine and aspartate aminotransferase levels were elevated at higher doses. Liver damage was seen only in rat tissue during histological examination. Other histological changes induced by PK1 included thymic and testicular atrophy, bone marrow depletion, gastrointestinal tract changes, and in the multiple-dose study an increase in nuclear size in the proximal tubules of the kidney (although no changes in urine were seen). Recovery from these effects was seen in rats at 59 days. The toxicities were generally typical of anthracyclines. This study recommended a PK1 dose of 20 mg/m^2 as a safe starting dose for phase I clinical trials.

Manufacture and Analytical Techniques

Advancing a polymer–drug conjugate into phase I and II trial typically requires several kilograms of product. This is needed for the validation of analytical techniques, formulation and stability assays, preclinical toxicology, and also to prepare sufficient vials for the first clinical studies. Over the last decade, the methodology for GMP manufacture and characterization of polymer–drug conjugates has become well established. The reactive polymer backbone and drug (or modified drug) are the two key intermediates. These may be sourced from companies with the specific expertise— an increasing number of specialty polymer companies have been established to meet the polymer need. Although residual impurities are typical of all manufactured drug substances, polymer conjugates bring an added complication of side products formed along the polymer chain or by polymer cross-linking.

A variety of synthetic routes may be adopted for a conjugate (e.g., the first and MAG-HPMA copolymer conjugates). Thus, it is important to define carefully the synthetic method and carefully define the potential polymeric side products. For example, nonspecific hydrolysis can occur during drug conjugation to HPMA copolymers by aminolysis reactions, leading to the introduction of a small number of monomers terminating in -COOH, and final stage aminolysis with 2-propanolamine leads to the introduction of 2-hydroxypropylamide–terminating units (Fig. 17.11). The following methods have been used to characterize polymer conjugates.

Identity

High-field (600 MHz) two-dimensional NOESY and TOCSY ^{1}H NMR has been successfully used to define

the identity of polymer–drug conjugates. In the case of FCE28068 and FCE28069 (84), it was possible to fully assign the protons by comparison with reference compounds and visualize the connection of doxorubicin with the polymer chain, and the D,L isomeric forms of Phe in the polymer–drug linker (84). Diagnostic signals for the alternative side chains terminating in -COOH and 2-hydroxyproylamide were also detected with the aid of model compounds. High-field NMR can also be used to detect contaminating solvents, free 2-propanolamine, free doxorubicin, and in the case of FCE28069, free galactosamine with great sensitivity (less than 0.1% in some cases). The bound galactosamine present in FCE28069 was found to present in the 4 isomeric α- and β-pyranose and furanose forms with α-pyranose form predominating.

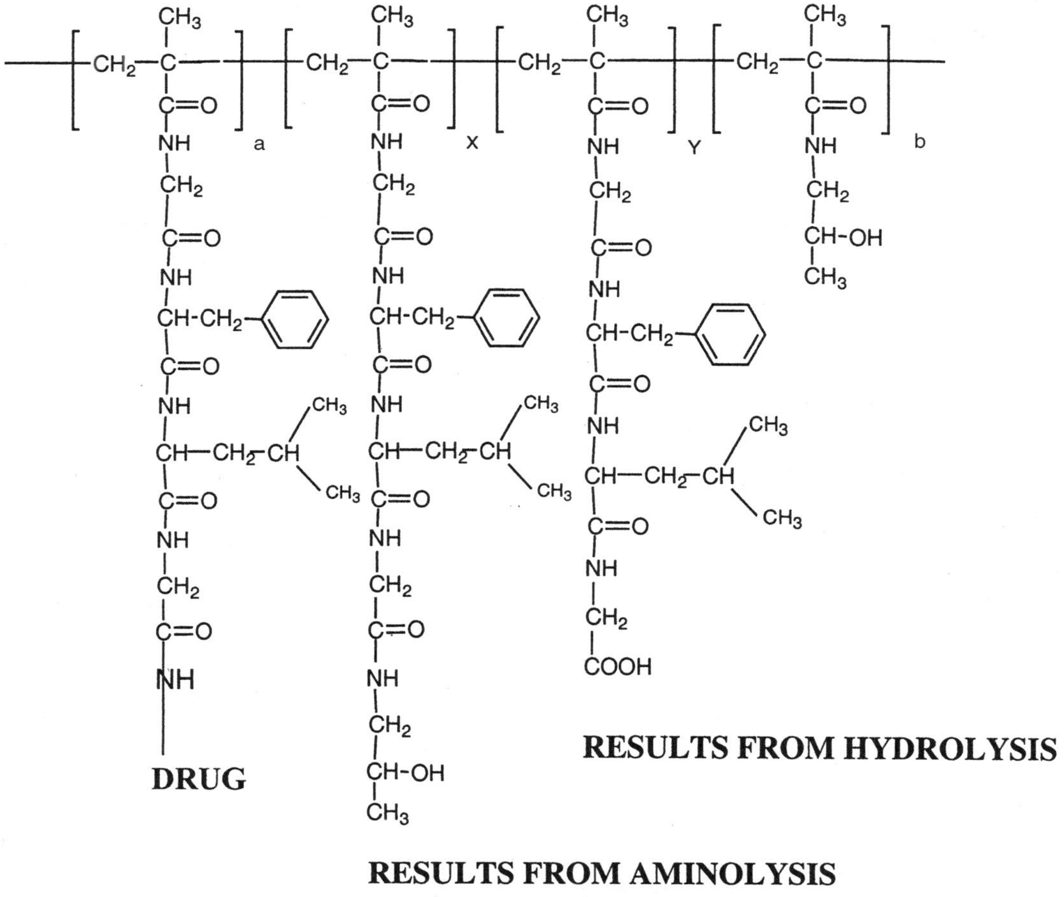

FIG. 17.11. Monomer structures (as impurities) introduced into N-(2-hydroxypropyl)methacrylamide (HPMA) copolymer structures during the aminolysis reaction.

Molecular Weight and Polydispersity

For any polymer–drug conjugate, it is essential to set an acceptable specification for batch molecular weight and polydispersity. For safety reasons, this is particularly important in the case of nonbiodegradable polymers because it is important to know the fraction (%) in any batch that would have a molecular weight higher than the renal threshold. Pharmacokinetics will be molecular-weight dependent and efficacy/toxicity will be influenced by major changes in these parameters. Gel-permeation chromatography techniques have been established using commercial columns to allow the construction of compound-specific universal calibrations to allow reproducible definition of these parameters for polymer anticancer conjugates (85,86). Molecular weight fractions of the polymer–drug of narrow polydispersity can be prepared to allow standardization of the technique and also for biological studies to ensure that the specification set is appropriate in terms of safety and efficacy. Thirteen fractions of the HPMA copolymer–paclitaxel conjugate PNU166945 and six fractions of the polymeric drug-carrier poly-HPMA were prepared, and they were characterized by size-exclusion chromatography, viscometry, and light scattering to give the molar mass distribution, intrinsic viscosity, and size dimensions. The presence of the drug considerably influences the conformation (87).

Content of Total and Free Drug

The ultraviolet (UV) extinction coefficient is often used in laboratory experiments to estimate total drug content of a conjugate. This is not advisable because it often changes after drug conjugation and the resultant inaccuracy would give a dangerous measure of clinical dose. Specialized HPLC techniques have been developed and are routinely used to determine these parameters (88,89). Free drug can be extracted from the conjugate in aqueous solution using an appropriate solvent, and then HPLC analysis allows direct quantitation. In the case of FCE28068, high polymer concentrations were used for the assay (5 mg/mL) to give better sensitivity (0.01% and 0.02%). The recovery of free doxorubicin was 97.7% (88).

To estimate total drug content, mild hydrolysis of the polymer conjugates has been used to liberate drug derivatives that also can also be quantified using HPLC. First, it is necessary to identify the optimum conditions for hydrolysis using a model compound. The release kinetics of drug derivative from the model and polymer are then compared, and finally the recovery is assessed by spiking. To estimate total doxo-

rubicin in FCE28068 and FCE28069, mild hydrolysis using 1N HCl at 50°C for 1.5 hours gave maximum conversion (more than 99% cleavage of the glycosidic bond and 96.9% recovery for the total doxorubicin content).

If the polymer–drug conjugate contains in addition a targeting group, it is necessary to validate methods for characterization of the targeting residue. HPLC techniques were also to assess the galactose content of FCE28069 (88). Derivatization with OPA led to poor HPLC results unless pretreatment with sodium borohydride was used to eliminate anomeric equilibrium and interconversion between the furanose, pyranose, and open forms of the sugar. Bound galactosamine in FCE28069 is only released from the polymer after heating under strongly acidic conditions (6N HCl), and this method was optimized using *N*-acetyl-D-galactosamine as a model.

Formulation of Polymer–Drug Conjugates

Despite their high solubility (approximately 5%), the dissolution rate of PK1 and PK2 is relatively slow (more than 30 minutes). Formulations studies with PK1 and PK2 (90) led to the conclusion that an optimized formulation contained surfactant (polysorbate 80) as a dissolution enhancer, a soluble filler like lactose, and a small amount of organic solvent (ethanol was used). Typically solutions of FCE28068 and FCE28069 (concentration ranging from 30–50 mg/mL conjugate) were filter sterilized and then freeze-dried. The resulting lyophilized cake could easily be reconstituted with water for injection or sodium chloride, and dissolution occurred in approximately 2 minutes.

TO THE FUTURE

Now that the concept of polymer–anticancer conjugates is becoming well established, many second-generation compounds are following. Of particular interest are the conjugates containing natural products and novel drugs that have yet to be accepted as clinical chemotherapy (91–93). Conjugation affords the possibility to abrogate unacceptable formulation problems and unacceptable clinical toxicity. More selective tumor delivery of very potent natural-product anticancer compounds can be achieved by polymer conjugation. An HPMA copolymer–TNP-470 conjugate is showing promise (94), suggesting a role of this approach in augmenting antiangiogenic activity. It is clear that a combination strategy will be needed to overcome the various stages in disease progression of those common solid tumors responsible for such high mortality in the population. Combinations of polymer conjugates and routine chemotherapy are already under clinical evaluation. As preclinical studies have also begun to explore the use of a combination of conjugates with radiotherapy (59), two-step administration of conjugates (e.g., polymer-directed enzyme polymer–prodrug therapy) (94, 95), use of the polymer platform to deliver a drug cocktail (selection of appropriate spacers allows the rate of release of each drug to be optimized) within the same tumor mass after a single injection, it will only be a matter of time before these concepts are also ready to enter clinical development. The lessons learned in the last two decades should accelerate this passage.

The author thanks the many colleagues and collaborators who brought the HPMA copolymer program into clinical development, the UK Cancer Research Campaign for supporting the program, and Tom Connors, Helmut Ringsdorf, and Federico Spreafico (Farmitalia Carlo Erba/Pharmacia), whose inspiration and support made possible the creation of this new class of anticancer agents.

A recent review of polymer therapeutics can be found in (96).

REFERENCES

1. Ringsdorf H. Structure and properties of pharmacologically active polymers. *J Polym Sci Symposium* 1975;51: 135–153.
2. Vasey P, Twelves C, Kaye S, et al. Phase I clinical and pharmacokinetic study of PKI (HPMA copolymer doxorubicin) first member of a new class of chemotherapeutics agents: drug-polymer conjugates. *Clin Cancer Res* 1999;5:83–94.
3. Matsumura Y, Maeda H. A new concept for macromolecular therapies in cancer chemotherapy: mechanism of tumoritropic accumulation of proteins and the antitumor agent SMANCS. *Cancer Res* 1986;6: 6387–6392.
4. Debruyne FM, Denis L, Lunglmayer G, et al. Long-term therapy with a depot luteinizing hormone-releasing hormone analogue (Zoladex) in patients with advanced prostatic carcinoma. *J Urol* 1988; 140:775–77.
5. Brem H, Sisi M, Brem S, et al. Placebo controlled trial of safety and efficacy of intraoperative controlled delivery by biodegradable polymers of chemotherapy. *Lancet* 1995;345:1008–1012.
6. Duncan R, Kopecek J. Soluble synthetic polymers as potential drug carriers. *Adv Polym Sci* 1984;57:51–101.
7. Duncan R Drug-polymer conjugates: potential for improved chemotherapy. *Anticancer Drugs* 1992;3:175–210.
8. Duncan R, Spreafico F. Polymer Conjugates: Pharmacokinetic considerations for design and development. *Clin Pharmacokinet* 1994;27:290–306.
9. Duncan R, Dimitrijevic S, Evagorou EG. The role of polymer conjugates in the diagnosis and treatment of cancer. *STP Pharm Sci* 1996;6:237–263.
10. Brocchini S, Duncan R. Pendent drugs, release from polymers. In: Mathiowitz E, ed. *Encyclopaedia of controlled drug delivery*, New York: John Wiley and Sons, 1999:786–816.
11. Kopecek J, Kopeckova P, Minko T, et al. HPMA copolymer-anticancer drug conjugates: design, activity and mechanism of action. *Eur J Pharm Biopharm* 2000;50:61–81.
12. Duncan R. Polymer–drug conjugates: targeting cancer. In: Muzykantov VR, Torchilin VP, eds. *Biomedical aspects of drug targeting*. New York: Kluwer Academic Publishers, 2002 *(in press)*.
13. Abuchowski A, Kazo GM, Verhoest CR, et al. Cancer therapy with chemically modified enzymes. I. Antitumour properties of polyethylene glycol-modified asparaginase conjugates. *Cancer Biochem Biophys* 1984; 7:175–186.
14. Danauser-Reidl S, Hausmann E, Schick H, et al. Phase-I clinical and pharmacokinetic trial of dextran conjugated doxorubicin (AD-70, DOX-OXD). *Invest New Drugs* 1993;11:187–195.
15. Duncan, R, Seymour LW, O'Hare KB, et al. Preclinical evaluation of polymer-bound doxorubicin. *J Control Release* 1992;19:331–346.
16. Duncan R, Seymour LCW, Scarlett L., et al. Fate of *N*-(2-Hydroxypropyl)methacrylamide copolymers with pendant galactosamine residues after intravenous administration to rats. *Biochim Biophys Acta* 1986; 880:62–71.
17. Julyan PJ, Ferry DR, Seymour LW, et al. Preliminary clinical study of the distribution of HPMA copolymer-doxorubicin bearing galactosamine. *J Control Release* 1999;57:281–290.
18. Seymour LW, Ferry DR, Anderson D, et al. Hepatic drug targeting: Phase I evaluation of polymer bound doxorubicin. *J Clin Oncol* 2002;20:1668–1676.
19. Meerum Terwogt JM, ten Bokkel Huinink WW, et al. Phase I clinical and pharmacokinetic study of PNU166945, a novel water soluble polymer-conjugated prodrug of paclitaxel. *Anticancer Drugs* 2001;12: 315–323.
20. Caiolfa VR, Zamal M, Fiorini A, et al. A. Polymer-bound camptothecin: Initial biodistribution and antitumour activity studies. *J Control Release* 2000;65: 105–119.
21. de Bono JS, Bissett D, Twelves C, et al. Phase I pharmacokinetic study of MAG-CPT (PNU 166148) a polymeric derivative of camptothecin. *Proceedings of the American Society of Clinical Oncology* 2000, 771.
22. Gianasi E, Wasil M, Evagorou EG, et al. HPMA copolymer platinates as novel antitumour agents: *in vitro* properties, pharmacokinetics and antitumour activity. *Eur J Cancer* 1999;3:994–1002.
23. Gianasi E, Buckley RG, Latigo J, et al. HPMA copolymers platinates containing dicarboxylato ligands. preparation, characterisation and *in vitro* and *in vivo* evaluation. *J Drug Target* 2002 *(in press)*.
24. Rice JR, Stewart DR, Safaei R, et al. Preclinical development of water-soluble polymer-platinum chemotherapeutics AP5280 and AP5286. In: *Proceedings of the 5th International Symposium on Polymer Therapeutics: From Laboratory to Clinical Practice, Cardiff, UK.* 2002:54.
25. Li C, Yu D, Newman R, et al. Complete regression well-established tumors using a novel water-soluble poly(L-

glutamic acid)-paclitaxel conjugate. *Cancer Res* 1998; 58:2404–2409.

26. J. Sludden AV, Boddy M.J, Griffin L, et al. Phase I and pharmacological study of CT-2103, a poly(L-glutamic acid)-paclitaxel conjugate. *Proceedings of American Association for Cancer Res* 2001;42:2883.

27. De Vries P, Kumar A, Heasley E, et al. C2103: A water soluble poly-L-glutamic acid(PG)-paclitaxel(TXL) conjugate has enhanced efficacy on MDR-1+human colon carcinoma cell line xenografts compared to free TXL. *Proceedings of American Association for Cancer Res* 2001;42:462.

28. De Vries P, Bhatt R, Stone I, et al. Optimisation of CT-2106: a water soluble poly-L-glutamic acid (PG)-camptothecin conjugate with enhanced in vivo antitumour efficacy. *Proceedings of AACR-NCI-EORTC International Conference* 2001:100.

29. Denis L, Hammond L, Hidalgo, et al. A phase I study of PEG-camptothecin (PEG-CPT) in patients with advanced solid tumours: a novel formulation with for an insoluble but active agent. *Proceedings of the American Society of Clinical Oncology* 2000;19:700

30. Greenwald RB, Pendri A, Bolikal D, et al. Highly water soluble taxol derivatives: 2-polyethylene glycol esters as potential prodrugs. *Bioorg Med Chem Lett* 1994;4: 2465–2470.

31. E. Kumazawa Y, Ochi N, Tanaka T, et al. DE-310, a novel macromolecular carrier system for the camptothecin analogue DX-8951f[I]:Its antitumour activities in the murine meth A solid tumour model. *Proceedings of the American Association for Cancer Res* 2001; 42:2023.

32. Ochi, Y, Kumazawa E, Nakata M, et al. DE-310, A novel macromolecular carrier for the camptothecin analogue DX-8951f[II]: Its antitumour activities in several model systems of human and murine tumours. *Proceedings of the American Association for Cancer Res* 2001;42:748.

33. Kopecek J, Bazilova H. Poly[N-(hydroxypropyl)methecrylamide]-I. Radical polymerisation and copolymerisation. *Eur Polym J* 1973; 9:7–14.

34. Flanagan PA, Duncan R, Rihova B, et al. Immunogenicity of protein-N-(2-hydroxypropyl)methacrylamide copolymer conjugates measured in A/J and B10 mice. *J Bioactive Compat Polym* 1990;5:151–166.

35. Kopecek J. Reactive copolymers of N-(2-hydroxypropyl)methacrylamide with N-methacryloylated derivatives of L-leucine and L-phenylalanine. *Macromol Chem* 1977;178:2169–2183.

36. Duncan R, Rejmanova P, Kopecek J, et al. Pinocytic uptake and intracellular degradation of N-(2-hydroxypropyl)methacrylamide copolymers. A potential drug delivery system. *Biochim Biophys Acta* 1981;678: 143–150.

37. Seymour LW, Duncan R, Strohalm J, et al. Effect of molecular weight (Mω) of *N*-(2-hydroxypropyl) methacrylamide copolymers on body distributions and rate of excretion after subcutaneous, intraperitoneal and intravenous administration to rats. *J Biomed Mater Res* 1987;21:1341–1358.

38. Pimm MV, Perkins AC, Duncan R., et al. Targeting of N-(2-hydroxypropyl)methacrylamide copolymer-doxorubicin conjugate to the hepatocyte galactose-receptor in mice: visualisation and quantification by gamma scintigraphy as a basis for clinical targeting studies. *J Drug Target* 1993;1:125–131.

39. Pimm M, Perkins AC, Strohalm J, et al. Gamma scintigraphy of the biodistribution of ^{123}I-labelled N-(2-hydroxypropyl) methacrylamide copolymer-doxorubicin conjugates in mice with transplanted melanoma and mammary carcinoma. *J Drug Target* 1996;3:375–383.

40. Duncan R, Kopeckova-Rejmanova P, Strohalm J, et al. Anticancer agents coupled to N-(2-hydroxypropyl) methacrylamide copolymers. 1. Evaluation of daunomycin and puromycin conjugates *in vitro*. *Br J Cancer* 1987;55:165–174.

41. Duncan R, Kopeckova P, Strohalm J, et al Anticancer agents coupled to N-(2-hydroxypropyl)methacrylamide copolymers. II. Evaluation of daunomycin conjugates *in vivo* against L1210 leukaemia. *Br J Cancer* 1988; 57:147–156.

42. Duncan R, Hume IC, Kopeckova P, et al. Anticancer agents coupled to *N*-(2-hydroxypropyl)methacrylamide copolymers, 3. Evaluation of adriamycin conjugates against mouse leukaemia L1210 *in vivo*. *J Control Release* 1989;10:51–63.

43. Duncan R, Cable HC, Lloyd JB, et al. Polymers containing enzymatically degradable bonds, 7. Design of oligopeptide side chains in poly [N-(2-hydroxypropyl)methacrylamide] copolymers to promote efficient degradation by lysosomal enzymes. *Macromol Chem* 1984;184:1997–2008.

44. Uchegbu, IF, Ringsdorf H, Duncan R. The lower critical solution temperature of doxorubicin polymer conjugates. *Proceedings of the International Symposium for Controlled Release of Bioactive Materials* 1996;23: 791–792.

45. Duncan R, Coatsworth JK, Burtles S. Preclinical toxicology of a novel polymeric antitumour agent: HPMA copolymer-doxorubicin (PK1). *Hum Exp Toxicol* 1998; 17:93–104.

46. Seymour LW, Ulbrich K, Strohalm J, et al. The pharmacokinetics of polymer-bound adriamycin. *Biochemical Pharmacology* 1990;39:1125–1131.

47. Cassidy J. PK1: results of phase I studies. In: *Proceedings of the 5th International Symposium on Polymer Therapeutics: From Laboratory to Clinical Practice, Cardiff, UK.* 2000:20.

48. Ashwell G, Harford J. Carbohydrate recognition systems of the liver. *Annu Rev Biochem* 1982;51:531–554.

49. Seymour LW, Ulbrich K, Wedge SR, et al. N-(2-Hydroxypropyl)methacrylamide copolymers targeted to the hepatocyte galactose-receptor: pharmacokinetics in DBA, mice. *Br J Cancer* 1991;63:859–866.

50. Ciaolfa VR, Frigerio E, Castelli MG, et al. HPMA-based tumour delivery: pharmacokinetics and antitumour activity of the first MAG-phe-leu-gly-CPT soluble derivative. *Proceedings of the American Association of Cancer Research* 2000;40:2923.

51. Schoemaker NE, Van Kesteren C, Rosingf H, et al. A Phase I and pharmacokinetic study of MAG-CPT, a water-soluble polymer conjugate of camptothecin. *Br J Cancer* 2002;87:608–614.

52. Schoemaker NE, Frigerio E, Fraier D, et al. High-performance liquid chromatographic analysis for the determination of a novel polymer-bound camptothecin derivative (MAG-camptothecin) and free camptothecin in human plasma. *J Chromatogr* 2001;763:173–183.

53. Duncan R, Hume IC, Yardley HJ, et al. Macromolecular prodrugs for use in targeted cancer chemotherapy: Melphalan covalently coupled to N-(2-hydroxypropyl) methacrylamide copolymers. *J Control Release* 1991; 16:121–136.

54. Rice JR, Stewart DR, Nowotnik DP. Enhanced antitumour activity of a new polymer-linked DACH-platinum complex. *Proceedings of the American Association for Cancer Research* 2002.

55. Hoes CJT, Potman W, Van Heeswijk WAR, et al. Optimisation of macromolecular prodrugs of antitumour antibiotic adriamycin. *J Control Release* 1985;2:205–213.

56. Shaffer SA, Baker Lee C, Nudelman E, et al. Metabolism of poly-L-glutamic acid (PG) paclitaxel (CT-2103); proteolysis by lysosomal cathepsin B and identification of intermediate metabolites. *Proceedings of the American Association of Cancer Research* 2002;2067.

57. Li C, Price JE, Milash, et al. Antitumour activity of poly(L-glutamic acid)-paclitaxel on syngeneic and xenografted tumours. *Clin Cancer Res* 1999;5:891–897.

58. Auzenne E, Donato NJ, Li C, et al. Superior therapeutic profile of poly-L-glutamic acid-paclitaxel copolymer compared with taxol in xenogeneic compartmental models of human ovarian carcinoma. *Clin Cancer Res* 2002;8:573–581.

59. Li C, Ke S, Wu Q-P, et al. Tumour irradiation enhances the tumour-specific distribution of poly(L-glutamic)-conjugates paclitaxel and its antitumour efficacy. *Clin Cancer Res* 2000;6:2829–2834.

60. Sabbatini P, Aghajanian C, Hensley M, et al. Early findings in a Phase I/II study of PG-paclitaxel (CT-2103) in recurrent ovarian or primary peritoneal cancer. *Proceedings of the 5th International Symposium on Polymer Therapeutics: Laboratory to Clinic Cardiff, UK.* 2002:20.

61. Bolton MG, Kudekla A, Cassidy J, et al. Phase I studies of PG-paclitaxel(CT-2103) as a single agent and in combination with cisplatin. *Proceedings of the 5th International Symposium on Polymer Therapeutics: Laboratory to Clinic Cardiff, UK.* 2002:20b.

62. Garzone PD, Mitchell P, Bolton MG, et al. Preliminary report of a phase I study of combination chemotherapy using CT-2103 and carboplatin in patients with solid tumors. *Proceedings of the American Society of Clinical Oncology* 2002:2161.

63. Kudelka AP, Verschraegen CF, Loyer E, et al. Preliminary report of a phase I study of escalating dose PG-paclitaxel (CT-2103) and fixed dose cisplatin in patients with solid tumors *Proceedings of the American Society of Clinical Oncology* 2002:2146.

64. Schulz J, Burris HA, Redfern C, et al. Phase II study of CT-2103 in patients with colorectal cancer having recurrent disease after treatment with a 5-fluorouracil-containing regimen. *Proceedings of the American Society of Clinical Oncology* 2002:2330.

65. Sabbatini P, Brown J, Aghajanian C, et al. A phase I/II study of PG-paclitaxel (CT-2103) in patients (pts) with recurrent ovarian, fallopian tube, or peritoneal cancer. *Proceedings of the American Society of Clinical Oncology* 2002:871.

66. Harper H, Marsland T, Mitchell P, et al. Phase II study of first line chemotherapy using CT-2103 in patients with non-small-cell lung cancer who are >70 years of age or who have PS = 2. *Proceedings of the American Society of Clinical Oncology* 2002:2685.

67. Greenwald RB. Drug delivery systems: anticancer prodrugs and their polymeric conjugates. *Expert Opin Ther Patents* 1997;7:601–609.

68. Greenwald RB. PEG-drugs: an overview. *J Control Release* 2001;74:159–171.

69. Greenwald RB, Gilbert CW, Pendri A, et al. Drug delivery systems: water soluble taxol 2-poly (ethylene glycol) ester prodrugs: design and in vivo effectiveness. *J Med Chem* 1996;39:424–431.

70. Greenwald RB, Pendri A, Conover CD, et al. Camptothecin-20-PEG ester transport forms: the effect of spacer groups on antitumour activity. *Bioorg Med Chem* 1998;6:551–562.

71. Greenwald RB, Choe YH, Conover CD, et al. Drug delivery systems based on trimethyl lock lactonisation:Poly(ethyleneglycol)prodrugs of amino-containing compounds. *J Med Chem* 2000;43:475–487.

72. Veronese FM, Harris JM, eds, Peptide and protein PEGylation. *Adv Drug Deliv Syst* 2002;54(4).

73. Sezaki H, Takakura Y, Hashida M. Soluble macromolecular carriers for delivery of antitumour agents. *Adv Drug Deliv Rev* 1989;3:247–266.

74. Schacht, E., Ruys, L., Vermeersch, J., et al. Use of polysaccharides as drug carriers: Dextran and inulin derivatives of procainamide. *Ann N Y Acad Sci* 1985;446:199–212.

75. Hreczuk-Hirst D, Chicco D, German L, et al. Dextrins as potential carriers for drug targeting: Tailored rates of dextrin degradation by introduction of pendant groups. *Int J Pharm* 2001;230:57–66.

76. Hreczuk-Hirst D, German L, Duncan R. Synthesis and characterisation of dextrin-doxorubicin conjugates: a new anticancer treatment. *Proceedings of the International Symposium of Controlled Release Bioactive Materials* 1999;26:1086–1087.

77. Przybylski M, Fell E, Ringsdorf H, et al. Pharmacologically active polymers. 17. Synthesis and characterisation of polymeric derivatives of the antitumour agent methotrexate. *Makromol Chem* 1978;179:1719–1733.

78. Seymour LW, Miyamoto Y, Brereton M, et al. Influence of molecular size on passive tumour-accumulation of soluble macromolecular drug carriers. *Eur J Cancer* 1995;5:766–770.

79. Duncan R, Pratten MK, Cable HC, et al. Effect of molecular size of ^{125}I-labelled poly(vinylpyrrolidone) on its pinocytosis by rat visceral yolk sacs and rat peritoneal macrophages. *Biochem J* 1980;196:49–55.

80. Sat YN, Burger AM, Fiebig HH,, et al. Comparison of vascular permeability and enzymatic activation of the polymeric prodrug HPMA copolymer-doxorubicin (PK1) in human tumour xenografts. *American Association for Cancer Res 90th Annual Meeting.* Philadelphia, PA; 1999:41.

81. Rihova B, Bilej M, Vetvicka, et al. R. Biocompatibility of N-(2-hydroxypropyl)methacrylamide copolymers containing adriamycin. Immunogenicity, and effect of haematopoietic stem cells in bone marrow *in vivo* and effect on mouse splenocytes and human peripheral blood lymphocytes *in vitro*. *Biomaterials* 1989;10:335–342.

82. Yeung TK, Hopewell JW, Simmonds RH, et al. Reduced cardiotoxicity of doxorubicin given in the form of N-(2-hydroxypropyl) methacrylamide conjugates: an experimental study in the rat. *Cancer Chemother Pharmacol* 1991;29:105–111.

83. Hopewell JW, Duncan R, Wilding D, et al. Modification of doxorubicin induced cardiotoxicity I. Preclinical studies of cardiotoxicity of PK2 : A novel polymeric antitumour agent. *Hum Exp Toxicol* 2001;20:461–470.

84. Pinciroli V, Rizzo V, Angelucci F, et al. Characterisation of two polymer–drug conjugates by ^{1}H-NMR: FCE

28068 and FCE 28069. *Magn Reson Chem* 1997;35: 2–8.

85. Mendichi R, Rizzo V, Gigli M, et al. Molecular characterisation of polymeric antitumour drug carriers by size exclusion chromatography and universal calibration. *J Liq Chromotogr Rel Technol* 1996;19:1591–1605.

86. Mendichi R, Rizzo V, Gigli M, et al. Molar mass distribution of a polymer–drug conjugate containing the antitumor drug paclitaxel by size exclusion chromatography and universal calibration. *J Liq Chromotogr Rel Technol* 1998;21:1295–1309.

87. Mendichi R, Rizzo V, Gigli M, et al. Dilute-solution properties of a polymeric antitumor drug carrier by size-exclusion chromatography, viscometry, and light scattering. *J Appl Polym Sci* 1998;70:329–338.

88. Configliacchi E, Razzano G, Rizzo V, et al. HPLC methods for the determination of bound and free doxorubicin and of bound and free galactosamine in methacrylamide polymer–drug conjugates. *J Pharm Biomed Anal* 1996;15:123–129.

89. Fraier D, Frigerio E, Pianezzola E, et al. A sensitive procedure for the quantitation of free and N-(2-hydroxypropyl)methacrylamide polymer-bound doxorubicin (PK1) and some of its metabolites, 13-dihydrodoxorubicin, 13-dihydrodoxorubicinone and doxorubicinone in human plasma and urine bt reverse phase HPLC with fluorometric detection. *J Pharm Biomed Anal* 1995;13: 625–631.

90. Cavallo, Adami M, Magrini R, et al. PK1/PK2 lyophilised formulations. HPMA doxorubicin conjugates with potentially improved antitumour activity. *Proceedings of the 1st World Meeting APGI/APV.* Budapest; 1995:843.

91. Searle F, Gac-Breton S, Keane R, et al. N-(2-hydroxypropyl)methacrylamide copolymer-6-(3-aminopropyl)-ellipticine conjugates, synthesis, characterisation and preliminary *in vitro* and *in vivo* studies. *Bioconj Chem* 2001;12:711–718.

92. Kasuya Y, Lu Z-R, Kopeckova P, et al. Influence of the structure of drug moieties on the *in vitro* efficacy of HPMA copolymer-geldanamycin derivative conjugates. *PharmRes* 2002;19:115–123.

93. Varticovski L, Lu Z-R, Mitchell K, et al. Water-soluble HPMA copolyme-wortmannin conjugate retains phosphoinositide 3-kinase inhibitory activity in vitro and in vivo. *J Control Release* 2001;74:275–281.

94. Satchi R, Connors TA, Duncan R. PDEPT: Polymer directed enzyme prodrug therapy I. HPMA copolymer-cathepsin B and PK1 as a model combination. *Br J Cancer* 2001;85:1070–1076.

95. Duncan R, Gac-Breton S, Keane R, et al. Polymer–drug conjugates, PDEPT and PELT: Basic principles for design and transfer from the laboratory to the clinic. *J Control Release* 2001;74:135–146.

96. Duncan R. The dawning era of polymer therapeutics. *Nature Rev Drug Disc* 2003;2:347–360.

18

Prodrug Drug Development and Retrometabolic Engineering

Daniel R. Budman

Experimental Therapeutics Section, Don Monti Division of Oncology,
North Shore University Hospital, New York University, Manhasset, New York 11030

The concept behind targeted drug development dates back to the last century with the theory of specificity of drug therapy as first promulgated as Dr. Paul Ehrlich's "magic bullet," which would affect only the disease process and not the patient (1). Despite millions of dollars and years spent in drug discovery, however, only approximately 400 targets are now available for pharmacologic intervention for all of medicine, with the promise of possibly 10,000 targets as an outgrowth of the genome project (2,3). As a result, there has been intense interest in the attempt to optimize the available drugs to make them more specific for their given targets and hopefully less damaging to normal tissue, thus leading to an enhanced therapeutic index. Many of these efforts have been devoted to chemical modifications of existing agents to enhance their pharmacokinetic or pharmacodynamic properties (Fig. 18.1) (4).

The choice of which starting structure to alter may depend upon the ease of synthesizing the starting compound, whether the structure can easily be modified, and whether the structure is proprietary to another company. In the event of any of these problems, the computational chemist may decide to data mine existing data banks of two-dimensional or three-dimensional chemical structures (5,6) to obtain a more practical starting compound, using the tertiary structure as a guide (Fig. 18.1). A *pharmacophore* is defined as the tertiary structure of the binding area of the drug to its target; a *scaffold* is the chemical structure of the pharmacophore. The computational chemist may suggest appropriate chemical modifications that will make the scaffold more stable or inert until the agent is metabolized, given that these procedures have been stored in databases by most pharmaceutical companies (7,8).

A *prodrug* can be defined as an active agent that has been chemically modified to be relatively inert in its manufactured form. When the prodrug is administered to the patient, it undergoes one or more metabolic steps (spontaneous or enzymatic induced) that result in generation of the active agent. Because many of the commercially available cytotoxic anticancer drugs are chemically labile in their active form, the majority of drugs used for treatment of cancer are prodrugs that require metabolic activation within the patient. Usually this metabolic step is a consequence of xenobiotic metabolism and uses the same enzymatic pathways that normally are used to degrade foreign substances (9).

The majority of the commercially available anticancer agents were discovered in their prodrug form. Only recently has there been increasing interest in rational synthetic chemical modification of existing anticancer agents to produce prodrugs that have altered pharmacokinetics or altered transport properties that may result in an enhanced therapeutic index. As a consequence, although prodrug synthesis became commonplace for many agents such as antibiotics in the early 1970s (10), except for alkylating agents, this approach was not pursued by the pharmaceutical industry until the 1990s. The early alkylating agents, such as nitrogen mustard, were reactive moieties with vesicant properties that led to the development of masked prodrugs requiring activation to make them better tolerated in the clinical setting. Cyclophosphamide, an alkylating agent, is an early example of designing a prodrug that is inert until it is metabolized (11,12).

Any prodrug must satisfy certain criteria: (a) it is a structural analog of the active agent; (b) an autolytic bond or metabolically sensitive side chain(s) is

Prodrug development

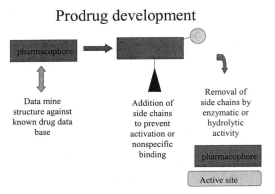

FIG. 18.1. Prodrugs are developed from a candidate compound or its active moiety.

present that allows the patient to convert the prodrug preferentially into the active compound; (c) the prodrug is chemically stable in formulation and when it is administrated to the patient; (d) the prodrug is not actively excreted prior to conversion; (e) other metabolites of the prodrug are not of enhanced toxicity to the patient; and (f) distribution of the prodrug and/or the active agent is able to reach the site of interest for therapeutic action.

The prodrug is not designed to target a given site but rather is formulated to overcome a deficiency noted in the parent compound (Table 18.1) (13). For example, an active drug may be relatively insoluble in aqueous solution, as is the case for etoposide. The addition of a phosphate moiety makes the drug water soluble, thus easing the task of intravenous administration (14–16). This approach is successful in humans because plasma phosphatases are able to efficiently convert the prodrug back into etoposide in the circulation (15). This

method has been applied in the generation of prodrugs of thiosemicarbazone with either phosphate groups or disulfide linkages (17) and combretastatin A-2 with phosphate groups (18). Paclitaxel is made more water soluble when it is formulated as an ester of malic acid, which degrades to the parent compound in human plasma (19). However, this effect is nonspecific in that the active drug does not concentrate within the tumor compared to normal tissue and no targeting effect occurs. A variety of enzymes have been used to activate anticancer drugs (Table 18.2) (10), but most common approaches include a carboxypepidase, an esterase, or a phosphatase.

Insertion of metabolizing enzymes by gene therapy into the target tissue [gene-directed enzyme/prodrug therapy (GDEPT)] has been suggested as a method to enhance the therapeutic index, but currently it remains of theoretical interest, with some ongoing human trials (20). A typical approach is the use of β-galactosidase inserted by gene therapy into a tumor model and then exposure of the cells to an agent such as N-[(4″RS)-4″-ethoxy-4″(1′″-O-β-D-galactopyranosyl)butyl] daunorubicin, which in a model system is 1,000-fold more cytotoxic in the presence of β-glactosidase and thus could offer targeting and an enhanced therapeutic index if the tumor expresses this enzyme (21).

A related concept is retrometabolic engineering. Chemical drug delivery, also known as *retrometabolic engineering,* is a term first defined by Dr. Nicholas Bodor to describe chemical modification(s) of an active agent that then becomes a prodrug. This new chemical entity ideally will undergo several metabolic steps, eventually resulting in enhanced concentration in the target tissue (22,23). As such, this approach potentially allows the pharmaceutical chemist to enhance the therapeutic index by having the active agent concentrate at the target site and not in normal host tissue. A corollary of this approach is a "soft drug," which is an agent that is active at the target site but is rapidly metabolized to inert substances at nontarget sites (24). The soft drug approach has not been actively pursued in cancer drug development.

TABLE 18.1. *Generation of a prodrug should enhance the biologic or pharmacokinetic properties of the initial candidate compound*

Goals of prodrug development
• Make biologically inert, stable agent that is converted into active agent
• Enhance
Absorption
Distribution (including central nervous system, if desired)
• Perturb metabolism
Change Cpmax, area under the curve, or terminal half-life of the active compound
Diminish metabolites which are toxic to the host
• Concentrate active agent in target (organ, tissue, tumor)

TABLE 18.2. *Enzymes that have been used to activate anticancer prodrugs (10)*

• Amidase	• β-Glucuronidase
• Azoreductase	• γ-Glutamyl transferase
• Carboxypeptidase	• Kinase
• Cytochrome P-450	• β-Lactamase
• Deaminase	• Nitroreductase
• Diaphorase	• Phosphatase
• Galactosidase	• Plasmin

TABLE 18.3. *Generation of new entities based upon a candidate compound must consider the problems similar to those of initial drug development*

Problems with the prodrug approach

- Poor "drug likeness" (rule of five)
- Low concentration at the target site
  Low penetration by the prodrug into the target site (factors: molecular size, lipophilicity, charge, amount of free drug)
  Inefficient conversion at the target site
  - Steric blocking by side chains
  - *In vitro* testing against a nonhuman enzyme with different affinity, not reflective of the human enzyme
  - Low levels of the appropriate enzyme
  - High K_m (low affinity for the converting enzyme)
  - pH not optimal for enzymatic activity
  High degrading metabolic activity at the target site

Prodrug design is further complicated in that preclinical *in vitro* and animal findings may not mimic the results in humans (Table 18.3). For example, screening of a new chemical entity for prodrug feasibility in an *in vitro* system may use nonhuman enzymes for activation, lack the appropriate enzyme at the target site, have an enzyme with low affinity for the prodrug expressed in humans, be active at a pH that is not characteristic of the actual tumor and diminishes the chemical conversion, or have a problem penetrating the tumor because of the size of the chemical entity and/or because of molecular charge (13). Polymorphism of enzyme activity or of expression (see Chapter 25) is a major concern for the pharmaceutical chemist, because heterogeneity of an enzyme needed for activation or metabolism will lead to suboptimal production of the active agent or to potentially rapid destruction of the active agent with lower concentration within the tumor (25–29). A polymorphism of the metabolizing enzyme also may lead to more toxic metabolites in some patients, as was seen with the cytotoxic agent amonifide (30). This may be compensated for by designing steric blockade of the metabolic site with additional substitutions. An additional concern in prodrug design is that the chemical entities arising from combinatorial chemistry or computer-aided design tend to be large insoluble molecules that may be difficult to change into a prodrug or to synthesize (31). Ease of synthesis, chemical stability, and ability to isolate pure compound are other concerns with prodrug design (32). Prodrug development must take into account that not only the active moiety but also the prodrug must

have "druglike" properties that allow the agent to be administered by a convenient route, with high absorption into the systemic circulation and a high volume of distribution so that there will not be a sanctuary [such as the central nervous system (CNS)] that allows the emergence of drug-resistant tumor clones. Computerized guidelines for selecting compounds with large volumes of distribution have been reliably estimated on the basis of human plasma protein binding; calculated lipophilicity on the basis of reverse phase, high-performance liquid chromatographic studies of candidate compounds not ionizable at pH 7.4 (33); and pK_a (negative log acidic dissociation constant) (34). Additional selection features used to distinguish a drug candidate acceptable for development include the general guidelines espoused by Lipinski et al. (31) (Table 18.4), which are based upon the computerized database of the World Drug Index. Increasing molecular weight is known to be an indicator of poor intestinal and CNS penetration. In the case of "rule of five" analysis, only 11% of active agents in the index had a molecular weight greater than 500 daltons (31). The calculated log P (35), which is a measure of lipophilicity, the number of hydroxyl and amino groups, and the number of hydrogen bond acceptors all served as discriminants to distinguish druglike molecules (31). The only exception to these filtering criteria is agents that act as substrates for transporter molecules (Table 18.4). Investigators at GlaxoSmithKline have suggested, based upon a rat model, that alternate criteria for estimating good oral absorption of a drug candidate are high molecular rigidity as reflected by ten or fewer rotatable bonds and a polar surface of 140 Å or less (32).

Solubility guides used by pharmaceutical chemists include a minimum thermodynamic solubility of 50 μg/mL (31). Conjugation of polyethylene glycol to a candidate drug such as paclitaxel has been used to enhance water solubility and plasma half-life and serves as another methodology of prodrug synthesis to enhance a pharmacologic property (36). Other studies have noted that the each addition of a pair of

TABLE 18.4. *"Classic" criteria of an effective drug based upon retrospective review*

Rule of five: a drug is marginal if it has

1. More than 5 H-bond donors
2. More than 10 H-bond receptors
3. Molecular weight >500 kDa
4. Calculated log P (lipophilicity) >5
5. Compounds that are substrate for transporter molecules are exceptions

hydrogen bonds formed with water reduces cell membrane permeability by one log, thus reducing CNS penetration, and that a molecular weight threshold of 400 to 600 daltons limits even very lipid soluble agents from CNS penetration (37). For example, the lipophilic vinca alkaloids vincristine and vinblastine have molecular weights of approximately 800 daltons but penetrate the CNS poorly, even though they have favorable log P values (38). Algorithms have been developed that allow prediction of the distribution of a candidate drug into the CNS (39).

Two basic mechanisms by which prodrugs potentially enhance the therapeutic index have been identified: (a) site-specific transport and (b) site-specific activation (13). These mechanisms are the basis of retrometabolic engineering in which a candidate drug is modified to take advantage of unique anatomic, biologic, or enzymatic features of the target. In the case of the former approach, the prodrug may be coupled to an antibody or carrier molecule (40) that allows the prodrug to be transported into an organ or a tumor target. The use of cytotoxics conjugated to ligands that are preferentially bound to tumor cells overexpressing the ligand receptor is an analogous example (41,42). Similar approaches with prodrugs not targeted to malignancies have been described for substitutions that use the amino acid, peptide (43), or glucose transporters (10). Many β-lactam antibiotics, angiotensin-converting enzyme inhibitors, and renin inhibitors are transported by peptide transporters (10). Investigations initially based upon the HIV-1 Tat domain, which is necessary for viral internalization into human cells, have led to the discovery of polyguanidine peptoid derivatives with six-methylene spacers that demonstrate active transport into cells and also can be used as carrier molecules (44).

The candidate drug may be coupled to a structure that prevents degradation or activation in tissue other than the target. An additional example of site-specific transport is the conjugation of sugar residues on corticosteroids to diminish absorption in the upper intestines, which allows the steroid to be concentrated in the colon (13). Sulfasalazine is also not absorbed in the upper intestinal tract and is hydrolyzed to release 5-aminosalicylic acid in the colon in an analogous manner (45). Site-specific transport may suffer from the same problems encountered with nonspecific prodrug formulation (Table 18.3) in that the resulting structure may exceed the optimal characteristics of a prodrug, may not be able to penetrate into a tumor spheroid because of size or charge, may not be internalized into the target cell, and may not be activated once it is internalized. An additional difficulty is that if the transport moiety is bound to both malignant and nonmalignant tissue, then even if the drug has higher affinity for the malignant tissue, the numerous low-affinity binding sites of nonmalignant tissue may bind the majority of the drug and lead to a loss of targeting function.

In the case of site-specific activation, the prodrug is preferentially activated at the target site by either enzymatic methods or hydrolytic cleavage. Site-specific activation may depend upon the local environmental characteristics of the tissue, such as the presence of hypoxia, low pH, or overexpression of enzymes (hydrolytic, P-450), which can be used to activate a prodrug (46–48). The design of bioreductive agents depends upon the formation of a prodrug that has a requirement for an oxygen-sensitive reductive event and thus is active in a hypoxic environment, leading to a reactive intermediate that is cytotoxic (49). Recently, paclitaxel has been conjugated to aromatic nitro groups, which degrade in hypoxic conditions to liberate free paclitaxel (50). A doxorubicin prodrug, N-[4-β-glucuronyl-3-nitrobenzyl-oxycarbonyl] doxorubicin, was demonstrated to be activated by β-gluconidase in a pH-dependent fashion, with the majority of cytotoxic effect seen at a pH of 6 (51). Another example of site-specific activation is designing a lipophilic prodrug that can penetrate into the CNS and then is metabolized to a charged form (hydrophilic) that cannot egress from the brain (8). The prodrug may need a linker group to connect the metabolic labile side chain because of steric considerations imposed by both the active agent and the enzyme used (52).

Retrosynthetic fragmentation of the World Drug Index of 36,000 compounds has identified unique building blocks of side chains that can be computer adapted to automated structure design (53), thus allowing *in silico* identification of prodrug candidates that may satisfy the requirements for targeting.

In most cases, amide or ester formation of side chains attached to the pharmacophore is used to generate the prodrug. This approach is a reflection of the numerous active esterases, identified in humans, that can degrade prodrugs (54). Esterases are known to vary among species and even among organs, are polymorphic, increase activity with age, and demonstrate temperature-dependent effects (55). An additional reason to consider an ester bond is that the modification does not result in formation of a chiral molecule, so isomerization is not a problem. Typical side groups of ester derivatives of an agent may include linear structures such as aliphatics, bulky groups such as aromatic substitutions, branched substituents, and cyclical structures such as lactones. Increasing steric hindrance around the ester moiety correlates with decreased enzymatic hydrolytic activity and has been

Retrometabolic Design

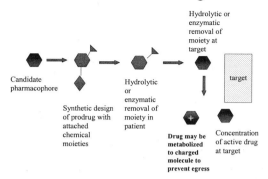

FIG. 18.2. Schema of the design of a prodrug to a target tissue or organ.

the basis of computer-aided design of side group structures (54). The inaccessible solid angle, which is the angle at which substitutions block access to a reaction site of the prodrug, has been modeled to provide a measure of the hydrolytic potential of a given substitution in drug design and thus the potential half-life in human plasma (54). This parameter thus offers an *in silico* method of selecting candidate carboxylic ester substitutions on a candidate drug prior to actual synthesis (54).

Other enzymes that have been exploited include amidases, carboxypeptidase (56), glycosidases, and kinases (57). The general schema of synthetic pathways is shown in Figure 18.2. Through either structure-activity design of candidate molecules or *in silico* techniques of drug design (58), the initial pharmacophore or drug is chemically modified with side chain structures that allow sequential metabolic degradation of an inactive or relatively inactive prodrug until it is restored to the active agent at the target tissue. The technique is predicated on the same principles as nonspecific prodrug design in that the required sequential metabolic steps are efficient, occur in the appropriate tissue, and do not result in toxic intermediates at the wrong site.

A preclinical approach to enhance tumor targeting by the use of overexpression of enzymes in tumor tissue is a prodrug of cytosine arabinoside coupled to a cleavable polyaminoacid. Enhancement of the therapeutic index occurs because the prodrug requires activation by plasmin, which is overexpressed in many tumors (52).

The best current example of retrometabolic engineering in oncology drug development is capecitabine, which presently is commercially available in many countries. This agent is a retrometabolically designed prodrug of 5-fluorouracil, which has high oral bioavailability (59) and by itself is not cytotoxic but must undergo several enzymatic steps to produce a cytotoxic agent (60–62). 5-Fluorouracil is poorly and erratically absorbed by the oral route and does not concentrate in tumor tissue. The prodrug doxifluridine (5′-DFUR) was generated to take advantage of the increased levels of the enzyme thymidine phosphorylase found in many tumors compared to normal tissue (63–65). 5′-DFUR requires thymidine phosphorylase to be converted into 5-fluorouracil, with the intention that this enzymatic effect would result in high levels of cytotoxic fluoropyrimidines and thus enhance the therapeutic index. However, 5′-DFUR also results in unacceptable gastrointestinal toxicity as thymidine phosphorylase also is present in intestinal tissue (66) and causes cardiac toxicity when administered intravenously (67). This agent is commercially available as an oral agent in Japan. Pharmaceutical chemists at Roche Japan then changed this agent to a nontoxic prodrug that could be administered via the oral route without causing dose-limiting toxicity at therapeutic dosages in animal models (60). The metabolic pathway of this agent is shown in Figure 18.3. The prodrug undergoes successive enzymatic steps to enhance oral absorption, prevent activation in intestinal tissue, and concentrate in tumor tissue by activation in the presence of increased levels of thymidine phosphorylase (62,68,69). The synthesis satisfies the criteria for targeted prodrug design in that the prodrug and the initial metabolites are only slightly cytotoxic, the level of active metabolite is found only at low levels in the circulating plasma (59,70), the penultimate drug is concentrated in the tumor tissue (68), and the major metabolic pathway is the desired activation pathway (Fig. 18.3). Of note, the common prodrug methodologies of using esterase and deaminase

Enzymatic activation of capecitabine

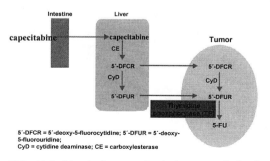

5′-DFCR = 5′-deoxy-5-fluorocytidine; 5′-DFUR = 5′-deoxy-5-fluorouridine;
CyD = cytidine deaminase; CE = carboxylesterase

FIG. 18.3. Metabolic steps in the retrometabolically designed prodrug capecitabine.

TABLE 18.5. *Targeted prodrug design*

Characteristics of chemical drug delivery systems

- Prodrug function with targeting on the basis of
  Carrier moiety (antibody, pegylation, side chains)
  Added moieties that are preferentially activated at
  the target site
  - By pH, enzymatic activity, autohydrolytic
    function
  - Resulting metabolism is the dominant form of
    chemical change of the prodrug

enzymes to metabolize the prodrug were used in the design of this drug with sequential activation steps (Table 18.5).

Methods to quantify a targeted effect by a prodrug are in development and described in Chapter 23. The general concepts that are useful in evaluating whether a given agent qualifies as a targeted drug with an enhanced therapeutic index are as follows.

Therapeutic index (TI) has been defined as

$$TI = \frac{MTTD}{MED}$$

where *MTTD* is the maximal tolerated dose and *MED* is the minimum effective dose (13). If a targeted and a nontargeted agent exist, the ratio of the targeted TI to the nontargeted TI can give a measure of the magnitude of the targeted effect. This approach is more feasible in animals in which host metabolic heterogeneity can be controlled and multiple experiments can be repeated for statistical validity. However, a related concept, the drug targeting index (DTI), which assumes that the biologic effect is a function of the

area under the time curve (AUC; concentration over time of exposure) of the active agent, can be defined as follows:

$$DTI = \frac{AUCr, ta/AUCt,ta}{AUCr,nta/AUCt,nonta}$$

where *AUCr,ta* is the concentration over time of the active targeted agent at the "response" site, *AUCt,ta* is the concentration over time of the targeted agent at the toxic site, *AUCr,nta* is the concentration over time of the nontargeted agent at the response site, and *AUCt,nta* is the concentration over time of the nontargeted agent at the toxic site (13). As imaging studies improve, these parameters can be better determined, even in clinical studies. A modification of this relationship can be made if a drug is administered as a prolonged infusion where AUC is approximately equivalent to the concentration at steady state C_{ss} so that the concentrations in the target can define the DTI (71).

The role of prodrug development and targeted therapy using small molecules in oncology is rapidly expanding. Understanding of the molecular mechanisms leading to targeted therapy and better understanding of the factors that control effective metabolism of a prodrug to an active compound remain under active development and are expected to assume a greater importance in the overview of pharmaceutical development. Development of more powerful preclinical computer-based algorithms will allow containment of prodrug development costs as generation of new analogs and new filtering mechanisms limits the need for formal structure-activity relationship studies of analogs in preclinical model systems.

REFERENCES

1. Drews J. Drug discovery: a historical perspective. *Science* 2000;287:1960–1964.
2. Sehgal A. Drug discovery and development using chemical genomics. *Curr Opin Drug Discov Devel* 2002;5:526–531.
3. Hopkins AL, Groom CR. The druggable genome. *Nat Rev Drug Discov* 2002;1:727–730.
4. Notari RE. Prodrug design. *Pharmacol Ther* 1981;14:25–53.
5. Lyne P. Structure-based virtual screening: an overview. *Drug Discov Today* 2002;7:1047–1055.
6. Cruciani G, Pastor M, Mannhold R. Suitability of molecular descriptors for database mining. A comparative analysis. *J Med Chem* 2002;45:2685–2694.
7. Kastenholz M, Pastor M, Cruciani G, et al. GRID/CPCA: a new computational tool to design selective ligands. *J Med Chem* 2000;10:3033–3044.
8. Bodor N, Buchwald P, Huang M-J. Computer-assisted design of new drugs based upon retrometabolic concepts. *SAR QSAR Environ Res* 1998;8:410–492.
9. Kwon CH. Metabolism-based anticancer drug design. *Arch Pharm Res* 1999;22:533–541.
10. Han HK, Amidon GL. Targeted prodrug design to optimize drug delivery. *AAPS Pharm Sci* 2000;2:E6.
11. Brock N, Gross R, Hohorst HJ, et al. Activation of cyclophosphamide in man and animals. *Cancer* 1971;27:1512–1529.
12. Cohen JL, Jao JY. Enzymatic basis of cyclophosphamide activation by hepatic microsomes of the rat. *J Pharmacol Exp Ther* 1970;174:206–210.
13. Kearney A. Review. Prodrugs and targeted drug delivery. *Adv Drug Deliv Rev* 1996;19:225–239.
14. Rose WC, Basler GA, Trail PA, et al. Preclinical antitumor activity of a soluble etoposide analog, BMY-40481-30. *Invest New Drugs* 1990;8[Suppl 1:]S25–S32.
15. Budman DR, Igwemezie LN, Kaul S, et al. Phase I evaluation of a water-soluble etoposide prodrug, etoposide phosphate, given as a 5-minute infusion on days 1, 3, and 5 in patients with solid tumors. *J Clin Oncol* 1994;12:1902–1909.

16. Mummaneni V, Kaul S, Igwemezie LN, et al. Bioequivalence assessment of etoposide phosphate and etoposide using pharmacodynamic and traditional pharmacokinetic parameters. *J Pharmacokinet Biopharm* 1996;24: 313–325.

17. Li J, Zheng L-M, King I, et al. Synthesis and antitumor properties of potent inhibitors of ribonucleotide reductase: 3-amino-4-methylpyridine-2-carboxaldehyde-thiosemicarbazone (3-Amp), 3-amino-pyridine-2-carboxaldehyde-thiosemicarbazone (3-Ap) and its water-soluble prodrugs. *Curr Med Chem* 2001;8:121–133.

18. Pettit GR, Moser BR, Boyd MR, et al. Antineoplastic agents 460. Synthesis of combretastatin A-2 prodrugs. *Anticancer Drug Des* 2001;16:185–193.

19. Damen EW, Wiegerinck PH, Braamer L, et al. Paclitaxel esters of malic acid as prodrugs with improved water solubility. *Bioorg Med Chem* 2000;8:427–432.

20. Greco O, Dachs GU. Gene directed enzyme/prodrug therapy of cancer: historical appraisal and future prospectives. *J Cell Physiol* 2001;187:22–36.

21. Bakina E, Farquhar D. Intensely cytotoxic anthracycline prodrugs: galactosides. *Anticancer Drug Des* 1999;14: 507–515.

22. Bodor N, Buchwald P. Drug targeting via retrometabolic approaches. *Pharmacol Ther* 1997;76: 1–27.

23. Bodor N. Recent advances in retrometabolic design approaches. *J Control Release* 1999;62:209–222.

24. Bodor N, Buchwald P. Soft drug design: general principles and recent applications. *Med Res Rev* 2000;20: 58–101.

25. Van Kuilenburg AB, Meinsma R, Zoetekouw L, et al. Increased risk of grade IV neutropenia after administration of 5-fluorouracil due to a dihydropyrimidine dehydrogenase deficiency: high prevalence of the IVS14 + 1g > a mutation. *Int J Cancer* 2002;101: 253–258.

26. Kham SK, Tan PL, Tay AH, et al. Thiopurine methyltransferase polymorphisms in a multiracial Asian population and children with acute lymphoblastic leukemia. *J Pediatr Hematol Oncol* 2000;24:353–359.

27. Daly AK, Hall AG. Pharmacogenetics of cytotoxic drugs. *Expert Rev Anticancer Ther* 2001;1:301–308.

28. Taub JW, Matherly LH, Ravindranath Y, et al. Polymorphisms in methylenetetrahydrofolate reductase and methotrexate sensitivity in childhood acute lymphoblastic leukemia. *Leukemia* 2002;16:764–765.

29. Krajinovic M, Labuda D, Mathonnet G, et al. Polymorphisms in genes encoding drugs and xenobiotic metabolizing enzymes, DNA repair enzymes, and response to treatment of childhood acute lymphoblastic leukemia. *Clin Cancer Res* 2002;8:802–810.

30. Kreis W, Chan K, Budman DR, et al. Clinical pharmacokinetics of amonafide (NSC 308847) in 62 patients. *Cancer Invest* 1996;14:320–327.

31. Lipinski C, Lombardo F, Dominy B, et al. Experimental and computational approaches to estimate solubility and permeability in drug discovery and development settings. *Adv Drug Deliv Rev* 2001;46:2–26.

32. Verber D, Johnson S, Cheng H-Y, et al. Molecular properties that influence the oral bioavailability of drug candidates. *J Med Chem* 2002;45:2615–2623.

33. Lombardo F, Shalaeva MY, Tupper KA, et al. ElogD(oct): a tool for lipophilicity determination in drug discovery. 2. Basic and neutral compounds. *J Med Chem* 2001;44:2490–2497.

34. Lombardo F, Obach RS, Shalaeva MY, et al. Prediction of volume of distribution values in humans for neutral and basic drugs using physicochemical measurements and plasma protein binding data. *J Med Chem* 2002;45: 2867–2876.

35. Moriguchi I, Hirono S, Nakagome I, et al. Comparison of reliability of log P values for drugs calculated by several methods. *Chem Pharm Bull* 1994;42:976–978.

36. Greenwald RB, Gilbert CW, Pendri A, et al. Drug delivery systems: water soluble Taxol 2′-poly(ethylene glycol) ester prodrugs—design and in vivo effectiveness. *J Med Chem* 1996;39:424–431.

37. Pardridge W. Transport of small molecules through the blood-brain barrier: biology and methodology. *Adv Drug Deliv Rev* 1995;15:5–36.

38. Greig NH, Soncrant TT, Shetty HU, et al. Brain uptake and anticancer activities of vincristine and vinblastine are restricted by their low cerebrovascular permeability and binding to plasma constituents in rat. *Cancer Chemother Pharmacol* 1990;26:263–268.

39. Abraham M, Chadha H, Mitchell R. Hydrogen bonding. 33. Factors that influence the distribution of solutes between blood and brain. *J Pharm Sci* 1994;83: 1257–1268.

40. Yang C, Tirucherai GS, Mitra AK. Prodrug based optimal drug delivery via membrane transporter/receptor. *Expert Opin Biol Ther* 2001;1:159–175.

41. de Groot FM, Damen EW, Scheeren HW. Anticancer prodrugs for application in monotherapy: targeting hypoxia, tumor-associated enzymes, and receptors. *Curr Med Chem* 2001;8:1093–1122.

42. Mitra AK, Dey S, Anand BS. Current prodrug strategies via membrane transporters/receptors. *Expert Opin Biol Ther* 2002;2:607–620.

43. Lepist EI, Kusk T, Larsen DH, et al. Stability and in vitro metabolism of dipeptide model prodrugs with affinity for the oligopeptide transporter. *Eur J Pharm Sci* 2000;11:43–50.

44. Wender P, Mitchell D, Pattabiraman K, et al. The design, synthesis, and evaluation of molecules that enable or enhance cellular uptake: peptoid molecular transporters. *Proc Natl Acad Sci U S A* 2000;97:13003–13008.

45. Azad Khan AK, Piris J, Truelove SC. An experiment to determine the active therapeutic moiety of sulphasalazine. *Lancet* 1977;2:892–895.

46. Mizen L, Burton G. The use of esters as prodrugs for oral delivery of beta-lactam antibiotics. *Pharm Biotechnol* 1998;11:345–365.

47. Patterson LH, McKeown SR, Robson T, et al. Antitumour prodrug development using cytochrome P450 (CYP) mediated activation. *Anticancer Drug Des* 1999;14:473–486.

48. Rauth AM, Melo T, Misra V. Bioreductive therapies: an overview of drugs and their mechanisms of action. *Int J Radiat Oncol Biol Phys* 1998;42:755–762.

49. Wilson W, Pruijn F. Hypoxia-activated prodrugs as antitumor agents: strategies for maximizing tumour cell killing. *Clin Exp Pharm Physiol* 1995;22:881–885.

50. Damen EW, Nevalainen TJ, van den Bergh TJ, et al. Synthesis of novel paclitaxel prodrugs designed for bioreductive activation in hypoxic tumour tissue. *Bioorg Med Chem* 2002;10:71–77.

51. Murdter TE, Friedel G, Backman JT, et al. Dose optimization of a doxorubicin prodrug (HMR 1826) in isolated perfused human lungs: low tumor pH promotes prodrug activation by beta-glucuronidase. *J Pharmacol Exp Ther* 2002;301:223–228.

52. Cavallaro G, Pitarresi G, Licciardi M, et al. Polymeric prodrug for release of an antitumoral agent by specific enzymes. *Bioconjug Chem* 2001;12:143–151.

53. Schneider G, Lee M-L, Stahl M, et al. De novo design of molecular architectures by evolutionary assembly of drug-derived building blocks. *J Computer Aided Mol Des* 2000;14:487–494.

54. Buchwald P, Bodor N. Structure-based estimation of enzymatic hydrolysis rates and its application in computer-aided retrometabolic drug design. *Pharmazie* 2000;55:210–217.

55. Buchwald P, Bodor N. Physiochemical aspects of the enzymatic hydrolysis of carboxylic esters. *Pharmazie* 2002;57:87–93.

56. Hamstra D, Page M, Maybaum J, et al. Expression of endogenously activated secreted or cell surface carboxypeptidase A sensitizes tumor cells to methotrexate-alpha-peptide prodrugs. *Cancer Res* 2000;60:657–665.

57. Denny WA. Prodrug strategies in cancer therapy. *Eur J Med Chem* 2001;36:577–595.

58. Bodor N. Retrometabolic drug design—novel aspects, future directions. *Pharmazie* 2001;56[Suppl 1]:S67–S74.

59. Reigner B, Blesch K, Weidekamm E. Clinical pharmacokinetics of capecitabine. *Clin Pharmacokinet* 2001;40:85–104.

60. Shimma N, Umeda I, Arasaki M, et al. The design and synthesis of a new tumor-selective fluoropyrimidine carbamate, capecitabine. *Bioorg Med Chem* 2000;8:1697–1706.

61. Ishikawa T, Utoh M, Sawada N, et al. Tumor selective delivery of 5-fluorouracil by capecitabine, a new oral fluoropyrimidine carbamate, in human cancer xenografts. *Biochem Pharmacol* 1998;55:1091–1097.

62. Budman DR. Capecitabine. *Invest New Drugs* 2000;18:355–363.

63. Fox SB, Westwood M, Moghaddam A, et al. The angiogenic factor platelet-derived endothelial cell growth factor/thymidine phosphorylase is up-regulated in breast cancer epithelium and endothelium. *Br J Cancer* 1996;73:275–280.

64. Nishimura G, Terada I, Kobayashi T, et al. Thymidine phosphorylase and dihydropyrimidine dehydrogenase levels in primary colorectal cancer show a relationship to clinical effects of 5′-deoxy-5-fluorouridine as adjuvant chemotherapy. *Oncol Rep* 2001;9:479–482.

65. Ackland SP, Peters GJ. Thymidine phosphorylase: its role in sensitivity and resistance to anticancer drugs. *Drug Resist Updat* 1999;2:205–214.

66. Di Bartolomeo M, Bajetta E, Somma L, et al. Doxifluridine as palliative treatment in advanced gastric and pancreatic cancer patients. *Oncology* 1996;53:54–57.

67. Olver IN, Reece PA, Bishop JF, et al. A phase I study of doxifluridine as a five-day stepped-dose continuous infusion. *Am J Clin Oncol* 1990;13:308–311.

68. Schuller J, Cassidy J, Dumont E, et al. Preferential activation of capecitabine in tumor following oral administration to colorectal cancer patients. *Cancer Chemother Pharmacol* 2000;45:291–297.

69. Morita T, Matsuzaki A, Suzuki K, et al. Role of thymidine phosphorylase in biomodulation of fluoropyrimidines. *Curr Pharm Biotechnol* 2001;2:257–267.

70. Budman DR, Meropol NJ, Reigner B, et al. Preliminary studies of a novel oral fluoropyrimidine carbamate: capecitabine. *J Clin Oncol* 1998;16:1795–1802.

71. Gibaldi M, Perrier D. *Pharmacokinetics,* 2nd ed. New York: Marcel Dekker, 1982.

19

Pharmacokinetics and Pharmacodynamics in Anticancer Drug Development

Chris H. Takimoto

University of Texas Health Science Center at San Antonio, Cancer Therapy and Research Center, San Antonio, Texas, 78229

INTRODUCTION

Recent scientific advances, such as high-throughput screening of novel molecules and the sequencing of the human genome, have led to the identification of thousands of promising new agents and therapeutic targets for anticancer therapy. Consequently, the drug development pipeline of new molecularly targeted anticancer agents is overflowing and easily exceeds the currently available resources for clinical testing of all promising new molecules. This places a premium on maximizing the efficiency of our clinical drug development program, a process that typically is complex and time consuming. One way to streamline these efforts is through the rigorous application and integration of pharmacokinetic and pharmacodynamic studies in the earliest stages of clinical drug development. Historically, early clinical trials of anticancer therapies have been conducted in a series of sequential, empirically designed, nonhypothesis testing studies that often are purely observational in nature (1). A more rational approach to early clinical development is to test the hypothesis that a drug's pharmacokinetic behavior is directly related to its pharmacodynamic endpoints, such as toxicity, efficacy, and effects on biologic markers. A comprehensive understanding of a drug's pharmacologic behavior can yield essential information for the rational design of the later stages of drug development. Ideally, the proactive utilization of this information can maximize the chances for a successful clinical development program.

This chapter outlines some of the basic principles of pharmacokinetics and pharmacodynamics, with a primary focus on clinically relevant concepts that can influence the drug development decision process. It is not intended as an introduction to basic pharmacokinetics and pharmacodynamics, nor is it meant to be a comprehensive review of clinical pharmacology. For that perspective, the reader is referred to more general discussions of clinical pharmacology (2–5). The emphasis for this discussion will be on an integrated approach to pharmacokinetics and pharmacodynamics in anticancer drug development.

Definitions

Clinical pharmacology can be broadly defined as the study of drugs in humans (2). The field of clinical pharmacology can be divided further into two major subdisciplines: pharmacokinetics and pharmacodynamics (2). Atkinson (2) defined *pharmacokinetics* as "the quantitative analysis of the process of drug absorption, distribution and elimination that determine the time course of drug action." Ratain (6) paraphrased the definition of pharmacokinetics as "what the body does to the drug." Classically, pharmacokinetics has involved the characterization of a drug's absorption, distribution, metabolism, and excretion (ADME) through measurements of drug concentration in accessible compartments over time. In contrast, *pharmacodynamics* is more directly related to drug mechanisms of action (2), and in practical terms it describes the relationship among drug dose, kinetics, and clinical effects, such as efficacy or toxicity. In simplified form, pharmacodynamics is "what the drug does to the body" (6).

Utility of Pharmacokinetics and Pharmacodynamics in Drug Development

The underlying principle of pharmacokinetic and pharmacodynamic analysis is that concentration-response relationships often are less variable than dose-response relationships for a given therapeutic agent (2). The theoretical basis for this assumption is that concentrations in measurable compartments are closely related to the concentrations of drug at the effective site of action. Thus, understanding the factors responsible for interpatient variability in drug kinetics can allow for the development of strategies to reduce this variability and thereby maximize therapeutic benefit in individual patients. The ultimate goal of pharmacokinetics and pharmacodynamics is to enhance a drug's therapeutic efficacy in the target population. A better understanding of a drug's pharmacologic behavior is a desirable objective for a drug development program; however, an even greater challenge is to optimally use this information in a clinically relevant manner to maximize the efficiency of the entire drug development process.

Characterization of a drug's pharmacokinetic behavior is clinically relevant for a variety of reasons (7). First, it provides a descriptive summary of a drug's behavior in a group of patients. Defining a pharmacokinetic model and the associated pharmacokinetic parameters is an excellent means to succinctly describe the behavior of a drug over time in a large population of patients. For example, a one-compartment, open, linear pharmacokinetic model with first-order elimination can describe a large amount of concentration versus time data. In addition, the coefficients of variation for the estimated mean values for the volume of distribution and elimination rate constant for this model can provide, at least in part, an estimate of the degree of interpatient variability in drug kinetics within the study population (6).

A second reason for defining pharmacokinetic behavior is to provide explanatory information (7). Pharmacokinetic analysis is a powerful tool for gaining insight into the basic physiologic processes that may modulate drug behavior. This can generate hypotheses about the underlying mechanisms responsible for drug distribution, elimination, or metabolism. Individual pharmacokinetic parameters can be correlated with important covariate factors within the population, such as age, gender, hepatic or renal function, pharmacogenetic variations in drug-metabolizing enzymes, concomitant medications, or body surface area (BSA). These factors may explain why pharmacokinetic variability exists within a population. Understanding population variability is a key goal for early pharmacologic studies of a new agent. For example, if drug clearance of a novel agent strongly correlates with creatinine clearance, then renal excretion may be hypothesized to be a major route of drug elimination (Fig. 19.1). The findings suggest that caution is warranted when administering such a drug to

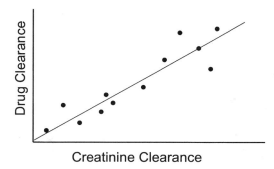

FIG. 19.1. Drug clearance versus creatinine clearance.

patients with impaired renal function. Furthermore, strong correlations among renal function, drug kinetics, and pharmacodynamic effects suggest that adaptive dosing, nomograms, or other individualized dosing strategies based upon estimated creatinine clearance may have potential clinical utility (8,9).

A third reason to define a drug's pharmacokinetic behavior is to provide predictive information (7). A model derived from a single pharmacokinetic experiment may accurately predict drug concentrations for vastly different doses and schedules of drug administration. For example, pharmacokinetic parameter estimates obtained after a single intravenous (IV) bolus of drug can be used to calculate the time and magnitude of steady-state drug concentrations following a prolonged continuous infusion of the same drug. For other drugs identified as having nonlinear pharmacokinetic behavior, it may be difficult to accurately predict the exact consequences of standard dose adjustments on the pharmacokinetics of a particular agent. Finally, more complex simulations of pharmacokinetic behavior and variability within a population can be used to forecast and evaluate different complex large-scale clinical trial designs, thus providing valuable information for further drug development (10). The expanded use of pharmacokinetic/pharmacodynamic clinical trial simulations has been heralded as a potentially revolutionary tool for rationally guiding drug development programs (11).

In contrast to the sometimes clinically obscure complexities of pharmacokinetic analysis, the direct clinical relevance of pharmacodynamic studies usually is obvious (12). The precise correlation between drug kinetics and biologic effects is the final step in understanding how drug administration relates to efficacy and toxicity endpoints. It is not possible to ascertain the clinical relevance of any pharmacokinetic measurement without a corresponding understanding of how kinetics relate to pharmacodynamic outcomes. In essence, a well-defined pharmacodynamic model strips away any variation in clinical outcome arising from pharmacokinetic variability. When a drug's kinetics are highly variable but its pharmacodynamics are highly consistent, then a target concentration strategy with therapeutic drug monitoring may be of substantial clinical benefit (13). Grochow (14) identified several drug characteristics that make an agent ideal for dose individualization strategies. These include agents with a large interindividual variability in drug elimination that also demonstrate robust exposure-response relationships that are closer than the dose-response relationships. If the primary clinical endpoints are not readily assessed as a basis for dose adjustment, then therapeutic drug monitoring of plasma drug concentrations may be a valuable guide to individualizing therapies. Relatively few practical examples of routine therapeutic drug monitoring exist in oncology, with high-dose methotrexate therapy the most notable exception (15).

It is important to recognize that clinical testing of anticancer agents provides unique challenges to the drug development scientist (16). First, phase I studies of anticancer agents are most often performed in patients and not in normal volunteers. The high toxicity and narrow therapeutic index of typical cytotoxic anticancer agents generally preclude extensive testing in normal volunteers. Furthermore, cancer patients are very heterogeneous (6) and may suffer from a variety of comorbidities, including malnutrition, liver metastases, extensive prior chemotherapy, prior radiation therapy, hypoalbuminemia, advanced age, or polypharmacy. Finally, the pharmacodynamics of most anticancer agents are complex, with long lag times of days or even weeks separating drug exposures from clinically relevant drug effects, such as myelosuppression or tumor response. Treating actual patients also raises special ethical issues for clinical trial study designs. Virtually all patients enter into experimental studies with some expectation and hope for therapeutic benefit. For example, once a recommended phase II dose has been determined, it may not be ethical to administered known subtherapeutic doses of drug to patients to formally test for dose proportionality using a crossover study design.

BASIC PHARMACOKINETIC PARAMETERS AND CONCEPTS

Clearance

Clearance probably is the single most important pharmacokinetic parameter for characterizing a drug's behavior, because clearance reflects all processes in the body that contribute to the elimination of drug over time. Total systemic drug clearance (CL) is the sum of all individual clearance processes ongoing in the body:

$$CL = CL_{renal} + CL_{hepatic} + CL_{other}, \qquad (1)$$

where CL_{renal} is renal clearance, $CL_{hepatic}$ is hepatic clearance, and CL_{other} is all other clearance processes. In clinical oncology, its relevance is enhanced because clearance is the only parameter that relates drug dose to the area under the curve AUC, which is a useful measure of systemic drug exposure. Thus, low clearance values are associated with increased systemic drug exposures and high AUC values. If $AUC_{0\text{-}INF}$ is the area under the concentration versus time curve from time zero extrapolated to infinity, then:

$$CL = Dose/AUC_{0\text{-}INF.} \qquad (2)$$

Clearance is also the most important parameter for designing long-term dosing regimens such as continuous drug infusions, because it is related to steady-state concentration C_{ss} by the formula:

$$CL = Infusion\ rate/C_{ss}. \qquad (3)$$

Clearance is not a rate; rather, it is defined as a volume cleared of drug per unit time. For a drug with dose-proportional kinetics, clearance is constant over any range of doses or concentrations.

In oncology, it is common practice to adjust drug doses based upon BSA. Although the uncritical implementation of this practice has been heavily criticized (17–26), it still is common to administer anticancer drugs in units of milligram per meter squared (mg/m^2). The rationale for BSA-based drug dosing is to achieve a uniform AUC in patients of all sizes when CL is dependent on BSA (Equation 2). Thus, careful examination of the relationship between clearance and BSA is important to perform early in drug development if a dosing scheme based upon BSA is contemplated. In actual practice, this correlation often is weak and does not always justify the use of doses based on BSA (mg/m^2) (25).

Elimination Half-life

The terminal elimination half-life is the amount of time required for half of an administered drug dose to be eliminated (13). It is an easily conceptualized pharmacokinetic parameter and, consequently, may be somewhat overemphasized in clinical applications. For example, a drug's terminal elimination half-life may or may not be clinically relevant for determining the proper time interval for drug dosing in actual practice. For example, drugs with active metabolites may have a biologic effect on half-lives that are much longer than the actual half-life of the administered agent. In addition, the development of highly sensitive analytical methods, such as mass spectroscopic detectors, has allowed for the characterization of very low concentrations of drug that may persist for prolonged periods after drug administration. These prolonged half-lives may be generated by the slow efflux of drug from deep tissue compartments or by release from tight binding sites, ultimately resulting in persistent but very low biologically inactive plasma drug concentrations (27). In such cases, the terminal elimination half-life may be less relevant than the shorter half-lives associated with drug concentrations in the biologically active range.

Half-lives can be readily estimated from compartmental or noncompartmental pharmacokinetic analyses. Often the terminal elimination rate constant is used to calculate the apparent half-life. In a well-designed pharmacokinetic study, if the final two or three terminal data points are obtained during the terminal linear elimination phase, then the slope of the log-linear concentration versus time plot is equivalent to the terminal elimination rate constant λ_z (28). This parameter is easily estimated from unweighted regression of the log-linear terminal elimination phase. Ideally the first and last data points for calculating the terminal elimination rate constant λ_z should differ in concentration by at least tenfold. In addition, these final measured drug concentrations must be greater than the measurement limit of the analytical assay. The terminal elimination rate constant is expressed in units of time^{-1}, and the half-life $t\frac{1}{2}$ can be calculated from the estimated λ_z using the formula:

$$t_{1/2} = ln(2)/\lambda_z = 0.693/\lambda_z. \qquad (4)$$

Note that the terminal elimination half-life is not a fundamental pharmacokinetic parameter because it is calculated from the estimated terminal elimination rate constant (13). The elimination rate constant is fundamentally related to volume of distribution of the central compartment and clearance by the formula:

$$CL = V_c \times \lambda_z. \qquad (5)$$

The terminal half-life is clinically useful for determining the time to reach steady state on a multidose schedule or during a continuous IV drug infusion (e.g., after four half-lives, drug concentrations will be 94% of the steady-state value).

Volume of Distribution

Volume of distribution is the pharmacokinetic parameter that relates the amount of drug in the body to the concentration in the measured compartment. Although it often is a clinically useful parameter, it does not necessarily correspond to an actual physiologic compartment. A number of different volumes of distribution are frequently reported in clinical pharmacologic studies, including volume of the central compartment V_c, volume of distribution at steady state V_{ss}, and volume of distribution during the terminal elimination phase V_{area} or V_z.

The *central volume of distribution V_c* is the constant of proportionality relating drug dose and the immediate postinfusion plasma drug concentration after a short IV bolus of drug. This parameter is clinically relevant because it allows for determination of maximum plasma concentration C_{max} immediately after IV drug bolus. It can be calculated using compartmental modeling techniques or by back extrapolation to estimate the maximal plasma concentration at time zero C_0.

For a single IV bolus:

$$V_c = Dose/C_0. \qquad (6)$$

For multiple doses:

$$V_c = Dose/(C_{postdose} - C_{predose}), \qquad (7)$$

where $C_{postdose}$ is the concentration immediately after the infusion and $C_{predose}$ is the drug concentration immediately prior to infusion.

The *volume of distribution at steady state V_{ss}* is the constant of proportionality relating the amount of drug in the body to the measured plasma concentration at steady state (29). This clinically useful parameter is independent of drug clearance, and it reflects the anatomic space occupied by the drug and relative amount of drug in the measured central compartments and the peripheral tissues at equilibrium. It does not require that actual steady-state concentrations be measured; instead, it can be estimated from information obtained after a single IV bolus of drug. However, the estimate of V_{ss} depends upon the assumption that drug is eliminated only from the central compartment and not from the peripheral or more slowly equilibrating sites. In a standard compartmental model, V_{ss} is defined by:

$$V_{ss} = V_1 + V_2 + \ldots + V_n, \qquad (8)$$

where n is the number of compartments in the model. In a noncompartmental analysis based upon statistical moment theory, V_{ss} can be calculated after a single IV bolus of drug using the following formula (29):

For a single bolus dose:

$$V_{ss} = Dose(AUMC)/(AUC)^2, \qquad (9)$$

where AUMC is the area under the first moment curve (concentration multiplied by time versus time plot) and AUC is the area under the concentration versus time curve. After a drug infusion, V_{ss} can be calculated as follows (29):

For a drug infusion:

$$V_{ss} = Dose(AUMC)/(AUC)^2 - [R_0T^2/2(AUC)], \quad (10)$$

where T is the duration of the infusion and R_0 is the dose rate of infusion. In general, a larger value for V_{ss} suggests widespread distribution, whereas a value of V_{ss} that approximates the plasma volume suggests an agent limited to the intravascular space.

The *terminal disposition volume of distribution V_z* is the constant of proportionality relating the amount of drug in the measured compartment during the terminal elimination phase. This term is clinically useful because it is the volume of distribution used to calculate the loading dose necessary to assure that average plasma drug concentrations never fall below the target mean steady-state concentration level. This volume term also is referred to as V_{area} and can be estimated from the following formula:

$$V_z = V_{area} = CL/\lambda_z = Dose/(\lambda_z \times AUC). \quad (11)$$

Area Under the Curve

The area under the concentration versus time curve is commonly used as an indicator of systemic drug exposure in oncology. As previously mentioned, it is related to clearance by drug dose (Equation 2). It is extremely useful in noncompartmental pharmacokinetic analyses as a tool for estimating other pharmacokinetic parameters such as clearance and volume of distribution at steady state (Equations 2, 9, and 10). Although some investigators have recommended deemphasizing AUC as a pharmacokinetic parameter in favor of clearance (30), it is still widely used as a measure of drug exposure in pharmacodynamic studies in oncology. The AUC can be directly estimated by simple numerical integration of the concentration versus time data. The most popular method of calculating the AUC is the linear trapezoidal rule or the log-linear trapezoidal rule with extrapolation to infinity (28).

Dose Proportionality

Dose proportionality is the condition in which drug concentrations in the measured compartment are strictly proportional to the dose of drug administered. Simply stated, if the dose of a drug is doubled, then the resulting plasma concentrations also are doubled (31,32). When dose proportionality is present, then parameters of drug exposure, such as AUC, steady-state plasma concentration C_{ss}, and maximum plasma concentration C_{max}, are directly proportional to drug dose.

In this situation, fundamental pharmacokinetic parameters such as volume of distribution, clearance, and rate constants are unchanged at different dose levels. Strictly speaking, drugs with linear pharmacokinetics also are dose proportional. Linear pharmacokinetics means that a drug's pharmacologic behavior can be described by a series of linear differential equations, such as those used to describe a multicompartmental model with first-order rate constants and elimination restricted to the central compartment.

Dose proportionality is clinically important because dose-proportional agents can be rationally dose adjusted in a predictable fashion. For drugs that lack dose proportionality, pharmacokinetic parameters such as clearance will demonstrate concentration dependence, time dependence, or both. In these situations, it often is difficult to predict the effect of dose changes on the resulting plasma drug concentrations. Non–dose-proportional agents are well described in the literature; the best-known examples are drugs with saturable Michaelis-Menten elimination processes, such as phenytoin (33). Other physiologic factors that can cause deviations from dose proportionality include saturable oral absorption, capacity-limited distribution, and saturable protein binding over relevant concentration ranges.

There are multiple ways to test for dose proportionality (28,31,32). One option is to perform weighted regression of the AUC or C_{max} versus dose level plot to see if the resulting line passes through the origin (28). Note that a simple regression line that fits the AUC versus dose plot but does not pass through the origin is not strictly linear (doubling the dose does not exactly double the AUC). More rigorous tests of dose proportionality include application of the power model (31) or analysis of variance (ANOVA) testing of the log-transformed CL or log-transformed dose-normalized (AUC/dose) values examined across various dose levels (28,31). In oncology, dose proportionality is commonly assessed in dose-escalating phase I dose trials, which often are the only opportunity to examine drug administration over a wide range of doses.

Protein Binding

Most drugs show some degree of binding to plasma proteins such as human serum albumin (34), α_1-acid glycoprotein (AAG) (35), or other macromolecular components in blood such as erythrocytes (36). Although free and bound drug are in equilibrium and thus vary in parallel, only the free fraction is thought to be biologically active. This unbound drug fraction equilibrates directly with the extravascular space and, theoretically, may be more closely related to drug concentrations in the biologically active effect compartment. Most bioanalytical assays measure only total drug concentrations and ignore the free drug fraction unless special procedures such as plasma ultrafiltration or equilibrium dialysis are used. The extent and variability in protein binding can directly affect a drug's pharmacokinetics (35), and interspecies differences in drug protein binding may complicate animal scale-up experiments (37). Furthermore, cancer patients may have accompanying disease states, such as renal or hepatic dysfunction, altered levels of circulating AAG, or hypoalbuminemia, which alter protein binding. Thus, protein binding may be an important source of interpatient variability in drug kinetics. Competitive drug displacement from plasma proteins was once thought to be a major mechanism of adverse drug interactions. However, most drug displacement protein binding interactions are not clinically relevant unless a concomitant interaction exists at the level of drug clearance (30,38).

Bioavailability

Historically, most anticancer therapies have been administered as IV agents. However, this trend may be changing as more chronically administered oral antitumor agents enter clinical development (39). For any extravascularly administered agent, bioavailability is an important pharmacokinetic parameter and another potential source of interpatient variability. Bioavailability F is defined as the fraction of an administered dose that reaches the systemic circulation compared with a reference route of administration. Typically, the reference standard for oral drug administration has been an IV infusion, which is arbitrarily given a bioavailability value of 1.0 (28). Under these conditions, oral bioavailability can range from 0 to 1.0, and it is defined using the formula:

$$F = dose(iv) \times AUC(oral)/[dose(oral) \times AUC(iv)], \quad (12)$$

where *dose(iv)* and *dose(oral)* are the IV and oral doses, respectively, and *AUC(oral)* and *AUC(iv)* are the oral and intravenous AUC values, respectively. Because the extent of absorption from the gut into the systemic circulation may vary, the actual dose entering the systemic circulation after oral administration is not known. This can complicate the estimation of pharmacokinetic parameters such as clearance or volume of distribution for orally administered agents. However, this may not be problematic because the summary pharmacokinetic parameters can easily be expressed as bioavailability-corrected factors (28). Thus, volume of

distribution is reported as V/F and clearance becomes CL/F, where F is the bioavailability. In many phase I pharmacokinetic studies of oral anticancer agents, formal estimates of bioavailability F are not routinely reported because it requires the administration of both oral and IV drugs in the same patient.

BASIC PHARMACODYNAMIC PARAMETERS AND CONCEPTS

In pharmacodynamic studies, clinical drug effects are modeled as a function of dose, drug concentrations, or other important kinetic parameters (6,40). Once pharmacokinetic variability has been accounted for, a pharmacodynamic model can explain how a particular degree of drug exposure correlates with clinical outcomes such as toxicity and/or efficacy. In a manner analogous to pharmacokinetic models, variability in pharmacodynamic relationships can be associated with patient covariates, such as age, gender, degree of prior chemotherapy, prior radiotherapy, and concomitant medications.

The parameters of drug exposure that have been most commonly utilized in oncologic pharmacodynamic studies are AUC and plasma drug concentrations such as C_{max} or C_{ss}. However, pharmacodynamic studies should not be constrained to testing only these parameters of drug exposure. Highly schedule-dependent agents may be better represented by models that define the time that drug concentrations remain above a particular threshold concentration, as has been identified for paclitaxel pharmacodynamics (41). The specific parameter used as the independent variable in a pharmacodynamic analysis will depend on the particular characteristics of the study drug.

The specific drug effects modeled in a pharmacodynamic analysis also will depend upon the agent being studied, the dose-limiting toxicities, and the nature of the study design. In anticancer phase I trials, the frequent occurrence of dose-limiting myelosuppression has led to numerous examples of pharmacodynamic models relating the absolute decrease in blood counts as a continuously modeled dependent variable to drug exposure (Fig. 19.2). This can be represented by a sigmoid maximum effect model that is described by the modified Hill equation (42):

$$Percent\ fall\ in\ blood\ counts = 100\% \times C^h/[C^h + (EC_{50})^h],$$

where C is the input parameter of drug exposure (often AUC or C_{ss}), EC_{50} is the value of C that produces a 50% decrease in drug counts, and h is the Hill con-

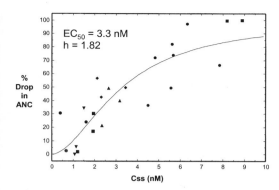

FIG. 19.2. Sigmoid maximum effect model described by the modified Hill equation parameters, where EC_{50} is the steady-state concentration C_{ss} value that produces a 50% decrease in drug counts, h is the Hill constant that is related to the degree of sigmoidicity of the exposure-effect curve, and ANC is the absolute neutrophil count.

stant, which is related to the degree of sigmoidicity of the exposure-effect curve. Nonlinear regression techniques can be used to estimate EC_{50} and h for any given data set. This general approach is readily applied to continuous outcome variables. However, many drug-related toxicities are graded on subjective toxicity scales defined by categorical (ordinal) variables and may require more complex statistical modeling to define pharmacokinetic relationships. For example, a logistic regression model may be necessary to predict the probability of developing grade 1 (minimal), grade 2 (mild), grade 3 (moderate), or grade 4 (severe) drug-related toxicities such as vomiting or diarrhea (43).

More complex mechanistic pharmacodynamic models of drug-related myelosuppression have been developed to describe and predict clinically important dose-limiting toxicities (44–47). These include models for paclitaxel- (45,47) and etoposide-induced neutropenia (46,47) that utilize compartmental indirect and population mixed effect modeling methods. These novel pharmacodynamic models are approaching the same level of sophistication seen in many complex pharmacokinetic models and ultimately may result in a greater understanding of clinically important drug effects. Finally, formal population pharmacodynamic models that incorporate key covariate effects such as age, gender, baseline conditions, prior therapy, and pharmacogenetic factors are still rare and need to be more fully explored (46). Nonetheless, these novel approaches to pharmacodynamic modeling remain a promising and exciting area of future research.

PHARMACOKINETIC/ PHARMACODYNAMIC STUDY DESIGN ISSUES

Collection and Quantitative Analysis of Pharmacokinetic Samples

The initial characterization of the full pharmacokinetic profile of a new drug typically requires a large number of time points, ranging from 15 to 20 blood samples obtained both during and after drug administration. The sampling period ideally should extend for up to five half-lives. The initial sampling scheme can be based upon extrapolation from preclinical studies testing. However, analysis of the initial pharmacokinetic samples should be performed as early as possible so that adjustments in sampling times can be implemented whenever necessary. Unexpectedly slow clearance may require the addition of several later time points to fully characterize all phases of drug kinetics. Guidelines for pharmacokinetic sample collection, processing, storage, and the pharmacokinetic analysis plan should be clearly outlined in the protocol document.

Clinical research support staff must be counseled on the proper methods for sample collection, processing, and storage conditions. Precise recording of drug doses, times of administration, and collection times are essential data for pharmacokinetic analysis. Blood samples should be drawn from venous puncture in the opposite extremity from the site of drug infusion whenever possible, and under no circumstances should blood be drawn from the same line or infusion device used to administer the drug. Proper flushing techniques to avoid administering miniature boluses of drug at the end of the infusion are important. Clinical research staff should be counseled that deviations from specified sampling times is not as problematic as failing to record the exact time of the actual blood draw.

Analyzing pharmacokinetic data assumes that one has a reliable validated bioanalytical assay to measure drug concentrations. The sensitivity of the assay may well dictate the times of sample collection at later time points. For a discussion of analytical methodology validation, the reader is referred to Chapter 14, which describes current good laboratory practices.

Pharmacokinetic and Pharmacodynamic Data Analysis

The two general approaches to analyzing concentration versus time data in a pharmacokinetic study are compartmental and noncompartmental data analysis. These two approaches differ in their underlying assumptions; however, either approach may be justifiable depending on the clinical circumstances. Examples of both methods can be found throughout the field of oncology.

Historically, *compartmental modeling* has been commonly used to analyze pharmacokinetic data sets. In the compartmental approach, the human body is represented by a vastly simplified series of compartments with rigid transfer constants (usually first-order) defining the movement of drug between these compartments over time. By convention, drug concentrations are measured in the central compartment, representing plasma or serum, with distribution into the tissues represented by the peripheral compartments. Standard box and arrows diagrams are easily converted into mathematical differential equations that describe the movement of drug between these various compartments over time (Fig. 19.3). Once these models are converted to mathematical statements, then data sets can be analyzed using nonlinear regression methods to estimate the specific parameters within the model. For example, the concentration in the central compartment after an IV bolus is represented by the formula:

$$C = (Dose/V_c) \, exp(-ke \cdot t). \qquad (13)$$

Solving this equation for a specific data set composed of concentration C and time t data yields parameter estimates for volume of distribution V_c and the elimination rate constant ke. In this case, dose is a known constant. Nonlinear regression analysis software programs specially designed for pharmacokinetic analysis include programs such as ADAPT II (48) or WinNonLin (Pharsight Corp., Mountain View, CA, USA). Proper weighting of data during nonlinear regression of pharmacokinetic data is essential because concentration measurement error rarely is homogeneous and varies with extremes of concentration. Formalized goodness of fit assessments and statistical tests can be used to evaluate the adequacy of different model types (49). Several excellent reviews on compartmental modeling have been published (7,42).

The compartmental approach to pharmacokinetic analysis has the dual advantages of being well accepted and of having a long history of application to pharmacokinetic systems. Its versatility and flexibility are evident in the types of simulations that can be performed using these models to predict pharmacokinetic behavior under conditions vastly different from the original data set. Formal pharmacokinetic models can serve as a basis for developing substantially more complex population covariate pharmacokinetic models and for clinical trial forecasting and simulation. Major disadvantages include the oversimplification of human physiology to a few homogeneous compartments and the complexity of the nonlinear regression process. Finally, a single specific "correct" model cannot always be identified because more than one model of equal complexity may be consistent with the existing data.

Compared to the compartmental approach, *noncompartmental pharmacokinetic analysis* (NCA) is based upon statistical moment theory and can be used to derive a number of descriptive pharmacokinetic parameters, such as clearance, volume of distribution at steady state, mean residence times, and terminal elimination rate constants. The NCA has grown in popularity as a method to summarize and describe basic pharmacokinetic data sets. It is an acceptable and entirely appropriate method for estimating pharmacokinetic parameters. Compared to standard compartmental modeling, NCA is mathematically less complex and relatively straightforward to implement. It also has the advantage of requiring fewer assumptions about the pharmacokinetic data. However, a NCA is less versatile in performing simulations. It sometimes is referred to as a *model-independent analytical method;* however, this is incorrect. Certain assumptions about drug behavior, such as terminal first-order elimination, still are required in NCA, but the strictness of these assumptions is less rigid than in a standard compartmental analysis. The reader is referred to several monographs for a more in-depth discussion of the NCA analytical approach (28,50,51).

SPECIAL TOPICS IN PHARMACOKINETICS AND PHARMACODYNAMICS

Population Pharmacokinetics

The ultimate goal of pharmacokinetic studies is to define a drug's pharmacokinetic behavior and variability within a large population of patients (52–54). Traditionally, this is performed using a classic "two-stage" pharmacokinetic analysis in which parameter

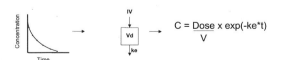

FIG. 19.3. Simple one-compartment, open model with intravenous bolus input is completely defined by two parameters: the volume of distribution (V) and the elimination rate constant (ke).

estimates for individual patients are pooled and characterized using summary statistics such as means, variances, and covariances. In these circumstances, the relative standard deviation or coefficient of variation (CV%) for each pharmacokinetic parameter is used as an indicator of the degree of interpatient variability within the population (6). However, this approach has significant limitations in that the true measures of interindividual variability are not defined separately from the random residual error. A more sophisticated and complex approach is to define a population pharmacostatistical model that simultaneously estimates interindividual and random residual variability within the population using a nonlinear mixed effect model. This can be implemented using software programs such as NONMEM (55). The power of this approach is the ability to incorporate key clinical covariates in the population pharmacokinetic model that help explain the variability of pharmacokinetic parameters. Other population approaches include nonparametric population modeling, which requires fewer assumptions about the distribution of parameters within the population (56).

Limited Sampling Strategies

Although a traditional well-designed pharmacokinetic study will require as many as 15 to 20 blood samples per patient, several methods have been developed to allow for pharmacokinetic parameter estimation based upon many fewer data points (57,58). Most of these approaches require the collection of a substantial amount of initial pharmacokinetic data before formalized limited sampling strategies can be developed (57). With sufficient prior information, as few as one to four blood samples can be used to estimate the pharmacokinetic parameters of interest. This approach may be of substantial value in later stages of drug development, such as during phase II or later studies when it is not feasible to perform extensive sampling on each patient participating in large multicenter clinical trials.

A variety of different methods for performing limited sampling exist. These range from multiple stepwise linear regression methods with fixed sampling times (57,59,60) to more flexible bayesian estimation schemes based upon known population parameters (57). Other approaches include D-optimality study designs that are readily implemented in the software program ADAPT II (61) or formalized sparse sampling data collection in a population mixed effect model as implemented in programs such as NONMEM (58).

Pharmacogenomics

Historically, the clinical effects generated by anticancer agents, such as toxicity and antitumor response, can vary greatly among individuals. This variability is due, in part, to pharmacogenetic variation in pharmacokinetics (drug absorption, distribution, metabolism, elimination) and pharmacodynamics (effects of drug at the molecular, cellular, and tissue level). McLeod and Evans (2) defined pharmacogenomics as the field of study of "the inherited nature of interindividual differences in drug disposition and effects." Pharmacogenomic studies have focused principally on inherited variations in the genes encoding drug-metabolizing enzymes (63,64). To date, about a half-dozen genetic polymorphisms (common genetic variants that occur with a frequency of 1% or greater) of drug-metabolizing enzymes known to affect anticancer drugs have been identified and characterized (65,66). Perhaps the best-known example in clinical oncology is the inherited deficiency of the enzyme thiopurine-S-methyltransferase (TPMT), which results in severe intolerance to thiopurine therapy (67,68). Another well-characterized clinically relevant pharmacogenetic syndrome in oncology is the inherited variation in dihydropyrimidine dehydrogenase (DPD) activity, the rate-limiting catabolic enzyme that metabolically degrades 5-fluorouracil (5-FU) (69). DNA alterations associated with DPD deficiency have been identified in rare cases of patients experiencing severe and fatal toxicity after treatment with standard doses of 5-FU (70).

Pharmacodynamic polymorphisms, such as inherited differences in drug targets (e.g., receptors, target enzymes), may be increasingly identified as important determinants of drug effect. For example, polymorphisms in the promoter region of the thymidylate synthase gene have been correlated with tumor response to 5-FU–based chemotherapy (71). Thus, knowledge of the genetic variation affecting drug disposition and drug efficacy potentially can identify patients who will respond more favorably to specific therapies. This is a growing and extremely important area of pharmacokinetics/pharmacodynamics. At present, it is unlikely that pharmacogenomic markers of drug metabolism can be identified prospectively in ongoing drug development programs. However, implementation of DNA banking protocols for later retrospective analysis of genetic features relevant to pharmacokinetic/pharmacodynamic properties is an important consideration for drug development programs. At the San Antonio Cancer Institute, whole

DNA blood samples are collected on a voluntary basis from patients entering early clinical trials at our institution. This DNA bank will facilitate future studies of inherited polymorphisms, testing the hypothesis that genetic variation can help explain differences in drug pharmacokinetics and pharmacodynamics in individual patients.

INTEGRATED PHARMACOKINETIC AND PHARMACODYNAMIC DRUG DEVELOPMENT PROGRAM

The full integration of pharmacokinetic/pharmacodynamic studies in a formal drug development must be flexible and specifically tailored for each individual agent under development. Nonetheless, some broad recommendations can be made for developing anticancer agents in general. These principles are outlined schematically in Fig. 19.4.

Much of the groundwork for later clinical pharmacokinetic/pharmacodynamic studies can be established in the preclinical phase of drug development.

Important milestones for this stage include the development and validation of analytical assays with sufficient sensitivity and reliability for performing pharmacokinetic studies. These can include assays for the administered compound and any associated metabolites. Efforts also can be directed toward validating pharmacodynamic endpoints by characterizing suitable surrogate markers for drug action. Application of these assays to animal models, such as human tumor xenografts in nude mice, provides the first information about pharmacokinetic/pharmacodynamic relationships in an intact organism. These experiments can provide valuable information for the design of first-time studies in humans.

Preclinical studies can include *in vitro* testing of drug metabolism using well-defined drug-metabolizing enzyme systems (72,73). These studies can provide valuable information about the specific pathways likely to be important for drug metabolism and elimination. When coupled with suitable quantitative analytical methods, they also can identify metabolites that may be searched for *in vivo*. *In vitro* metabolic

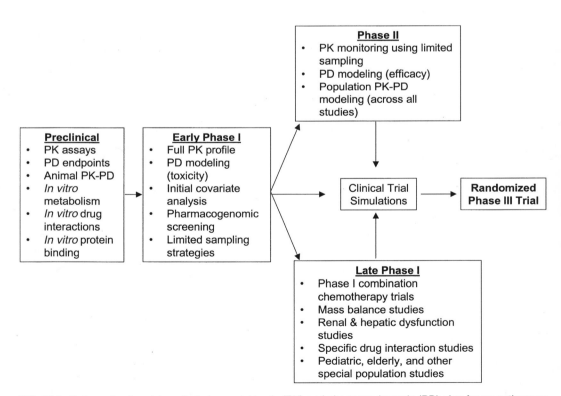

FIG. 19.4. Schematic of an integrated pharmacokinetic (PK) and pharmacodynamic (PD) plan for an anticancer drug development program.

studies have grown in importance as a technique to identify potentially relevant drug interactions caused by competition for common drug-metabolizing enzymes, such as CYP3A4 (72). In addition, *in vitro* protein binding studies performed prior to clinical testing can provide early clues to the relative extent of distribution of a novel agent.

As the important bridge from preclinical to clinical studies is crossed, the first-time phase I trial in humans is the most common time to obtain detailed pharmacokinetic information about a new molecular entity. These labor-intensive pharmacologic studies ideally are performed at institutions with extensive pharmacokinetic experience in this area. Summary descriptive pharmacokinetics for a group of patients in a phase I study can provide the first indication of the degree of kinetic variability of a new agent. Covariate correlation analyses can highlight important factors that underlie this variability within the study population. Because escalation to dose-limiting toxicity is a hallmark of a traditional phase I study design, pharmacodynamic modeling of toxicity endpoints is commonly conducted at this stage. These pharmacodynamic studies ideally should focus on defining the extent of variability in pharmacokinetics/pharmacodynamics observed at the clinical relevant recommended phase II dose (6). In the ideal program, phase I pharmacokinetic studies should incorporate pharmacogenomic screening in the study design. Although important genetic polymorphisms may not be known prior to the initiation of these early trials, the ability to retrospectively analyze data is a valuable tool for any rational drug development program. Finally, the information obtained in these early, intensive pharmacokinetic studies can be used to develop optimal and limited sampling strategies that can readily be applied to pharmacokinetic monitoring of clinical studies in later stages of development.

After completion of the single-agent phase I trials, the most common next step in the clinical development of most anticancer agents is widespread clinical efficacy testing in phase II studies performed in patients with specific types of tumors. Typically, these trials are larger than a traditional phase I study and may be conducted at multiple institutions. The total number of patients entering into the drug development program can increase substantially from this point forward. As the number of patients and participating centers increase, the fiscal and logistical difficulties in performing extensive pharmacokinetic sampling may grow prohibitive. An extensive phase II clinical testing program may be better suited for limited or sparse sampling strategies to further ex-

pand the pharmacokinetic database. Because phase II studies are designed to demonstrate meaningful antitumor activity, pharmacodynamic modeling at this stage may place a greater emphasis on efficacy endpoints. Pooled data from all the pharmacokinetic studies performed to date can be formally analyzed in population pharmacokinetic studies. Nonlinear mixed effect modeling can characterize the magnitude and sources of kinetic variation within the population. Finally, comprehensive population pharmacokinetic/pharmacodynamic models developed at this stage can serve as the basis for early clinical trial forecasting and simulations that assist in the design of larger, more resource-intense randomized phase III trials.

Simultaneously with phase II testing, a new anticancer agent may undergo expanded phase I testing in specialized pharmacokinetic trials. These can include combination phase I studies that administer a novel experimental agent with other standard anticancer therapies rationally selected because of pharmacologic synergistic activity. Alternatively, a new agent may be combined with standard treatments in common use for specific disease types such as lung, colon, or breast cancer, depending upon the tumor types targeted in drug development. A phase I trial of any new drug concentration ideally should include pharmacokinetic monitoring to define potential drug interactions in the new treatment regimen.

Other specialized studies include the initiation of formal mass balance studies that define the total excretion of an experiment agent in urine, feces, and other bodily fluids over time. These studies typically are performed in carefully controlled settings with radioactively labeled drug. Mass balance studies, combined with information from other early pharmacokinetic trials, can precisely define the major routes of drug elimination and may define the need for additional specialized studies. For example, a drug that is largely excreted unchanged in the urine will need to be carefully examined in pharmacokinetic studies in patients with renal dysfunction. In contrast, a hepatically metabolized drug or one undergoing biliary excretion should be examined in formal studies in patients with liver dysfunction. Careful pharmacokinetic monitoring is imperative in these organ dysfunction studies. Finally, if the growing body of clinical information identifies potential drug interactions, then a formalized drug interaction study can be performed with the compound of interest (74). Other pharmacokinetic studies that may be desirable include pediatric phase I studies and specialized studies in geriatric or other specialized populations and disease states. This phase of drug development may temporally overlap with other phases of drug development and may even stretch into the postmarketing period.

The final and most resource-intense phase of drug development is the randomized phase III trial. Consequently, the growing field of clinical trial forecasting and simulation based upon pharmacokinetic/pharmacodynamic modeling may offer the greatest benefit immediately prior to this stage of drug development. Ideally, this involves the maximal utilization of all prior pharmacologic information collected to date. Formalized simulations of various study designs and possible outcomes can be explored in detail. If the results are favorable, then this stage culminates in the initiation of a randomized phase III clinical trial, most often the penultimate step in a successful registration program.

CONCLUSION

Anticancer drug development is a complex and risky business. The potential pitfalls are many, and the cold hard fact is that most agents in development will fail. The promise and potential of new molecularly targeted agents are great, however, and the responsibility for bringing these agents into the clinic as expeditiously as possible lies with the current cadre of drug development scientists. A proactive, integrated pharmacokinetic/pharmacodynamic plan is the cornerstone for a rational and efficiently designed drug development program.

REFERENCES

1. Meibohm B, Derendorf H. Pharmacokinetic/pharmacodynamic studies in drug product development. *J Pharm Sci* 2002;91:18–31.
2. Atkinson AJ. Introduction to clinical pharmacology. In: Atkinson AJ, Daniels CE, Dedrick RL, et al., eds. *Principles of clinical pharmacology*. San Diego, CA: Academic Press, 2001:1–6.
3. Gibaldi M, Perrier D. *Pharmacokinetics,* 2nd ed. New York: Marcel Dekker, 1982:445–449.
4. Gibaldi M. Introduction to pharmacokinetics. In Gibaldi M, ed. *Biopharmaceutics and clinical pharmacokinetics,* 4th ed. Philadelphia: Lea & Febiger, 1991:1–13.
5. Roland M, Tozer TN. *Clinical pharmacokinetics: concepts and applications,* 3rd ed. Baltimore: Williams & Wilkins, 1995.
6. Ratain MJ, Mick R. Principles of pharmacokinetics and pharmacodynamics. In Schilsky RL, Milano GA, Ratain MJ, eds. *Principles of antineoplastic drug development and pharmacology, vol 9.* New York: Marcel Dekker, 1996:123–141.
7. Bourne DWA. *Mathematical modeling of pharmacokinetic data.* Lancaster: Technomic, 1995:95–110.
8. Calvert AH. Dose optimisation of carboplatin in adults. *Anticancer Res* 1994;14:2273–2278.
9. Calvert AH. A review of the pharmacokinetics and pharmacodynamics of combination carboplatin/paclitaxel. *Semin Oncol* 1997;24:S2-85–S2-90.
10. Aarons L, Karlsson MO, Mentre F, et al. Role of modelling and simulation in Phase I drug development. *Eur J Pharm Sci* 2001;13:115–122.
11. Holford NH, Kimko HC, Monteleone JP, et al. Simulation of clinical trials. *Annu Rev Pharmacol Toxicol* 2000;40:209–234.
12. Ratain MJ, Schilsky RL, Conley BA, et al. Pharmacodynamics in cancer therapy. *J Clin Oncol* 1990; 8:1739–1753.
13. Atkinson AJ. Clinical pharmacokinetics. In: Atkinson AJ, Daniels CE, Dedrick RL, et al., eds. *Principles of clinical pharmacology*. San Diego, CA: Academic Press, 2001:9–20.
14. Grochow LB. Individualized dosing of anticancer drugs and the role of therapeutic monitoring. In: Grochow LB,

Ames MM, eds. *A clinician's guide to chemotherapy: pharmacokinetics and pharmacodynamics.* Baltimore: Williams & Wilkins, 1998:3–16.
15. Ackland SP, Schilsky RL. High-dose methotrexate: a critical reappraisal. *J Clin Oncol* 1987;5:2017–2031.
16. Leventhal BG, Wittes RE. *Research methods in clinical oncology.* New York: Raven Press, 1988.
17. Grochow LB, Baraldi C, Noe D. Is dose normalization to weight or body surface area useful in adults? *J Natl Cancer Inst* 1990;82:323–325.
18. Reilly JJ, Workman P. Normalisation of anti-cancer drug dosage using body weight and surface area: is it worthwhile? A review of theoretical and practical considerations. *Cancer Chemother Pharmacol* 1993;32: 411–418.
19. Slone TH. Body surface area misconceptions. *Risk Anal* 1993;13:375–377.
20. Gurney H. Dose calculation of anticancer drugs: a review of the current practice and introduction of an alternative. *J Clin Oncol* 1996;14:2590–2611.
21. Dobbs NA, Twelves CJ. What is the effect of adjusting epirubicin doses for body surface area? *Br J Cancer* 1998;78:662–666.
22. Frazier DL, Price GS. Use of body surface area to calculate chemotherapeutic drug dose in dogs: II. Limitations imposed by pharmacokinetic factors. *J Vet Intern Med* 1998;12:272–278.
23. Egorin MJ. Horseshoes, hand grenades, and body-surface area-based dosing: aiming for a target. *J Clin Oncol* 2003;21:182–183.
24. Felici A, Verweij J, Sparreboom A. Dosing strategies for anticancer drugs: the good, the bad and body-surface area. *Eur J Cancer* 2002;38:1677–1684.
25. Sawyer M, Ratain MJ. Body surface area as a determinant of pharmacokinetics and drug dosing. *Invest New Drugs* 2001;19:171–177.
26. Ratain MJ. Dear doctor: we really are not sure what dose of capecitabine you should prescribe for your patient. *J Clin Oncol* 2002;20:1434–1435.
27. van Groeningen CJ, Pinedo HM, Heddes J, et al. Pharmacokinetics of 5-fluorouracil assessed with a sensitive mass spectrometric method in patients on a

dose escalation schedule. *Cancer Res* 1988;48:6956–6961.

28. Noe DA. Noncompartmental pharmacokinetic analysis. In: Grochow LB, Ames MM, eds. *A clinician's guide to chemotherapy: pharmacokinetics and pharmacodynamics.* Baltimore: Williams & Wilkins, 1998: 515–530.

29. Perrier D, Mayersohn M. Noncompartmental determination of the steady-state volume of distribution for any mode of administration. *J Pharm Sci* 1982;71:372–373.

30. Holford NH. Input from the deep south compartment. a personal viewpoint. *Clin Pharmacokinet* 1905;29: 139–141.

31. Gough K, Hutchison M, Keene O, et al. Assessment of dose proportionality: report from the statisticians in the pharmaceutical industry/pharmacokinetics UK joint working party. *Drug Information J* 1995;29:1039–1048.

32. Smith BP, Vandenhende FR, DeSante KA, et al. Confidence interval criteria for assessment of dose proportionality. *Pharm Res 2000;*17:1278–1283.

33. Ludden TM. Nonlinear pharmacokinetics: clinical implications. *Clin Pharmacokinet 1991;*20:429–446.

34. Mick R, Ratain MJ. Modeling interpatient pharmacodynamic variability of etoposide. *J Natl Cancer Inst* 1991;83:1560–1564.

35. Stewart CF, Zamboni WC. Plasma protein binding of chemotherapeutic agents. In: Grochow LB, Ames MM, eds. *A clinician's guide to chemotherapy: pharmacokinetics and pharmacodynamics.* Baltimore: Williams & Wilkins, 1998:55–66.

36. Hinderling PH. Red blood cells: a neglected compartment in pharmacokinetics and pharmacodynamics. *Pharmacol Rev* 1997;49:279–295.

37. Kosa T, Maruyama T, Otagiri M. Species differences of serum albumins: I. Drug binding sites. *Pharm Res* 1997;14:1607–1612.

38. Benet LZ, Hoener BA. Changes in plasma protein binding have little clinical relevance. *Clin Pharmacol Ther* 2002;71:115–121.

39. Takimoto CH. The clinical pharmacology of the oral fluoropyrimidines. *Curr Probl Cancer* 2001;25:134–213.

40. Lowe ES, Balis FM. Dose-effect and concentration-effect analysis. In: Atkinson AJ, Daniels CE, Dedrick RL, et al., eds. *Principles of clinical pharmacology.* San Diego, CA: Academic Press, 2001:235–244.

41. Kearns CM, Gianni L, Egorin MJ. Paclitaxel pharmacokinetics and pharmacodynamics. *Semin Oncol* 1995; 22:16–23.

42. Gabrielsson J, Weiner D. *Pharmacokinetic and pharmacodynamic data analysis, concepts and applications,* 2nd ed. Stockholm: Swedish Pharmaceutical Press, 1997.

43. Ratain MJ. Therapeutic relevance of pharmacokinetics and pharmacodynamics. *Semin Oncol* 1992;19:8–13.

44. Rosner GL, Muller P. Pharmacodynamic analysis of hematologic profiles. *J Pharmacokinet Biopharm* 1994; 22:499–524.

45. Karlsson MO, Molnar V, Bergh J, et al. A general model for time-dissociated pharmacokinetic-pharmacodynamic relationship exemplified by paclitaxel myelosuppression. *Clin Pharmacol Ther* 1998;63:11–25.

46. Karlsson MO, Port RE, Ratain MJ, et al. A population model for the leukopenic effect of etoposide. *Clin Pharmacol Ther* 1995;57:325–334.

47. Minami H, Sasaki Y, Saijo N, et al. Indirect-response model for the time course of leukopenia with anticancer drugs. *Clin Pharmacol Ther* 1998;64:511–521.

48. D'Argenio DZ, Schumitzky A. A program package for simulation and parameter estimation in pharmacokinetics. *Comp Prog Biomed* 1979;9:115–134.

49. Yamaoka K, Nakagawa T, Uno T. Application of Akaike's information criterion (AIC) in the evaluation of linear pharmacokinetic equations. *J Pharmacokinet Biopharm* 1978;6:165–175.

50. Gillespie WR. Noncompartmental versus compartmental modelling in clinical pharmacokinetics. *Clin Pharmacokinet* 1991;20:253–262.

51. Foster DM. Noncompartmental vs. compartmental approaches to pharmacokinetic analysis. In: Atkinson AJ, Daniels CE, Dedrick RL, et al., eds. *Principles of clinical pharmacology.* San Diego, CA: Academic Press, 2001:75–92.

52. Miller R. Population pharmacokinetics. In: Atkinson AJ, Daniels CE, Dedrick RL, et al., eds. *Principles of clinical pharmacology.* San Diego, CA: Academic Press, 2001:113–119.

53. Mandema JW, Verotta D, Sheiner LB. Building population pharmacokinetic—pharmacodynamic models. I. Models for covariate effects. *J Pharmacokinet Biopharm* 1992;20:511–528.

54. Sambol NC, Sechaud R. The population approach: description and applications to anticancer agents. In: Grochow LB, Ames MM, eds. *A clinician's guide to chemotherapy: pharmacokinetics and pharmacodynamics.* Baltimore: Williams & Wilkins, 1998:531–549.

55. Beal SL, Sheiner LB. *NONMEM user's guides.* San Francisco, CA: University of California, 1989.

56. Jelliffe R, Schumitzky A, Van Guilder M. Population pharmacokinetics/pharmacodynamics modeling: parametric and nonparametric methods. *Ther Drug Monit* 2000;22:354–365.

57. van Warmerdam LJ, ten Bokkel Huinink WW, Maes RA, et al. Limited-sampling models for anticancer agents. *J Cancer Res Clin Oncol* 1994;120:427–433.

58. Sallas WM. Development of limited sampling strategies for characteristics of a pharmacokinetic profile. *J Pharmacokinet Biopharm* 1995;23:515–529.

59. Ratain MJ, Staubus AE, Schilsky RL, et al. Limited sampling models for amonafide (NSC 308847) pharmacokinetics. *Cancer Res* 1988;48:4127–4130.

60. Ratain MJ, Vogelzang NJ. Limited sampling model for vinblastine pharmacokinetics. *Cancer Treat Rep* 1987; 71:935–939.

61. D'Argenio DZ. Optimal sampling times for pharmacokinetic experiments. *J Pharmacokinet Biopharm* 1981;9:739–756.

62. McLeod HL, Evans WE. Pharmacogenomics: unlocking the human genome for better drug therapy. *Annu Rev Pharmacol Toxicol* 2001;41:101–121.

63. Nebert DW. Polymorphisms in drug-metabolizing enzymes: what is their clinical relevance and why do they exist? *Am J Hum Genet* 1997;60:265–271.

64. Flockhart DA. Clinical pharmacogenetics. In: Atkinson AJ, Daniels CE, Dedrick RL, et al., eds. *Principles of clinical pharmacology.* San Diego, CA: Academic Press, 2001:158–165.

65. Boddy AV, Ratain MJ. Pharmacogenetics in cancer etiology and chemotherapy. *Clin Cancer Res* 1997;3: 1025–1030.

66. Krynetski EY, Evans WE. Pharmacogenetics of cancer therapy: getting personal. *Am J Hum Genet* 1998;63: 11–16.

67. Weinshilboum RM, Sladek SL. Mercaptopurine pharmacogenetics: monogenic inheritance of erythrocyte thiopurine methyltransferase activity. *Am J Hum Genet* 1980;32:651–662.

68. Relling MV, Hancock ML, Rivera GK, et al. Mercaptopurine therapy intolerance and heterozygosity at the thiopurine S-methyltransferase gene locus. *J Natl Cancer Inst* 1999;91:2001–2008.

69. Diasio RB, Johnson MR. The role of pharmacogenetics and pharmacogenomics in cancer chemotherapy with 5-fluorouracil. *Pharmacology* 2000;61:199–203.

70. Ridge SA, Sludden J, Wei X, et al. Dihydropyrimidine dehydrogenase pharmacogenetics in patients with colorectal cancer. *Br J Cancer* 1998;77:497–500.

71. Villafranca E, Okruzhnov Y, Dominguez MA, et al. Polymorphisms of the repeated sequences in the enhancer region of the thymidylate synthase gene promoter may predict downstaging after preoperative chemoradiation in rectal cancer. J *Clin Oncol* 2001; 19:1779–1786.

72. Thummel KE, Wilkinson GR. In vitro and in vivo drug interactions involving human CYP3A. *Annu Rev Pharmacol Toxicol* 1998;38:389–4301998.

73. Iwatsubo T, Hirota N, Ooie T, et al. Prediction of in vivo drug metabolism in the human liver from in vitro metabolism data. *Pharmacol Ther* 1997;73:147–171.

74. Huang SM, Lesko LJ, Williams RL. Assessment of the quality and quantity of drug-drug interaction studies in recent NDA submissions: study design and data analysis issues. *J Clin Pharmacol* 1999;39:1006–1014.

PART 6

Clinical Studies

20

Allometric Scaling

Predicting Pharmacokinetic Parameters of Drugs in Humans from Animals

Iftekhar Mahmood

Division of Clinical Trial Design and Analysis, Office of Therapeutic Research and Review, Clinical Pharmacology and Toxicology Branch (HFD-579), Center for Biologics Evaluation and Research, Food & Drug Administration, Rockville, Maryland 20852

Interspecies scaling frequently is used to predict pharmacokinetic parameters from animals to man during drug development and is becoming a useful tool, especially for selection of the first-time dose in humans (1). Interspecies scaling to predict pharmacokinetic parameters in humans can be performed by two approaches: (i) physiologically based pharmacokinetic (PB-PK) models; and (ii) empirical allometric approaches.

PB-PK models mathematically describe the disposition of a drug in the body based on organ blood flow and organ volumes. In a PB-PK model, it is assumed that a drug will be distributed in compartments that represent actual organs and tissues. A number of factors, such as blood flow rate to a given organ, blood to tissue partition coefficient, and diffusion of drug between blood and tissue, generally influence the uptake of drug in these organs. PB-PK models are difficult to validate experimentally in animals because a large number of tissue samples is required at many time points after drug administration. Furthermore, it is almost impossible to validate PB-PK models in humans. Therefore, PB-PK models have found only limited use in drug discovery and development. This approach is costly, mathematically complex, and time consuming. On the other hand, the allometric approach, although empirical, is less complicated and easier to use than the physiologically based method.

Allometry is based on the assumption that there are anatomic, physiologic, and biochemical similarities among animals, and these similarities can be expressed mathematically by the allometric equation. The allometric approach is based on the power function, as the body weight from several species is plotted against the pharmacokinetic parameter of interest on a double log scale. The power function can be written as follows:

$$Y = aW^b, \qquad (1)$$

where Y is the parameter of interest, W is the body weight, and a and b are the coefficient and exponent of the allometric equation, respectively. The log transformation of Equation 1 is represented as follows:

$$\log Y = \log a + b \log W, \qquad (2)$$

where $\log a$ is the y-intercept, and b is the slope.

The allometric equation has also been used to establish a relationship between body weight and physiologic parameters such as liver weight, liver blood flow, kidney weight, kidney blood flow, and glomerular filtration rate of several species, including humans (2).

The three pharmacokinetic parameters, clearance (CL), volume of distribution, and elimination half-life $t_{\frac{1}{2}}$, are most frequently predicted in humans from animals. The following sections describe different allometric approaches to predict the aforementioned pharmacokinetic parameters in humans from animal data.

CLEARANCE

Clearance can be defined as the fixed volume of blood or plasma cleared of drug per unit of time (3). Clearance can be estimated by Equation 3:

$$\text{Clearance} = \frac{\text{Dose}}{\text{AUC(0-infinity)}} \qquad (3)$$

where AUC is the area under the plasma or blood concentration versus time curve calculated by the trapezoidal rule and then extrapolated to infinity (3).

The predicted human clearance can be used for the selection of first-time dosing in humans. Therefore, considering the importance of clearance, over the years many investigators have worked extensively to improve the predictive performance of allometry for clearance.

A survey of the literature (2) indicates that simple allometry (Equation 1 or 2) alone is not adequate to predict clearance in humans from animal data. Therefore, over the years many different approaches have been proposed to improve the predictive performance of allometry for clearance. These approaches can be summarized as follows.

Simple Allometry

This approach is based on Equation 1 or 2, where one plots the clearance of several species against the body weight of the species.

Maximum Lifespan Potential

This approach is based upon the concept of neoteny (4), where the clearance is predicted on the basis of species weight and maximum lifespan potential (MLP).

$$CL = a(MLP \times \text{Clearance})^b/8.18 \times 10^5, \qquad (4)$$

where 8.18×10^5 (in hours) is the MLP value in humans.

MLP (in years) is calculated from Equation 5 as described by Sacher (5):

$$\text{MLP (years)} = 185.4(BW)^{0.636}(W)^{-0.225}, \qquad (5)$$

where brain weight (BW = 1.53) and body weight (W = 70) are in kilograms.

Although Boxenbaum and Dilea (1) describe neoteny as a trivial biologic phenomena with no real relationship to the phase I oxidative metabolism of drugs, MLP is a useful tool that can be used to predict clearance in humans under specific conditions.

Two-term Power Equation

Boxenbaum and Fertig (6) suggested this approach, which uses a two-term power equation based on brain weight and body weight to predict intrinsic clearance of drugs that are primarily eliminated by phase I oxidative metabolism.

$$CL = A(\text{body weight})^b(\text{brain weight})^c, \qquad (6)$$

where A is the coefficient, and b and c are the exponents of the allometric equation.

Product of Brain Weight and Clearance

In order to improve the predictive performance of allometry for clearance, Mahmood and Balian (7,8) suggested the use of the product of brain weight and clearance.

$$CL = (BW \times \text{Clearance})^b/1.53, \qquad (7)$$

where brain weight (BW) and body weight (W) are in kilograms.

These four methods to predict the clearance of drugs were evaluated by Mahmood and Balian (7). The authors used at least three animal species (human data were not included in the scaling) in their analysis and concluded that all four methods would predict clearance with different degrees of accuracy. However, these approaches could not be used indiscriminately, and for all practical purposes it is necessary to identify the suitability of a given approach. In a separate study, Mahmood and Balian (8) evaluated three methods (except the two-term power equation) to predict the clearance of 40 drugs in humans from data obtained from at least three animal species. In this study, the exponents of clearance ranged from 0.35 to 1.39. From this study the authors concluded that there are specific conditions under which only one of the three methods can be used for reasonably accurate prediction of clearance:

1. If the exponent of the simple allometry lies between 0.55 to 0.70, simple allometry will predict clearance more accurately than CL × MLP or CL × BW.
2. If the exponent of the simple allometry lies between 0.71 and 1.0, the CL × MLP approach will predict clearance better compared to simple allometry or CL × BW.
3. If the exponent of the simple allometry is 1.0 or greater, the product of CL and BW is a suitable approach to predict clearance in humans compared to the other two methods.
4. If the exponents of the simple allometry are greater than 1.3, it is possible that the prediction of clearance from animals to man may not be accurate even using the approach of CL × BW, and if the exponents of simple allometry are below 0.55, the predicted clearance may be substantially lower than the observed clearance.

This "rule of exponents" is not rigid, however, and there will be some exceptions where this rule may not work. Furthermore, caution should be applied when the exponents of simple allometry are on the borderline (0.99 vs 1.0).

Interspecies scaling is generally conducted on pharmacokinetic parameters obtained after intravenous administration. Because most drugs are given orally, it is essential that interspecies scaling also should be performed after oral administration. Mahmood (9) evaluated the interspecies scaling for a wide variety of drugs to predict oral clearance in humans. The exponents of the allometry ranged from 0.286 to 1.573. The author concluded that oral clearance can be predicted with the same degree of accuracy as systemic clearance, provided the rule of exponents is used.

Incorporation of *In Vitro* Data in *In Vivo* Clearance

In order to improve the prediction of clearance in humans from animal data, many investigators have suggested the incorporation of *in vitro* clearance data in *in vivo* clearance (10–12). Although this approach has not been thoroughly tested, a limited number of studies indicate that the approach may be of some value in allometric scaling. In a systematic study, Lave et al. (11) compared several methods (simple allometry, product of clearance and brain weight, and *in vitro/in vivo* method) to predict clearance of ten extensively metabolized drugs. The *in vitro* intrinsic clearance (from the liver microsomes or hepatocytes) was combined with the *in vivo* animal clearance and then *in vivo* human clearance was predicted using the allometry. The authors concluded that the integration of *in vitro* data in the allometric approach improved the prediction of human clearance compared with the

approach of simple allometry or the product of brain weight and clearance.

Reanalysis of Lave's data (11) by Mahmood (13) indicated that the normalization of clearance by MLP (as required based on the exponents of the simple allometry) for some of the drugs studied could have produced the same results as seen when *in vitro* clearance was incorporated in the *in vivo* clearance (13). Mahmood pointed out that application of the product of brain weight and clearance was inappropriate because the exponents of the simple allometry for all ten drugs studied by Lave et al. (11) were less than 1 (Table 20.1).

There are numerous limitations of the *in vitro* approach. One major disadvantage of the *in vitro* approach is the need to measure the *in vitro* clearance, which is time consuming. It is not known how well the *in vitro* approach will predict clearance if a drug is partly metabolized and partly renally excreted. There is only limited experience with the *in vitro/in vivo* approach; therefore, extensive work is needed in this direction before one can clearly establish the advantage and accuracy of the *in vitro* approach in predicting clearance of drugs over other existing methods.

In a separate study, Mahmood (14) examined if the predicted clearance of a drug in humans from *in vitro* human liver microsomes is comparable with the predicted clearance in humans obtained by allometric scaling. In a comparative study of 16 drugs, hepatic clearances of these drugs were predicted using human liver microsomes. Allometric scaling was performed using at least three animal species and the rule of exponents as described by Mahmood and Balian (8). The results of this study indicated that the use of human liver microsomes to predict hepatic clearance

TABLE 20.1. *Observed and predicted clearance (mL/min) in humans using the rule of exponents or* in vitro *data*

Drugs	Exponent	Obs CL	Pred CL[a]	Percent error	Pred CL[b]	Percent error
Antipyrine	0.93	32	116	263	18	44
Bosentan	0.56	259	294	14	126	51
Caffeine	0.58	140	98	30	98	30
Mibefradil	0.90	490	630	29	265	46
Midazolam	0.77	770	483	37	1190	55
Mofarotene	0.73	770	112	85	441	43
Ro24-6173	0.71	840	420	50	392	53
Propranolol	0.82	910	896	2	700	23
Theophylline	0.92	43	34	21	65	51
Tolcapone	0.65	189	189	0	147	22

Percent error = (Observed − Predicted)* 100/Observed.
[a]Based on the rule of exponents (maximum lifespan potential was used when the exponent was >0.70).
[b]Incorporating in vitro data.
Obs CL, observed clearance; Pred CL, predicted clearance.

TABLE 20.2. *Percent error in prediction of clearance using simple allometry, the rule of exponents, and the in vitro approach using human liver microsomes*

Drugs	SA	RE	Well stirred		Parallel tube	
			Q = 1500	Q = 825	Q = 1500	Q = 825
Diazepam	3208	1692	1423	1154	1639	1419
Warfarin	1000	100	1485	1425	1519	1500
Quinidine	416	6	68	34	95	66
Propafenone	194	11	122	27	143	34
Sildenafil	25	25	10	25	3	10
Metoprolol	21	21	45	58	34	47
Tolcapone	4	4	11	15	7	10
Theophylline	7	7	92	91	92	91
Dofetilide	100	100	59	60	58	59
Citalopram	234	36	27	6	43	27
Propranolol	16	16	47	13	75	3
Cyclophosphamide	214	32	154	99	200	150
Ethinyl estradiol	111	19	230	96	294	118
Troglitazone	122	5	175	119	222	172
Tirilazad	13	13	146	38	159	42
Tacrolimus	403	10	43	NA	30	NA

Q (in mL/min); Q = 1500 (liver blood flow); Q = 825 (plasma flow).
Percent error = (Observed − Predicted)* 100/Observed.
NA, not applicable; RE, rule of exponents; SA, simple allometry.
From Mahmood I. Prediction of clearance in humans from in vitro liver microsomes and allometric scaling. A comparative study of the two approaches. *Drug Metab Drug Interact* 2002;19:49–64, with permission.

in humans would provide unreliable predictions. On the other hand, the prediction of clearance in humans using allometric scaling combined with the rule of exponents provided comparatively accurate and reliable prediction of clearance in humans (Table 20.2).

Human liver microsomes contain different cytochrome P-450 isozymes, which are responsible for the metabolism of drugs. Mahmood (15) attempted to determine if there was a systematic trend that could indicate that the clearance of a drug metabolized by a particular isozyme could be predicted with reasonable accuracy. In his analysis, Mahmood (15) used 27 drugs metabolized by different isozymes. The clearances of these drugs were predicted using the rule of exponents. The results of this study indicated that knowledge of a particular isozyme would not provide a guide for the failure or success of allometry for the prediction of clearance.

Protein Binding

Because there is considerable variability in plasma protein binding among species, it is conceivable that one should be able to predict the unbound clearance in humans from animal data. However, a systematic study in this direction was lacking until Mahmood (16) compared the total and unbound clearance of a wide variety of drugs to determine whether unbound clearance of a drug could be predicted more accurately than

total clearance and if there was any real advantage to predicting unbound clearance. The author concluded that the correction for protein binding does not necessarily improve the prediction of clearance in humans from animals (Table 20.3). The analysis also indicated that the prediction of unbound clearance might be more erratic than the prediction of total clearance. Mahmood's conclusion was further strengthened by the study of Bjorkman and Redke (17). In their study, the authors used five anesthetic drugs and reported that application of the rule of exponents helped to improve the prediction of clearance but that the correction for protein binding introduced comparatively more error in the prediction of clearance.

Important Considerations for Prediction of Clearance of Drugs in Humans

The following salient features of the allometry for prediction of clearance should be kept in mind during the process of interspecies scaling.

1. The exponents of simple allometry have no physiologic meaning. Normalization of clearance by MLP or brain weight is a mathematical manipulation that may not be related with the physiology of the species used in the scaling. As the exponents of the simple allometry become larger, the predicted clearance becomes comparatively higher than the

observed clearance. The predicted clearance values will be in order of Simple allometry > MLP × CL > Brain weight × CL.

2. The exponents of clearance for a given drug are not universal and will depend on the species used in the allometric scaling (8).

3. The application of MLP and the product of brain weight and clearance should not be limited to the extensively metabolized drugs; rather, these two approaches are equally applicable to drugs that are eliminated by the renal route.

4. One should avoid using the fixed exponent of 0.75 for clearance. The exponents of allometry vary widely and, due to this variability in the exponents, the use of a fixed exponent will produce errors in the prediction of clearance for drugs.

5. The prediction of clearance from animals to humans may require a minimum number of species. Mahmood and Balian (18) concluded that three or more species (excluding humans) are required for reliable prediction of clearance. Although sometimes two species may provide a good prediction of clearance, the reliability of such predictions on a regular basis is doubtful.

6. Interspecies scaling of drugs for the prediction of clearance in humans may be complicated due to renal secretion or biliary excretion. The difficulty in predicting clearance of renally secreted and biliary excreted drugs was demonstrated by Mahmood et al. (19,20). Whereas the total clearance often renally secreted drugs could not be predicted reasonably well (30% difference between observed and predicted clearance), the prediction of renal clearance was improved by normalizing the renal clearance by a "correction factor" for animals that exhibited renal secretion. The correction factor was obtained by adjusting the glomerular filtration rate, kidney blood flow, body weight, and kidney weight of a given species. For the biliary excreted drugs, Mahmood and Sahajwalla (20) also used a correction factor obtained by adjusting the bile flow rate based on the body weight of the species. Using Mahmood and Balian's rule of exponents and combining it with the correction factor, a substantial improvement in the prediction of clearance for biliary excreted drugs was obtained.

7. The impact of plasma protein binding on allometric scaling has been overemphasized, and the concept that prediction of unbound clearance is superior to prediction of total clearance is more of a theoretical nature rather than of a practical value. There is no real advantage to predicting unbound clearance over total clearance.

8. Scaling can become unpredictable for drugs whose clearances are greater than the liver blood flow.

TABLE 20.3. *Observed versus predicted total and unbound clearance (mL/min) in humans*

Drug	Exponent	Total clearance			Exponent	Unbound clearance		
		Obs CL	Pred CL	Percent error		Obs CL_u	Pred CL_u	Percent error
Cefpiramide	0.442	18	27	50	0.638	486	224	54
Recainam	0.482	502	477	5	0.526	580	656	13
Dofetilide	0.498	331	312	6	0.521	836	717	14
Cefoperazone	0.577	71	76	7	0.733	402	118	71
Tamsulosin	0.594	48	814	1596	0.742	4800	1778	63
Cefmetazole	0.634	112	173	54	0.701	745	509	32
Cefotetan	0.641	30	99	230	0.597	336	311	7
Moxalactam	0.651	82	73	11	0.672	206	151	27
Propranolol	0.674	850	716	16	1.020	13281	29022	119
Sildenafil	0.680	420	568	35	0.534	10500	3348	68
Cefazolin	0.731	53	39	26	0.648	408	270	34
Diazepam	0.787	26	466	1692	0.998	813	3085	279
Susalimod	0.792	5	35	600	0.865	1923	10000	420
Troglitazone	0.801	172	169	2	0.987	182800	347400	90
Quinidine	0.805	330	285	14	1.081	2538	1538	39
Morphine	0.882	1600	1428	11	0.891	2462	1789	27
Theophylline	0.905	55	54	2	0.797	94	75	20
Valproic acid	0.950	11	60	445	1.148	212	126	41
Meloxicam	1.102	12	9	25	1.068	3000	484	84
GV150526	1.196	6	132	2100	0.906	300000	163100	46

Percent error = (Observed − Predicted* 100/Observed.
Obs CL, observed clearance; Pred CL, predicted clearance.

The scaling will become even more complicated if the clearance of a drug in animals is higher than the liver blood flow but lower than in humans. At this time, no solution is available for such drugs.

VOLUME OF DISTRIBUTION

Like clearance, volume of distribution is an important pharmacokinetic parameter. The volume of distribution of the central compartment V_c is used to relate plasma concentration at time zero C_0 of a drug and the amount of drug X in the body (21):

$$X = V_c \times C_0. \tag{8}$$

A small V_c (<3 L) indicates that most of the drug is in the plasma, whereas a large V_c (>7 L) means the drug is present in high concentrations in the extravascular space.

The volume of distribution at steady state V_{ss} can be estimated from Equation 9:

$$V_{ss} = \frac{\text{Dose} * \text{AUMC}}{\text{AUC}^2} = CL * MRT, \tag{9}$$

where

$$MRT \text{ is mean residence time} = \frac{\text{AUMC}}{\text{AUC}}, \tag{10}$$

where AUC and AUMC are the area under the curve and the area under the moment curve, respectively.

The volume of distribution by area V_{area}, also known as V_z, can be obtained from Equation 10:

$$V_z = \text{Clearance}/\beta \tag{11}$$

where β is elimination rate constant.

There is a good correlation between body weight and volume of distribution among species. Generally the exponents of volume revolve around 1.0, which indicates that body weight and volume are directly proportional. There are, however, examples where the exponents of some drugs deviated from 1.0 and were found to be as low as 0.58 (22). Unlike clearance, volume can be predicted with reasonable accuracy using only two species (18).

Although the literature indicates that V_c, V_{ss}, and V_z are predicted indiscriminately in humans from animals, Mahmood (23) showed that V_c can be predicted with more accuracy than V_{ss} or V_z. Furthermore, there is no practical application of V_{ss} or V_z for selection of the first-time dose to humans.

V_c can play an important role in establishing the safety or toxicity for first-time dosing in humans. Because an administered dose is always known, the predicted V_c can be used to calculate plasma concentration of a drug at time zero C_0 after intravenous administration. This initial plasma concentration may provide an index of safety or toxicity. Furthermore, V_c also can be used to predict half-life, if clearance is known ($t^{\frac{1}{2}} = 0.693 V_c/CL$).

ELIMINATION HALF-LIFE AND MEAN RESIDENCE TIME

Half-life is not directly related to the physiologic function of the body; rather, it is a hybrid parameter. It is difficult to visualize that one can establish a relationship between body weight and half-life $t\frac{1}{2}$. Like clearance, the allometric exponents of half-life vary widely. In his evaluation, Mahmood (23) noted that the exponents of half-life of drugs (n =18) varied from −0.066 to 0.547. In some cases, the predicted half-life values were far off from the observed values. Because of the poor correlation between half-life and body weight and the uncertainty in the predictive performance of allometry for half-life, some indirect approaches have been proposed.

Bachmann (24), Mahmood and Balian (7), and Obach et al. (12) used Equation 12 to predict the half-lives of several drugs:

$$t_{\frac{1}{2}} = \frac{0.693 V}{CL}. \tag{12}$$

Although this approach appeared to be suitable and predicted the half-life of drugs reasonably well, an important requirement of this approach is that one must obtain reasonable predictions of both CL and volume.

Another indirect approach to predict half-life was suggested by Mahmood (23). In this approach, first MRT was predicted by allometry and then the predicted MRT was used to predict half-life in humans using Equation 13:

$$t_{\frac{1}{2}} = \frac{MRT}{1.44}. \tag{13}$$

A better correlation between body weight and MRT compared to body weight and half-life was found. Like half-life, the exponents of MRT varied from −0.260 to 0.385. The predicted half-life values were reasonably close to the observed values. The results of this study indicated that the MRT approach to predict half-life probably is the best approach.

Although Equations 12 and 13 are only true for a one-compartment model, both of these equations for prediction purposes also may be used in a multicompartment system. It should be emphasized that one does not need a very accurate estimate of half-life because its practical application for the selection of first-time dosing to humans is limited. Information on predicted half-life from animal data can, however, be used to design the blood sampling scheme for the first human pharmacokinetic study.

PREDICTION OF PLASMA CONCENTRATIONS USING SPECIES-INVARIANT TIME METHODS AND PHARMACOKINETIC CONSTANTS

In chronologic time, as the size of the animals increases their heart beat and respiratory rates decrease. However, on a physiologic time scale, regardless of their size all mammals have the same number of heart beats and breaths in their lifetime. The physiologic time can be defined as the time required to complete a species-independent physiologic event. Thus, in smaller animals the physiologic processes are faster and the lifespan is shorter.

The physiologic time can be obtained by transforming chronologic time into a species-invariant time. Dedrick et al. (25) were first to apply the concept of species-invariant time to methotrexate disposition in five mammalian species after intravenous administration. The transformation of chronologic time to physiologic time was achieved as follows:

$$y\text{-axis} = \frac{\text{concentration}}{(\text{Dose}/W)}, \qquad (14)$$

$$x\text{-axis} = \frac{\text{time}}{W^{0.25}}, \qquad (15)$$

where W is body weight.

By transforming chronologic time to physiologic time, the plasma concentrations of methotrexate were superimposable in all species. The authors termed this transformation *equivalent time.*

Boxenbaum (26) refined the concept of equivalent time by introducing two new units of pharmacokinetic time: kallynochrons and apolysichrons. Kallynochrons and apolysichrons are transformed time units in an elementary Dedrick plot and a complex Dedrick plot, respectively.

Although many investigators have used the concept of species-invariant time in their allometric analysis (27–29), a direct comparison of allometric approaches with species invariant time has not been systematically evaluated. Mahmood and Yuan (30) compared empirical allometric approaches with species-invariant time methods using equivalent time, kallynochron, apolysichron, and dienetichrons. Clearance, volume of distribution, and elimination half-life of ethosuximide, cyclosporine and ciprofloxacin were predicted using allometric approach as well as species invariant time methods. The results of this study indicated that species in-

variant time method does not necessarily provide an improvement over conventional allometric approach, e.g., both simple allometry and species invariant time methods gave almost similar results. The authors also noted that the equivalent time approach does not predict plasma concentrations or pharmacokinetic parameters as accurately as elementary or complex Dedrick plots. The reason may be that the exponent of elimination half-life of drugs is not always 0.25. The exponents of half-life for ethosuximide, cyclosporine, and ciprofloxacin in this study were 0.47, −0.24, and 0.04, respectively.

The allometric approach has been used to predict plasma concentrations of a drug (using pharmacokinetic constants) from animals to humans, and these predicted concentrations were used to estimate pharmacokinetic parameters in humans.

Equation 16 represents a two-compartment pharmacokinetic model after intravenous administration.

$$C = Ae^{-\alpha t} + Be^{-\beta t}, \qquad (16)$$

where A and B are the intercepts on the y-axis of a plasma concentration versus time plot, and α and β are the rate constants for the distribution phase and elimination phase, respectively.

Mordenti (31) and Swabb and Bonner (32) predicted the plasma concentrations of ceftizoxime and aztreonam, respectively, in humans from animal data using pharmacokinetic constants (Equation 16). Although the approach was successfully applied for ceftizoxime and aztreonam, a systematic study of the suitability of this approach in predicting pharmacokinetic parameters was lacking. In a study conducted by Mahmood (33), the predicted pharmacokinetic parameters of six drugs were compared using either pharmacokinetic constants or conventional allometric approach. Pharmacokinetic constants (A and B) and the rate constants (α and β) derived from at least three animal species were plotted as a function of body weight as described in Equation 1. The allometric equation thus generated was used to predict pharmacokinetic constants in man. From these pharmacokinetic constants, plasma concentrations were predicted in man according to Equation 16. The results of the study, like the species-invariant time method, indicated that the use of pharmacokinetic constants to predict pharmacokinetic parameters does not necessarily provide an improvement over the conventional allometric approach. Like the species-invariant time method, the pharmacokinetic constant approach may provide some information about plasma concentrations of a drug, but the accuracy of the method for the prediction of plasma concentrations in man may be questionable.

TABLE 20.4. *Predicted and observed maximum tolerated dose (mg/kg) in humans using simple allometry or the maximum lifespan potential approach*

	Exponents	Obs MTD	Pred SA	1/3 Pred	Ratio	Pred MLP	1/3 Pred	Ratio	Steps[a]
Amethopterin	0.733	0.41	0.27	0.09	4.56	0.12	0.04	10.25	6
6-Mercaptopurine	0.802	27.00	17.5	5.83	4.63	8.50	2.83	9.53	6
5-Fluorouracil	0.805	15.00	8.6	2.87	5.23	4.20	1.40	10.71	6
Floxuridine	0.798	40.00	30.7	10.23	3.91	15.00	5.00	8.00	5
Nitrogen mustard	0.805	0.20	0.19	0.06	3.16	0.10	0.03	6.00	4
Nitromin	0.658	2.00	1.91	0.64	3.14	1.91	0.64	3.14	2
L-Phenylalanine	0.636	0.20	0.27	0.09	2.22	0.27	0.09	2.22	2
Alanine mustard	0.753	0.90	0.86	0.29	3.14	0.45	0.15	6.00	4
Cytoxan	0.830	10.00	13.44	4.48	2.23	6.60	2.20	4.55	3
Thiotepa	0.710	0.20	0.52	0.17	1.15	0.25	0.08	2.40	2
Myleran	0.887	0.70	3.95	1.32	0.53	1.90	0.63	1.11	1
Actinomycin D	0.849	0.02	0.026	0.01	2.31	0.01	0.003	6.00	4
Mitomycin C	0.775	0.20	0.37	0.12	1.62	0.20	0.07	3.00	2
Mithramycin	0.952	0.03	0.11	0.04	0.82	0.05	0.02	1.80	1
9H-Purine	0.780	5.00	4.95	1.65	3.03	2.40	0.80	6.25	4
Imidazole	0.707	10.00	24.2	8.07	1.24	12.10	4.03	2.48	2
Ammonium	0.894	42.00	66.8	22.27	1.89	33.50	11.17	3.76	3
Pactamycin	0.432	0.45	0.03	0.01	45.00	0.03	0.01	45.00	>8
Glycine	0.690	155.40	34.8	11.60	13.40	34.80	11.60	13.40	7
Tylocrebrine	0.477	1.92	0.27	0.09	21.33	0.27	0.09	21.33	>8
Acetophenone	0.998	550.00	855	285.00	1.93	429.00	143.00	3.85	3
Cytosine 1 B-D	0.718	7.00	13.5	4.50	1.56	6.80	2.27	3.09	2
Hydrazine	0.996	30.00	75.6	25.20	1.19	36.80	12.27	2.45	2
Phosphorodimidic	0.627	2.70	3.94	1.31	2.06	3.94	1.31	2.06	2
Urea	0.763	1.50	2.95	0.98	1.53	1.41	0.47	3.19	2

Maximum lifespan potential (MLP) was applied when the exponent of the simple allometry was >0.70.
[a]Modified Fibonacci scheme for escalation of dosage.
MTD, maximum tolerated dose; Obs, observed; Pred, predicted; SA, simple allometry.
From Mahmood I. Interspecies scaling of maximum tolerated dose (MTD) of anticancer drugs: relevance to starting dose for phase I clinical trials. *Am J Ther* 2001;8:109–116, with permission.

PREDICTION OF MAXIMUM TOLERATED DOSE

In phase I clinical trials, estimation of a starting dose in humans is an important step and remains a challenge. A conservative low-dose approach will result in a subtherapeutic or ineffective dose, whereas aggressive dose escalation may produce toxicity. Certain classes of drugs (e.g., anticancer drugs) are so toxic that for ethical reasons they cannot be given to healthy subjects. Therefore, predicting maximum tolerated dose (MTD) in humans from animal data may be useful. For anticancer agents, generally one tenth of the LD_{10} (the dose that kills 10% of the experimental animals) in mice or one third of the toxic dose level (TDL) in the dog (in mg/m²) is used as the starting dose in phase I clinical trials (34). There is no consensus regarding the best approach for estimating the starting dose, and controversy persists in this direction. Over the years, different investigators have reached different conclusions. For example, Goldsmith et al. (35) reported that using one third of the TDL would have produced significant toxicity in the patients for 5 of 30

drugs. The authors suggested that for a safe starting dose in phase I clinical trials, not only toxicology data from dog and monkey, but also data from rat, mice, and tumor-bearing mice, should be included. Homan (36) concluded that there was a 5.9% probability of exceeding the human MTD if the starting dose in clinical trials were one third of the TDL of large animal species (dog or monkeys). Rozencwig et al. (34) suggested that one sixth of LD_{10} in the mouse and one third of TDL in the dog corresponds to an acceptable dose in humans, provided both preclinical and clinical data are obtained under identical schedules and compared on a mg/m² basis. Mice and dogs may provide different information for a given drug, but combining data from both species can be helpful in determining the starting dose in humans for phase I clinical trials (34).

Using 25 anticancer drugs, Mahmood (37) evaluated if MTD can be predicted from animals to humans. The analysis was carried out to compare the predictive performance of two different approaches of allometry for prediction of MTD in humans from animal data. The two approaches to predict MTD in humans in this analysis were the use of (1) a fixed exponent of 0.75

and the LD_{10} in mice and (2) LD_{10} or MTD data from at least three animal species (interspecies scaling). Allometric scaling was performed using the body weight of the species, and human data were not included in the study. The results of the study indicated that MTD can be predicted more accurately using interspecies scaling than using a fixed exponent of 0.75. Like clearance, it was noted that MLP can be used to improve the prediction of MTD for some drugs. MLP was applied when the exponents of simple allometry was greater than 0.70. The author suggested that one third of the predicted MTD from interspecies scaling can be used as a starting dose in humans. This approach may save time and avoid many unnecessary steps to attain MTD in humans (Table 20.4).

MODIFIED CONTINUAL REASSESSMENT METHOD

Once a starting dose has been determined, a dose escalation scheme must be selected. There is no defined rule for the selection of an optimal or efficient escalation scheme for drugs. In general, five to eight dose escalation steps are generally acceptable. In the early 1990s, O'Quigley and Chevret (38) proposed and evaluated the continual reassessment trial design [continual reassessment model (CRM)]. Because this early version was considered aggressive, Faries (39) proposed a modified version of CRM. Despite the modification, there are some shortcomings with the CRM. For example, the CRM requires an initial guess of the MTD. Furthermore, the starting dose based on one tenth of LD_{10} in mice may be conservative and time consuming. Using the interspecies scaling technique (body surface area vs MTD), Mahmood (40) predicted the MTD in humans. Once MTD was predicted in humans, the predicted MTD value was used as an initial starting dose and to provide a dose escalation scheme for subsequent doses in a continual reassessment trial design. Based on the analysis, Mahmood proposed that the second dose may be an increment of 50% over the first dose and the third dose can be a 20% or 30% increment over the second dose. Us-

TABLE 20.5. *Escalation steps for 25 anticancer drugs based on allometric scaling and continual reassessment method*

Drug	Observed MTD	Predicted MTD	1st Dose	2nd Dose	3rd Dose	Ratio 1st	Ratio 2nd	Ratio 3rd
Amethopterin	28	20	7	10	16	0.25	0.37	0.56
6-mercaptopurine	1848	1217	420	630	954	0.23	0.34	0.52
5-fluoroucil	1027	607	209	314	476	0.20	0.31	0.46
Floxuridine	2738	2200	759	1139	1724	0.28	0.42	0.63
Nitrogen mustard	14	15	5	8	12	0.37	0.55	0.84
Nitromin	137	149	51	77	117	0.38	0.56	0.85
L-phenylalanine	14	18.8	6	10	15	0.46	0.70	1.05
Alanine mustard	62	64	22	33	50	0.36	0.53	0.81
Cytoxan	685	575	198	298	451	0.29	0.43	0.66
Thiotepa	14	37	13	19	29	0.93	1.36	2.07
Myleran	48	160	55	83	125	1.15	1.73	2.61
Actinomycin D	1.4	1.6	0.6	0.8	1.3	0.39	0.59	0.90
Mitomycin C	14	31	11	16	24	0.76	1.15	1.74
Mithramycin	2.1	4	1.4	2	3.1	0.66	0.95	1.49
9H-purine	342	395	136	204	310	0.40	0.60	0.91
Imidazole	685	1695	585	877	1329	0.85	1.28	1.94
Ammonium	2875	2485	858	1286	1948	0.30	0.45	0.68
Pactamycin	31	2.1	0.7	1.1	1.6	0.02	0.04	0.05
Glycine	10,637	2495	861	1292	1956	0.08	0.12	0.18
Tylocrebrine	131	19	7	10	15	0.05	0.08	0.11
Acetophenone	37,648	32,478	11,208	16,812	25,457	0.30	0.45	0.68
Cytosine 1 B-D	479	978	338	506	767	0.70	1.06	1.60
Hydrazine	2056	2874	992	1488	2253	0.48	0.72	1.10
Phosphorodimidic	184	260	90	135	204	0.49	0.73	1.11
Urea	103	169	58	87	132	0.57	0.85	1.29

Second dose is 1.5 times the first dose. Third dose was calculated using a 20% probability according to the equation: Third dose = [Second dose + ln{0.2/1 − 0.2}/β] + Second dose. Ratio = first, second, third dose/observed maximum tolerated dose.

From Mahmood I. Application of preclinical data to initiate the modified continual reassessment method for maximum tolerated dose-finding trials. *J Clin Pharmacol* 2001;41:19–24, with permission.

ing this dosing scheme (20% increment over the second dose), at least 15 of 25 anticancer drugs achieved 70% of the observed human MTD within three steps (Table 20.5).

CONCLUSION

Although interspecies scaling has become an important tool during drug discovery, many old and untested theories persist. Views such as correction for protein binding, fixed exponent of 0.75 for clearance and 0.25 for half-life, and incorporation of *in vitro* data in *in vivo*

clearance are of little practical value. Because the most important objective of allometric scaling is to select a safe and tolerable dose for first-time administration to humans, it is essential that scaling be done with proper understanding and practical considerations. Many external factors, such as experimental design, species, analytical errors, and physicochemical properties of drugs (renal secretion, biliary excretion, and clearance greater than the liver blood flow) may have an impact on allometric scaling; therefore, sound scientific judgment and experience in allometric scaling are essential before any interpretation of data is performed.

REFERENCES

1. Boxenbaum H, Dilea C. First-time-in-human dose selection: allometric thoughts and perspectives. *J Clin Pharmacol* 1995;35:957–966.
2. McNamara PG. Interspecies scaling in pharmacokinetics. In: Welling PG, Tse FLS, Dighe SV, eds. *Pharmaceutical bioequivalence.* New York: Marcel Dekker, 1999;267–300.
3. Gibaldi M. Noncompartmental pharmacokinetics. In: *Biopharmaceutics and clinical pharmacokinetics,* 3rd ed. Philadelphia: Lea & Febiger; 1984:17–28.
4. Boxenbaum H. Interspecies pharmacokinetic scaling and the evolutionary-comparative paradigm. *Drug Metab Rev* 1985;15:1071–1121.
5. Sacher G. Relation of lifespan to brain weight and body weight in mammals. In: Wolstenholme GEW, O'Connor M, eds. *CIBA Foundation colloquia on aging.* London: Churchill, 1959:115–133.
6. Boxenbaum H, Fertig JB. Scaling of antipyrine intrinsic clearance of unbound drug in 15 mammalian species. *Eur J Drug Metab Pharmacokin.* 1984;9:177–183.
7. Mahmood I, Balian JD. Interspecies scaling: predicting pharmacokinetic parameters of antiepileptic drugs in humans from animals with special emphasis on clearance. *J Pharm Sci* 1996;85:411–414.
8. Mahmood I, Balian JD. Interspecies scaling: predicting clearance of drugs in humans. Three different approaches. *Xenobiotica* 1996;26:887–895.
9. Mahmood I. Interspecies scaling: predicting oral clearance in humans. *Am J Ther* 2002;9:35–42.
10. Houston B. Utility of in vitro drug metabolism data in predicting in vivo metabolic clearance. *Biochem Pharmacol* 1994;47:1469–1479.
11. Lave TH, Dupin S, Schmitt C, et al. Integration of in vitro data into allometric scaling to predict hepatic metabolic clearance in man: application to 10 extensively metabolized drugs. *J Pharm Sci* 1997;86:584–590.
12. Obach RS, Baxter JG, Liston TE, et al. The prediction of human pharmacokinetic parameters from preclinical and in vitro metabolism. *J Pharmacol Exp Ther* 1997;283:46–58.
13. Mahmood I. Integration of in-vitro data and brain weight in allometric scaling to predict clearance in humans: some suggestions. *J Pharm Sci* 1998;87:527–529.
14. Mahmood I. Prediction of clearance in humans from in vitro human liver microsomes and allometric scaling. A comparative study of the two approaches. *Drug Metab Drug Interact* 2002;19:49–64.
15. Mahmood I. Interspecies scaling: is a priori knowledge of cytochrome P450 isozymes involved in drug metabolism helpful in prediction of clearance in humans from animal data? *Drug Metab Drug Interact* 2001; 18:135–147.
16. Mahmood I. Interspecies scaling: role of protein binding in the prediction of clearance from animals to humans. *J Clin Pharmacol* 2000;40:1439–1446.
17. Bjorkman S, Redke F. Clearance of fentanyl, alfentanil, methohexitone, thiopentone and ketamine in relation to estimated hepatic blood flow in several animal species: application to prediction of clearance in man. *J Pharm Pharmacol* 2000;52:1065–1074.
18. Mahmood I, Balian JD. Interspecies scaling: a comparative study for the prediction of clearance and volume using two or more than two species. *Life Sci* 1996;59:579–585.
19. Mahmood I. Interspecies scaling of renally secreted drugs. *Life Sci* 1998;63:2365–2371.
20. Mahmood I, Sahajwalla C. Interspecies scaling of biliary excreted drugs. *J Pharm Sci* 2002;91:1908–1914.
21. Shargel L, Yu ABC. Multicompartment models. In: *Applied biopharmaceutics and pharmacokinetics,* 3rd ed. Norwalk, CT: Appleton and Lange, 1992:61–76.
22. Boxenbaum H, Ronfeld R. Interspecies pharmacokinetic scaling and the Dedrick plots. *Am J Physiol* 1983; 245:R768–R774.
23. Mahmood I. Interspecies scaling: predicting volumes, mean residence time and elimination half-life. Some suggestions. *J Pharm Pharmacol* 1998;50:493–499.
24. Bachmann K. Predicting toxicokinetic parameters in humans from toxicokinetic data acquired from three small mammalian species. *J Appl Toxicol* 1989;9: 331–338.
25. Dedrick RL, Bischoff KB, Zaharko DZ. Interspecies correlation of plasma concentration history of methotrexate (NSC-740). *Cancer Chemother Rep* 1970; 54[Pt 1]:95–101.
26. Boxenbaum H. Interspecies scaling, allometry, physiological time and the ground plan of pharmacokinetics. *J Pharmacokinet Biopharm* 1982;10:201–207.
27. Hutchaleelaha A, Chow H, Mayersohn M. Comparative pharmacokinetics and interspecies scaling of amphotericin B in several mammalian species. *J Pharm Pharmacol* 1997;49:178–183.
28. Lave T, Saner A, Coassolo P, et al. Animal pharmacokinetics and interspecies scaling from animals to man of

lamifiban, a new platelet aggregation inhibitor. *J Pharm Pharmacol* 1996;48:573–577.

29. Mehta SC, Lu DR. Interspecies pharmacokinetic scaling of BSH in mice, rats, rabbits, and humans. *Biopharm Drug Dispos* 1995;16:735–744.

30. Mahmood I, Yuan R. A comparative study of allometric scaling with plasma concentrations predicted by species invariant time methods. *Biopharm Drug Dispos* 1999; 20:137–144.

31. Mordenti J. Pharmacokinetic scale-up: accurate prediction of human pharmacokinetic profiles from human data. *J Pharm Sci* 1985;74:1097–1099.

32. Swabb E, Bonner D. Prediction of aztreonam pharmacokinetics in humans based on data from animals. *J Pharmacokinet Biopharm* 1983;11:215–223.

33. Mahmood I. Prediction of clearance, volume of distribution and half-life by allometric scaling and by plasma concentrations predicted by pharmacokinetic constants: a comparative study. *J Pharm Pharmacol* 1999;51: 905–910.

34. Rozencwig M, Von Hoff DD, Staquet MJ, et al. Animal toxicology for early clinical trials with anticancer agents. *Cancer Clin Trials* 1981;4:21–28.

35. Goldsmith MA, Slavik M, Carter SK. Quantitative prediction of drug toxicity in humans from toxicology in small and large animals. *Cancer Res* 1975;35: 1354–1364.

36. Homan ER. Quantitative relationship between toxic doses of antitumor chemotherapeutic agents in animals and man. *Cancer Chemother Rep* 1972;3:13–19.

37. Mahmood I. Interspecies scaling of maximum tolerated dose (MTD) of anticancer drugs: relevance to starting dose for phase I clinical trials. *Am J Ther* 2001;8:109–116.

38. O'Quigley J, Chevret S. Methods for dose finding studies in cancer clinical trials: a review and results of Monte Carlo study. *Stat Med* 1991;10:1647–1664.

39. Faries D. Practical modifications of the continual reassessment method for phase I cancer clinical trials. *J Biopharm Stat* 1994;4:147–164.

40. Mahmood I. Application of preclinical data to initiate the modified continual reassessment method for maximum tolerated dose-finding trials. *J Clin Pharmacol* 2001;41:19–24.

21

Phase I Clinical Trial Design

Lawrence V. Rubinstein* and Richard M. Simon*

Biometric Research Branch, National Cancer Institute, Bethesda, Maryland 20892-7434

The objective of a phase I trial is to determine the appropriate dosage of an agent or combination to be taken into further study and to provide initial pharmacologic and pharmacokinetic studies. At this stage of testing, it is generally assumed that increased dose is associated with increased chance of clinical efficacy; therefore, the phase I trial is designed as a dose escalation study to determine the maximum tolerable dosage (MTD), which is the maximum dose associated with an acceptable level of dose-limiting toxicity (DLT; usually defined as grade 3 or greater toxicity, except grade 3 neutropenia unaccompanied by either fever or infection) (1). This MTD then is taken into further testing. Because evaluation of efficacy is generally not the objective of a phase I trial, it is not necessary to restrict to a patient population homogeneous with respect to disease or even to restrict to patients with measurable disease (for which tumor response is determinable). It is important, however, to exclude patients with impaired organ function, who may be more prone to serious toxicity. The fundamental conflict in phase I trials is between escalating too fast so as to expose patients to excessive toxicity and escalating too slow so as to deny patients the opportunity to be treated at potentially efficacious dose levels (2). Phase I trials for compounds or biologics in which toxicity is not expected and determination of the MTD is not the objective are discussed later in this chapter.

The first problem in a phase I trial is deciding on a safe, but not overly conservative, initial dose for the trial. If the agent is new to clinical testing, this must be based on animal studies. It has been determined that the dose (defined in milligrams per meters squared of body surface area) associated with 10% lethality in mice ($MELD_{10}$) can be predicted to be roughly equivalent to the human MTD (3). This approach is derived from the concept of "allometric scaling" (4,5). Toxicity as a function of body weight or surface area is assumed to be roughly constant across species. The initial dose for the phase I trial is taken to be one tenth the $MELD_{10}$ or, if smaller, one third the LD_{10} (associated with 10% lethality) in the beagle dog (6). The use of a second species has been shown to be necessary, because in approximately 20% of about 90 reviewed drugs, mouse data alone were insufficient to safely predict the human MTD (7). US investigators generally use the dog as the second species, whereas European investigators generally use the rat, with equivalent safety (7). The next problem is to define dose increments for the subsequent dose levels, and it is here that the various phase I trial designs part company.

STANDARD PHASE I DESIGN

The "standard" phase I design uses a set of decreasing Fibonacci dose level increments proposed by Schneiderman (8), currently taken to be 100%, 67%, 50%, 40%, and 33% thereafter (2). These increments are added to each dose level to give the succeeding level. In other words, the second dose level is 100% greater than the first, the third is 67% greater than the second, and so forth. The purpose is to allow more aggressive dose escalation for the initial levels, which are expected to be sufficiently removed from the MTD for this to be safe. If the $MELD_{10}$ accurately predicted the human MTD, only five to six such dose escalations would be necessary to complete a "standard" phase I design. Unfortunately, this is often not the case (9).

The "standard" rule governing dose escalation from one level to the next relies on no assumptions concerning the shape of the dose-toxicity curve or the potential for cumulative toxicity; therefore, the decision to escalate to the next dose level is based solely on toxicity results from the first-course administration of the current level. The dose escalation

---

* The authors contributed equally and are listed alphabetically.

TABLE 21.1. *Dose escalation rules for the standard phase I trial*

Outcome: No. DLT Among No. Patients	*Action:* Escalate, suspend, or halt dose escalation
0 DLT among 3 patients	Escalate dose for next cohort of 3 patients
1 DLT among 3 patients	Treat next cohort of 3 patients at the same dose
>1 DLT among 3 patients	Halt dose escalation: treat total of 6 patients at previous dose to determine MTD[a]
1 DLT among 6 patients	Escalate dose for next cohort of 3 patients
>1 DLT among 6 patients	Halt dose escalation: treat total of 6 patients at previous dose to determine MTD[a]

[a] MTD: highest dose for which no more than 1 of the 6 treated patients exhibits dose-limiting toxicity (DLT).

rules (Table 21.1) proceed as follows, escalating in cohorts of three to six patients per dose level (1). Three patients are treated at the current dose level. If at least two patients are observed to have DLT, the prior dose level is defined as the MTD (unless only three patients have been treated at that level, in which case it is the tentative MTD). If none of the three patients is observed to have DLT, the dose level is escalated one step for the next cohort of three patients, and the process continues as described earlier. If exactly one of the three patients treated show DLT, three additional patients are treated at the current dose level. If none of these additional three patients shows DLT, the dose level is escalated for the next cohort of three patients, and the process continues; otherwise, the prior dose level is defined as the MTD (unless only three patients have been treated at that level, in which case it is the tentative MTD). A tentative MTD becomes final when a total of six patients are treated with fewer than two showing DLT.

The statistical operating characteristics of this approach are as follows (Table 21.2). If at least two of three patients treated at a particular dose show DLT, we can conclude with 90% confidence that the true probability of DLT at that dose is greater than 20%. (In other words, as shown in Table 21.2, unless the

true probability of DLT at that dose is at least 20%, the probability of at least two of three patients exhibiting DLT is less than 10%.) On the other hand, if none of three patients shows DLT, we can conclude with 90% confidence that the true probability of DLT is less than 55%. (Again, as shown in Table 21.2, unless the true probability of DLT is less than 55%, the probability of none of three patients exhibiting DLT is less than 10%.) In the interest of efficiency, we accept either of these situations as sufficient to halt or continue escalation after treating only three patients at the current level. Allowing for expansion to six patients in case one of the initial three patients shows DLT, the dose escalation rule gives 91% probability that dose escalation will not halt at doses associated with DLT probability less than 10%, and it gives 92% probability that escalation will not proceed beyond doses associated with DLT probability in excess of 60% (Table 21.2). The process of approaching the MTD from below, in successive steps, further protects against defining an MTD associated with excessive toxicity. Table 21.2 plus simulations (10, 11) show that, for a wide variety of dose-toxicity curves, the probability is approximately 85% to 90% that the defined MTD will be associated with DLT probability of approximately 10% to 45%.

TABLE 21.2. *Probabilities of halting or continuing dose escalation for various probabilities of DLT associated with dose level for the standard phase I design*

True probability of DLT for dose level	0.05	0.1	0.2	0.3	0.4	0.5	0.6	0.7
Probability of halting dose escalation after accruing either 3 or 6 patients (>1 DLT)[a]	0.03	0.09	0.29	0.51	0.69	0.83	0.92	0.97
Probability of continuing escalation after only 3 patients (0 DLT)[b]	0.86	0.73	0.51	0.34	0.22	0.13	0.06	0.03
Probability of halting escalation after only 3 patients (>1 DLT)[b]	0.01	0.03	0.10	0.22	0.35	0.50	0.65	0.78

[a] This row gives probabilities of halting dose escalation, at a given dose, if the true probability of dose-limiting toxicity (DLT) for that dose level is as indicated.

[b] These rows gives probabilities of continuing or halting dose escalation after accruing only 3 patients, at a given dose, if the true probability of DLT for that dose level is as indicated. We see that, in all cases, the cohort will be limited to 3 patients with at least 50% probability, and for the more extreme DLT probabilities (0.05 or 0.7) the cohort will be expanded to 6 patients with 20% probability.

The primary criticisms of the standard phase I design (1,10,12,13) are as follows:

1. It does not target a particular probability of DLT to be associated with the MTD, and, in practice, the DLT rate associated with the defined MTD will be somewhat dependent on the DLT rates of the various dose levels.
2. The MTD definition is unnecessarily imprecise in that it does not make adequate use of all the available first-course toxicity data.
3. The dose escalation is unnecessarily slow, leading to treatment of excessive numbers of patients at dose levels less likely to be efficacious.

Storer (13) proposed defining the MTD by fitting all the first-course toxicity data to a logistic dose-toxicity curve (a sigmoidal curve that maps dose levels to associated DLT rates, for example, Equation 1, discussed in more detail later) and letting the MTD be the dose level associated with the targeted DLT rate (usually 20% to 30%), thus addressing criticisms 1 and 2 of the standard design. To address criticism 3, he suggested escalating the dose in single-patient cohorts until DLT is observed, at which point dose escalation would revert to the standard design.

CONTINUAL REASSESSMENT METHOD

O'Quigley et al. (12) extended the modeling idea of Storer (13) by proposing the use of a dose-toxicity model to guide the dose escalation, as well as to define the MTD. First, a statistical model, such as Equation 1, which relates dose to probability of DLT, is defined. Using a bayesian statistical approach (14), the free parameter α of the model initially is given a "prior" probability distribution such that the model maps the dose levels to probabilities of DLT in accord with investigator expectations. O'Quigley et al. (12) proposed that each successive patient in the phase I trial be treated at the expected MTD, according to the current state of the model, and that the model be immediately "updated" [that the "posterior" distribution of the free parameter be recalculated, according to Bayes' theorem (14)] by incorporating first-course toxicity data obtained from each successive patient. They proposed that when the sample size reached a preset limit of 20 to 25, the MTD be calculated from the final state of the dose-toxicity model.

Original Form of the Continual Reassessment Method

O'Quigley et al. (12) designated the above approach the continual reassessment method (CRM). It can be made clearer by examining use of the following one-parameter logistic model, proposed by Goodman et al. (10) for defining the probability of DLT p_i at the ith dose level, in conjunction with CRM:

$$p_i = e^{3+a \cdot x_i}/(1 + e^{3+a \cdot x_i}) \qquad (1)$$

By the methods of Goodman et al. (10) the investigators first define an increasing set of dose levels (indexed by i) to be used in the phase I trial. The investigators provide initial expectations of the probabilities of DLT (the p_is) at those doses. The initial ("prior") distribution of the parameter α is taken to be the standard exponential distribution with mean and variance equal to one. The x_i values are determined by Equation 1 by letting α be equal to one (its mean according to the initially given exponential distribution) and by letting the p_is be the initial expectations of the investigators. [For example, Goodman et al. (10) give x_i values of -5.9, -5.2, -4.3, -3.6, -3.0, and -2.15, to correspond to prior expectations for DLT rate p_i of 0.05, 0.1, 0.2, 0.35, 0.5, and 0.7.] The substantial uncertainty of the investigators' initial expectations is represented by the variability associated with the initial distribution of α. For example, using the prior distribution, the dose initially associated with an expected DLT rate of 20% has a 33% probability of actually being associated with a DLT rate in excess of 75%, and it has a 20% probability of being associated with a DLT rate less than 5%. (In other words, the initial state of the model reflects that the investigators' initial guess at an MTD could actually be either a very toxic dose or a very nontoxic dose, both with reasonably high probability.) As each successive patient is treated, the distribution of α is recalculated according to Bayes' theorem (14) to reflect the new toxicity data and the greater certainty associated with the dose-toxicity relationship. Equation 1, with α having this recalculated "posterior" distribution, eventually reflects the dose-toxicity pattern actually observed in the phase I trial, with substantially less uncertainty associated with the predicted DLT rates p_i.

O'Quigley et al. (12,15) suggested fixing the sample size of a CRM-based phase I trial at 20 to 25 patients. At the termination of the trial, the MTD is defined to be the dose associated with the target DLT rate (usually 15% to 25%), according to the final state of the dose-toxicity model (according to Equation 1, for example, letting α be the mean of its final "posterior" distribution). O'Quigley (16) gives simulations to demonstrate the accuracy of the confidence interval for the rate of DLT at the chosen MTD (for sample size 20). O'Quigley et al. (12,15) argued that CRM addresses the serious concerns associated with the standard phase I design, given earlier. They noted that use of a dose-toxicity model allows the investigators to target a specific DLT rate to be associated with the MTD, and it allows all of the first-course toxicity to be incorporated in defining the MTD. They stressed the importance of treating each patient at a sufficiently high dose to offer the hope of an effect, and they asserted that treating each patient at the currently estimated MTD avoids systematic undertreatment of patients, without involving significantly increased risk of DLT (compared to the standard design), according to their simulations (15).

Amendments and Alterations of the Continual Reassessment Method

Based on their simulations, Korn et al. (11) argued that CRM did, in fact, significantly increase the DLT risk to patients, compared to the standard design. They demonstrated that CRM tended, with substantially increased probability, to treat patients at doses higher than the MTD, even at doses two or more levels higher, where DLT could be not only more frequent but also more serious. This was seen to be a result of treating each successive patient at the currently estimated MTD. In particular, the initial patients were to be treated thus, despite the fact that the initial state of the dose-toxicity model might often reflect the uncertainty of the investigators with respect to the clinical toxicity of the untested agent.

Concerns such as these resulted in a number of proposed alterations to the original CRM. Goodman et al. (10) suggested that dose escalation begin at the standard initial dose (usually the $MELD_{10}$) and that it proceed, at most, one dose step at a time (although they did not give guidance as to how these dose steps should be defined). They presented simulations to demonstrate that this approach avoided the increased DLT risk associated with the original CRM while preserving the advantages of greater efficiency and accuracy. Babb et al. (17) suggested that, rather than treat patients at the dose expected to yield the targeted rate of DLT (which gives 50% likelihood of exceeding the targeted MTD, according to the dose-toxicity model), patients should be treated at the dose associated with 25% likelihood of exceeding the MTD, according to the current state of the model. They presented simulations to demonstrate that this approach also avoided the increased DLT risk of the original CRM while preserving efficiency and accuracy. Finally, in answer to concerns about attempting to define an initial dose-toxicity model without clinical experience, Potter (18) suggested that the initial stage of the phase I trial proceed in a standard fashion (escalating from the start-

ing dose with successive 50% dose increments) until DLT is observed. At that point, a dose-toxicity model would be constructed, based on the trial data only. Patients then would be treated at the currently estimated MTD, based on the model. The trial would terminate when 18 patients had been treated, with at least four instances of DLT, and with at least nine patients treated subsequent to the initial such instance.

All of these alterations were accompanied by a retreat from single-patient cohorts, as originally suggested by O'Quigley et al. (12,15), to three-patient cohorts. This was prompted, in part, by the practical consideration relating to the usual brisk accrual to phase I trials but also, more importantly, by the desire to achieve greater safety with the accumulation of more first-course toxicity data between successive updates of the dose-toxicity model.

ACCELERATED TITRATION DESIGNS

Accelerated titration designs attempt to improve several aspects of conventional designs. (i) With standard designs many patients are treated at doses well below the biologically active level, minimizing the opportunity for antitumor response. (ii) Many phase I trials using the standard design take a long time to complete. (iii) Conventional designs select a dose for the population of patients, and there is no attempt to tailor doses to individual patients. (iv) Conventional designs provide little information about interpatient variability, cumulative toxicity, or the steepness of the dose-toxicity relationships.

Accelerated titration designs are characterized by: (i) a rapid initial escalation phase; (ii) intrapatient dose escalation; and (iii) analysis of results using a model that incorporates parameters for intrapatient variation in toxic effects, cumulative toxicity, and steepness of dose-toxicity effects. The analytic model incorporates data from all courses of therapy and for graded toxicity levels.

Rapid Acceleration Phase

Simon et al. (1) defined several accelerated titration designs and compared them to a standard design (called design 1). Design 1 differs from the standard phase I design described earlier only in that Simon et al. (1) used fixed 40% dose steps because it was believed that there is not real justification for the standard Fibonacci approach.

Design 2 uses single-patient cohorts per dose level during the accelerated phase with 40% dose increments. When the first instance of first-course DLT or the second instance of first-course intermediate toxicity is observed, the cohort for the current dose level is expanded to three patients and the trial reverts to use of design 1 for further cohorts. *Intermediate toxicity* can be defined in a protocol-specific manner. Simon et al. (1) used any grade 2 toxicity that was considered treatment related as intermediate toxicity.

Design 3 is similar to design 2 in that single-patient cohorts are used during the accelerated phase. With design 3, however, double dose steps are used during the accelerated phase. Two 40% dose steps corresponds to approximately a doubling of the actual dose. The accelerated phase ends, as with design 2, when the first instance of first-course DLT or the second instance of first-course intermediate toxicity occurs. After that, design 1 is used for all further cohorts.

Design 4 is similar to design 3 in that single-patient cohorts and double dose steps are used during the accelerated phase. Design 4 differs from design 3 only in the criterion used for triggering the end of the accelerated phase. With designs 2 and 3, the accelerated phase ends with the first instance of first-course DLT or the second instance of first-course intermediate toxicity. With design 4, the trigger is the first instance of any-course DLT or the second instance of any-course intermediate toxicity. Hence, design 4 may stop the accelerated phase earlier than design 3.

Intrapatient Dose Escalation

Accelerated titration designs were designed to permit dose escalation in subsequent courses for a patient who remains in the study and has no evidence of toxicity at the dose used during the current course. The rule used was that if less than intermediate-level toxicity is observed for a patient during a course, then the dose is escalated for the next course if that patient stays in the study. If intermediate-level toxicity occurs, then the dose stays the same for the next course if that patient stays on study. If DLT occurs, then the patient generally goes off the study; if not, then the dose is reduced. For design 2, single dose steps are used for intrapatient dose changes. For designs 3 and 4, double dose steps are used for intrapatient dose changes during the accelerated phase and single dose steps subsequently. The accelerated titration designs were evaluated by computer simulation both with and without intrapatient dose escalation.

Model-Based Analysis

Because accelerated titration designs use graded toxicity results and multicourse treatment results, the information yield can be greater than for conventional or CRM designs. The model used by Simon et al. (1)

was based on measuring the worst toxicity experience by each patient during each course of treatment, that is, the model does not consider separate toxicity for each organ system separately but takes the maximum over the organ systems and records that worst toxicity separately for each course of treatment for each patient. The toxicity for patient i in course j is determined by Equation 2:

$$\log (d_{ij} + \alpha D_{ij}) + \beta_i + \varepsilon_{ij} \qquad (2)$$

where d_{ij} denotes the dose received by patient i in course j, and D_{ij} denotes the cumulative dose received by patient i up to but not including course j. For the first course, D_{ij} is zero for all patients. α is a cumulative toxicity parameter, and $\alpha = 0$ represents no cumulative toxicity. All logarithms are natural logarithms. The β_i terms represent interpatient variability in toxic effects. The term is the same for all courses of treatment of patient i but its value differs among patients. The β_i values are taken as independent draws from a normal distribution with zero mean and variance σ^2_β. Hence, the model has a single parameter σ^2_β that reflects the amount of interpatient variability in susceptibility to toxicity. The ε_{ij} terms are the random variations that reflect the uncontrolled sources of variation other than dose that influence the toxic response for a given patient. These are taken as independent draws from a normal distribution with zero mean and variance σ^2_β.

In addition to the three parameters α, σ^2_β, and σ^2_ε, there are several parameters for converting the quantitative value of Equation 2 into a graded level of toxicity. Values of Equation 2 less than K_1 correspond to less than intermediate toxicity. Values between K_1 and K_2 correspond to intermediate toxicity, values between K_2 and K_3 correspond to DLT, and values greater than K_3 correspond to life-threatening toxicity. If one does not wish to distinguish DLT from life-threatening toxicity, then only K_1 and K_2 are needed, so there are five to six parameters to be estimated from the data. This model is a generalization of the $K_{\mathbf{max}}$ model of Sheiner et al. (19) and of the model of Chou and Talalay (20).

Given the data of the grade of toxicity (worst over organ systems) for each course of each patient, the method of maximum likelihood is used to estimate the model parameters. Splus software for fitting the parameters is available at *http://linus.nci.nih.gov/~brb*. That web site also contains an Excel macro for managing dose assignments to patients during Accelerated Titration Design trials. The macro assists investigators in quality control of the dose assignment process and provides a convenient way of recording dose assignments in a systematic manner that makes the data available for subsequent analysis.

Simon et al. (1) fit model 2 to data from 20 phase I trials. Only three of the trials showed any evidence of cumulative toxicity ($\alpha > 0$). The estimates of α for the other trials were zero or very close to zero. The trials varied substantially in the other parameters and thus provide a broad range of experience for evaluation of the accelerated titration designs.

Evaluation of Performance

Simon et al. (1) evaluated the performance of accelerated titration designs by simulating phase I data based on the 20 sets of parameters estimated from the 20 real trials that they studied. For each of the 20 sets of parameters, they generated data for 1,000 phase I trials and applied each of their designs to the simulated data. Figure 21.1 shows the average number of patients per trial used by each of the designs. For each design, the average is taken over the same 20,000 simulated data sets generated from the sets of parameters derived from the 20 actual trials analyzed. Results for eight designs are shown. Designs 1 to 4 are as described earlier. The designs labeled with B use intrapatient dose escalation if the toxicity in the previous course is less than intermediate. Designs labeled with A do not permit intrapatient dose escalation.

Design 1A corresponds to the standard design, although it does not use Fibonacci dose steps. Design lB is the standard design augmented to permit intrapatient dose escalation. As can be seen in Figure 21.1, the average number of patients is much greater for the standard design 1A or lB than for any of the accelerated titration designs. The average number of patients is somewhat less for designs 3 and 4 that use double

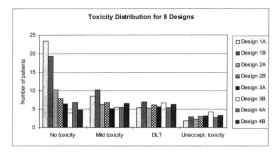

FIG. 21.2. Toxicity distributions for eight designs.

dose steps compared to design 2. Although the average differences are not great, the differences for individual trials can be, that is, for a trial in which the starting dose is very low relative to the dose at which intermediate toxicity is expected, designs 2 and 3 will require substantially fewer patients.

Figure 21.1 also shows the average number of patient cohorts used by each design. The average is lowest for designs 3 and 4 that use double dose steps. Although the difference in average number of cohorts is not large, the difference in average time to complete the trials will be much shorter for designs 2 to 4 if patients are not instantaneously available because the accelerated phase of those designs requires only one patient per cohort.

Figure 21.2 shows the average number of patients experiencing each level of toxicity as their worst toxicity during their treatment on the trial. With the standard design, an average of 23 patients experience less than intermediate toxicity (labeled "no toxicity" in Fig. 21.1). These patients are undertreated. For design 2B the average number of undertreated patients is about eight, and for designs 3B and 4B the number is less than five. This major reduction in the number of undertreated patients is achieved with very small increases in the average number of patients experiencing DLT or unacceptable toxicity with the accelerated titration designs.

The accelerated titration designs without intrapatient dose escalation (designs 2A, 3A, and 4A) performed quite well with regard to reduction in average number of patients and reduction of number of undertreated patients. They do not, however, provide patients accrued early in the trial a full opportunity to be treated at a therapeutic dose. They are also less effective in situations where interpatient variability in susceptibility to toxicity is large. These designs may be attractive, however, when there is concern about cumulative toxicity. It is worth noting, in this regard, that analysis of the 20 phase I trials used for evalua-

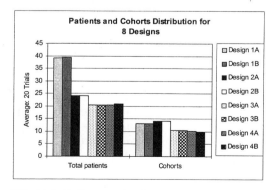

FIG. 21.1. Patients and cohorts distribution for eight designs.

tion of these designs revealed no evidence of ill effect from intrapatient dose escalation and led the investigators to conclude that "cumulative toxicity does not appear to be a valid reason to prohibit intrapatient dose escalation, as it occurs rarely" (7).

Accelerated titration designs can dramatically reduce the number of patients accrued to a phase I trial. They also can substantially shorten the duration of the phase I trial. They provide much greater information than other designs with regard to cumulative toxicity, interpatient variability, and steepness of the dose-toxicity curve. They also provide all patients entered in the trial a maximum opportunity to be treated at a therapeutic dose.

PHARMACOKINETICALLY GUIDED DOSE ESCALATION

An entirely different approach to the problem of safely accelerating the dose in phase I studies was proposed by Collins et al. (2). They presented a retrospective analysis of anticancer agents demonstrating that, for the most part, toxicity was not a function of administered drug dosage but rather was a function of AUC, which is the area ($C \times T$) under the curve of plasma drug concentration (C) measured over time of exposure (T). Therefore, they proposed a "pharmacokinetically guided dose escalation" (PGDE) scheme that involved targeting the AUC associated with the mouse LD_{10} (rather than the $MELD_{10}$ itself).

Initial Pharmacokinetically Guided Dose Escalation Proposal of Collins et al.

The initial PGDE scheme of Collins et al. (2) involved escalating to an MTD by targeting a maximal tolerated AUC and proceeded as follows:

1. Determine the mouse LD_{10}, and the associated mouse AUC, of the new agent.
2. Treat the initial cohort of three patients at one tenth $MELD_{10}$, as is standard, and measure the average (human) AUC over this cohort of patients.
3. Escalate the doses for subsequent cohorts of three patients according to the distance to the target AUC (that which is associated with the $MELD_{10}$), according to one of the following two rules:
   A. First escalation step increases the initial dose by a factor equal to the square root of the ratio of the target AUC to the AUC associated with the initial dose, and subsequent escalation steps follow the Fibonacci scheme.
   B. Escalation steps are by a factor of two until the AUC is 40% of the target AUC, and subsequent escalation steps follow the Fibonacci scheme.

Retrospective analyses by Collins et al. (2) indicated that the sample sizes of phase I trials could be reduced by 20% to 50% by using the PGDE scheme.

The efficiency of PGDE relies on the assumption that drug toxicity is really a function of drug AUC and that equivalent AUC for human and mouse will result in equivalent toxicity. Furthermore, the underlying assumption is that the mouse LD_{10} roughly equals the human MTD, with both doses measured as a function of body surface area (in mg/m^2) because, in general, the two doses yield roughly equivalent AUC levels for the two species. However, as noted by Collins et al. (2), there are important exceptions to this rule. For example, the MTD of doxorubicin in humans is five-fold higher than the $MELD_{10}$ because the clearance rate of doxorubicin is much higher in man than in the mouse, leading to a much smaller AUC in man for the equivalent dose. This sort of situation leads to a striking advantage for PGDE because the smaller than expected AUC for the first dose will result in escalation of the initial dose step(s). Other situations, also noted by Collins et al. (2), on the other hand, may lead to problems for PGDE. For some drugs, there is a drug concentration threshold for action and a necessary minimum exposure time above that threshold. For such drugs, the relation between mouse toxicity and human toxicity is complicated by the fact that, in general, the smaller species experiences a higher initial drug concentration and a shorter half-life (4). Thus, if the threshold is high and the necessary exposure time short, the mouse may experience much more serious toxicity for equivalent AUC (or equivalent dose). Likewise, if the threshold is low and the necessary exposure time long, the human may experience much more serious toxicity. For other drugs, there is a marked difference between the two species with regard to target cell sensitivity, again rendering mouse drug dose or AUC nonpredictive of the human MTD.

Reception and Status of Pharmacokinetically Guided Dose Escalation

The European Organization for Research and Treatment of Cancer (EORTC) published a generally positive review of PGDE (21). However, the EORTC (21) also reiterated the cautions given by Collins et al. (2), and it added some of its own, in particular, the following:

1. For pharmacokinetic measures to translate across species, the preclinical conditions (in particular, the route of administration) should match the anticipated clinical conditions.

2. Metabolism of active (and toxic) agents in humans, but not in mice, may complicate the use of the AUC (for the drug alone) to predict toxicity across the species.
3. Plasma drug concentration is really a surrogate measure for target tissue drug concentration, so if the relationship between the two is not equivalent for the two species, it may not be predictive of toxicity.
4. Despite these cautions, the EORTC review (21) of PGDE was positive.

The EORTC review (21) concluded by noting that "the worldwide experience to date reveals no example in which the use of PGDE would introduce a greater risk to patients than the procedures currently employed. In many cases the new procedures would lead to a more efficient dose escalation." The EORTC reiterated the initial Collins PGDE scheme and proposed that it be evaluated prospectively.

A later review by Collins et al. (22) reviewed the role of prospective application of PGDE concepts to eight consecutive trials sponsored by the National Cancer Institute. For three of the drugs, development was reported to be too far advanced for impact from the PGDE project. For two (merbarone and deoxyspergualin), preclinical data demonstrated that a continuous infusion schedule would reduce toxicity and allow use of a substantially higher initial phase I dose (for hexamethyline bisacetamide [HMBA] preclinical data also enabled a higher initial dose), which Collins et al. (22) claimed to be an extension of the PGDE concepts. For the remaining two (flavone acetic acid and piroxantrone), phase I dose escalation was accelerated according to the PGDE scheme. Collins et al. (22) also noted the use of a related concept, that is, AUC measurements to individually adapt patient dosage, particularly in cases where there is wide variation in AUC among patients receiving the same dose. They noted the use of this "adaptive control" approach in the development of regimens for etoposide and HMBA.

As PGDE continued to be used, problems arose, some of which were successfully addressed and some not. Gianni et al. (23) reported on the discovery, in the course of a phase I trial of I-Dox, that it metabolized (in the human but not in the mouse) to the active and toxic agent I-Doxol, which attained plasma concentrations tenfold those of the original drug. PGDE was eventually utilized successfully in this trial, based on the combined AUC of I-Dox plus I-Doxol, in the human, equated to the AUC of I-Dox in the mouse. Fuse et al. (4) argued that new agents often can be classified into one of two types. For type I drugs (including alkylating agents and some antitumor antibiotics), toxicity is a function of AUC; therefore, PGDE can be advantageously used. For type II drugs (antimetabolites and vinca alkaloids), toxicity is a function of exposure time, rather than AUC, and the use of PGDE is not possible.

Another situation that makes it impossible to use PGDE is the presence of large interpatient variability in AUC for the same administered dose. The advantage of using AUC, as opposed to dose, is based on the assumption that interspecies variation in AUC is high (particularly between the mouse and the human) but intraspecies variation (for both mice and men) is low, so equivalent doses will result in predictable AUC levels for the two species (although not equivalent). Conley et al. (24) reported that for HMBA, the variability of AUC was very high among patients in the phase I trial receiving equivalent doses. In this case, the use of adaptive control was possible because AUC, although variable, proved to be predictive of toxicity. On the other hand, for CI-941, Foster et al. (25) reported that not only was the AUC quite variable, but also AUC was no more predictive of toxicity than was the administered dose. For this drug, neither PGDE nor adaptive control, based on individual AUC measures, would be useful.

Collins (26) sums up the present state of PGDE. Despite encouraging reports on its success in the United States, Europe, and Japan, in the end investigators find the requirement of real-time pharmacokinetic monitoring to be a drawback. Collins (26) concludes that although such pharmacokinetics could prove useful, because of this attitude "PGDE has failed to be widely accepted, and has generally faded from regular use." Similarly, Newell (9) noted that the common failure to collect pharmacodynamic data and data relating to biologic efficacy against the intended targets of new agents is seen as a serious failure by the preclinical investigators involved in drug development.

PHASE I DESIGNS FOR NONTOXIC THERAPEUTICS

Certain types of therapeutics are not expected to be toxic in the dose range used. Some molecularly targeted drugs and therapeutic vaccines are of this type. Conventional phase I designs are not suitable for such drugs because there is no interest in the MTD. Nevertheless, there may be uncertainty about the appropriate dose to use for clinical development. Resolving this uncertainty may not be possible, however, in the context of small three to six patients per cohort studies used for cytotoxics (27,28). Much larger studies may be required, depending on the specific objectives.

Pharmacokinetics Designs

A pharmacokinetics-based design generally can be accomplished with a limited number of subjects. One determines a target serum concentration based on pre-clinical or *ex vivo* studies. For molecularly targeted drugs, the target concentration is chosen to maximally inhibit the target. The phase I trial then includes **n** patients for each of several dose levels. The serum concentration of the active metabolite is measured and the dose chosen that best achieves the target concentration. The target concentration is often a steady-state level or a concentration integrated over time (C $\times$ T). In some cases the target concentration may be determined based on *ex vivo* studies using tissue obtained from subjects in the trial but prior to treatment.

The sample size **n** may be derived in the following manner. Suppose one wishes to estimate the mean concentration associated with each dose so that the estimate is within $100\gamma\%$ of the true mean with high confidence $1 - \alpha$. If the serum concentration measurements are normally distributed with constant coefficient of variation **cv** and if the coefficient of variation is known, then the required sample size is as follows:

$$n = (z_{1 - \alpha/2} \, cv/\gamma)^2 \qquad (3)$$

where $z_{1 - \alpha/2}$ is the $100(1 - \alpha/2)$nd percentile of the standard normal distribution. A confidence level of 90% corresponds to the z value of 1.645. If the coefficient of variation is 0.5 and we want to be within 25% of the mean ($\gamma = 0.25$), then we obtain **n** = 11 patients per dose level. If the accuracy of the assay is greater and there is little interpatient variability in pharmacokinetics, then we might have a smaller coefficient of variability. If $cv = 0.25$, then with the other parameters the same as given earlier, the equation indicates that only three patients per dose level are required. Equation 3 is actually an underestimate of the number of patients required in most circumstances because it assumes that the coefficient of variation is known and does not account for the variability in estimation of the **cv** from the data. In general, the $z_{1 - \alpha/2}$ term should be replaced by the corresponding percentile of the **t** distribution with degrees of freedom equal to *(n − 1)* times the number of dose levels to be studied.

For some clinical trials, even a reasonable estimate of the coefficient of variation may not be known in advance. In such a case the **cv** probably should be estimated based on an initial cohort of patients treated at a fixed dose. After estimating the **cv,** the sample size per cohort can be determined from Equation 3 for use with the subsequent patients. Because toxicity is not expected, it is best to randomize subsequent patients among the dose levels to be studied.

Minimal Biologically Active Dose

One may define biologic activity based on inhibition of a molecular target, or based on an immunogenic response, and attempt to identify the smallest dose that is biologically active. Table 21.3 shows the probability of no biologic response in **n** patients as a function of the true responsibility. If one wants a dose at which the response probability is at least 30%, then after observing no responses in seven patients it would be appropriate to escalate to the next dose level. Simon's optimal two-stage phase II designs can also be used to distinguish a response probability of some uninteresting level p_o (e.g., 0.05) from a promising level p_1 (e.g., 0.30) (29). Unless p_1 is much greater than p_o, however, the required number of patients will be much larger than for cytotoxic phase I trials (Table 21.4).

Korn et al. (27) defined a sequential procedure for finding a biologically active dose, although not necessarily the minimal active dose. During an initial accelerated phase they treat one patient per dose level until a biologic response is seen. After the first response is seen, they treat cohorts of three to six patients per dose level. With zero to one biologic response among the three patients at a dose level, they escalate to the next level for the next cohort of patients. With two or three responses from the three pa-

TABLE 21.3. *Finding the minimum active dose*

Probability of biologic response	No. of patients treated at dose	Probability of no biologic responses
0.20	11	0.09
0.25	9	0.08
0.30	7	0.08
0.40	5	0.08
0.50	4	0.06

TABLE 21.4. *Optimal two-stage designs*

Target response rate (p_1)	First-stage sample size (N_1)	Maximum sample size (N)	No. of responses required for activity (A)	Probability of early termination
20%	12	37	4	.54
25%	9	24	3	.63
30%	7	21	3	.70
35%	6	12	2	.74

$p_0 = 5\%$

tients, they expand the cohort to a total of six patients. With five or six biologic responses from the six patients, they declare that dose level to be the biologically active level and terminate the trial. With fewer than five biologic responses from the six patients, a new cohort of three patients is accrued at the next higher dose level, etc. Korn et al. (27) describe some of the statistical properties of this sequential design.

Determining the Presence of a Dose-Response Relationship and Characterizing the Relationship

Trying to determine whether there is a relationship between dose and biologic response involves comparing response rates or response distributions for patients at different dose levels. If designed properly, such trials require larger sample sizes. For example, suppose that biologic response is binary and one wishes to plan a study of two dose levels and test whether the biologic response rates differ at the two levels. If the true response probabilities at the two dose levels are 50% and 90%, then 20 patients treated at each dose level are required for a one-sided statistical significance of 0.10 and a statistical power of 0.90 (27). Larger sample sizes are required to detect smaller differences. Using more than two dose levels allows one to treat somewhat fewer patients at each dose level, but the total number of patients required to detect a dose-response relationship will actually be much larger than if only two dose levels are tested. This is because the two most extreme dose groups are the most informative for detecting a dose-response relationship.

Trying to characterize the shape of the dose-biologic response relationship or finding an optimum biologic dose (OBD) is an even more ambitious objective than a two-dose comparison of biologic response rates. It is rarely practical in a phase I study unless there is an accurate quantitative assay of biologic response with little intrapatient or interpatient variability in assay results.

Trials using biologic response endpoints are complicated by issues of assay adequacy and access to biologic tissues. Because of the difficulties of accessing tumor tissue, some studies have used normal tissue in which the molecular target is highly expressed (30). Thus, one strategy for phase I study of molecularly targeted drugs is to compare dose levels with regard to biologic response in accessible normal tissue using an optimized highly reproducible assay. The use of normal tissue may serve to reduce interpatient variability.

If use of normal tissue for assessing biologic response is not acceptable or if a highly reproducible assay is not available, trying to characterize an OBD probably is not feasible. In such cases it probably would be better to optimize the dose level using clinical response as the endpoint. It probably would require more patients and more time to characterize the OBD than to compare dose levels with regard to clinical response. Such studies can either use tumor shrinkage or time to progressive disease as the clinical endpoint. The studies are best conducted as randomized trials, but the type I error level α need not be set stringently at the conventional 5% level. Several investigators, such as Budde and Bauer (31) and Chen and Simon (32) have developed designs that can be used for clinical trials with dose-response objectives.

FURTHER CONSIDERATIONS

Several other alternative phase I designs have been proposed for special situations. For drugs with variable dose effect based on a patient's baseline characteristic (initial white blood count, in particular), Mick and Ratain (33) suggested using a dose-toxicity model that incorporated this additional variable to define both the MTD and the dose escalation schema. For phase I studies of drug combinations, Korn and Simon (34) point out that there may be a wide variety of combined MTDs involving different drug proportions. They provide guidance in arriving at a favorable combination, from a dose-intensity perspective, as well in designing the combined dose escalation schema.

Phase I studies in children are generally performed after an adult MTD has been established, and dose escalation begins at 80% of the adult dose to minimize undertreatment (35). In the past, phase I studies have routinely excluded elderly patients because of the assumption that they are inherently more susceptible to toxicity. Cascinu et al. (36) review the results of a comparison of toxicity seen in 120 elderly patients compared with that seen in 120 nonelderly patients with similar clinical features and receiving the same chemotherapeutic regimens. They report that the chemotherapeutic regimens yield similar benefits and similar toxicities for both groups. They conclude that chronologic age is a weak predictor of either toxicity or failure to respond.

Except for phase I studies of nontoxic therapeutics, which we have discussed at length, there usually is little attempt to assess the efficacy of the therapy in the phase I trial. Sometimes the MTD cohort is expanded to approximately ten patients to further assess toxicity. In these cases, care should be taken to not overinterpret any responses seen or, more importantly, lack of response. Phase II trials of efficacy are significantly larger than ten patients and still give only crude indications of response rate. Moreover, a total of ten patients without response is generally insufficient evidence upon which to reject the potential efficacy of an agent. Most importantly, the patient population of phase I trials is generally not as favorable as that of phase II trials with respect to the likelihood of seeing tumor response.

The last decade has witnessed a dramatic change in the design and practice of phase I trials. A study of the phase I trials conducted at M.D. Anderson Cancer Center between 1991 and 1993 (37) concluded that all used standard designs, with 23% of the patients treated at less than 50% of the determined MTD. In contrast, all participants in a 1998 colloquium on new phase I designs (38) agreed that they no longer used standard phase I designs routinely, that dose escalation with one-patient cohorts in the initial stages of phase I trials had become frequent and was apparently safe, and that all of the commonly used newer methods are generally preferable to the standard phase I design.

REFERENCES

1. Simon RM, Freidlin B, Rubinstein LV, et al. Accelerated titration designs for phase I clinical trials in oncology. *J Natl Cancer Inst* 1997;89:1138.
2. Collins JM, Zaharko DS, Dedrick RL, et al. Potential roles for preclinical pharmacology in phase I clinical trials. *Cancer Treat Reports* 1986;70:73.
3. Grieshaber CK, Marsoni S. The relation of preclinical toxicology to findings in early clinical trials. *Cancer Treat Reports* 1986;70:65.
4. Fuse E, Kobayashi T, Inaba M, et al. Prediction of the maximal tolerated dose (MTD) and therapeutic effect of anticancer drugs in humans: integration of pharmacokinetics with pharmacodynamics and toxicodynamics. *Cancer Treat Rev* 1995;21:133.
5. Mahmood I, Balian JD. The pharmacokinetic principles behind scaling from preclinical results to phase I protocols. Clin Pharmacokin 1999;36:1.
6. Leventhal BG, Wittes RE. *Research methods in clinical oncology.* New York: Raven Press, 1988.
7. Arbuck SG. Workshop on phase I study design—Ninth NCI/EORTC New Drug Development Symposium. *Ann Oncol* 1996;7:567.
8. Schneiderman MA. Mouse to man: statistical problems in bringing a drug to clinical trial. In: *Proceedings of the Fifth Berkeley Symposium on Mathematical Statistics and Probability.* Berkeley, CA: University of California Press, 1967:855.
9. Newell DR. Pharmacologically based phase I trials in cancer chemotherapy. *Hematol Oncol Clin North Am* 1994;8:257.
10. Goodman SN, Zahurak ML, Piantadosi S. Some practical improvements in the continual reassessment method for phase I studies. *Stat Med* 1995;14:1149.
11. Korn EL, Midthune D, Chen TT, et al. A comparison of two phase I trial designs. *Stat Med* 1994;13:1799.
12. O'Quigley J, Pepe M, Fisher L. Continual reassessment method: a practical design for phase I clinical trials in cancer. *Biometrics* 1990;46:33.
13. Storer BE. Design and analysis of phase I clinical trials. *Biometrics* 1989;45:925.
14. Lindley DV. Bayesian inference, In: Kotz S, Johnson NL, eds. *Encyclopedia of statistical sciences, volume 1.* New York: John Wiley & Sons, 1982:197.
15. O'Quigley J, Chevret S. Methods for dose finding studies in cancer clinical trials: a review and results of a Monte Carlo study. *Stat Med* 1991;10:1647.
16. O'Quigley J. Estimating the probability of toxicity at the recommended dose following a phase I clinical trial in cancer. *Biometrics* 1992;48:853.
17. Babb J, Rogatko A, Zacks S. Cancer phase I clinical trials: efficient dose escalation with overdose control. *Stat Med* 1998;17:1103.
18. Potter DM. Adaptive dose finding for phase I clinical trials of drugs used for chemotherapy of cancer. *Stat Med* 2002;21:1805.
19. Sheiner LB, Beal SL, Sambol NC. Study designs for dose ranging. *Clin Pharmacol Ther* 1989;46:63.
20. Chou TC, Talalay P. Generalized equations for the analysis of inhibitions of Michaelis-Menten and higher-order kinetic systems with two or more mutually exclusive and nonexclusive inhibitors. *Eur J Biochem* 1981;115:207.
21. EORTC Pharmacokinetics and Metabolism Group. Pharmacokinetically guided dose escalation in phase I clinical trials: commentary and proposed guidelines. *Eur J Clin Oncol* 1987;23:1083.
22. Collins JM, Grieshaber CK, Chabner BA. Pharmacologically guided phase I clinical trials based upon preclinical drug development. *J Natl Cancer Inst* 1990;82:132.
23. Gianni L, Vigano L, Surbone A, et al. Pharmacology and clinical toxicity of 4′-iodo-4′-deoxydoxorubicin: an example of successful application of pharmacokinetics to dose escalation in phase I trials. *J Natl Cancer Inst* 1990;82:469.
24. Conley BA, Forrest A, Egorin MJ, et al. Phase I trial

using adaptive control dosing of hexamethylene bisac-etamide. *Cancer Res* 1989;49:3436.

25. Foster BJ, Newell DR, Graham MA, et al. Phase I trial of the anthrapyrazole CI-941: prospective evaluation of a pharmacokinetically guided dose-escalation. *Eur J Cancer* 1992;28:463.

26. Collins JM. Innovations in phase I trial design: where do we go next? *Clin Cancer Res* 2000;6:3801.

27. Korn EL, Rubinstein LV, Hunsberger SA, et al. Clinical trial designs for cytostatic agents and agents directed at novel molecular targets. In: Adjei AA, Buolamwini JK, eds. *Strategies for discovery and clinical testing of novel anticancer agents.* Elsevier, Amsterdam, 2004 (in press).

28. Simon RM, Steinberg SM, Hamilton M, et al. Clinical trial designs for the early clinical development of therapeutic vaccines. *J Clin Oncol* 2001;19:1848.

29. Simon RM. Optimal two-stage designs for phase II clinical trials. *Control Clin Trials* 1989;10:1.

30. Albanell J, Rojo F, Averbuch S, et al. Pharmacodynamic studies of the epidermal growth factor receptor inhibitor ZD1 839 in skin from cancer patients: histopathologic and molecular consequences of recseptor inhibition. *J Clin Oncol* 2002;20:110.

31. Budde M, Bauer P. Multiple test procedures in clinical dose finding studies. *J Am Stat Assoc* 1989;84:792.

32. Chen TT, Simon R. A multiple decision procedure in clinical trials. *Stat Med* 1994;13:431.

33. Mick R, Ratain MJ. Model-guided determination of maximum tolerated dose in phase I clinical trials: evidence for increased precision. *J Natl Cancer Inst* 1993;85:217.

34. Korn EL, Simon R. Using the tolerable-dose diagram in the design of phase I combination chemotherapy trials. *J Clin Oncol* 1990;8:374,.

35. Smith M, Bernstein M, Bleyer WA, et al. Conduct of phase I trials in children with cancer. *J Clin Oncol* 1998;16:966.

36. Cascinu S, Del Ferro E, Catalano G. Toxicity and therapeutic response to chemotherapy in patients aged 70 years or older with advanced cancer. *Am J Clin Oncol* 1996;19:371.

37. Smith TL, Lee JJ, Kantarjian HM, et al. Design and results of Phase I cancer clinical trials: three-year experience at M.D. Anderson Cancer Center. *J Clin Oncol* 1996;14:287.

38. Eisenhauer EA, O'Dwyer PJ, Christian M, et al. Phase I clinical trial design in cancer drug development. *J Clin Oncol* 2000;18:684.

22

Phase I Trial Design

Considerations in the Pediatric Population

Elizabeth Fox and *Peter C. Adamson

*Pharmacology & Experimental Therapeutics Section, Pediatric Oncology Branch, National Cancer
Institute, Bethesda, Maryland 20892; and *Division of Clinical Pharmacology & Therapeutics, The
Children's Hospital of Philadelphia, Philadelphia, Pennsylvania 19104*

The development of new agents for children with cancer is critically important. The rate of improvement in survival for children with cancer made over the past 4 decades will not continue without the successful identification and development of novel therapeutic agents for pediatric malignancies.

The conduct of drug development and associated correlative studies in children may have clinical and scientific impact beyond the pediatric cancer population. Clinical trials in childhood cancer not only have resulted in decreased mortality but have defined many of the principles of anticancer therapy used today in both children and adults. Evidence that combination chemotherapy can cure cancer was first demonstrated in childhood leukemia more than 40 years ago. The success of a multimodality treatment approach (chemotherapy with surgery and/or radiation therapy) for chemosensitive solid tumors was first demonstrated in Wilms' tumor. Many advances in bone marrow and stem cell transplantation also were realized initially in pediatric patients. More recently, the efficacy of biologic agents in tumors was demonstrated with the use of retinoic acid in pediatric patients, not only in the treatment of acute promyelocytic leukemia (1) but in children with advanced stage neuroblastoma (2).

Cooperative group and multiinstitutional trials have been critical to the advances in cancer therapy. In 1955, the Children's Cancer Study Group (CCSG) was the first cooperative group formed by the National Institutes of Health (NIH) for the treatment of childhood cancers. It later became known as the Children's Cancer Group (CCG). Disease-specific groups, including the National Wilms' Tumor Study Group (NWTS) and the Intergroup Rhabdomyosarcoma Study Group (IRS), were also were created. In 1980, pediatric institutions in the Southwest Oncology Group and Cancer and Leukemia Group B formed the Pediatric Oncology Group (POG) (3,4). Through clinical trials, these groups improved the overall survival of children with leukemia from less than 5% in 1960 to greater than 70% in 1990, and survival in children with solid tumors improved from approximately 28% to greater than 70% in this same period. For children diagnosed with cancer between 1974 and 1992, the 5-year survival for all cancers increased from 55% to greater than 70% (Fig. 22.1). Recently, the CCG, POG, IRS, and NWTS merged into the Children's Oncology Group (COG), which is now the largest pediatric cooperative group internationally.

In comparison to adults with cancer, the incidence of pediatric cancers is fortunately low (Fig. 22.2), with ten cases of childhood cancer per 100,000 diagnosed annually. Each year in the United States there are approximately 12,500 new cases of childhood cancer (5). Importantly, more than 50% of pediatric patients with newly diagnosed cancer are enrolled in cooperative group trials, compared to approximately 2% of adults with cancer. Despite the low incidence of pediatric malignancies, the high enrollment in clinical trials, and the improvements in overall survival, the number of years of life lost to childhood cancer is four to five times greater than adult malignancies (Fig. 22.3).

The goal of front-line therapy for children with cancer is cure. For many types and stages of childhood cancer, this goal has in large part been realized. For some pediatric cancers, such as stage I to II

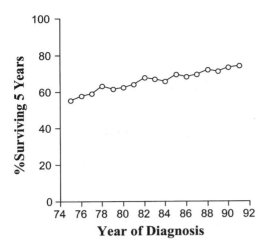

FIG. 22.1. Five-year survival for children (0–14 years old) with cancer from 1975 through 1990. Dramatic increases in survival are due, in part, to clinical trials for children with cancer.

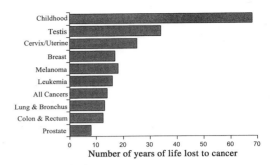

FIG. 22.3. Despite the low incidence of pediatric malignancies, the high enrollment in clinical trials, and the improvements in overall survival, the number of years of life lost to childhood cancer is four to five times greater than adult malignancies.

Hodgkin disease or Wilms' tumor, the survival rate is greater than 90%. For other solid tumors and high-risk hematologic malignancies, success has come with the advent of dose-intense multimodality therapies. The acute toxicity experienced by childhood cancer patients today and the late effects of modern therapy unique to growing children are substantial. In a recent front-line treatment protocol for rhabdomyosarcoma (IRS-III Study), 1,062 patients were treated with one of seven regimens. More than 80% of the patients experienced at least one toxicity that was severe, life-threatening, or fatal. Twenty-two of the 32 deaths during the study were from sepsis during neutropenia. Other treatment-related causes of death included cardiotoxicity, metabolic complica-

tions, radiation toxicity, adult respiratory distress syndrome, central nervous system toxicity, and hemorrhage during thrombocytopenia. This is the current standard therapy for childhood rhabdomyosarcoma, a standard that pediatric oncologists, families, and patients do not consider a mark of truly successful treatment (6). Similarly, late effects of therapy for childhood cancer, including alkylator-induced infertility, epipodophyllotoxin-associated secondary leukemia, and anthracycline-induced cardiotoxicity, must be decreased or eliminated.

The major improvements in survival have not been shared by all children with cancer. Pediatric oncology research has shifted focus to the subgroups of children with cancer who continue to have a poor outcome. These include patients with high-grade gliomas, metastatic sarcomas, advanced-stage neuroblastoma, Philadelphia chromosome-positive leukemia, and infants with leukemia. The outcome for these patients, coupled with the acute and late effects of current therapy, underscores the need for new agents and treatment approaches for children with cancer.

New anticancer agents developed for adult cancer must be carefully and independently tested in childhood cancer because of differences in both the tumor biology and the developmental stage of the patient population. Scaling of adult doses for children based on body weight or surface area does not account for developmental changes that may affect drug disposition and tissue/organ sensitivity. The clearance of vincristine is an example (Fig. 22.4). In clinical trials, infant and adult patients appeared to be more susceptible to vincristine-induced peripheral neuropathy. Pharmacokinetic analysis revealed that vincristine clearance normalized to body surface area varies with age. Children clear vincristine more rapidly than adults; therefore, when receiving the same dose normalized to body surface area, children will have lower

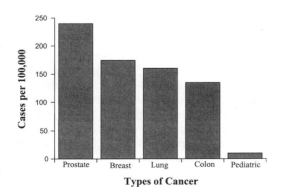

FIG. 22.2. Comparison of the incidence of cancer per 100,000 persons for common adult malignancies and all pediatric cancers. The incidence of all types of childhood cancer is a fraction of the adults diagnosed with prostate, breast, lung, or colon cancer.

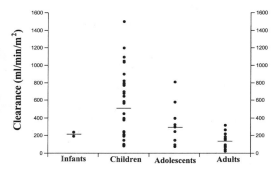

FIG. 22.4. Comparison of vincristine clearance normalized to body surface area in infants, children, adolescents, and adults. Infants are at greater risk of developing neurotoxicity when dosed based on body surface area. (Adapted from Crom W, de Graaf SS, Synold T, et al. Pharmacokinetics of vincristine in children and adolescents with acute lymphocytic leukemia. *J Pediatr* 1994;125:642–649; and Sagar Sethi V, Jackson DV Jr, White DR, et al. Pharmacokinetics of vincristine sulfate in adult cancer patients. *Cancer Res* 1981;41:3551–3555, with permission.)

plasma concentrations than adults (7–9). Differences in end-organ sensitivity may differ between children and adults, as has been observed with retinoids. The maximum tolerated dose (MTD) and dose-limiting toxicity (DLT) of all-*trans*-retinoic acid and 9-*cis*-retinoic acid are age dependent (Table 22.1), with young children being more susceptible to neurotoxicity than older children and adults (10–13).

In this chapter we review approaches to the unique challenges of pediatric cancer drug development, from preclinical through early-stage clinical trials. Additionally, the ethical and regulatory considerations for the study of new anticancer agents in children are presented.

PRECLINICAL DRUG DEVELOPMENT

Many of the cytotoxic agents in use today were identified through a large-scale screening process at the National Cancer Institute (NCI). The initial screening program that began in 1955 relied on L1210 and P388 murine leukemia *in vivo* models. In 1985 an *in vitro* screening program for pure compounds and natural products was implemented, and by 1990 it was fully operational as the NCI 60-cell panel (NCI-60). The 60 human tumor cell lines used in this *in vitro* cytotoxicity screening are exclusively adult histologies (14). Anticancer drugs identified in this process, such as topotecan, are active in adult and childhood cancers. Compounds recently prioritized by the NCI-60 screen include the proteosome inhibitor PS-341, flavopiridol, MGI-114, depsipeptide, and UCN-01. The clinical value of these new agents currently is being investigated in clinical trial in adults and, a select number are being investigated in children (15). Because the NCI-60 panel screen does not include pediatric histologies, its utility for prioritizing new agents for pediatric drug development is limited (16). The challenges are further compounded by the fact that activity in adult cancers does not necessarily predict activity in childhood cancer. This was observed with paclitaxel, a taxane that is highly effective in ovarian, breast, non–small cell lung, and head and neck cancer (17) but has not demonstrated significant activity in a spectrum of pediatric solid tumors (18,19).

In an effort to fill the void in the screening of new agents for pediatric tumors, a number of investigators have developed xenograft models of pediatric malignancies. Such models include rhabdomyosarcoma (20), neuroblastoma (21,22), osteosarcoma (23), pediatric brain tumors (24–26), peripheral neuroectodermal tumors, and leukemia (27,28). Rhabdomyosarcoma and neuroblastoma xenografts have been found to be predictive for clinical activity of topoisomerase 1 inhibitors (20,21), and the rhabdomyosarcoma xenograft model has been predictive of melphalan activity in patients (29). To date, 22 new agents have been tested in one or more pediatric tumor xenografts, but until a coordinated and consis-

TABLE 22.1. *Maximum tolerated dose and dose-limiting toxicity of retinoids in adults and children*

	≤12 Years	>12 Years	Adult
All-*trans*-retinoic acid			
MTD	60 mg/m²/d	90 mg/m²/d	150 mg/m²/d
DLT	Pseudotumor cerebri	Headache, pseudotumor cerebri	Dermatologic
9-*cis*-retinoic acid			
MTD	35 mg/m²/d	85 mg/m²/d	140 mg/m²/d
DLT	Pseudotumor cerebri	Headache, pseudotumor cerebri	Headache, diarrhea, dermatologic

DLT, dose-limiting toxicity; MTD, maximum tolerated dose.

tent approach is adopted, the role of such models in pediatric drug development will remain unclear (30).

Other models, including transgenic mouse models of juvenile myelomonocytic leukemia (31), other leukemias, neuroblastoma (32), gliomas, medulloblastoma, and rhabdomyosarcoma, have been used. Xenograft and transgenic mouse models may be more sensitive in identifying agents that induce apoptosis, alter cell cycle, or are antiangiogenic and thus may become increasingly important as cytostatic or molecularly targeted agents are developed in childhood cancer. Transgenic animals may be particularly useful if they are engineered with a molecular defect in a pathway of malignant transformation that a drug can target.

At the present time, a comprehensive approach to preclinical drug development does not exist for pediatric tumors. To begin to address this, the NCI and COG Phase 1 Consortium recently conducted a workshop on preclinical testing for pediatric anticancer agent development to identify and evaluate existing models and discuss the establishment of a program for preclinical testing in pediatrics. Results of this symposium detail the current state of the art in pediatric preclinical models (30).

The number of agents available for testing in humans is increasing, but the number of pediatric patients eligible for early clinical trials remains relatively small. Therefore, agents must be carefully selected for development in childhood cancers. As described earlier, only a limited number of pediatric preclinical models have been successfully utilized for drug prioritization; thus, other criteria factor heavily into agent selection for pediatric drug development. Factors for selection include agents with a novel mechanism of action, a unique resistance profile, or improved toxicity profile. Additionally, agents may be selected because of favorable pharmacologic properties, such as good penetration across the blood–brain barrier, good bioavailability of an oral formulation, or a formulation that alters the distribution and toxicity profile. Promising agents that show activity in early adult trials are also prioritized for pediatric development.

New challenges in preclinical drug development have arisen as the cytotoxicity paradigm of anticancer drugs shifts to a molecularly target-based approach. As investigators in pediatric oncology develop *in vitro* and *in vivo* models for drug development, it will be important to characterize these models at the genetic and protein levels to better understand the role of specific targets in pediatric malignant disease.

PEDIATRIC CLINICAL DRUG DEVELOPMENT

In the United States, the majority of clinical trials in children, and virtually all phase III randomized trials, are coordinated by members of the COG, which provides a unified scientific goal, data collection, and reporting. Similar cooperative groups exist in the United Kingdom and Europe. The COG encompasses 235 institutions in the United States, Canada, and Australia and currently is treating more than 40,000 children with cancer. A select subset of 21 institutions within the COG conduct pediatric phase I trials.

Pediatric Phase I Clinical Trials

Adult and pediatric phase I studies are similar in that both determine a recommended phase II dose, often the MTD, as their primary objective and use DLT as the primary endpoint. Similar to adult studies, MTD is defined as the dose immediately below the dose where two or more patients of six enrolled patients experience a DLT. Toxicity is graded according to the Common Toxicity Criteria version 2 or the recently developed Common Terminology Criteria for Adverse Events version 3 (available at *http://ctep.info. nih.gov*). For cytotoxic agents, DLT typically is defined as any nonhematologic toxicity that is greater than or equal to grade 3, grade 4 neutropenia for longer than a specified duration of time (e.g., 5 days), or grade 4 thrombocytopenia. Children are eligible for phase I trials if their disease is refractory to standard therapy or no standard curative therapy exists.

Adequate organ function and performance status are important requirements for children entering onto a phase I trial. Age-specific performance scales have been developed for pediatric studies. For children 10 years or younger, performance status is estimated using the Lansky scale, which measures age-appropriate activities, such as time engaged in active play. The Karnofsky scale can be used for children older than 10 years (33).

Pharmacokinetic studies are an integral component of early clinical trials in children. Attention must be given to blood sample volume, because the total blood volume that can be safely obtained is limited in small children. Fortunately, with modern assays utilizing sensitive and specific detectors such as liquid chromatography with tandem mass spectrometry, sample volume is no longer a limiting factor. The importance of performing pharmacokinetics studies in children cannot be overemphasized, because significant differences in drug disposition, including volume of distribution and drug clearance, occur as a function of growth and development. Additionally, pharmacokinetics studies in phase I trials define the interpatient variability of systemic exposure, allow for comparison of systemic exposure and toxicity between adult and pediatric patients, identify agents with saturable clearance mechanisms, and help provide for a rational selection of schedules of drug administration (34).

Dose escalation strategies in pediatric phase I trials differ from those used in adults. The starting dose in an adult phase I trial typically is one tenth the dose lethal to 10% of a cohort of mice (1/10 MELD$_{10}$) (35) or one tenth the MTD in the most sensitive animal species. Dose escalation classically has proceeded via a modified Fibonacci scheme in which the first dose escalation is 100% of the starting dose and subsequent dose levels are increased by 67%, 50%, 40%, and 33%. Multiple dose levels often are evaluated before biologic activity is observed. Other dose escalation schema, including the continual reassessment model, endeavor to make adult phase I trials more efficient by accelerating the dose escalation scheme to treat fewer patients at lower dose levels in which the likelihood of a response is low. In pediatrics, the starting dose for a phase I trial is often 80% of the adult MTD. This greatly increases the likelihood that pediatric patients are exposed to biologically active doses. Dose escalation usually is in fixed 30% increments, with studies usually requiring fewer than five dose levels (36).

Other dose escalation strategies have been used successfully in pediatric phase I trials. One study design of individualized dosing to treat patients closer to the MTD was used in a phase I study of continuous infusion topotecan in children with recurrent acute leukemia. In this study, target systemic topotecan exposure was established using a severe combined immune deficiency (SCID) mouse model. In children enrolled on the trial, steady-state topotecan lactone concentrations (Css) were measured within the first 24 hours of the continuous infusion and the dose was adjusted to achieve the target concentration. The maximum tolerated systemic exposure was 4.0 ng/mL and the exposure-limiting toxicity was mucositis at 5.3 ng/mL. A significant relationship between topotecan lactone Css and the severity of mucositis was observed. Responses were noted at the Css comparable to those producing responses in the SCID mouse model (37).

The importance of performing phase I trials in children and not relying on adult data is exemplified by the unpredictable association between the adult and pediatric MTD (Fig. 22.5). In the 1970s, for the majority of agents, the MTDs determined in pediatric phase I studies were greater than the adult MTD by 10% to 200%. However, in the 1990s the majority of

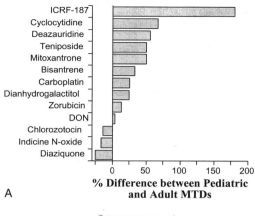

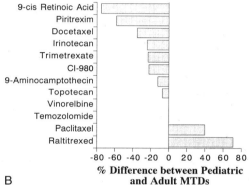

FIG. 22.5. Percent difference in the maximum tolerated dose (MTD; in mg/m^2) for investigational agents evaluated in phase I trials in pediatric and adult populations. Trials were conducted in the 1970s **(A)** and the 1990s **(B)**. The unpredictable association between adult and pediatric MTD is a strong rationale for conducting phase I trials separately in adult and pediatric populations.

agents had MTDs that were 10% to 80% lower than the adult MTD. This may reflect differences in the pharmacokinetics of the agents; however, it is more likely due to the increased dose intensity of prior treatment regimens for childhood cancers.

Initial therapies for childhood cancer are intense and delivered with curative intent. If a patient's tumor is refractory or recurs, many pediatric patients are treated with second-line or "salvage regimens" or high-dose therapy with stem cell support prior to enrolling in phase I studies. Therefore, the patient may be less tolerant of therapy and tumors may be more refractory to therapy when the child is enrolled in a phase I study. The impact of prior therapy is demonstrated in the phase I trial of docetaxel in children with refractory solid tumors. In the initial phase I study of docetaxel administered as a 1-hour infusion, the MTD was 125 mg/m^2 and the DLT was neutropenia; however, thrombocytopenia was mild. Three of the four patients who responded were treated with doses greater than 100 mg/m^2 (38). A second phase I study was completed using filgrastim granulocyte colony stimulating factor (G-CSF) support. In this study the MTD was 185 mg/m^2, which was 50% higher than the MTD of docetaxel alone in children and 85% higher than the recommended adult dose. The DLT was a generalized erythematous desquamating skin rash and myalgias (39).

Pediatric phase I studies have been performed safely for more than 3 decades. In a review of studies conducted by St. Jude Children's Research Center or the Pediatric Oncology Group since 1967, a total of 577 children with leukemia or solid tumors were enrolled in 27 phase I trials. The mortality due to direct toxicity of the investigational agent was 2.4% and the overall response rate was 5.9%. Progressive disease was responsible for the majority of deaths of patients enrolled in these trials (78%) (40). A more recent report examined pediatric phase I clinical trials of antineoplastic agents to identify trends in response and toxicity over time. A total of 1,606 children with cancer were enrolled in 56 single-agent phase I trials between 1978 and 1996. Death and response rates of evaluable patients for the periods 1978 to 1984, 1985 to 1989, and 1990 to 1996 are given in Table 22.2. The overall response rate was 7.9%. Death occurred in 7% of all enrolled patients, and only 0.7% of patients experienced a death related to drug toxicity (41). This supports the concept that well-designed phase I clinical trials do not expose children to unacceptable risk of fatal toxicity and offer hope for a therapeutic effect.

Pediatric Phase II Clinical Trials

Phase II trials are similar in both pediatric and adult populations. The primary objective of phase II trials is to define the spectrum of antitumor activity for a new agent administered at the optimal dose and schedule determined in a phase I trial. Phase II trials are restricted to patients with specific histologic types of cancer, which are selected based on activity of the drug in preclinical cancer models, the mechanism of action of the drug, and activity observed in phase I trials. For conventional cytotoxic drugs the endpoint in a phase II trial is response, which is measured as the percent decrease in size of the tumor compared to the pretreatment tumor size. Therefore, patients enrolled on conventional phase II trials must have measurable tumor that is refractory to standard therapy.

A number of phase II clinical trial designs have emerged, but most attempt to determine whether a new drug has a sufficient level of antitumor activity to warrant testing in a randomized trial to evaluate efficacy. Traditional phase II trials are uncontrolled and incorporate an early stopping rule in an attempt to minimize the number of patients enrolled if the drug turns out to be inactive. For example, using the optimum two-stage design (42) and assuming type I and II error probabilities of 0.10, if a response rate of 25% would justify further clinical development of a new drug, then nine patients with the specified type of cancer would be entered during the first stage of accrual. If no response were observed in the first nine patients, then the trial is terminated. If one or more patients experience a response, then accrual continues up to a total of 24 patients, and two or more responses in the 24 patients would be consistent with a response rate 25% or greater. Trials with this two-stage design may require suspension of enrollment after accrual to the first stage is complete until response data have been collected. For cytotoxic agents, response can be evaluated over a relatively short time (weeks to months).

To avoid problems of acquired drug resistance in tumors and decreased tolerance in heavily pretreated patients, phase II trials ideally are conducted in untreated patients. However, most childhood cancers are curable with standard therapy instituted at initial diagnosis. Therefore, phase II trials in children usually specify that patients are eligible if their tumors did not respond to standard therapy. Standard therapy in childhood malignancies tends to be dose intensive and may result in a decreased tolerance to investigational agents in a phase II setting. To eliminate the impact of prior therapy, some phase II evaluations in children have been conducted prior to definitive standard therapy as an "experimental window" or "upfront

TABLE 22.2. *Risk and benefit of phase I trials in children*

Year	Evaluable patients	Death rate (%)		Response rate (%)
		Overall	Toxic	
1978–1984	293	6.0	0.9	5.5
1985–1989	535	8.3	0.5	6.0
1990–1996	620	6.6	0.9	10.3

phase II window" (43). These trials are conducted in pediatric patients with poor prognosis, and examples include the development of ifosfamide in children and adolescents with metastatic osteosarcoma (44) or unresectable rhabdomyosarcoma (45).

The potential to identify active agents using an upfront window initially was demonstrated with the development of melphalan in rhabdomyosarcoma. In a conventional phase II trial, melphalan had a response rate of 1 of 13 patients. Because of compelling activity in a mouse rhabdomyosarcoma xenograft model, a phase II window trial was conducted and yielded 10 of 13 partial responses during the 6-week window of melphalan in previously untreated patients with rhabdomyosarcoma (29). In a subsequent study, melphalan was administered in combination with vincristine, and although the combination had an excellent response rate (complete remission plus partial remission) of 78% (51/65) the 3-year failure-free survival was 20% for patients who received melphalan plus vincristine compared to 30% failure-free survival in patients treated with conventional therapy (46).

Ethical issues with "phase II window" designs include the potential for delays in conventional chemotherapy, the possibility of progressive disease during the window period, and the possibility that toxicity from the investigational agent may prevent administration of full doses of conventional agents. In light of these concerns, performing up-front phase II window studies is becoming less common.

ETHICAL AND REGULATORY CONSIDERATIONS

Children are afforded additional research protections that must be considered when designing and performing pediatric clinical trials. In addition to the guidelines that apply to the conduct of research in both adults and children detailed in Chapter 33, we review here issues specific to the pediatric population.

In 1947 the Nuremberg Code defined ethical and legal requirements for experimentation based on informed voluntary consent of the individual. Because children cannot give informed consent, the Nuremberg Code, if taken literally, excludes them from participating in clinical research trials (47,48). The Declaration of Helsinki (1964, revised 1975, 1983, 1989, 1996) opened the door to research involving children by permitting their parents or legal guardians to give consent. In 1974 the National Commission for Subjects of Biomedical and Behavioral Research convened and ultimately produced the Belmont Report (1979), which delineates the ethical principles and guidelines for the protection of human subjects in

biomedical research. The commission introduced the concepts of permission, assent, and deliberate objection. In 1995 the Academy of Pediatrics furthered the distinction between informed consent, permission, and assent, stating that only persons who have full decision-making capacity and legal empowerment can give informed consent. Parents or guardians provide informed permission, and a child can only offer assent (49). In 1981 the Code of Federal Regulations 45CFR46: Protection of Human Subjects instituted regulations governing the protection of all subjects in federally funded research. This included composition, function, and procedures of institutional review boards (IRBs), as well as general requirements for informed consent. In 1983, 45CRF46 was amended (45CRF46 Subpart D) to include additional protections for children.

The National Commission for Subjects of Biomedical and Behavioral Research also delineated various degrees of risk involved in research and the prospect of direct benefit for the patients involved. The three categories are minimal risk, minor increment above minimal risk, and more than a minor increment above minimal risk. IRBs may approve a clinical trial that presents greater than minimal risk only if it offers the prospect of direct benefit to the individual child, and (a) the risk is justified by the anticipated benefit to the subjects; (b) the relation of the anticipated benefit to the risk is at least as favorable to the subjects as that presented by available alternative approaches; and (c) adequate provisions are made for soliciting the assent of the children and permission of their parents or guardians. Almost all pediatric phase I cancer trials are approved by IRBs under 45CFR46.405 (and the related United States Food and Drug Administration (FDA) 21CFR50.52) as greater than minimal risk with the prospect of direct benefit.

The potential for direct benefit to children participating in a pediatric phase I trial extend beyond the complete and partial response rate, which, similar to adults, averages only approximately 5% (50,51). An additional fraction of patients also experience stable disease. Moreover, patients and families participating in phase I trials receive increased attention by the health care team involved in the clinical trial. Most importantly, although not curative, such trials provide a source of hope for families of children with refractory cancer.

Concerns about the ethical issues of children as research subjects coupled with the technical difficulty of conducting research in children, the relative scarcity of children with cancer (small market share for any drug), and regulations regarding labeling of drug for use in children have hampered pediatric cancer drug development. The FDA made efforts to encourage pharmaceutical companies to include labeling for use in children during the drug development process. Section 111 of the FDA Modernization Act (FDAMA) of 1997 states that if a drug has market exclusivity based on a patent or marketing license, the exclusivity can be extended by 6 months for the submission of pediatric data to the FDA. The 1998 Final Pediatric Rule mandated that if a drug is under review by the FDA and the disease the drug is intended to treat exists in both pediatric and adult populations, pediatric studies must be performed. It is mandatory but only applies to drugs intended to treat diseases that are similar in adult and pediatric populations. Only a limited number of pediatric malignancies are likely to be considered the same in children and adults. Incentives (extension of marketing exclusivity) for submission of pediatric data stipulated by FDAMA may improve the number of new agents available for evaluation in children (52), but the ultimate impact of this legislation for children with cancer is not yet known.

FUTURE CHALLENGES

The rapidly accumulating knowledge of the molecular pathogenesis of cancer provides new targets for drug discovery and development. This has resulted in a shift from an empirical random screening of cytotoxic anticancer agents to a more rational and mechanistic, target-based approach. Drugs that validate the molecularly targeted approach to anticancer drug development include tretinoin (all-*trans*-retinoic acid), which targets the PML-RAR fusion protein in acute promyelocytic leukemia (1,53), and imatinib mesylate (STI-571, Gleevec™), which targets the BCR-ABL fusion protein in chronic myelogenous leukemia (54,55) and the mutated KIT receptor in gastrointestinal stromal tumors (56). The clinical development of target-based anticancer drugs will require fundamental changes to the traditional clinical trial design and endpoints that have been used for conventional cytotoxic drugs. In the phase I and II setting, traditional endpoints (toxicity and response) may not be suitable for more selective, cytostatic target-based agents, and these endpoints may be replaced by biologic or pharmacokinetic

endpoints to define the optimal dose and the therapeutic effect of the drug on its target.

At present, a number of clinical trials for target-based agents are open in the COG. The objectives of these trials couple traditional phase I endpoints of toxicity and pharmacokinetics with biologically relevant endpoints such as receptor phosphorylation. For example, a pediatric phase I trial of gefitinib (Iressa™), an oral inhibitor of the epidermal growth factor receptor (EGFR) tyrosine kinase, is currently accruing patients. EGFR is a major component of growth factor-induced proliferation of cells. EGFR expression has been observed in pediatric malignancies including neuroblastoma, rhabdomyosarcoma, and high-grade gliomas. The pediatric phase I trial of gefitinib will determine the MTD of gefitinib, but it also will determine the drug's effects on surrogate markers of biologic activity, including the effects on EGFRs in epithelial cells obtained from buccal smears, on serum vascular endothelial growth factor, and on matrix metalloproteinase MMP-2 and MMP-9 concentrations.

In addition to challenges in adapting clinical trial design for target-based therapy, the development of target-based agents in children with cancer poses unique challenges. Because histology and embryology differ in most adult and pediatric malignancies, pediatric targets may differ. Unique targets, such as the EWS-FLI 1 fusion transcript in Ewing's sarcoma, exist and may be potential targets for therapy. Because the number of pediatric patients is small, it is unlikely that the pharmaceutical industry will develop independent programs developing drugs targeting pediatric malignancies. Cooperative efforts of academic centers, government support, and industry likely will be required to develop agents targeting unique pediatric targets.

Although pediatric drug development trials present additional challenges to laboratory and clinical investigators, the importance of such research is high. The expertise to safely and efficiently conduct such research is present at a number of academic centers internationally. More targeted therapy and less toxic therapy are the goals of current efforts. Current research will build upon the impressive track record in pediatric oncology achieved since the introduction of chemotherapy for the treatment of childhood leukemia more than 50 years ago.

REFERENCES

1. Tallman M, Andersen JW, Schiffer CA, et al. All-trans-retinoic acid in acute promyelocytic leukemia. *N Engl J Med* 1997;337:1021–1028.
2. Matthay K, Villablanca JG, Seeger RC, et al. Treatment of high-risk neuroblastoma with intensive chemotherapy, radiotherapy, autologous bone marrow transplant, and 13-cis-retinoic acid. *N Engl J Med* 1999;341:1165–111173.
3. Bleyer WA. The US Pediatric Cancer Clinical Trials Programmes: international implications and the way forward. *Eur J Cancer* 1997;33:1439–1447.
4. Pratt C. Pediatric clinical trials. *Oncologist* 1996;1: 169–172.

5. Ries L, Smith MA, Gurney JG et al. *Cancer incidence and survival among children and adolescents: United States SEER Program 1975–1995.* Bethesda, MD: National Cancer Institute, SEER Program, 1999, NIH Publication No. 99-4649.

6. Crist W, Gehan EA, Ragab AH, et al. The Third Intergroup Rhabdomyosarcoma Study. *J Clin Oncol* 1995; 13:610–630.

7. Crom W, de Graaf SS, Synold T, et al. Pharmacokinetics of vincristine in children and adolescents with acute lymphocytic leukemia. *J Pediatr* 1994;125:642–649.

8. Sagar Sethi V, Jackson DV Jr, White DR, et al. Pharmacokinetics of vincristine sulfate in adult cancer patients. *Cancer Res* 1981;41:3551–3555.

9. Gidding C, Meeuwsen-deBoer GJ, Koopmans P, et al. Vincristine pharmacokinetics after repetitive dosing in children. *Cancer Chemother Pharmacol* 1999;44: 203–209.

10. Smith M, Adamson PC, Balis FM, et al. Phase I and pharmacokinetic evaluation of all-trans-retinoic acid in pediatric patients. *J Clin Oncol* 1992;10:1666–1673.

11. Mahmoud H, Hurwitz CA, Roberts WM, et al. Tretinoin toxicity in children with acute promyelocytic leukemia. *Lancet* 1993;342:1394–1395.

12. Lee J, Newman RA, Lippman SM, et al. Phase I evaluation of all-trans retinoic acid in adults with solid tumors. *J Clin Oncol* 1993;11:959–966.

13. Adamson P, Pitot HC, Balis FM, et al. Variability of oral bioavailability of all-trans retinoic acid. *J Natl Cancer Inst* 1993;85:993–996.

14. Boyd M. The NCI in vitro anticancer drug discovery screen: concept, implementation, and operation, 1985–1995. In: Teicher B, ed. *Anticancer drug development guide: preclinical screening, clinical trials, and approval.* Totowa, NJ: Humana Press, 1996:23–42.

15. Johnson J, Monks A, Hollingshead MG, et al. Preclinical aspects of cancer drug discovery and development. In: Chabner B, Longo DL, eds. *Cancer chemotherapy & biotherapy.* Philadelphia: Lippincott, Williams & Wilkins, 2001:17–36.

16. Weitman S, Carlson L, Pratt CB. New drug development for pediatric oncology. *Invest New Drugs* 1996; 14:1–10.

17. Rowinsky E. Update on the antitumor activity of paclitaxel in clinical trials. *Ann Pharmacother* 1994; 28[Suppl 5]:S18–S22.

18. Hurwitz C, Strauss LC, Kepner J, et al. Paclitaxel for the treatment of progressive or recurrent childhood brain tumors: a pediatric oncology phase II study. *J Pediatr Hematol Oncol* 2001;23:277–281.

19. Harris M, Hurwitz C, Sullivan JG, et al. Taxol in pediatric solid tumors: a Pediatric Oncology Group (POG) phase II study (POG#9262). *Proc Am Soc Clin Oncol* 1999;18:563a(abst 2170).

20. Houghton P, Cheshire PJ, Hallman JD, et al. Efficacy of topoisomerase I inhibitors, topotecan and irinotecan, administered at low dose levels in protracted schedules to mice bearing xenografts of human tumors. *Cancer Chemother Pharmacol* 1995;36:393–403.

21. Kretschmar C, Kletzel M, Murray K, et al. Upfront phase II therapy with Taxol and topotecan in untreated children (>365 days) with disseminated (INSS stage 4) neuroblastoma: a Pediatric Oncology Group study. *Med Pediatr Oncol* 1995;25:243(abst).

22. Khanna C, Jaboin J, Drakos E, et al. Biologically relevant orthotopic neuroblastoma xenograft models: primary adrenal tumor growth and spontaneous distant metastasis. *In Vivo* 2002;16:77–86.

23. Meyer W, Houghton JA, Houghton PJ, et al. Development and characterization of pediatric osteosarcoma xenografts. *Cancer Res* 1991;50:2781–2785.

24. Friedman H, Colvin OM, Ludeman SM, et al. Experimental chemotherapy for human medulloblastoma. *Cancer Res* 1986;46:2827–2833.

25. Friedman H, Colvin OM, Skapek SX, et al. Experimental chemotherapy of human medulloblastoma. *Cancer Res* 1988;48:4189–4195.

26. Hare C, Elion GB, Houghton PJ, et al. Therapeutic efficacy of the topoisomerase I inhibitor, 7-ethyl-10-(4-[1-piperidono]-piperidino)-carbonyloxy-camptothecin against pediatric and adult central nervous system tumor xenografts. *Cancer Ther Pharmacol* 1997;39:187–191.

27. Uckun F, Manivel C, Arthur D, et al. In vivo efficacy of B43 (anti-CD19)-pokeweed antiviral protein immunotoxin against human pre-B cell acute lymphoblastic leukemia in mice with severe combined immunodeficiency. *Blood* 1992;79:2201–2214.

28. Jansen B, Uckun FM, Jaszcz WB, et al. Establishment of a human t(4;11) leukemia in severe combined immunodeficient mice and successful treatment using anti-CD19 (B43)-pokeweed antiviral protein immunotoxin. *Cancer Res* 1992;52:406–412.

29. Horowitz M, Etcubanas E, Christensen ML, et al. Phase II testing of melphalan in children with newly diagnosed rhabdomyosarcoma: a model for anticancer drug development. *J Clin Oncol* 1988;6:308–314.

30. Houghton P, Adamson PC, Blaney S, et al. Testing of new agents in childhood cancer preclinical models: meeting summary. *Clin Cancer Res* 2002;8:3646–3657.

31. Jacks T, Shih TS, Schmitt EM, et al. Tumor predisposition in mice heterozygous for a target mutation in Nf1. *Nat Genet* 1994;7:353–361.

32. Weiss W, Alape K, Mohapatra G, et al. Targeted expression of MYCN causes neuroblastoma in transgenic mice. *EMBO J* 1997;16:2985–2995.

33. Lansky S, List MA, Lansky LL, et al. The measurement of performance in childhood cancer patients. *Cancer* 1987;60:1651–1656.

34. Smith M, Bernstein M, Bleyer WA, et al. Conduct of phase I trials in children with cancer. *J Clin Oncol* 1998;16:966–978.

35. Grieshaber C, Marsoni S. Relation of preclinical toxicology to findings in early clinical trials. *Cancer Treat Reports* 1986;70:65–72.

36. Vassal G, Pein F, Goyette A, et al. Development of new anticancer agents in children: methodology, difficulties, and strategies. *Ann Pediatr* 1994;41:477–484.

37. Furman W, Baker SD, Pratt CB, et al. Escalating systemic exposure of continuous infusion topotecan in children with recurrent acute leukemia. *J Clin Oncol* 1996;14:1504–1511.

38. Blaney S, Seibel NL, O'Brien M, et al. Phase I trial of docetaxel administered as a 1-hour infusion in children with refractory solid tumors: a collaborative Pediatric Branch, National Cancer Institute and Children's Cancer Group Trial. *J Clin Oncol* 1997;15:1538–1543.

39. Seibel N, Blaney SM, O'Brien M, et al. Phase I trial of docetaxel with filgrastim support in pediatric patients with refractory solid tumors: a collaborative Pediatric Oncology Branch, National Cancer Institute and Children's Cancer Group Trial. *Clin Cancer Res* 1999;5:733–737.

40. Furman W, Pratt CB, Rivera GK. Mortality in pediatric

phase I clinical trials. *J Natl Cancer Inst* 1989;81: 1193–1194.

41. Shah S, Weitman S, Langevin AM, et al. Phase I therapy trials in children with cancer. *J Pediatr Hematol Oncol* 1998;20:431–438.

42. Simon R. Optimal two-staged designs for phase II clinical trials. *Control Clin Trials* 1989;10:1–10.

43. Ungerleider R, Ellenberg SS, Berg SL. Cancer clinical trials: design, conduct, analysis, and reporting. In: Pizzo P, Poplack DG, eds. *Principles and practice of pediatric oncology*. Philadelphia: Lippincott Williams & Wilkins, 2002:465–488.

44. Harris M, Cantor AB, Goorin AM, et al. Treatment of osteosarcoma with ifosfamide: comparison of response in pediatric patients with recurrent disease versus patients previously untreated: a Pediatric Oncology Group study. *Med Pediatr Oncol* 1995;24:87–92.

45. Pappo A, Ercubanas E, Santana VM, et al. A phase II trial of ifosfamide in previously untreated children and adolescents with unresectable rhabdomyosarcoma. *Cancer* 1993;71:2119–2125.

46. Breitfeld P, Lyden E, Raney RB, et al. Ifosfamide and etoposide are superior to vincristine and melphalan for pediatric metastatic rhabdomyosarcoma when administered with irradiation and combination chemotherapy: a report from the Intergroup Rhabdomyosarcoma Study Group. *J Pediatr Hematol Oncol* 2001;23: 225–233.

47. Koren G. Informed consent in pediatric research. In: Koren G, ed. *Textbook of ethics in pediatric research*. Malaber, FL: 1993, Krieger Publishing, 1994.

48. Grodin M, Alpert JJ. Children as participants in medical research. *Pediatr Clin North Am* 1988;35:1389–1401.

49. Susman J, Dorn LD, Fletcher JC. Participation in biomedical research: the consent process as viewed by children, adolescents, young adults, and physicians. *J Pediatr* 1992;121:547–552.

50. Decoster G, Stein G, Holdener EE. Response and toxic deaths in phase I clinical trials. *Ann Oncol* 1990;1: 175–181.

51. von Hoff D, Turner J. Response rates, duration of response, and dose response effects in phase I studies of antineoplastics. *Invest New Drugs* 1991;9: 115–122.

52. Hirschfeld S, Shapiro A, Dagher R. Pediatric oncology: regulatory initiatives. *Oncologist* 2000;5:441–444.

53. Sun G, Ouyang RR, Chen SJ, et al. Treatment of acute promyelocytic leukemia with all-trans retinoic acid: a five-year experience. *Chin Med J (Engl)* 1993;106:743–748.

54. Druker B, Sawyers CL, Kantarjian H, et al. Activity of a specific inhibitor of the BCR-ABL tyrosine kinase in the blast crisis of chronic myeloid leukemia and acute lymphoblastic leukemia with the Philadelphia chromosome. *N Engl J Med* 2001;344:1038–1042.

55. Druker B, Talpaz M, Resta DJ, et al. Efficacy and safety of a specific inhibitor of the BCR-ABL tyrosine kinase in chronic myeloid leukemia. *N Engl J Med* 2001; 344:1031–1037.

56. van Oosterom A, Judson I, Verweij J, et al. Safety and efficacy of imatinib (STI571) in metastatic gastrointestinal stromal tumours: a phase I study. *Lancet* 2001; 358:1421–1423.

23

Measurements of Endpoints in Phase I Drug Design

Toxicity versus Alternatives

Jerry M. Collins and *Merrill J. Egorin

*Laboratory of Clinical Pharmacology, Food and Drug Administration, Rockville, Maryland 20857;
and *Departments of Medicine and Pharmacology, University of Pittsburgh Cancer Institute,
Pittsburgh, Pennsylvania 15213*

The entry of a novel molecule into human beings for the first time is unquestionably an exciting event, yet this stage of drug development does not generally attract much attention. Some features of a phase I study are constant, but almost every investigator is inclined to reengineer a few design factors. Recent efforts to redesign the entire drug development process place additional scrutiny on phase I. Although the science generated via the discovery and development process can be dazzling, the "art" of phase I trials requires continual focus on safety and the need to acquire information that will facilitate subsequent evaluations of therapeutic potential.

We begin a first-in-human study not only with high expectations, but also with a large amount of preclinical data. How do we effectively use this prior information? For example, we would like to test the new drug for its mechanism of action, but how often do we know such information at an early stage, or even for drugs that we use everyday?

Most readers automatically associate "phase I" with first-in-human studies. More generally, phase I studies also occur throughout development to evaluate the influence of specific factors such as renal or hepatic impairment, drug–drug interactions, sex, race/ethnicity, food, and changes in dosage forms. Previously, all subjects in phase I studies of anticancer drugs were patients with cancer. Currently, when the toxicologic properties of the drug are suitable, healthy volunteers are being used in phase I studies for evaluation of the specific factors mentioned, as well as testing the feasibility of attaining target concentrations. There are occasional differences observed between volunteers and patients, but generally the results are similar.

The focus of this chapter is primarily on studies in patients with cancer, which is the population that permits an extension of our traditional goals toward studies that test hypotheses about mechanisms of drug actions and effects, that is, "proof-of-concept" studies. Although the primary goal of phase I studies is to evaluate safety in humans, there is always an element of therapeutic intent when patients are the subjects. Realistically, there is only a low probability of success in many settings, but our obligation is to maximize that chance and document any responses.

For drugs with a narrow therapeutic index, variability in the delivery of systemic exposure is always a key issue. Although variability in exposure has been encountered often in the development of intravenous therapy, we currently are facing a new set of challenges due to the emphasis upon oral delivery. Also, many drugs now have been developed for chronic daily use, compared to the previous model of dosing once every 3 or 4 weeks.

EFFICIENCY FACTORS: STARTING DOSE AND DOSE ESCALATION

Although determination of a safe dosing regimen must be the outcome of a phase I investigation, all parties involved in a phase I study have a desire for efficient determination of a dose and schedule that might optimize benefit to patients. A compelling humanitarian motivation underlies the participation of patients, investigators, and pharmaceutical sponsors. Of course, there are also various forms of self-interest. Individuals volunteer with the desire to gain whatever slim opportunity might be available in a desperate situation. No one's career or economic prospects are enhanced by lengthy phase I trials. Thus, a primary aim of improved phase I designs should be to move quickly toward bioactive doses.

Regardless of the details for phase I trial design, the two essential elements for a first-in-human study are the starting dose and the dose escalation scheme. The criteria for choosing a starting dose are somewhat dependent on the phase I trial endpoints. For the traditional determination of the maximum tolerated dose (MTD) in humans, the choice of starting dose will be based upon MTD in animal studies. If the goal is to reach a specific plasma concentration, then the reference values for starting the phase I study will be doses that produced the target concentration in animals. In all cases, the actual starting dose in humans would be reduced compared with the reference dose in animals, in order to provide a safety margin for interspecies differences in either kinetics, including metabolism or dynamics.

Selection of the starting dose is caught in a conflict between a desire for safety (leading to a cautious choice) versus an interest in efficiency. Efficiency has many dimensions, including the desire to provide therapeutic opportunity, and can stimulate a more aggressive choice of starting dose.

The same conflicts exist for the escalation scheme. Once the current dose level has been demonstrated to be safe, increasing the dose to the next higher level is clouded by uncertainty about the steepness of the dose-toxic response curve. The size of dose increase could be prespecified in the protocol, or it might be tied to feedback from ongoing evaluation of the endpoints.

Recently, there has been an appreciation of the linkage between choices for starting dose and escalation rate. In particular, the combination of a cautious starting dose with a very conservative escalation rate can lead to trials that are so lengthy that no one's interests are served.

Experience with the accelerated titration (1) and continual reassessment methods (2) for dose escalation have improved phase I trials in a number of important ways. It is particularly noteworthy that fewer patients are exposed to completely inactive doses because of two innovations: (i) reducing the cohort size at early stages from three patients to one; and (ii) encouraging intrapatient escalation of doses.

TOXICITY AS AN ENDPOINT

Although there are an increasing number of exceptions, the dominant emphasis for anticancer drugs has been placed upon defining the MTD as an endpoint of the phase I study. Because the therapeutic index for anticancer drugs is so narrow and because the disease is life threatening, the concept of MTD has played a central role in phase I studies of these drugs. For the types of anticancer agents that have been available for exploration, there has been little choice other than the MTD.

As we have moved into an era in which we have focused upon targets for which maximum effect might be reached below the level of an MTD and have used modulators that possess no intrinsic antitumor activity in themselves, we have sought alternative endpoints. Indeed, there are already several classes of molecules that have undergone clinical evaluation for which the MTD was not determined and/or not relevant to the drug's use.

Fortunately, there is ample precedent for alternatives to the MTD in areas outside oncology. Careful clinical monitoring for adverse events is always an essential element for first-in-human studies, regardless of the therapeutic discipline or the nominal endpoint of a phase I investigation. It also is recognized that there is considerable value in exploring doses above the target value during the first-in-human study (3). The controlled clinical setting of a phase I study provides the safest opportunity to determine when adverse experiences are likely and the nature of these events. The goal is not to push the dose to the MTD but to understand the safety margin of the doses selected for the initial set of follow-up studies of therapeutic activity.

As a practical matter, if subsequent studies of activity indicate that the desired target value is inadequate and suggest that higher doses would be helpful, then the supporting safety evaluation for higher doses would already be available without delay. Further, knowledge of the safety profile can guide the approach to accidental overdoses or a variety of circumstances equivalent to an overdose, including genetically based impairments in clearance pathways or drug–drug interactions.

BEYOND TOXICITY: WHEN TO STOP DOSE ESCALATION?

What is the impact of this new approach of alternative endpoints upon phase I designs? Specifically, what is the endpoint for dose escalation? As the MTD fades in importance, what replaces it? As shown in Figure 23.1,

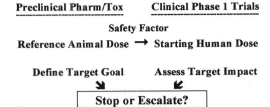

FIG. 23.1. Target-guided dose selection. The starting dose for phase I testing is determined as a fraction of a reference dose in animal toxicology studies. As an alternative to the fixed procedure for increasing doses, the decision to stop or escalate could be based on the impact on the target by the current drug dosage compared with target goals defined in preclinical studies.

the process for target-guided phase I investigations is rather straightforward. We might even give it a name: "target-guided dose selection." But how is the indicator target selected, and how is a value determined that would serve as a goal? In the following sections, we address the strengths and weaknesses of some specific approaches, but it is important to recognize upfront that there are some overall limitations. Schellens and Ratain (4) comment upon exposure targets, but their remarks should be appreciated more generally: "Desirable exposure levels in patients have to be based on preclinical pharmacokinetic and pharmacodynamic experiments, using artificial tumor models that poorly represent the biologic complexity of real life."

HOW DO WE SELECT THE TARGET AND ITS VALUE?

The most likely alternative endpoints are listed in Table 23.1. Determination of drug exposure (plasma concentration) has frequently been a secondary objective in phase I studies of anticancer drugs. In the majority of cases in which MTD has not been the primary endpoint, plasma concentration of drug has served as the alternative endpoint. A target concentration is defined from studies in vitro or in animals. Doses are escalated until plasma concentrations reach this target level. Plasma concentrations usually are reliable as a measure of extracellular drug delivery but

TABLE 23.1. *Candidate endpoints*

Concentration of drug in plasma
Concentration of drug in tumor
Impact on target in white blood cells
Impact on target in tumor
Noninvasive imaging

are completely uninformative about variations in the intrinsic sensitivity of the tumor to a particular drug.

For drugs that are highly bound to plasma proteins, an adjustment must be made so that comparisons are based upon unbound drug, as discussed later in this chapter. When the target concentration is defined by experiments *in vitro*, the concentration versus time profile in the incubation media must be checked to determine if adjustments are needed because of factors such as instability of the drug in culture or loss of drug due to binding to the incubation apparatus.

From time to time, it seems appealing to some investigators to obtain biopsies and analyze drug concentration within the tumor. Generally, such exercises do not yield any useful information unless they are part of an organized effort that obtains a sufficient number of samples for comparative evaluations. Of course, if the goal were to determine the effect of transport processes upon how much drug enters the tumor and how long it stays, then such a strategy would be sensible. When extensive nonspecific tissue binding occurs, the interpretation of concentration data is more difficult.

Circulating blood cells are highly accessible and frequently used as a source for cellular investigations. For leukemic cells, this strategy can provide a direct window to intracellular target events. In a study of fludarabine as a modulator of cytarabine, Gandhi et al. (5) reported that the optimal dose was lower than the MTD in leukemic patients.

Because of the inaccessibility of most solid tumors, some studies have examined normal peripheral white blood cells (WBCs) as a convenient source of material for biochemical or molecular evaluations. This strategy provides some qualitative indication of bioactivity, but it is catastrophic for cases in which WBC response is more sensitive than tumor response. In this worst case scenario, escalation of the drug is prematurely terminated, prior to achieving sufficient action at the tumor target. For example, Spiro et al. (6) reported that the average dose of O6-benzylguanine (O6-BG), which inactivates alkyltransferase, in WBC was substantially lower than that required for inactivation in tumors. Further, they did not find a direct relationship between alkyltransferase activity in WBC and tumors. Thus, WBCs certainly are convenient but not necessarily relevant as surrogates for tumors.

A major effort to utilize noninvasive imaging as a supplement or replacement for biopsies of tumors currently is underway. In the recent and ongoing phase I evaluations of antiangiogenic agents, dose escalation is being assisted via monitoring of blood flow/perfusion by both magnetic resonance imaging (MRI) and positron emission tomography (PET) (7,8).

PHASE I AS AN EXTENSION OF DISCOVERY PROCESS

As suggested in Table 23.2, monitoring of targets can provide information that links phase I back to the discovery stage or forward to the design of phase II trials. Indeed, if information can be obtained about the response of the target at various doses or concentrations, then we could consider initial human studies as a continuing extension and validation of the discovery process.

For "accessible" targets such as blood pressure or heart rate, monitoring of biomarkers is not a new concept for phase I investigations. Many highly relevant oncologic biomarkers are locked inside tumor tissue. Although the study of Spiro et al. (6) demonstrated the payoff from systematically obtaining biopsies, the overall success rate of such a strategy has been inadequate for most drug development programs.

The techniques of noninvasive imaging are just beginning to be utilized to permit real-time monitoring of oncologic targets that previously were considered to be inaccessible, such as various regions of the human brain in situ. The precedents established in the development of neuropharmacologic agents, where imaging studies during initial trials have played a key role (9), can give us the confidence to proceed further in application of imaging techniques to the development of anticancer drugs (10).

TABLE 23.2. *Information desired from target monitoring*

- Does treatment effect change at the desired target? (Discovery)
- What is the dose-concentration-response curve at the target? (phase II design)
- What is the duration of effect at the target? (phase II design)

It is encouraging to note the example of $[^{18}F]$-fluorodeoxyglucose (FDG) as a PET probe in patients with gastrointestinal stromal tumors (GIST) who are treated with imatinib (Gleevec^{TM}; ST-571). The PET imaging results quickly and consistently predicted positive or negative outcomes before conventional measures of response were able to find changes. As illustrated in Figure 23.2 and summarized by Demetri et al. (11): "In all patients with a response, the $[^{18}F]$-FDG uptake in the tumor had decreased markedly from base line as early as 24 hours after a single dose of imatinib. Increases in tumor-related glycolytic activity, activity at new sites, or both were seen in all patients with disease progression. PET results correlated with subsequent evidence of a response or progression on CT [computed tomography] or MRI.

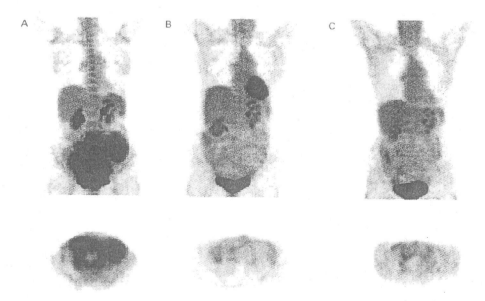

FIG. 23.2. Reduction of ^{18}F-fluorodeoxyglucose (FDG) uptake in gastrointestinal stromal tumor during imatinib therapy. **A:** Pretreatment uptake. **B:** Uptake after 1 month of therapy. **C:** Uptake after 16 months of continuous therapy. (Adapted from Demetri GD, von Mehren M, Blanke CD, et al. Efficacy and safety of imatinib mesylate in advanced gastrointestinal stromal tumors. *N Engl J Med* 2002;347:472–480, with permission.)

On the other hand, it is a discouraging that $[^{18}F]$-FDG is the only probe of tumor status that is widely available. It is relatively nonspecific in that it is a global indicator of tumor metabolic rate. Probes for imaging that intend to monitor processes across the full spectrum of targets, both as broad indicators of tumor function (such as FDG) and at the level of specific enzymes or transporters, are under development. The set of new approaches to PET imaging includes probes for deoxyribonucleic acid (DNA) synthesis as an index of proliferation (e.g., 3′-fluoro-thymidine), hormone receptors (e.g., $[^{18}F]$-fluoroestradiol), enzyme inhibition, amino acid uptake, and various approaches to evaluate drug transporters in context of multidrug resistance (10).

Regardless of whether our assessment tools are invasive biopsies or noninvasive imaging techniques, we want to know if the drug has an impact on the desired target. The evaluation can be very broad or very specific. If inhibition of an enzyme is the presumed mechanism of action, then we want to know residual activity and/or percentage inhibition by the drug. If our goal is to study a multifactorial process such as proliferation or apoptosis, then we either focus upon the step that we desire to effect or evaluate the overall impact on the process, that is, change in proliferation or apoptosis.

This type of utilization for these probes represents the extension of the discovery process into the clinic. If we cannot monitor the effect of the drug on the tumor, then we resort to conventional empirical development if development is continued.

SHIFTING THE BOUNDARY BETWEEN PHASE I AND PHASE II

Determination of safety will always be a necessary part of phase I trials, and work should continue on fine tuning the efficiency of attaining this goal. However, the study of toxicity without consideration of antitumor activity is inherently unsatisfying. As it becomes more common to seek proof-of-concept or mechanistic evaluations during phase I, an increased emphasis on demonstrating therapeutic activity, the usual domain for phase II study, looms on the horizon.

By monitoring a target biomarker, both proof-of-concept and dose determination might be achieved simultaneously. Further, by enrolling in the trial patients who have favorable expression profiles of the target, an "enriched" population is obtained that has a higher likelihood of response if the therapeutic concept has merit. This blurring of the traditional lines of demarcation between clinical phases of drug development has its pitfalls and disorienting aspects, but

also it presents exciting new opportunities for all stakeholders in drug development.

Once we have a tool to assess drug effect, we can explore the last two questions in Table 23.2. From the viewpoint of drug delivery, the two most important specifications for a phase II protocol design are the dose (or series of doses) and the dosing interval. The range of doses investigated during a phase I trial provides a superb opportunity to define dose-response relationships, for example, for extent of inhibition of target enzyme activity. The time course of recovery of enzyme activity provides an indication of the length of duration of effect at the target and can guide selection of a practical frequency of dosing.

For most phase I studies of anticancer drugs, the population has included any patient with cancer without proven therapeutic alternatives. Of course, there have always been isolated trends to extrapolate activity profiles from preclinical data and to conduct disease-specific studies, with a blurring of phase I and phase II goals. There are some pitfalls to this approach, but this trend can only be expected to accelerate. By monitoring the target, both proof-of-concept and dose determination might be achieved simultaneously.

Once again, we turn to imatinib as a prototype for specialized first-in-human trials. Due to the distinctive staging criteria in the chronic myelogenous leukemia trial (12), patients in this phase I study were even more homogeneous than most phase II populations. Because responses occurred at doses less than those associated with dose-limiting toxicity, the initial dose ranging could be driven by response rates instead of a search for the MTD. Because responses actually occurred, there is the additional issue of evaluating whether duration of response would be longer at higher doses, even if response rates were similar.

Most gratifying, nearly all patients in this study derived direct benefit. This trial had the substantial advantages of well-defined phenotypic and molecular targets, as well as convenient access to the leukemic cells for direct observation. The challenge for solid tumor trials is to find ways to translate targeting concepts into molecular and functional assays suitable for clinical application.

MONITORING PLASMA CONCENTRATION

Strategies for dose escalation are covered elsewhere in this book. Among the possibilities is the pharmacologically guided dose escalation (PGDE) scheme. In many ways, PGDE is a precursor to a more general target-guided dose selection, and we can learn from its successes and failures.

The PGDE design is based upon a straightforward hypothesis that there is a direct link between pharmacokinetics and drug effect. When comparing animal and human doses, expect equal toxicity for equal drug exposure (13). A fundamental principle of clinical pharmacology is that drug effects are caused by circulating concentrations of the unbound ("free") drug molecule and are less tightly linked to the administered dose.

Immediately after introduction of the PGDE design, there was an initial surge of trials that produced encouraging reports from Europe (14), Japan (15), and the United States (16). Over time, investigators became discouraged by the need to provide relatively rapid feedback from the laboratory to the clinic regarding assays of drug in plasma, and they turned to methods that did not require plasma concentrations, for example, those that relied upon statistical (continual reassessment method) and/or individual titration (empirical toxicity monitoring). Consequently, PGDE has failed to be widely accepted and has generally faded from regular use. Perhaps the lack of enthusiasm for real-time monitoring of a target concentration will also limit some uses of target-guided dose selection.

One legacy from the PGDE era is a comparison of limiting doses in humans versus mice (16). The doses used for this comparison were normalized for body surface area (e.g., 100 mg/m^2). (*Note:* Whereas contemporary analyses find no advantage to normalizing doses to body surface area in adult humans, it is quite helpful for cross-species comparisons.) There are two principal conclusions from an evaluation of these data, as shown in Figure 23.3: (i) There is enormous scatter in the ratio of human-to-murine tolerable doses. Thus, although murine doses may seem to give reasonable predictions for acceptable human doses on the average, there is no predictive consistency that could be relied upon for any specific drug about to enter phase I study. (ii) The drug exposure [area under the curve (AUC)] ratio at approximately equitoxic doses has much less variability, indicating that pharmacokinetic differences account for almost all of the differences observed for toxic doses between humans and mice.

As mentioned earlier, it is the unbound drug that is generally the pharmacologically active species. Therefore, when target concentrations are defined based upon plasma concentrations in animals or concentrations in media for cell culture, differences in binding between plasma of animals and humans, or between plasma in humans and culture media, need to be considered (17).

Strategies to modulate drug resistance are among the major applications of target concentrations. For this class of drugs, target concentrations usually are based upon reversal of resistance in cell culture systems that have relatively low amounts of binding capacity compared with plasma. Thus, stopping the dose escalation of the modulating agent at a target concentration, in the absence of toxicity, can be problematic. Alternatively, even if the modulating drug produces dose-limiting toxicity, monitoring of total drug concentrations in plasma can produce a false conclusion that drug delivery was adequate for further testing. Two examples follow.

A phase I study investigated the antibiotic novobiocin as a resistance reversal agent for the topoisomerase II agent etoposide (18,19). *In vitro* studies had demonstrated that novobiocin, at 100 μg/mL, reversed resistance to etoposide. Patients were administered doses of novobiocin that could achieve and

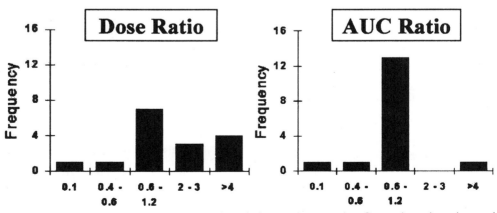

FIG. 23.3. Survey of acute toxicity of anticancer drugs in humans versus mice. Comparisons based upon dose **(left)** exhibit more scatter than those based on drug exposure (AUC) **(right).** (Adapted from Collins JM, Grieshaber CK, Chabner BA. Pharmacologically-guided Phase I trials based upon preclinical development. *J Natl Cancer Inst* 1990:82:1321–1326, with permission.)

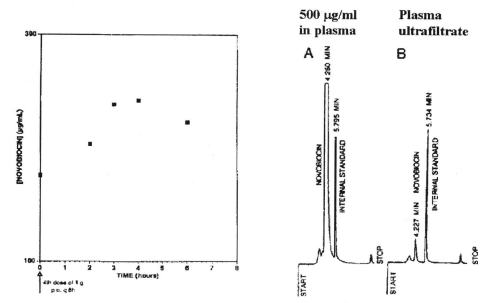

FIG. 23.4. Plasma concentrations of novobiocin in plasma from a patient who ingested 1 g novobiocin every 8 hours for 96 hours to reverse resistance to etoposide. The target concentration for novobiocin was 100 μg/mL. **Left:** The target was readily achieved for total drug concentration in plasma. **Right:** The unbound drug concentration failed to reach the target value. (Based on data from Zuhowski EG, Gutheil JC, Egorin MJ. Rapid and sensitive high-performance liquid chromatographic assay for novobiocin in human serum. *J Chromatogr B Biomed Appl* 1994;655:147–152.)

maintain plasma concentrations well in excess of the 100 μg/mL target (Fig. 23.4), yet there was no evidence of reversal of resistance to etoposide. One potential explanation for this finding and for why the study was discontinued was the fact that novobiocin was 99% protein bound in plasma but only 40% protein bound in tissue culture medium supplemented with fetal bovine serum. As a consequence, concentrations of active (unbound) novobiocin were 60 times greater in cell culture than in plasma containing similar total concentrations of novobiocin.

A similar set of events occurred with the investigation of megestrol acetate, a steroid hormone. A phase I study determined that, at doses of megestrol that were tolerable in combination with vinblastine, total megestrol concentrations were achieved and sustained at values sufficient to reverse resistance to vinblastine in cell culture (20). However, the maximum unbound concentrations of megestrol in plasma were 25-fold lower than in cell culture, and the authors concluded that reversal of resistance was unlikely because increasing the oral dose of megestrol failed to increase circulating plasma concentrations (saturable absorption).

It often is difficult to sort out the many reasons why a drug fails to act similarly in humans as in animal models. For equal doses, differences in plasma AUC

(drug exposure) values simply indicate differences in total body clearance. Renal elimination and metabolic elimination are the major contributors to total body clearance. Renal clearance tends to exhibit only small differences across species, whereas there are many examples of interspecies differences in metabolism. Furthermore, across many drug categories, metabolism is quantitatively more important than renal elimination. Therefore, more emphasis on interspecies differences in drug metabolism could improve phase I studies. We have tools that are not yet fully used in an optimal manner, especially metabolism data for interspecies differences and finding active and/or toxic metabolites. The next two sections provide specific examples of the impact of monitoring metabolism during early human studies.

INTERSPECIES DIFFERENCES IN DRUG METABOLISM

Gianni et al. (21) conducted a first-in-human study of the anthracycline iododeoxydoxorubicin (I-Dox). As shown in Table 23.3, at equitoxic doses, there was four-fold greater exposure to the parent drug in mice and 13-fold greater exposure to the hydroxylated metabolite (I-Dox-ol) in humans. Thus, there was a 50-fold difference in the relative AUC exposure ratios

TABLE 23.3. *Area under the curve values in plasma for iododeoxydoxorubicin (I-Dox) and its metabolite (I-Dox-ol) in mouse and human equitoxic doses*

Compound	Mouse (μM · h)	Human (μM · h)
I-Dox	5.0	0.3
I-Dox-ol	1.2	4.0

Data from Gianni L, Vigano L, Surbone A, et al. Pharmacology and clinical toxicity of 4'-1000-4'-deoxydoxorubicin: an example of successful application of pharmacokinetics to close escalation in Phase I trials. *J Natl Cancer Inst* 1990;82:469–477.

(metabolite-to-parent drug) for humans and mice. This extreme example of an interspecies difference in drug metabolism was comparable to studying one molecule (the parent) in mice and then (unintentionally) studying a different molecule (the metabolite) in humans. Because the metabolite I-Dox-ol has similar bioactivity to the parent, these exposure comparisons also reflect pharmacologic response.

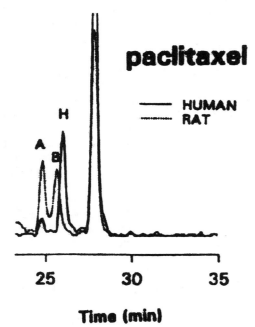

FIG. 23.5. Comparison of *in vitro* paclitaxel metabolism by hepatic microsomes from rats and humans. The major human metabolite, corresponding to the high-performance liquid chromatography peak ("H"), was not formed by rats. (Adapted from Jamis-Dow CA, Klecker RW, Katki AG, et al. Metabolism of Taxol by human and rat liver in vitro: a screen for drug interactions and interspecies differences. *Cancer Chemother Pharmacol* 1995;6:107–114, with permission.)

Whereas the difference in metabolite exposure was quantitative for I-Dox, Figure 23.5 illustrates a qualitative interspecies difference in paclitaxel metabolism (22). The principal metabolite formed in humans (peak "H", 6-α-hydroxy-paclitaxel) was not produced by rat microsomes. This example illustrates the potential of *in vitro* studies to discover interspecies differences in metabolism. In most cases, it is no longer necessary (and not advisable) to wait for *in vivo* phase I studies to discover such differences! It is important to note that this paclitaxel metabolite had less than 10% of the molar activity of the parent drug. Further, once clinical studies were underway, it could be shown that exposure to metabolite was far lower than to parent. Thus, overall, the parent paclitaxel dominates the bioactivity profile.

ACTIVE METABOLITES

The development of O6-BG has been mentioned with respect to determination of its impact at the target. It also provides an interesting example of the role of an active metabolite in prolonging pharmacologic effect. O6-BG itself is directly active, but it has a short half-life and modest exposure in the body, as shown in Figure 23.6. Thus, maintaining effective concentrations for more than a few hours would be difficult. However, Friedman et al. (23) demonstrated that 8-oxo-O6-BG, the active metabolite with similar potency to the parent molecule, not only achieves 18-fold greater exposure than the parent but also has greater persistence due to a longer half-life.

During first-in-human studies with the investigational anticancer drug penclomedine, it was found that exposure to parent drug concentrations was very brief (24). A metabolite, demethylpenclomedine, was discovered unexpectedly to have more than 100-fold greater exposure than the parent drug and to accumulate throughout the course of a 5-day treatment cycle (Fig. 23.7). Because the parent drug and its metabolite have about equal activity, any therapeutic benefit would be based upon the overwhelmingly higher metabolite exposure. On the other hand, the acute toxicity of the parent molecule limits not only its own direct exposure but also the amount of secondary exposure to the active metabolite. Thus, the penclomedine case clearly demonstrates the danger of not knowing which molecules are circulating in the body. If this type of information is determined early enough in drug development, the metabolite can be selected to replace the parent molecule as the lead development candidate.

The history of the contemporary antihistamine fexofenadine (Allegra[R]) is remarkably similar to that of demethylpenclomedine but has a much higher profile.

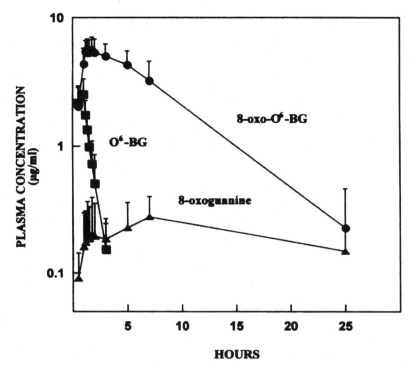

FIG. 23.6. Plasma profiles of O6-benzylguanine (O6-BG), its active metabolite 8-oxo-O6-BG, and an inactive metabolite 8-oxoguanine. (Adapted from Friedman HS, Pluda J, Quinn JA, et al. Phase I trial of carmustine plus O6-benzylguanine for patients with recurrent or progressive malignant glioma. *J Clin Oncol* 2000;18:3522–3528, with permission.)

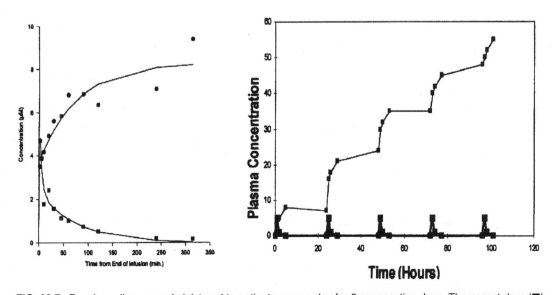

FIG. 23.7. Penclomedine was administered to patients once a day for 5 consecutive days. The parent drug (■) disappeared rapidly from plasma, whereas the demethyl metabolite (•) accumulated over the course of therapy. (Adapted from Hartman NR, O'Reilly S., Rowinsky EK, et al. Murine and human in vivo penclomedine metabolism. *Clin Cancer Res* 1996;2:953–962, with permission.)

Originally, terfenadine (Seldane^R) was marketed and was a highly successful product, but it subsequently was withdrawn from the market. In early clinical studies, it was not appreciated that the major source of clinical benefit was its metabolite fexofenadine. It became obvious that the metabolite should have been the lead compound only after cardiotoxicity subsequently was discovered for the parent drug but not the metabolite, and only under conditions in which the biotransformation was inhibited.

CONCLUDING COMMENTS

The price of a poorly designed phase I study is readily measured in terms such as excessive length, too many patients treated at homeopathic doses, or a dose recommendation for phase II study that is too high and disrupts further development while it is adjusted downward.

The hidden costs are harder to gauge. If the recommended phase II dose is too low, then the antitumor activity may be underestimated. There also are hidden costs if we fail to uncover substantial intersubject variability. As we move toward alternative phase I endpoints, our lack of experience is likely to produce some false-negative results as part of the price for more rapid discovery of the true positives.

We can envision the ideal phase I trial as a program that seeks answers to a series of increasingly detailed questions (Table 23.4). Our first priority is the assessment of drug delivery via the circulation to the tumor. If we have a target plasma concentration, it is obvious that we want to know if delivery is adequate. Even in the absence of a prespecified target concentration, information about systemic drug exposure will provide insight about variability in drug delivery within the population. In addition to our interest in the parent drug, this is the first opportunity to learn about the metabolite profile *in vivo*.

As we have learned more about various transport processes in tumors, we recognize that even with consistent systemic exposure there can be variations in the amount of drug uptake by tumors and retention of drug in adequate amounts for a sufficient duration of time. Thus, our next priority may be to assess drug in the tumor. Of course, as mentioned earlier, we need to keep in mind that there are difficulties in obtaining

TABLE 23.4. *Hierarchy of questions*

Does the drug
1. Circulate to tumor in adequate concentrations?
2. Accumulate in tumor adequately?
3. Have antitumor effect?

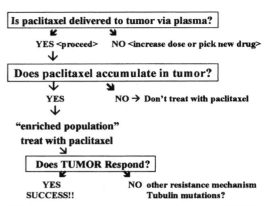

FIG. 23.8. Conceptual flowchart for target-guided drug development, using paclitaxel as an example.

and interpreting these drug accumulation data, either via biopsies or noninvasive imaging.

The final question (any antitumor effect?) jumps over the boundary that previously separated phase I from phase II. At this stage, we are not assessing the ultimate value of the drug, but we are trying to gain an early indication if the drug has the intended mechanism of action. If there are objective responses, we seek to link these outcomes to variation in drug action on the target.

Using paclitaxel as an example, Figure 23.8 provides a schematic approach to data collection and decision making in phase I investigations. At the time of paclitaxel's development, substantial efforts were invested in the first stage, monitoring of paclitaxel concentration in plasma (systemic drug exposure). Unfortunately, no specific target concentration was prospectively defined; thus, the data were observational and not suitable for decision making.

Due to concern about resistance of tumors to paclitaxel based upon overexpression of efflux pumps, the second question (does drug accumulate in tumor?) is highly relevant. If the technology had been in place, the drug accumulation may have provided some insight into the mechanism of successes and failures for individual patients or across tumor types. Ravert et al. (25) have reported that positron-labeled paclitaxel is feasible. This tool has arrived too late for drug development, but it may assist individual patient management. If successful, it would serve as a stimulus to give probe development a higher priority in earlier stages of development.

Fortunately, occasional antitumor responses were observed during phase I studies of paclitaxel. We did not have the tools to understand the mechanisms and therefore relied upon traditional phase II trials to determine an empirical profile of the types of tumors that responded, that is, breast and ovarian studies were positive; colon was negative. We need more experience with phase II studies that are stratified by molecular targets rather than by organ site, but obtaining the preliminary information during phase I studies should be part of the strategy.

Even with extensive preparation for a target-guided approach to phase I trials, there will always be some surprises. For paclitaxel, the interplay among doses, schedules, and toxicity profiles was not anticipated. The increased dose intensity of the weekly schedule was not associated with severe toxicity as would be predicted from toxicities linked with doses administered every 3 weeks. For the every-3-week schedule, the expression of toxicity shifts from neurotoxicity to myelosuppression to mucositis as the length of the infusion stretches from 3 hours to 24 hours to 96 hours. There has been no obvious therapeutic advantage to any particular duration of infusion.

Phase I trials often are not considered the most glamorous part of drug development. However, we have witnessed an exciting progression from empirical determination of dose-limiting toxicity to concentration-oriented designs to monitoring of molecular targets, and culminating in dramatic proof-of-concept for the imatinib trials in chronic myelogenous leukemia and GIST. We should not underestimate the amount of effort required to bring more of these examples to fruition. Nonetheless, in addition to our longstanding motivations for efficient phase I trials, we now are further stimulated by a spectacular demonstration of the rewards.

REFERENCES

1. Simon R, Freidlin B, Rubinstein L, et al. Accelerated titration designs for Phase I clinical trials in oncology. *J Natl Cancer Inst* 1997;89:1138–1147.
2. O'Quigley J, Pepe M, Fisher L. Continual reassessment method: a practical design for phase 1 clinical trials in cancer. *Biometrics* 1990;46:33–48.
3. Cutler NR, Sramek JJ. Investigator perspective on MTD: practical application of an MTD definition—has it accelerated development? *J Clin Pharmacol* 2000;40:1184.
4. Schellens JH, Ratain MJ. Endostatin: are the 2 years up yet? *J Clin Oncol* 2002;20:3758–3760.
5. Gandhi V, Estey E, Du M, et al. Minimum dose of fludarabine for the maximal modulation of 1-beta-D-arabinofuranosylcytosine triphosphate in human leukemia blasts during therapy. *Clin Cancer Res* 1997;3:1539–1545.
6. Spiro TP, Gerson SL, Liu L, et al. O6-benzylguanine: a clinical trial establishing the biochemical modulatory dose in tumor tissue for alkyltransferase-directed DNA repair. *Cancer Res* 1999;59:2402–2410.
7. Taylor JS, Tofts PS, Port R, et al. MR imaging of tumor microcirculation: promise for the new millennium. *J Magn Reson Imaging* 1999;10:903–907.
8. Libutti SK, Choyke P, Carrasquillo JA, et al. Monitoring responses to antiangiogenic agents using noninvasive imaging tests. *Cancer J Sci Am* 1999;5:252–256.
9. Fowler JS, Volkow ND, Wang G-J, et al. PET and drug research and development. *J Nucl Med* 1999;40:1154–1163.
10. Collins JM. PET and drug development. In: Wahl RL, ed. *Principles and practice of positron emission tomography*. Philadelphia: Lippincott, Williams & Wilkins, 2002;411–419.
11. Demetri GD, von Mehren M, Blanke CD, et al. Efficacy and safety of imatinib mesylate in advanced gastrointestinal stromal tumors. *N Engl J Med* 2002;347:472–480.
12. Vastag B. Leukemia drug heralds molecularly targeted era. *J Natl Cancer Inst* 2000;92:6–8.
13. Collins JM, Zaharko DS, Dedrick RL, et al. Potential roles for preclinical pharmacology in Phase I trials. *Cancer Treat Rep* 1986;70:73–80.
14. Newell DR. Pharmacologically based phase I trials in cancer chemotherapy. *Hematol Oncol Clin North Am* 1994;8:257–275.
15. Fuse E, Kobayashi S, Inaba M, et al. Application of pharmacokinetically guided dose escalation with respect to cell cycle phase specificity. *J Natl Cancer Inst* 1994;82:1321–1326.
16. Collins JM, Grieshaber CK, Chabner BA. Pharmacologically-guided Phase I trials based upon preclinical development. *J Natl Cancer Inst* 1990;82:1321–1326.
17. Collins JM, Klecker RW Jr. Highly-bound drugs: interspecies, intersubject, and related comparisons. *J Clin Pharmacol* 2002;42:971–975.
18. Murren JR, DiStasio SA, Lorico A, et al. Phase I and pharmacokinetic study of novobiocin in combination with VP-16 in patients with refractory malignancies. *Cancer J* 2000;6:256–265.
19. Zuhowski EG, Gutheil JC, Egorin MJ. Rapid and sensitive high-performance liquid chromatographic assay for novobiocin in human serum. *J Chromatogr B Biomed Appl* 1994;655:147–152.
20. Matin K, Egorin MJ, Ballesteros MF, et al. Phase I and pharmacokinetic study of vinblastine and high-dose megestrol acetate. *Cancer Chemother Pharmacol* 2002; 50:179–185.
21. Gianni L, Vigano L, Surbone A, et al. Pharmacology and clinical toxicity of 4'-iodo-4'-deoxydoxorubicin: an example of successful application of pharmacokinetics to dose escalation in Phase I trials. *J Natl Cancer Inst* 1990;82:469–477.
22. Jamis-Dow CA, Klecker RW, Katki AG, et al. Metabolism of Taxol by human and rat liver in vitro: a screen for drug interactions and interspecies differences. *Cancer Chemother Pharmacol* 1995;6:107–114.
23. Friedman HS, Pluda J, Quinn JA, et al. Phase I trial of carmustine plus O6-benzylguanine for patients with recurrent or progressive malignant glioma. *J Clin Oncol* 2000;18:3522–3528.
24. Hartman NR, O'Reilly S, Rowinsky EK, et al. Murine and human in vivo penclomedine metabolism. *Clin Cancer Res* 1996;2:953–962.
25. Ravert HT, Klecker RW Jr, Collins J, et al. Radiosynthesis of [11C]paclitaxel. *J Label Compounds Radiopharm* 2002;45:471–477.

24

Tumor Response Evaluation in Clinical Trials

RECIST

A. Dimitrios Colevas

Investigational Drug Branch, NCI/CTEP, Rockville, Maryland 20892

INTRODUCTION AND HISTORICAL PERSPECTIVE

Change in tumor size in response to a therapeutic intervention is a useful indicator of therapeutic benefit only if that change can be associated with a clinically relevant outcome, such as survival, cure, or change in quality of life. Tumor shrinkage per se should not be used to define the clinical utility of an anticancer therapy. Response assessment of an experimental intervention is properly used to determine whether further investigation of the intervention is warranted. In most cases, tumor response as a primary endpoint is only appropriate in early clinical trials. In definitive trials, tumor response should not be used as a primary endpoint as a surrogate for clinical benefit. Tumor response may aid patients and physicians in the overall benefit assessment of a particular anticancer intervention, but the distinction between use of response as part of an assessment of clinical benefit and that benefit assessment itself should not be blurred.

The definitions of response and progression for solid tumors historically have been expressed as the percentage change from baseline in tumor measurement. One must keep in mind, however, that the cutoffs chosen to distinguish partial response (PR) and disease progression (PD) from stable disease (SD) are arbitrary. Historically, definitions of complete response (CR) have been straightforward, as the absence of all evaluable disease is self-evident. Assessment of PD and PR is complicated by both arbitrary cutoffs and evaluation of individual lesions versus cumulative tumor bulk assessment. The percentage cutoffs chosen in the era before computerized tomography (CT) were largely based on investigators' impressions of what linear measurement changes represented unequivocal changes in tumor mass.

Traditionally, CR rates have been regarded the most important indication of effectiveness of chemotherapy, although PR rates are regarded as useful in the early clinical development of agents. The importance placed on response versus stabilization is historically linked to the era in which most therapies were cytotoxic. In the future, the paradigm of objective tumor shrinkage as a threshold necessary to move forward with oncology drug development may be rendered irrelevant as improved screening and diagnostic procedures allow for early detection of disease and cytostatic agents begin to populate the oncologists' armamentarium.

Clinical trials traditionally have reported CR and PR rates separately (1). The basis for stressing the relevance of CRs is the observation made in bacteria by Luria and Delbruck (2) in 1943 and subsequently applied to cancer cells by Goldie and Coldman (3) in 1979 that survival after exposure to a chemical or biologic agent was related to the spontaneous mutation rate of the organism rather than acquired resistance caused by exposure to a particular agent. Therefore, a reduction of tumor volume by 50% associated with the initial doses of an agent, although impressive in terms of physical or radiologic examination, would be associated with approximately one log cell kill. In terms of a clinically detectable tumor of 10^9 cells, a 50% reduction in volume would still leave at least 10^8 cells that would be inherently resistant to the agent for multiple spontaneous mutations occurring some time before or during exposure to the agent. For most human cancers, regrowth due to repopulation of a large number of resistant clones after chemotherapy-induced death of sensitive clones is sufficiently brief that it is difficult to demonstrate clinical benefit from a 50% reduction in tumor mass. Furthermore, it has been recognized for decades that precise and reproducible determination of responses defined by a decrease in tumor volume of less than 50% is virtually impossible (4).

Leukemia and lymphoma response assessments traditionally have been made using criteria significantly different than those used for solid tumors. Recently, response criteria for chronic lymphocytic leukemia, acute myeloid leukemia, Hodgkin disease, and non-Hodgkin lymphoma have been published (5–9). This chapter focuses on the evolution of response evaluation for solid tumors.

By the early 1970s, reporting of response data on oncology clinical trials, although not standardized globally, was moving in the direction of coalescent cooperative group guidelines for trials performed within any given group. A survey of criteria used by the Central Oncology Group (COG), Eastern Cooperative Oncology Group (ECOG), Southwest Oncology Group (SWOG), and Southeastern Cancer Study Group (SEG) during this era revealed that although response criteria across these organizations were similar, they were not identical (Table 24.1) (10). Investigators were concerned that these differences in tumor response assessment might explain, in part, the different response rates of identical regimens conducted at different centers. It was in this era that the standard of integration of the products of bidimensional measurement emerged.

By the late 1970s the clinical trialist community accepted the need for the development of one worldwide standard for evaluating and reporting outcomes from clinical trials. On the initiative of the World Health Organization (WHO), Committees on the Standardization of Reporting Results of Cancer Treatment (WHO criteria) were convened in 1977 and 1979 to codify a set of recommendations concerning reporting results of oncology clinical trials (11). This ecumenical effort included representatives from the European Organization for Research and Treatment of Cancer (EORTC), The United States National Cancer Institute (NCI), The International Union Against Cancer (UICC), and several national cooperative cancer groups. The WHO committee based their response criteria on guidelines proposed by the US Breast Cancer Task Force and those proposed for breast cancer by the UICC. The guidelines were meant to be minimal requirements that left investigators leeway to collect any additional data deemed relevant. The WHO criteria stipulated that evaluation of the disease should include description of the measurability of the disease, with lesions being described according to one of the following categories: measurable, bidimensional; measurable, unidimensional; or nonmeasurable but evaluable. Bidimensionally measurable lesions were to be measured by ruler or caliper using metric units,

by multiplying the longest diameter by the greatest perpendicular diameters. Although these criteria were developed prior to the advent of CT, they did address nonroentgenographic studies such life-size liver scans. Unidimensionally measurable disease included any lesion measurable by rulers or calipers and included mediastinal widening noted on chest x-ray film if subtracted from premorbid mediastinal width. Pelvic and abdominal masses and lymphangitic or confluent multinodular lung masses were considered nonmeasurable but evaluable, again largely a function of the pre-CT era of tumor assessment. Chemical and biologic markers were not to be used routinely to evaluate response unless specifically specified in individual protocols. For the most part, WHO criteria harmonized the response criteria systems that had evolved over the prior decade (Table 24.2). The WHO criteria included definitions for measurable disease and types of measurability, definition of response duration, how to measure lesions bidimensionally (longest axis, and then greatest perpendicular axis), and specification of how to integrate changes in multiple lesions to derive overall response. Still missing were criteria specifically outlining which lesion sites should be included and determination of extent of disease (number of lesions) to be evaluated for response assessment. The definition of measurability was vague and did not stipulate minimal size requirement for measurability, although many groups adopted a 1-cm minimum.

The WHO definition of PD of measurable disease has been debated, based on the reading of the original Miller paper (12). Whereas some have parsed the definition into three segments (PD1: 25% or greater increase in tumor area, PD2: 25% or greater increase in one lesion, PD3: appearance of a new lesion), most have reported PD using only the first and last of these criteria, ignoring the single lesion in favor of the summed change in area.

The WHO criteria were accepted for the next 2 decades as the world standard for solid tumor response assessment, with only intermittent minor variations introduced primarily to assist in response assessment of tumors in which a serum marker could be used to assess for antitumor activity prior to radiographic or physical examination changes, for example, α-fetoprotein and human chorionic gonadotropin levels in germ cell tumors and prostate-specific antigen in prostate cancer (13,14).

Technologic advancement was a major impetus to the reconsideration of response criteria for solid tumors in the 1980s and 1990s. In this era, response assessment shifted dramatically from primarily a clinical and conventional x-ray–based assessment to an

TABLE 24.1. *Response criteria for cooperative group trials circa 1970s*

Measured lesion response (4-week duration required in all groups)	COG	ECOG	SWOG	SEG
CR (complete response)	Complete disappearance of all objective evidence of tumor	Complete disappearance of all lesions and recalcification of skeletal lesions	Disappearance of all clinical evidence of active tumor; reossification of lytic lesions; absence of pain	No evidence of disease except for persistence of bone defects
PR (partial response)	≥50% decrease in the sum of the product of the diameters	≥50% decrease in the product of the largest diameters and/or partial reossification of lytic lesions	≥50% decrease in the sum of the products of the diameters; improvement in the skeleton; hypercalcemia controlled without aid	Good: ≥50% decrease in both diameters of all measured lesions or ≥75% reduction in the sum of the products. Fair: ≥25% decrease in both diameters of all measured lesions or ≥50% reduction in the sum of the products. Lytic lesions assymptomatic; do not increase in size
IMP (improvement)			Some reduction but <50%; disappearance or steady state of skeletal lesions on roentgenogram	
NC (no change)	Increase or decrease, 50% in sum of products or diameters	Decrease of <50% or increase <25% in sum of products of diameters; stable osseous lesions	Failure to improve with no obvious progression	Improvement in symptoms; lesions stable or with growth arrested after initiating therapy
PROG (progression)	50% increase in sum of products of diameters; new lesion size	25% increase over original measurements of product of diameters; new lesions; progression of osteolytic lesions	50% increase of any measured lesion; new lesion; uncontrolled hypercalemia and/or clearly progressive skeletal involvement	25% increase in the product of diameters of any lesion; new lesion

(continued)

TABLE 24.1. *Continued*

Measured lesion response (4-week duration required in all groups)	COG	ECOG	SWOG	SEG
Progression after a response	Increase in the sum of the products over the minimal size, which represents 25% return to original size; new lesion	50% increase in product of diameters over minimal size; new lesion	50% increase in product of diameters of any measured lesion from minimal size; new lesion; reappearance of lesion after a CR; hypercalcemia; new or progressive skeletal involvement; abnormal clinical or laboratory observations secondary to disease	Any existing tumor progresses or new lesion appears
Response duration				
PR	Time of 50% decrease to relapse	Time of 50% decrease to relapse	Time of 50% decrease to relapse	Time of response to relapse
CR	Time of NED to relapse	Includes time in PR	Includes time in PR	Includes time in PR

Reprinted from Davis HL Jr, Multhauf P, Klotz J. Comparisons of Cooperative Group evaluation criteria for multiple-drug therapy for breast cancer. *Cancer Treat Rep* 1980;64:507–517, with permission.

ultrasound-, CT-, or magnetic resonance imaging (MRI)-based assessment. For example, assessment of hepatomegaly by clinical examination was replaced by CT imaging of the liver, rendering response rates based upon the former obsolete (4). These new technologies permitted much more quantifiable and verifiable assessments. For the first time, true volumetric assessment became a reality rather than an estimate based on extrapolation from unidimensional or bidimensional assessments. The ease with which response assessments could be reviewed, however, led to the realization that despite the use of more precise tools, wide variability in response rates for the same or similar therapies continued to be reported.

Comparisons of assessments using newer imaging modalities demonstrated nearly as wide a variability as had been reported in the literature historically (15,16). What emerged was recognition that the method of evaluation of the image was as important as the choice of imaging modality. Associations among evaluation intervals, response rates, and durations of remission became transparent with the availability of easily reviewed imaging data. The variance in re-

sponse interpretation as a function of lesion size also emerged as a significant issue, especially when defining PD, where the difference from baseline necessary to define a change was only 25% when there is a one in four chance of erroneously reporting PD (17).

A second impetus to the development of new response criteria was the realization that what and how lesions should be used to evaluate responses had not been adequately delineated. What was considered measurable versus nonmeasurable was not applied consistently; therefore, the definition of evaluable lesion varied substantially. Minimum size for evaluation and extent of evaluation (how many lesions should be evaluated in any one subject) had not been defined. Some groups defined PD according to a change in any one lesion, whereas others used a more integrated approach in an attempt to consider the overall tumor bulk as the primary determinant of PD.

With the emergence of the ability to image and measure tumors in two and three dimensions, investigators realized that this added information came with an increased burden of labor. Several groups set themselves to the task of comparison of unidimensional, bidimensional, and volumetric assessments tumor response. If we accept the premise that an antitumor agent kills a fixed proportion of cancer cells (2,3), then the absolute number of cancer cells killed by a therapy depends upon the number, and therefore the mass, of cells at the time of exposure to the therapy. In other words, the effectiveness of an anticancer therapy is proportional to the log of the number of cells killed and, therefore, is proportional to the reduction in tumor volume. In the case of a relatively spherical tumor, this tumor volume can easily be related to either unidimensional or bidimensional tumor measurements, as shown in Fig. 24.1 (18). Additionally, perpendicular diameters of a tumor mass are not independent variables with respect to response to therapy. Intuitively one can see that if a fixed number of tumor cells in a tumor mass are destroyed by an anticancer agent, then there is no reason to assume that the resultant loss of volume would be polarized, that is, that there would be a greater proportional shrinkage along one axis versus another. Additionally, it has been known for decades that there is a high degree of correlation between the length of a tumor's maximum diameter and the greatest perpendicular diameter, and that the diameter is a poor estimate of tumor volume only when the tumor's length is greater than twice its width (19–21).

TABLE 24.2. *World Health Organization response evaluation guideline*

Type of lesion	CR (complete response)	PR (partial response)	NC (no change)	PD (progressive disease)
Measurable Bidimensional (BD)	Disappearance of all known disease determined by two observations not less than 4 weeks apart	BD: ≥50% decrease in the sum of the products of the perpendicular diameters of the lesions	Neither a 50% decrease as defined in PR nor 25% increase as defined in PD in one or more measurable lesions	BD: ≥25% increase in the sum of the products of the perpendicular diameters of the lesions
Unidimensional (UD)		UD: ≥50% decrease in linear tumor measurement *and* no appearance of new lesions, no progression of any one lesion		UD: ≥25% increase in linear tumor measurement *or* appearance of any new lesion
Nonmeasurable	Complete disappearance of all known disease for at least 4 weeks	Estimated decrease in tumor size of ≥50% for at least 4 weeks	Estimated change in tumor to be neither a 50% decrease as defined in PR nor 25% increase as defined in PD in one or more measurable lesions	Estimated ≥25% increase in tumor measurement *or* appearance of new lesions
Bone metastases	Complete disappearance of all lesions on x-ray film or scan for at least 4 weeks	Partial decrease in size of lytic lesions; recalcification of lytic lesions; decreased density of blastic lesions for at least 4 weeks.	No change sufficient to define PR or PD; must be applied only after at least 8 weeks on therapy	Inrease in size to existent lesions *or* appearance of new lesions
Overall response	Progression at any site denotes disease progression, despite responses at other sites. All sites must achieve CR for overall CR assignment. There must be greater number of sites assigned either PR or CR than NC to merit overall PR assignment.			

Constructed from data in Miller A, Hoogstraten B, Staquet M, et al. Reporting results of cancer treatment. *Cancer* 1981;47:207–214, with permission.

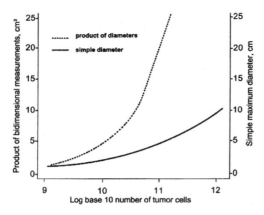

FIG. 24.1. Relationships between change in the number of tumor cells in a spherical tumor and simple maximum diameter and bidimensional product measurements. (From James K, Eisenhauer E, Christian M, et al. Measuring response in solid tumors: unidimensional versus bidimensional measurement. *J Natl Cancer Inst* 1999;91:523–528, with permission.)

RESPONSE EVALUATION CRITERIA IN SOLID TUMORS (RECIST) CRITERIA

The EORTC, NCI, and National Cancer Institute of Canada Clinical Trials Group (NCIC) established the Response Evaluation Criteria In Solid Tumors (RECIST) working group in 1994 to review the various existent criteria for solid tumor treatment response evaluation. A task force drafted a new set of criteria, known as the RECIST criteria, modeled largely on the WHO criteria. The drafts of the RECIST criteria underwent several iterations, and the effort resulted in a final draft presented at a consensus meeting in 1998 that included representatives from academia, governmental research, the pharmaceutical industry, and regulatory authorities. These guidelines were first presented to the oncology community at the 1999 annual meeting of the American Society for Clinical Oncology and published in the *Journal of the National Cancer institute* in February 2000 (22). A quick reference to the RECIST is available on-line at *http://ctep.info.nih.gov/guidelines/recist.html*. A web-based forum for addressing questions to the members of the RECIST working party is available at *http://www.eortc.be/recist/*.

Baseline Evaluation

RECIST codifies the WHO terms "measurable" and "nonmeasurable" to describe all tumor lesions, explicitly recommending avoidance of the term "evaluable." Any lesion accurately measurable as 20 mm or greater in at least one dimension by conventional techniques, including physical examination, chest x-ray film, MRI, or conventional CT, and 10 mm or greater by spiral CT is measurable. All smaller lesions; lesions that

TABLE 24.3. *RECIST measurement specifications*

Measurement modality	Requirements	Notes
Physical examination	20-mm minimum	Measurable by ruler or caliper
Chest radiograph	20-mm minimum	
Conventional computed tomography	20-mm minimum	Two contiguous 10-mm slices
Spiral computed tomography	10-mm minimum	Two contiguous 5-mm reconstructions
Magnetic resonance imaging	20-mm minimum	
Ultrasound/endoscopy/laparoscopy	Discouraged	Subjective; irreproducible for independent review
Tumor markers	Not routine	Must be normal for CR
Pathology	Not routine	Rare utility in distinguishing PR from CR (e.g., germ cell tumor)
Metabolic scanning (e.g., positron emission tomography, technetium, bone scan)	Discouraged	False-positive scans common

CR, complete response; PR, partial response.
Based on data from Therasse P, Arbuck SG, Eisenhauer EA, et al. New guidelines to evaluate the response to treatment in solid tumors. European Organization for Research and Treatment of Cancer, National Cancer Institute of the United States, National Cancer Institute of Canada. *J Natl Cancer Inst* 2000;92:205–216, with permission.

are not accurately measurable using the techniques mentioned, including bone, leptomeningeal, pericardial, lymphangitic, and inflammatory breast lesions; ascites; and thoracic effusions are nonmeasurable (22).

Trials whose primary endpoint is response should be restricted to patients with at least one measurable lesion (Table 24.3). Lesions must be measured within 4 weeks before initiation of treatment, and subsequent lesion measurements are to be measured using the same modality and same technique. In the case of chest x-ray film, if the baseline examination is a posteroanterior projection, all subsequent chest x-ray films should use the same projection. In the case of CT, the window setting, reconstruction algorithm, slice volume, and use of contrast should be identical. In the case of MRI, the signal weight, contrast, and magnetic strength should be identical.

Every patient who enrolls in a trial whose primary endpoint is response should have prospectively defined baseline target lesions. Target lesions must be measurable and should be representative of all organ involvement. Target lesions are chosen based on their size and suitability for repeated diameter assessment. A maximum of five lesions per organ and a total of ten lesions should be identified as target lesions. All other lesions, measurable and not measurable, should be noted at baseline and at every subsequent response evaluation.

RECIST LESION RESPONSE CRITERIA

The RECIST tumor response criteria are reminiscent of the WHO criteria in that the overall response assessment is based on integration of both measurable and nonmeasurable lesion change. The major difference is that the RECIST criteria use a one-dimensional measurement of each of the target lesions to generate a sum diameter, whereas WHO uses the sum of the bidimensional product of each measurable lesion. According to RECIST, target lesions may be only a subset of all measurable lesions. If there are more than ten measurable lesions, some of them will necessarily be excluded from the rigorous quantitative assessment required for target lesion response. Additionally, the percentage change from baseline used to define PR or PD differs between WHO and RECIST criteria (Table 24.4). If one considers the volumetric difference resulting from a diameter change or an area (bidimensional product) change in an idealized tumor mass, the 30% change cutoff for RECIST and 50% cutoff for WHO PR criteria correspond to the same volume change, namely, 65% (23). However, the 20% increase in diameter (RECIST) does not correspond to the 25% area (WHO) cutoff for definition of PD (Table 24.5). The RECIST working group intentionally raised the threshold for PD definition in order to address the concerns of erroneously declaring a PD in the case of

TABLE 24.4. *Measurable lesion (WHO) and target lesion (RECIST) and nontarget lesion (RECIST) response criteria*

Response	WHO measurable lesions	RECIST target lesions	RECIST nontarget lesions
Complete response (CR)	Complete disappearance of all disease	Complete resolution of all target lesions	Disappearance of all lessions and normal tumor maker level
Partial response (PR)	At least 50% reduction in sum of product of the longest diameter and the greatest perpendicular diameter	At least 30% reduction in sum of longest diameters.	No criteria; cannot be coded as PR
No change or stable disease (SD)	Neither PR nor PD	Neither PR nor PD	Persistent lesion(s) or abnormal tumor marker
Progressive disease (PD)	>25% increase in sum of product of the longest diameter and the greatest perpendicular diameter or new lesion	>20% increase in sum of longest diameters	New lesion or unequivocal progression of existing lesion

TABLE 24.5. *Relationship between change in diameter, cross-sectional area, and volume of a tumor, assuming a uniform change in size*

	Diameter	Area	Volume
Response	Decrease	Decrease	Decrease
	30%	50%	65%
	50%	75%	87%
Progression	Increase	Increase	Increase
	12%	25%	40%
	20%	44%	73%
	25%	56%	95%
	30%	69%	120%

From Sohaib SA, Turner B, Hanson JA, et al. CT assessment of tumour response to treatment: comparison of linear, cross-sectional and volumetric measures of tumour size. *Br J Radiol* 2000;73: 1178–1184, with permission.

true SD while simultaneously addressing the concerns of waiting too long to declare PD (17,24).

RECIST and WHO differ considerably in terms of evaluation of nontarget and nonmeasurable lesions, respectively. As mentioned earlier, RECIST explicitly includes the possibility of measurable lesions in the nontarget category; therefore, reanalysis of response data captured according to WHO using the RECIST criteria is possible only if lesion-by-lesion data are available. Unlike WHO, RECIST does not attempt to define PRs for nontarget lesions. Instead, RECIST limits response assignment of nontarget lesions to only three categories. CR is the disappearance of all nontarget lesions and normalization of tumor markers. Incomplete response/stable disease is the persistence of any nontarget lesion or abnormal tumor marker level. PD is unequivocal progression of nontarget lesions or appearance of new lesions (22). The absence of the PR category in the RECIST criteria represents an attempt to remove the subjective component from the definition of PR (Table 24.6).

RECIST OVERALL RESPONSE CRITERIA

The overall response assessment made according to RECIST is weighted to assessment of the target lesions. Unlike the WHO criteria, the overall PR assessment in RECIST is primarily based on the quantitative assessment of target lesion response within the context of no overt progression of nontarget lesions. In theory this might increase the reported overall PR rate when using the RECIST criteria versus WHO, because diminution of nonmeasurable lesions is not a requirement in the former criteria in order to assess an overall PR. Weighting PR assessment on target lesions, however, would favor the reproducibility of PR rates when response assessments are reviewed and would tend to minimize the difference in PR assignment across trial sites as less weight is placed on subjective, nonquantifiable response assessment.

RECIST RESPONSE CONFIRMATION AND DURATION

Response confirmation by repeated imaging or clinical examination over time serves two purposes. First, it diminishes the random error associated with single measurements, just as measurements of multiple tumor masses at any one time diminish the contribution of any one erroneous measurement. These errors may result from the expected variability introduced when capturing images of smaller tumors when CT slice thickness

TABLE 24.6. *RECIST criteria for overall responses for all possible combinations of tumor responses in target and nontarget lesions with or without the appearance of new lesions*

Target lesions	Nontarget lesions	New lesions	Overall response
CR	CR	No	CR
CR	Incomplete response/SD	No	PR
PR	Non-PD	No	PR
SD	Non-PD	No	SD
PD	Any	Yes or no	PD
Any	PD	Yes or no	PD
Any	Any	Yes	PD

CR, complete response; PD, progressive disease; PR, partial response; SD, stable disease.
From Therasse P, Arbuck SG, Eisenhauer EA, et al. New guidelines to evaluate the response to treatment in solid tumors. European Organization for Research and Treatment of Cancer, National Cancer Institute of the United States, National Cancer Institute of Canada. *J Natl Cancer Inst* 2000;92;205–216, with permission.

is a significant fraction of the tumor mass diameter or may be the result of inaccurate measurement of a lesion on a radiographic film. Second, confirmation of response over a period of time adds clinical meaning to a response assignment. The duration of response may be more clinically relevant than the volumetric quantity of a response. The RECIST criteria specify that when reporting response data, a distinction must be made between confirmed and unconfirmed responses, and that repeat assessments for confirmation should be performed no less than 4 weeks apart, although individual protocols might specify longer intervals.

The duration of overall response is defined as the time between first documentation of a CR or PR and documentation of PD, taking as reference for PD the smallest tumor measurements recorded after initiation of the trial. For example, in the case of a patient whose tumor is assigned a CR, any detectable tumor subsequent to achievement of that CR would define PD for the purposes of overall response duration, even if the tumor bulk is less than baseline and would be assigned a PR relative to baseline. The duration of stable disease is measured beginning at the start of treatment until PD, taking as reference for PD definition the smallest measurements recorded after treatment initiation.

RECIST RESPONSE REVIEW AND RESULT REPORTING

Relevant experts not involved with the clinical trial should review all response data. Ideally this review should consist of review of primary research documentation, including the patients' files and unaltered radiographic images. It is probable that in the future, images will be electronically transmitted to independent data monitoring centers for review in order to render definitive independent response assessments. Such a centralized and standardized approach will reduce both random and systematic errors in response assessment, as well as facilitate the development of databases with which results of future subsequent trials may be compared.

The RECIST criteria specify that all study patients must be assessed for treatment response and assigned to one of the following categories: (i) CR, (ii) PR, (iii) SD, (iv) PD, (v) early death from malignant disease, (vi) early death from toxicity, (vii) early death from other cause, or (ix) unknown. All patients who meet the eligibility criteria should be assigned a treatment response, and all analyses and conclusions should be based on evaluation of data from all of these patients without regard to errors in treatment, patient withdrawal, and protocol violations. Intention-to-treat analysis protects against introduction of bias. Al-

though further analysis based on patient subsets may be performed, conclusions drawn from these analyses should be viewed as exploratory and potentially biased, and in general they should not be used to address the primary endpoint of a trial.

RECIST ANALYSES

The authors of the RECIST criteria retrospectively evaluated how closely the RECIST and WHO approaches to response assessment matched each other (22). Evaluation of data from 4,613 patients enrolled in 14 trials demonstrated congruence of both PR and CR rates using WHO and RECIST criteria. Evaluation of PD in a subset of 794 patients from six trials demonstrated a slight difference in PD rates, with PD occurring slightly more often in WHO analysis. Of the 8.1% of patients who had different dates of PD using the two criteria, the vast majority (7.3%) experienced earlier PD according to WHO criteria. Attempts to examine the extent of the time difference in PD were not possible using the data sets available.

Other groups have subsequently conducted similar comparisons of WHO versus RECIST criteria. A retrospective evaluation of breast cancer patients in Japan demonstrated that 30% of patients eligible for tumor response assessment according to a WHO variant were not eligible by the RECIST criteria and that there were some discrepancies in PR and CR rates, primarily based on the exclusion of small lesions and bone lesions in the RECIST analysis (25). Another retrospective study of 255 patients with gastric cancer demonstrated that a large number of patients enrolled in the trial using the WHO criteria would have no target lesions by RECIST criteria, 20% because they had only nonmeasurable lesions. Of the 171 WHO measurable lesions, only 51% were 20 mm or greater (26). Using a cutoff of 10 mm instead of 20 mm for the RECIST criteria, they found response rates according to the two criteria to be nearly identical. A French group retrospectively compared WHO and RECIST criteria in 91 patients undergoing treatment for metastatic colorectal cancer (12). In this patient population the response rate according to the common version of WHO (no PD2) was slightly lower than the rate according to RECIST (22% vs 28%), whereas the PD rates were virtually identical.

Although the comparative data between WHO and RECIST are limited and virtually all are retrospective, several observations seem to hold true. The 20-mm minimum size definition for target lesions according to RECIST excludes some patients who otherwise would have had measurable lesions by the WHO criteria. As expected, the liberal definition of PD according to RECIST often leads to a lower rate of PD than when WHO criteria are used. Overall, however, the two systems seem to be remarkably congruent with respect to response assignment.

SUMMARY

The RECIST criteria represent a refinement of the WHO criteria without deviating from the meaning and concepts of response and progression embodied in the WHO criteria. Major innovations of RECIST include the incorporation of summed one-dimensional tumor measurements, specification of target lesions by restriction to measurable lesions greater than 20 mm (10 mm for spiral CT), restriction of quantitation of tumor burden to no more than ten lesions, elimination of subjective assessment of nonmeasurable lesions for PR assessment, emphasis on quantitative values for overall response assessment, and emphasis on use of quantitative auditable imaging as the primary mode of response assessment.

The RECIST criteria are not a means by which the clinical utility of anticancer agents should be measured; therefore, we cannot ask that it be validated as a predictor of survival or quality-of-life improvement. The strength of RECIST is in the tool's rigorous circumscription of tumor response evaluation. RECIST was born in the era of precise solid tumor measurement championed by CT and antitumor therapy championed by cytotoxic agents. It is likely that as tools used to measure biologic activity and noncytotoxic anticancer agents move to the fore of oncology, another paradigm of antitumor activity evaluation will be needed to supplement these criteria.

REFERENCES

1. Chu E, DeVita VTJ. Principles of cancer management: chemotherapy. In: DeVita VTJ, Hellman S, Rosenberg S, eds. *Cancer: principles and practice of oncology,* 6th ed. Philadelphia: Lippincott, Williams & Wilkins, 2001: 293.
2. Luria S, Delbruck M. Mutations of bacteria form virus sensitivity to virus resistance. *Genetics* 1943;28:491–511.
3. Goldie JH, Coldman AJ. A mathematic model for relating the drug sensitivity of tumors to their spontaneous mutation rate. *Cancer Treat Rep* 1979;63:1727–1733.
4. Moertel CG, Hanley JA. The effect of measuring error on the results of therapeutic trials in advanced cancer. *Cancer* 1976;38:388–394.
5. Cheson BD, Horning SJ, Coiffier B, et al. Report of an international workshop to standardize response criteria for non-Hodgkin's lymphomas. NCI Sponsored International Working Group. *J Clin Oncol* 1999;17:1244.
6. Cheson BD, Cassileth PA, Head DR, et al. Report of the National Cancer Institute-sponsored workshop on definitions of diagnosis and response in acute myeloid leukemia. *J Clin Oncol* 1990;8:813–819.
7. Cheson BD, Bennett JM, Grever M, et al. National Cancer Institute-sponsored Working Group guidelines for chronic lymphocytic leukemia: revised guidelines for diagnosis and treatment. *Blood* 1996;87:4990–4997.
8. Cheson BD, Bennett JM, Kantarjian H, et al. Report of an international working group to standardize response criteria for myelodysplastic syndromes. *Blood* 2000;96: 3671–3674.
9. Lister TA, Crowther D, Sutcliffe SB, et al. Report of a committee convened to discuss the evaluation and staging of patients with Hodgkin's disease: Cotswolds meeting. *J Clin Oncol* 1989;7:1630–1636.
10. Davis HL Jr, Multhauf P, Klotz J. Comparisons of Cooperative Group evaluation criteria for multiple-drug therapy for breast cancer. *Cancer Treat Rep* 1980;64: 507–517.
11. Miller A, Hoogstraten B, Staquet M, et al. Reporting results of cancer treatment. *Cancer* 1981;47:207–214.
12. Trillet-Lenoir V, Freyer G, Kaemmerlen P, et al. Assessment of tumour response to chemotherapy for metastatic colorectal cancer: accuracy of the RECIST criteria. *Br J Radiol* 2002;75:903–908.
13. Rowland RG. Serum markers in testicular germ-cell neoplasms. *Hematol Oncol Clin North Am* 1988;2:485–489.
14. Bubley GJ, Carducci M, Dahut W, et al. Eligibility and response guidelines for phase II clinical trials in androgen-independent prostate cancer: recommendations from the Prostate-Specific Antigen Working Group. *J Clin Oncol* 1999;17:3461–3467.
15. Warr D, McKinney S, Tannock I. Influence of measurement error on assessment of response to anticancer chemotherapy: proposal for new criteria of tumor response. *J Clin Oncol* 1984;2:1040–1046.
16. Labianca R, Pancera G, Dallavalle G, et al. Response evaluation as the key-point in results interpretation. *Tumori* 1997;83[1 Suppl]:S73–S76.
17. Lavin PT, Flowerdew G. Studies in variation associated with the measurement of solid tumors. *Cancer* 1980; 46:1286–1290.
18. James K, Eisenhauer E, Christian M, et al. Measuring response in solid tumors: unidimensional versus bidimensional measurement. *J Natl Cancer Inst* 1999;91: 523–528.
19. Gurland J, Johnson RO. Case for using only maximum diameter in measuring tumors. *Cancer Chemother Rep* 1966;50:119–124.
20. Spears CP. Volume doubling approach to tumor measurement. *J Clin Oncol* 1985;3:1563.
21. Spears CP. Volume doubling measurement of spherical and ellipsoidal tumors. *Med Pediatr Oncol* 1984;12: 212–217.
22. Therasse P, Arbuck SG, Eisenhauer EA, et al. New guidelines to evaluate the response to treatment in solid tumors. European Organization for Research and Treatment of Cancer, National Cancer Institute of the United States, National Cancer Institute of Canada. *J Natl Cancer Inst* 2000;92:205–216.

23. Sohaib SA, Turner B, Hanson JA, et al. CT assessment of tumour response to treatment: comparison of linear, cross-sectional and volumetric measures of tumour size. *Br J Radiol* 2000;73:1178–1184.

24. Hilsenbeck SG, Von Hoff DD. RESPONSE: re: measure once or twice—does it really matter? *J Natl Cancer Inst* 1999;91:1780A–1781A.

25. Kimura M, Tominaga T. Outstanding problems with response evaluation criteria in solid tumors (RECIST) in breast cancer. *Breast Cancer* 2002;9:153–159.

26. Yoshida S, Miyata Y, Ohtsu A, et al. Significance of and problems in adopting response evaluation criteria in solid tumor RECIST for assessing anticancer effects of advanced gastric cancer. *Gastric Cancer* 2000;3:128– 133.

25

Pharmacogenetics and Cancer Chemotherapy

Hany Ezzeldin and Robert B. Diasio

Department of Pharmacology and Medicine, Division of Clinical Pharmacology, Comprehensive Cancer Center, University of Alabama at Birmingham, Birmingham, Alabama 35294

There is increasing evidence of the important role of genetics in determining drug response (both drug efficacy and drug toxicity) and particularly in accounting for the variability in drug response from individual to individual [1,2].

There is perhaps no class of therapeutic agents that is so dramatically affected by subtle genetic changes as the cancer chemotherapy agents [3]. The basis for this finding derives from the fact that these drugs are characterized by a relatively "narrow therapeutic window," with the difference between the mean therapeutic efficacious dose (ED_{50}) and the mean toxic dose (TD_{50}) being relatively slight. This is particularly true with the cytotoxic cancer chemotherapy drugs, which are inherently toxic to normal host cells, such that small changes in the level of drug or active metabolite can result in clinically obvious increased toxicity. Even slight changes in the structure of the genes responsible for critically important steps in metabolism of these drugs can result in alterations in how quickly the drug is metabolized, leading to increased levels of drug or metabolite, which in turn may result in toxicity greater than typically seen or possibly a difference in drug efficacy. The term *pharmacogenetics* has been used to describe the differences in drug response or toxicity that can result from an inherited trait where changes in the gene coding for a specific protein (e.g., a drug-metabolizing enzyme, transporter, or drug target) lead to major changes in the qualitative or quantitative function of that protein [1].

With sequencing of the human genome almost complete and function of the various genes now being clarified, there is increasing recognition of the considerable variability that may exist even at the level of the single nucleotide [4]. Increasingly, it may be possible to associate drug response information with these structural changes using newer, more rapid, sequencing methods. This has given rise to the relatively new discipline of pharmacogenomics [5], an area that is of major interest for the pharmaceutical industry and those interested in drug development [6].

In this chapter we review several specific examples of how genetic changes can alter the pharmacology of cancer chemotherapy agents, accounting for several of the more commonly recognized pharmacogenetic syndromes associated with cancer chemotherapy agents. In addition we highlight the potential role of pharmacogenomics in the future of cancer chemotherapy.

RECOGNIZING THE POSSIBILITY OF A PHARMACOGENETIC SYNDROME

What characteristics lead one to suspect a pharmacogenetic syndrome? Over the years they have changed as genetic methods have evolved. In the past the focus relied almost entirely on phenotypic observations at the clinical level. Typically this was limited to assessment of an individual patient's clinical response (efficacy) or toxicity to a drug compared to that of other individuals in the same population. In contrast, more recently there has been increasingly a genotypic focus. With near completion of the human genome sequence, today's emphasis has shifted to associating relatively easily detectable changes at the level of the deoxyribonucleic acid (DNA) sequence with both altered drug response and toxicity.

In actual fact, a combined (phenotypic and genotypic) approach is most useful when evaluating the possibility of a pharmacogenetic syndrome. Following is a list of several of the current methods that can be used to evaluate a pharmacogenetic syndrome [7].

Clinical Presentation

For cancer chemotherapy drugs, it typically has been the appearance of unexpected toxicity (during the initial clinical evaluation: history, physical examination, or routine laboratory tests) that is out of proportion to the administered drug dose that leads to suspicion of a pharmacogenetic syndrome (3). As noted earlier, this presentation typically is due to an alteration in the function of a critical drug-metabolizing enzyme with resultant disturbance in the levels of a drug characterized by a relatively low therapeutic index. Often the excess drug or metabolites may produce a clinical presentation with symptoms, signs, or laboratory tests suggestive of an overdose due to the presence of a relatively greater amount of drug (or metabolite).

Pharmacokinetics

One of the most important methods that traditionally has been used to confirm the suspected relationship between genetics and altered drug metabolism has been pharmacokinetics (2,7). Most commonly it is used to determine if the levels of drug or key metabolite(s) are elevated. This can be attempted initially by quantitating the levels of drug or key metabolite in plasma (serum), urine, or tissue. However, one may fail to detect the presence of elevated drug or metabolite levels if the plasma/serum, urine, or tissue samples are not appropriately timed in relation to when the drug was administered. A more useful approach is to administer a known dose of drug under controlled testing conditions, such that plasma/serum, urine, and/or tissue samples are collected and assessed over time for drug and potentially metabolite levels. One of the dangers of using this approach with cancer chemotherapy agents is that there is a potential risk of serious toxicity. Therefore, a test dose of drug may be utilized to lessen the safety risk. A particularly useful sensitive approach has been to administer a radioactive tracer dose of drug to permit not only accurate quantitation of drug but also quantitation of the various drug metabolites that may permit delineation of the actual step of drug metabolism that is altered (see next section). This approach has been used successfully in characterizing the pharmacologic consequences of dihydropyrimidine dehydrogenase (DPD) deficiency (8).

Identifying the Altered Step in Drug Metabolism

From a scientific perspective, it is of interest to know which step in drug metabolism is altered and therefore responsible for the altered drug or metabolite levels that cause the pharmacogenetic syndrome. The availability of drug and metabolite levels, together with pharmacokinetic data, can provide some insight into which site in the metabolic pathway is affected (a good example of this approach was used in the initial evaluation of DPD deficiency, see later) (8). Studies in animal models may provide guidance with regard to probing the metabolic pathway, as well provide a clue as to which tissue can be accessed for detecting the pharmacogenetic syndrome clinically (2). Subsequent clinical studies then can be undertaken. Although drug-metabolizing enzymes often are localized mainly in the liver, biopsy of this site is an invasive procedure that is best avoided if possible. Other potentially accessible tissues, such as peripheral blood mononuclear (PBM) cells or fibroblasts, may be useful for identifying which enzyme in the metabolism of the drug is altered, even if these tissues are not the primary site of drug metabolism. The available tissue then can be analyzed for enzyme activity, with enzyme kinetic analysis performed to provide insight into the biochemical basis of the enzyme deficiency, e.g., lower substrate affinity (increased K_m) or decreased maximal velocity (decreased V_{max}) (2) suggesting the possibility of a pharmacogenetic syndrome.

Family Studies (Pattern of Inheritance)

Although direct administration of a test dose of drug to family members often is used with drugs from other therapeutic classes, this approach cannot be justified ethically with cancer chemotherapy drugs in healthy noncancer patients because of the inherent risk of many of these drugs. Other phenotypic tests, such as assessment of drug-metabolizing enzyme activity or occasionally determination of the level of substrate for the enzyme in question, may be used in family members to clarify the pattern of inheritance.

Following identification and confirmation of the particular metabolic defect in the affected patient, studies can be undertaken in family members to determine the pattern of inheritance (2,7). This can provide insight on whether the defect is an autosomal or sex chromosomal inherited trait and whether there is a dominant, codominant, or recessive pattern of inheritance.

With elucidation of the human genome and functional assignment of enzyme activity to a particular gene, it is becoming possible at a relatively early point in pharmacogenetic investigations to conduct molecular studies in family members to unequivocally delineate the inheritance of a specific gene (4–6). Techniques that can unequivocally identify a specific sequence or mutation, such as allele-specific polymerase chain reaction (PCR)-based methods, should make this relatively easy to evaluate in the near future (9).

Population Studies

In the evaluation of a pharmacogenetic syndrome, it is important to assess the frequency of the altered trait within the general population. As with the family studies discussed earlier, this can utilize either phenotypic or genotypic tests. The frequency of individuals carrying a particular allele can be characterized using the Hardy-Weinberg equation to estimate the likely number of homozygous (both for the wild-type allele and the mutant allele) and heterozygous individuals in the general population (7). With the recent availability of the human genome sequence and more importantly the assignment of function to a particular gene (i.e., a specific protein or, in this case, a drug-metabolizing enzyme associated with a particular sequence) (4–6), it is more likely that we will increasingly utilize genotypic tests at an early point in the evaluation of a new pharmacogenetic syndrome. This should allow the collection of more accurate data not only on the frequency of homozygotes and heterozygotes of a particular allele but also on the identification of multiple alleles. The existence of multiple alleles associated with a pharmacogenetic syndrome now is recognized to be common (see examples following). Thus, it is useful in these early population studies to understand the relative frequency of the various alleles associated with the specific pharmacogenetic syndrome.

Following an assessment of phenotypic and genotypic markers in the general population, it may be useful to undertake surveys of the pharmacogenetic trait (phenotypic survey) or its associated alleles (genotypic survey) in specific populations. Thus, it may be of interest to survey populations with regard to race and ethnicity, as well as patients having specific types of cancer (10). Of particular relevance are studies of populations of patients being treated with a particular chemotherapy agent. This provides clinically useful information for determining the risk of the pharmacogenetic syndrome in the cancer patient population at risk.

Screening Tests

Ultimately the goal is to develop methods that can be used to screen individuals prior to the administration of chemotherapy to avoid the risk of a pharmacogenetic syndrome. This is particularly true for cancer chemotherapy, in which affected individuals may suffer life-threatening toxic consequences and in which the genetic abnormality is not a rare event. The availability of such screening tests should permit the physician to potentially modify the drug dose prior to administration and thus avoid the risk of toxicity. Ideally these tests should be user friendly, easy to perform, sensitive, specific, rapid, and inexpensive. Also important is the ability to perform these tests in easily accessible tissues, such as red blood cells (RBCs), plasma, or urine, as opposed to the need to perform an invasive procedure (e.g., tissue biopsy) that would be impractical for widespread use and would pose an unnecessary risk to the individual being tested. As noted earlier, both phenotypic and genotypic tests can be used for this purpose. With certain phenotypic tests, such as determination of substrate concentration (for a drug-metabolizing enzyme) or quantitation of enzymatic activity in which the factor being measured also is present normally, it is necessary to determine the "normal" distribution of these markers in a study using a large number of subjects (see previous section on Population Studies), after which a discrimination point (separating normal and abnormal individuals) can be determined (3,7). It should be noted that although genotypic tests are being used more frequently today, the diagnosis will be missed if the test for the specific allele responsible for the pharmacogenetic syndrome is not performed. Because many of the pharmacogenetic syndromes associated with cancer chemotherapy (see later) may be caused by more than one mutant allele, it becomes important to reconsider the use of functional (phenotypic) assays as part of the overall workup. This has led to frequent use of phenotypic and genotypic tests together in screening for pharmacogenetic syndromes.

PHARMACOGENETIC SYNDROMES IMPORTANT IN CANCER

Over the past several years there has been an increasing appreciation of the association of cancer chemotherapy with pharmacogenetics (3,11,12) and what is now known as pharmacogenomics (4). Several of the well-characterized pharmacogenetic syndromes recognized to be associated with several of the commonly used cancer chemotherapy agents are discussed in this chapter.

THIOPURINE METHYLTRANSFERASE DEFICIENCY

Introduction

Thiopurine methyltransferase (TPMT) deficiency was the first of the pharmacogenetic syndromes associated with cancer chemotherapy to be described at the clinical, pharmacokinetic, population, and genetic levels (13). Because the associated drugs 6-mercaptopurine (6-MP) and 6-thioguanine (6-TG) are used in a relatively small fraction of oncology patients essentially restricted to acute leukemias (14–16) and many of these subjects are pediatric patients with childhood acute lymphoblastic leukemia (14,15), there has been relatively limited appreciation of this pharmacogenetic syndrome by the adult medical oncology community until recently. In addition to affecting the antileukemic drugs 6-MP and 6-TG, TPMT deficiency can affect the 6-MP prodrug azathioprine (AZA), which is used in the management of systemic lupus erythematosus (SLE), rheumatoid arthritis, autoimmune hepatitis, and inflammatory bowel disease, in dermatologic conditions, and in solid organ transplant rejection (17,18).

Metabolic Regulation

Methylation is an important phase II metabolic reaction of many drugs and xenobiotics, including the thiopurine chemotherapeutic drugs (13). Thiopurine methyltransferase (also known as TPMT, thiopurine *S*-methyltransferase, EC 2.1.1.67) is one of several methyltransferases responsible for methylation, using *S*-adenosyl-L-methionine (Ado-Met) as the methyl group donor. The thiopurine drugs 6-MP, 6-TG, and AZA are metabolized, in part, by *S*-methylation catalyzed by the cytoplasmic *S*-adenosyl-L-methionine–dependent enzyme TPMT (19,20). Thiopurines are useful drugs, but unfortunately they have a relatively narrow therapeutic index and life-threatening toxicity, including occasional fatal myelosuppression, after administration of standard doses (13,14).

6-MP, 6-TG, and AZA are inactive prodrugs and require metabolism to thioguanine nucleotides (TGNs) in order to exert cytotoxicity (21–23). The transformation of inactive thiopurines to the active TGN metabolites involves multiple enzymes and is initiated by hypoxanthine guanine phosphoribosyltransferase (22). Alternatively, thiopurines can be inactivated via oxidation by xanthine oxidase or methylation by TPMT to the inactive thiouric acid or methylmercaptopurine, respectively (24,25). An alternative mechanism for cytotoxicity is achieved by the formation of a potent inhibitor of de novo purine synthesis via the *S*-methylation of 6-thioinosine 5′-monophosphate by TPMT (Fig. 25.1) (21,22,26). In hematopoietic tissues, xanthine oxidase is negligible, leaving TPMT as the only inactivation pathway (27). During the 1980s the steady increase in knowledge of the biochemistry and regulation of TPMT in human tissues was paralleled by an increasing understanding of the metabolism of thiopurine drugs. It was demonstrated that levels of TGNs measured in the erythrocytes correlated with both thiopurine therapeutic efficacy and toxicity, e.g., myelosuppression (28). However, the variable response of pa-

tients treated with standard doses of thiopurine drugs and their different RBC TGN concentrations was unexplained.

Importance of TPMT in Thiopurine Metabolism

TPMT is a catabolic enzyme important in the metabolism of the cancer chemotherapy drug 6-MP (16,21–26). Figure 25.1 shows the reaction catalyzed by TPMT, as well as its central position in the metabolism of thiopurine drugs. Although TPMT was one of the first enzymes associated with a pharmacogenetic presentation shown to be relevant to cancer chemotherapy, knowledge of the polymorphic nature of the enzyme did not come from an initial investigation of an unusual clinical presentation but from an investigation of the methylation reaction (25). Although obviously important in the metabolism of thiopurine drugs, its primary role in the metabolism of endogenous compounds remains unclear.

Clinical Presentation

The clinical presentation of TPMT deficiency is now well characterized (29–31). Patients who are completely deficient in TPMT activity typically present with evidence of severe hematologic toxicity, with leukopenia, thrombocytopenia, and anemia after exposure to any of the drugs metabolized by this enzyme. The leukopenia can be life threatening, with rare deaths reported when patients who were completely deficient in TPMT activity received a standard dose of thiopurine drug (32). Patients who are heterozygotes for the mutant TPMT alleles and have partial TPMT activity (between normal and completely deficient) typically have less toxicity.

In childhood acute lymphoblastic leukemia, the durations of treatment for homozygous wild-type and heterozygous patients do not differ. However, in one patient with a homozygous mutant TPMT genotype, the duration of maintenance treatment was reduced by 53% due to severe toxicity from 6-MP (17). In another study, a full dose of 6-MP was tolerated by heterozygous and homozygous wild-type patients for 65% and 84% weeks of therapy, respectively, for a period of 2.5 years of treatment, whereas two homozygous TPMT-deficient patients in the same study tolerated the full dose of 6-MP for only 7% of weeks. In wild-type, heterozygous, and homozygous mutant individuals, 6-MP dosage had to be decreased to prevent toxicity in 2, 16, and 76% weeks of treatment, respectively (33).

Furthermore, TPMT polymorphism has been implicated in other dramatic consequences of 6-MP

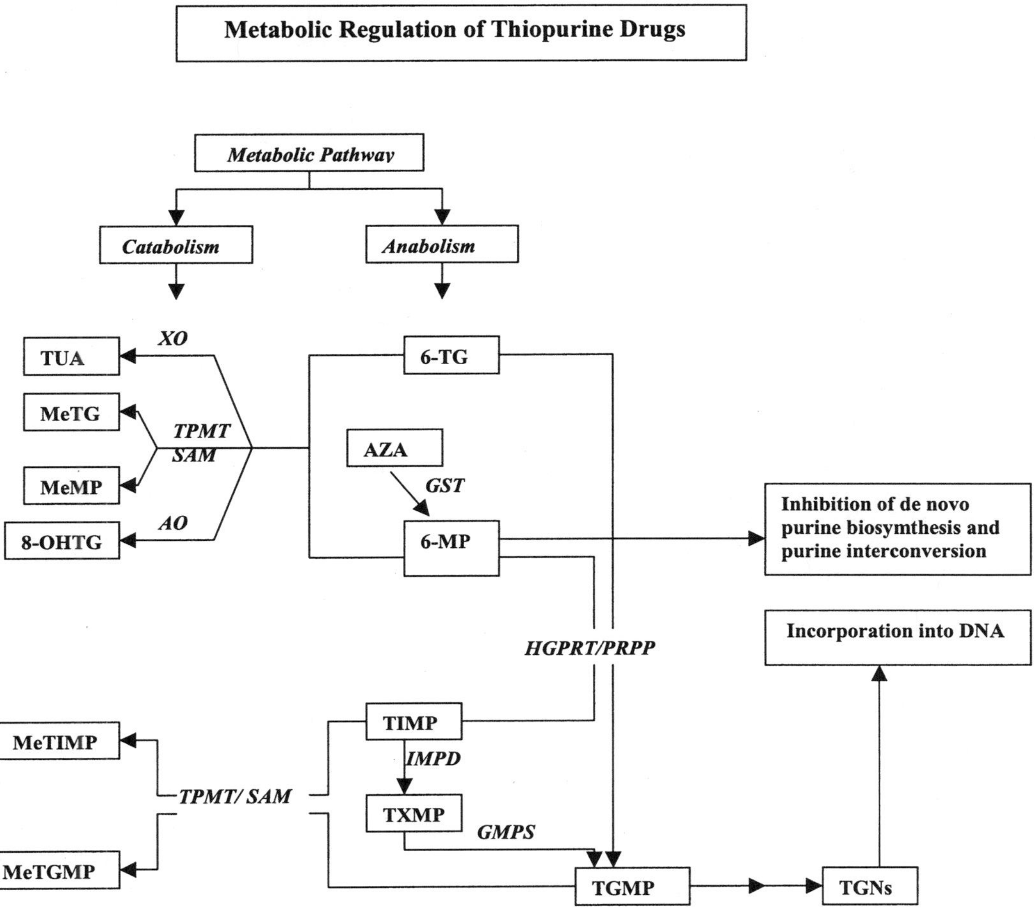

FIG. 25.1. Metabolic regulation of thiopurine drugs. The anabolic pathway leads to activation of thiopurine drugs by conversion into thioguanine nucleotides, which are incorporated into DNA. An alternative pathway is shown through the inhibition of purine biosynthesis by the active metabolite of thiopurine drugs. In the catabolic pathway, more drug is shunted toward the formation of methylated inactive metabolites by the enzyme thiopurine methyltransferase, which regulates the bioavailability of the active thioguanine nucleotides (TGNs) in target cells and thereby competes with the activation pathway. In addition, thiopurine drugs could be inactivated by xanthine oxidase into thiouric acid or transformed into 8-hydroxythioguanine by the enzyme aldehyde oxidase (AO). AZA, azathioprine; GMPS, guanosine monophosphate synthase; GST, glutathione-*S*-transferase; HGPRT, hypoxanthine guanine phosphoribosyltransferase; IMPD, inosine monophosphate dehydrogenase; MeMP, methylmercaptopurine; MeTG, methylthioguanine; MeTGMP, methylthioguanine monophosphate; MeTIMP, methylthioinosine monophosphate; 6-MP, 6-mercaptopurine; 8-OHTG, 8-hydroxythioguanine; PRPP, 5-phosphoribosyl-1-pyrophosphate; SAM, S-adenosine-L-methionine; 6-TG, 6-thioguanine; TGMP, thioguanosine monophosphate; TGNs, thioguanine nucleotides; TIMP, thioinosine monophosphate; TPMT, thiopurine methyltransferase; TUA, thiouric acid; TXMP, thioxanthine monophosphate; XO, xanthine oxidase.

therapy. It was reported that TPMT-deficient or heterozygous patients treated with topoisomerase inhibitors and thiopurines are at risk for developing secondary acute myeloid leukemia after treatment (34,35), and patients treated with 6-MP while receiving cranial irradiation are at higher risk for developing secondary brain tumors (36).

In 67 patients with rheumatic diseases (mostly rheumatoid arthritis), TPMT genotype identified patients who are at risk for toxicity after the administration of AZA (37). Five of six patients heterozygous for mutant TPMT alleles had to discontinue therapy after 1 month of starting treatment due to low leukocytic count. The sixth patient did not comply with AZA therapy (37). Patients with wild-type TPMT received therapy for a median of 39 weeks, whereas patients who were heterozygous for mutant TPMT alleles received therapy for a median of 2 weeks. Three Japanese patients with rheumatic disease and the mutant TPMT allele (TPMT*3C) (Table 25.1) discontinued AZA because of leukopenia (38), and four wild-type patients (12%) developed unexplained leukopenia (38).

In a multifactorial disease such as SLE, the detection of mutant TPMT genotype appeared to predict adverse effects after treatment with AZA. In 120 patients treated with AZA for SLE, mutant TPMT alleles were identified in seven patients (5.8%) (39). TPMT*3A homozygous genotype was identified in one patient who developed severe marrow aplasia; three patients with heterozygous mutations appeared to tolerate the medication. Five patients with wild-type TPMT alleles had unexplained leukopenia, suggesting that the TPMT genotype in SLE patients does not account for all cases of myelosuppression after administration of AZA (39).

It should be noted that individuals with high or high-normal TPMT activity may present with a clinical course suggesting that they are relatively resistant to 6-MP or 6-TG because a greater proportion of the drug is efficiently catabolized. These patients may fail to achieve a remission after antileukemia therapy with 6-MP or 6-TG (32). After demonstrating elevated TPMT activity in such patients, a decision can be made to treat these patients with an increased dose of 6-MP or 6-TG (40).

Diagnosing TPMT Deficiency

To investigate the underlying causes of individual variation in the pathway of thiopurine biotransformation and its possible correlation with individual differences in drug toxicity and/or therapeutic efficacy, in the early 1960s Remy (19) initiated studies on the TPMT enzyme that catalyzed the biotransformation of the inactive thiopurines to the active TGN in rodent tissue. Since then, methylation was reported to be a metabolic pathway for thiopurine drugs in humans (41), and attempts were made to assess the TPMT enzyme activity responsible for the methylation of thiopurine drugs. It was not until the

TABLE 25.1. *Variant alleles of the TPMT gene*

	TPMT allele	Exon	Nucleotide change reference	Amino acid change	Associated enzyme activity** (reference)	Expression of TPMT activity relative to wild type/(reference)
	TPMT*1	1–10	—	—	Normal	Normal
	TPMT*1S	7	T474C (74)	Silent mutations	Normal	
		5	C339T (74)			
1	TPMT*2	5	G238C (65)	80 Ala → Pro	Low (65)	>100-fold reduction (64)
2	TPMT*3A	7	G460A (68)	154 Ala → Thr	Low (68)	>200-fold reduction (64)
		10	A719G (68)	240 Tyr → Cys		
3	TPMT*3B	7	G460A (68)	154 Ala → Thr	Low (72)	Reduction (64,71)
4	TPMT*3C	10	A719G (68)	240 Tyr → Cys		
5	TPMT*3D	5	G292T (74)	96 Glu → Stop	Not measured	Not evaluated
		7	G460A (68)	154 Ala → Thr	Low (72)	Reduction
		10	A719G (68)	240 Tyr → Cys		
6	TPMT*4	i − 9	G>A (66, 70)	Intron/exon splice site	Low (74)	Not evaluated
7	TPMT*5	4	T146C (66)	49 Leu → Ser	Intermediate (66)	Not evaluated
8	TPMT*6	8	A539T (66)	180 Tyr → Phe	Intermediate (66)	Not evaluated
9	TPMT*7	10	T681G (69)	227 His → Glu	Intermediate (69)	Not evaluated
10	TPMT*8	10	G644A (73)	215 Arg → His	Intermediate (73)	Not evaluated
11	TPMT*1A	1 (O-ORF)	C(−178)T (74)	—	Intermediate (74)	Not evaluated
12	—	3 (O-ORF)	T(−30)A (74)	—	Intermediate (74)	Not evaluated
13	—	i − 3	T114A (74)	—	Intermediate (74)	Not evaluated
14	—	i − 3	A(−101)T (74)	—	Intermediate (74)	Not evaluated
15	—	i − 4	T35C (74)	—	Intermediate (74)	Not evaluated
16	—	i − 4	G98T (74)	—	Intermediate (74)	Not evaluated
17	—	i − 5	C58T (74)	—	Intermediate (74)	Not evaluated

*O-ORF, sequence in exons outside open reading frame.
**Based on analysis data from healthy blood donors (81,82); <2 nmol 6-methylthioguanine/g Hb/h = deficient; 2-23.5 nmol 6-methylthioguanine/g Hb/h= intermediate; >23.5 nmol 6-methylthioguanine/g Hb/h= wild type), i, intron.

late 1970s, however, that TPMT activity was first assayed and studied in human tissue (RBC) (42). Use of RBC, which is an easily accessible tissue, made it possible to develop a clinical test that demonstrated a correlation between RBC TPMT activity and enzyme activity at sites of thiopurine metabolism, such as the liver, kidney, and lymphocytes, in large population samples (24,43–45). Those extensive studies led to a steady increase in the understanding of the biotransformation of thiopurine drugs in humans and demonstrated that thiopurines undergo metabolic activation to 6-thioguanine nucleotides (6-TGNs) (23). Levels of 6-TGNs measured in the RBC were correlated with both thiopurine therapeutic efficacy and toxicity (e.g., myelosuppression) (28).

Interestingly, studies indicated that patients with very high TPMT activity displayed decreased therapeutic efficacy after administration of standard doses of thiopurine drugs. The possibility that the level of TPMT activity was increased during chronic drug therapy was considered because the level of RBC enzyme activity decreased by 25% after termination of drug treatment. This suggests that enzyme activity was increased during chronic therapy (40). Furthermore, clinical studies have confirmed repeatedly the association of very low TPMT activity with thiopurine toxicity (46). This was confirmed by studies indicating that high TPMT activity inactivates more drug via the methylation pathway, decreasing the bioavailability of cytotoxic TGNs (21,22). Conversely, high TGN concentrations have been detected in the tissues of TPMT-deficient patients, including RBCs (29,47), after administration of thiopurine drugs. Thus, the accumulation of knowledge about thiopurine clinical pharmacology indicated that the higher the level of TPMT activity, the lower the 6-TGN levels in the RBCs. There must be an additional factor that is responsible for individual variations in 6-TGN concentrations. The unexplained variations in individual response (life-threatening thiopurine toxicity) after the administration of standard doses of thiopurine have been attributed to a defective level of TPMT activity (31,40,48). These earlier studies led to the introduction of TPMT enzyme activity assay as a standard clinical test at some referral centers (49), thus representing one of the first pharmacogenetic tests performed in clinical practice.

Pharmacologic Consequences of TPMT Inhibition

The alteration in TPMT activity can have profound effects in patients given 6-MP. If TPMT activity is relatively low, then more 6-MP theoretically is available.

However, pharmacokinetic studies have demonstrated that this may not be reflected in plasma concentrations (50). A much better assessment can be made by quantitating RBC TGN concentrations, which are predictive of toxicity when relatively elevated. At the same time it has been suggested that if decreased 6-TGN concentrations may predict failure to respond and could provide the rationale for increasing the dose of 6-MP to individualize therapy (51).

Drug Interactions

Clinically significant drug interactions were discovered during the biochemical characterization of TPMT, where benzoic acid derivatives such as salicylic acid were found to be potent inhibitors of the TPMT enzyme (52,53). Such drug interaction could have a major impact on thiopurine toxicity and/or therapeutic efficacy. Drug interaction may account for some of the observed individual variations in response after the administration of standard doses of thiopurine drugs (54) by potentially altering the enzyme phenotype. Interactions were documented between thiopurines and TPMT inhibitors such as the aminosalicylic acid derivatives (used to treat inflammatory bowel disease) (55,56), and sulfasalazine and other aminosalicylic acid derivatives have been shown to be potent *in vitro* inhibitors of recombinant human TPMT (57).

Clinical Management

For patients with low TPMT who were not screened and received a standard dose of thiopurine for leukemic therapy, the most reasonable management approach is aggressive supportive care with management of anemia, bleeding, and particularly infection.

As noted earlier, patients who are found on testing to have TPMT levels above the normal range may be considered for a higher dose of 6-MP to ensure effective control of leukemia.

Molecular Basis of TPMT Deficiency

After genetically decreased TPMT activity in RBCs and life-threatening thiopurine-induced toxicity were identified (24), molecular studies into the mechanisms underlying the phenotypic differences in TPMT enzyme activity were undertaken. The human kidney TPMT enzyme was purified and characterized, the partial amino acid sequence was identified (20,58), and the TPMT complementary (cDNA) was cloned (59). Northern blot analysis showed that the messenger ribonucleic acid (mRNA) for the enzyme is expressed in many human tissues (60), suggesting that TPMT function extends beyond the biotransformation of thiopurine drugs (61). TPMT was found to be encoded by a 27-kb gene represented by ten exons on human chromosome 6p22.3 (21,22,62,63). Eight of the TPMT exons encode the 28-kDa protein. Exon 2 was observed in one of 16 human liver cDNA samples during initial cloning but has not been detected in most analyses (18). However, the presence of a processed pseudogene for TPMT that was located on the long arm of chromosome 18 complicated initial attempts to clone the gene using the human TPMT cDNA (60). DNA contamination of RNA preparations could lead to amplification of this intronless pseudogene during reverse transcription-polymerase chain reaction (RT-PCR) to study TPMT, which could be mistaken for a variant mRNA species. To avoid amplifications of the TPMT-processed pseudogene, use of primers that include at least one intron-based primer is recommended. The use of anchored PCR techniques made it possible to map the active gene to chromosome 6, which was cloned from a chromosome 6-specific cosmid library, thus avoiding the processed pseudogene on chromosome 18 (63).

Knowledge of the TPMT gene structure allowed the rapid flow of information on the molecular basis for the common genetic polymorphism that regulated the trait at the level of enzyme activity. Two single nucleotide polymorphisms (SNPs), one located on exon 7 and the other on exon 10, altered the encoded amino acid, were present in the most common variant allele for low TPMT activity in Caucasians (TPMT*3A), and were associated with decreased levels of immunoreactive TPMT protein during transient expression in COS-1 cells (63). This was attributed to the increased degradation rate of the variant TPMT protein encoded by this allele, probably through a proteosome-mediated mechanism (64).

A number of variant TPMT alleles have been detected, all of which involved SNPs and most of them lying within the cDNA open reading frame (ORF) that resulted in missense or nonsense codons (Table 25.1) (65,66). The altered TPMT activity predominantly resulted from SNPs (66,67), as evidenced by low-to-intermediate enzyme activity in those patients and as proven by expression studies of these inactivating mutations. Three of the TPMT alleles (TPMT*2, TPMT*3A, and TPMT*3C) accounted for 80% to 95% of intermediate or low enzyme activity in patient studies (64,66–70). Expression of the mutant allele TPMT*2 (G238C, 80 Ala→Pro) (65) in a yeast heterologous expression system led to greater than 100-fold reduction in TPMT activity relative to wild-type cDNA despite a comparable level of mRNA expression (64). Expression of the second and more prevalent mutant allele TPMT*3A (G460A, 154 Ala→Thr and A719G, 240 Tyr→Cys) (68), in yeast or COS-1 cells, led to more than 200-fold reduction in TPMT activity and immunodetectable protein compared to wild-type cDNA (64). Heterologous expression in yeast established that the mutant TPMT proteins encoded by TPMT*2 and TPMT*3A alleles had an enhanced rate of proteolysis, showing degradation half-lives of approximately 15 minutes for both mutant proteins versus 18 hours for the wild type (64). In addition, the mutant TPMT proteins encoded by TPMT*3B and TPMT*3C have shown an enhanced proteolysis rate when expressed in mammalian cells (71) that correlated with measured low activities of the protein in individuals who inherited these alleles (72). The molecular mechanism(s) underlying the variable enzyme activity associated with the mutant alleles TPMT*4–8 (Table 25.1) has not been fully elucidated for these variants. TPMT*4 (G→A transition at the intron 9-exon 10 junction disrupts the final nucleotide of the intron at the 3′ acceptor splice site sequence (66,70). TPMT*5 (T146C, 49 Leu→Ser) was identified in a heterozygous individual of undefined ethnicity who had intermediate TPMT activity (66). TPMT*6 (A539T, 180 Tyr → Phe) was identified in a Korean subject with intermediate activity (66). TPMT*7 (T681G, 227His → Glu) was identified in a single European subject with intermediate TPMT activity (69). TPMT*8 (G644A, 215 Arg → His) has been identified in one heterozygous African-American individual with intermediate activity (73).

These studies demonstrated that the level of RBC TPMT activity (enzyme phenotype/trait) is controlled by genetic polymorphism in the TPMT gene. Approximately 89% of the Caucasian population studied was homozygous for a gene(s) that resulted in high activity; 11% were heterozygous and had intermediate activity; and one of every 300 subjects was homozygous for the trait of low-level RBC TPMT activity.

TPMT Promoter

The identified variant alleles in the ORF of the TPMT gene were associated with intermediate and low TPMT enzyme activity in patients with thiopurine toxicity (65,66,68–70,74) and with variable expression levels of the protein (64,72). The wide range of enzyme activity measured in the different subjects with high TPMT enzyme activity was attributed to effects of inheritance (75), although they are not fully understood. These observations led to the search for possible additional molecular genetic mechanisms that might be involved in upregulation and/or downregulation of TPMT enzyme function. The outcome of this search was the discovery of functional polymorphisms within the 5′ flanking region of TPMT.

Studies in the 5′ flanking region of TPMT demonstrated that it was GC rich (76) but lacked the canonical TATA box and the CCAAT sequence, typically located near the site of transcription initiation with a series of potential Sp1 binding sites (63). This illustrated that the transcription factor Sp1 is an important transactivator of the TPMT promoter (77). Results of 3′ truncation analysis of the TPMT promoter demonstrated that the sequence upstream from the transcription start sites [one major and two closely located minor transcription start points were identified in HepG2 cells (77)] is sufficient for a high level of constitutive transcriptional activity. These studies revealed the presence of a positive regulatory element within the region $+34$ to $+60$. The 5′ truncation analysis of the TPMT promoter revealed important positive regulatory elements in regions -85 to -75 and -68 to -51, which contain binding sites for transcription factors Sp1 and Egr-1. Gradual truncations of these regions led to gradual reduction in TPMT promoter activity (77).

Subsequent studies demonstrated that the 5′ flanking region of TPMT included a polymorphic variable number tandem repeat (VNTR). Five alleles were reported (76) in which a 17- to 18-bp element were repeated four to eight times (76,78). Larger studies confirmed that TPMT VNTR*4 and *5 were the most common alleles in Caucasians, with repeat numbers that varied from three to nine (76,79). An inverse relationship was reported between the sum of repeat units and level of RBC TPMT activity (to a much smaller extent in comparison to the effects of ORF-based SNPs) (78,79). Reporter gene constructs confirmed this relationship (78). The modulatory role of the TPMT VNTR was further supported by the detection of two additional VNTR alleles, *V3 and *V9 (79). Linkage disequilibrium between the VNTR allele *V5 and TPMT *3A was noted (79). However, this relationship was not confirmed by a subsequent study in which the genotype *V4/*V4 had a lower activity than *V4/*V5 (78). It was postulated recently that the number of motifs within the VNTR internal structure, rather than the number of tandem repeats, is a probable factor that modulates TPMT enzyme activity (80). The clinical importance of such a mechanism proposed to play a role in modulating the level of TPMT activity remains to be elucidated.

Intronic Sequence Variations

Intronic sequence variations were identified in introns 3, 4, 5, and 9. Although sequence variations in

introns 3 [T114A and A(-101)T] (74), 4 [T35C and G98T] (74), and 5 (C58T) (74) have been detected in patients with varying enzyme activities ranging from low to intermediate, their contribution to the trait of the TPMT enzyme activity and expression of the protein is not fully understood [based on analysis of healthy blood donors, where less than 2 nmol 6-methylthioguanine per gram hemoglobin per hour is deficient; 2 to 23.5 nmol is intermediate, and greater than 23.5 nmol is wild type (81,82)]. However, the SNP found at the TPMT intron 9-exon 10 splice junction (G→A) disrupted the canonical sequence found at splice sites, which resulted in activation of a cryptic splice site within intron 9 and a significant decrease in the level of TPMT mRNA (70) (see Table 25.1 for a list of reported polymorphisms and/or mutations).

Genotype-Phenotype Correlation

Based on population studies, the genotype of the most common TPMT alleles (TPMT*2, TPMT*3A, or TPMT*3C) correlated with the enzyme phenotype and proved that these alleles are acceptable genetic predictors for the TPMT enzyme phenotype in patients treated with thiopurine drugs. Similar population studies illustrated that patients heterozygous for these alleles had intermediate enzyme activity and those who were homozygous were TPMT deficient (67). Compound heterozygotes (TPMT*2/*3A, TPMT*3A/*3C) also showed a deficient TPMT enzyme trait (67). However, genotype-phenotype discrepancies were noted within both the homozygous wild-type and heterozygous groups, showing a high degree of variability in TPMT enzyme activity. High TPMT enzyme activity was detected in some individuals who were heterozygous, whereas some homozygous wild-type subjects had an intermediate phenotype. This might be due to the fact that the alleles associated with regulating TPMT enzyme activity detected thus far do not account for 100% of encountered variations in the RBC TPMT enzyme activity (75), suggesting that other factors such as promoter polymorphisms or motifs within the VNTR or drug interactions contribute to the observed genotype-phenotype discrepancies.

Pattern of Inheritance

Family studies performed early in the course of the investigation of TPMT deficiency demonstrated that TPMT activity is inherited as an autosomal codominant trait (83). Individuals who were normal were hypothesized initially to be homozygous for a wild-type allele; those who were completely deficient were thought to be homozygous for a mutant allele; and those with intermediate activity were thought to be heterozygotes, with one allele having altered TPMT activity and one allele being wild type.

Population Studies

Epidemiologic studies have shown variations in the frequency and distribution patterns of mutant TPMT alleles among different ethnic populations (Table 25.2). The relationship between TPMT genotype and phenotype for the TPMT variant alleles has been clearly defined for the most common mutant alleles identified in Caucasians, (TPMT*2, TPMT*3A, and TPMT*3C) (67,84). The TPMT*2 allele represented 0.2% to 0.5% of all alleles in Caucasian populations and proved to be the least common of the three alleles (37,67,84–88). TPMT*3A was the most common, with a frequency of 3.2% to 5.7%, followed by TPMT*3C, with an allele frequency of 0.2% to 0.8% (37,67,84–88). In West-African populations the frequency of TPMT mutations was 2.4% for TPMT*3C, followed by TPMT*3A (0.8%) and TPMT*2 (0.4%) (Table 25.2) (73). In African populations the TPMT*3C allele was the most common: 9.2% to 10.9% heterozygous and 0.5% homozygous (Table 25.2) (86,88). In a southwest Asian population (Indian and Pakistani) TPMT*3C was not detected. In this population the TPMT*3A mutant allele displayed a frequency of 2% (heterozygotes) (84). It was postulated that this allele was either not present in the Asian population or was present at a very low frequency (63,89).

Using the RBC assay to assess TPMT activity, studies demonstrated that there was a trimodal pattern in several of the populations tested, including healthy otherwise "normal" individuals as well as patients with leukemia. It is estimated that 10% of Caucasians and 10% of African Americans in the United States are likely to have intermediate TPMT activity (i.e., heterozygotes), with approximately one in 300 of these individuals having profound TPMT deficiency (i.e., homozygotes for a mutant allele) (46). Complicating the interpretation of TPMT activity in population studies is the fact that TPMT activity can be influenced by many factors, including patient age, renal function, dosing of thiopurine drug, and tissue source (29,42).

Additional population studies demonstrated the distribution of TPMT activity in RBCs was trimodal, with 90% having high activity, 10% having intermediate activity, and 0.3% having low or no detectable enzyme activity (22,62,90). Other clinical reports confirmed that low TPMT activity is associated with thiopurine toxicity (46). The initial observation that genetically low TPMT activity was associated with an increased risk of drug toxicity (31) was confirmed by studies reporting disorders as diverse as acute lymphoblastic leukemia, dermatologic disease, rheumatoid arthritis, and autoimmune hepatitis. Subsequently, additional studies reported the association between genetically decreased TPMT activity and life-threatening thiopurine-induced myelosuppression (29,91–94).

In parallel with the clinical studies described earlier there was a rapid advance in research investigating the molecular mechanisms underlying individual phenotypic differences in TPMT enzyme activity. Examination of the different expression patterns of inherited TPMT enzyme traits also has been accelerated by advances in DNA and RNA technology and bioinformatics.

TABLE 25.2. *Thipurine-S-methyltransferase (TPMT) allele frequency in different ethnic populations*

Ethnic population	n	TPMT*2%	TPMT*3A%	TPMT*3C%	Reference
Ghanian	217	0	0	7.6	88
Kenyan	101	0	0	5.4	86
Thai	75	0	0	5.3	96
African American	248	0.4	0.8	2.4	73
Chinese	192	0	0	2.3	85
Japanese	553	0	0	1.5	95
French Caucasian	191	0.5	5.7	0.8	87
British Caucasian	199	0.5	4.5	0.3	88
American Caucasian	282	0.2	3.2	0.2	73
Southwest Asian	99	0	1	0	85

Screening for TPMT Deficiency

Rapid and relatively inexpensive assays developed for detection of the three most common signature mutations in TPMT gene will identify 80% to 95% of all mutant alleles (66,67). These include the use of allele-specific PCR or PCR-restriction fragment length polymorphism and recently the introduction of denaturing high-performance liquid chromatography as a rapid and sensitive robust method for the detection of known (common) or unknown variants in the TPMT gene, which may be extended to include the detection of the VNTR in the promoter 5′ flanking region (67,73,74,85,86,88,95–97).

Concluding Remarks

One of the benefits of TPMT pharmacogenetic studies for clinical practice has been to permit oncologists to individualize therapy for patients receiving thiopurine drugs. Knowledge of the TPMT genotype of an individual patient can help predict the efficacy and/or toxicity of thiopurine drugs after administration of standard doses. For patients homozygous for a specific TPMT mutant allele, the risk of having a poorer outcome was greater (17), whereas individuals heterozygous for a mutant TPMT allele were at lesser risk during the course of treatment. These latter individuals were able to have longer durations of maintenance treatment (33), which were not feasible for patients homozygous for the allele associated with low TPMT enzyme activity (17).

DIHYDROPYRIMIDINE DEHYDROGENASE DEFICIENCY

Introduction

DPD deficiency is a pharmacogenetic syndrome associated with severe, potentially life-threatening toxicity after the administration of 5-fluorouracil (5-FU) or a related drug (8). DPD deficiency currently is considered one of the most important pharmacogenetic syndromes associated with cancer chemotherapy because of the following reasons: (i) worldwide, 5-FU is one of the most widely used cancer chemotherapy drugs for treatment of several of the more common malignancies (colorectal cancer, breast, and skin), with an estimated 2,000,000 patients receiving the drug each year (98); and (ii) DPD deficiency, unlike many of the other pharmacogenetic syndromes, has been associated with death (99).

Metabolic Regulation

DPD is the initial and rate-limiting step in pyrimidine catabolism. It is responsible for converting the naturally occurring pyrimidines uracil and thymine to dihydrouracil and dihydrothymine, respectively, as well as the cancer chemotherapy antimetabolite drug 5-FU to dihydrofluorouracil (Fig. 25.2) (100). DPD (also known as dihydrouracil dehydrogenase, dihydrothymine dehydrogenase, uracil reductase, or EC1.3.1.2) requires the cofactor NADPH to donate two hydrogen atoms in this enzyme reaction, in which the double bond in the pyrimidine ring structure is removed. In studies at the cellular (101) and clinical (102) levels, it has been demonstrated to have a critical position in the overall metabolism of 5-FU and responsible for conversion of greater than 85% of clinically administered 5-FU to 5-fluorodihydrouracil (an inactive metabolite) in an essentially irreversible enzymatic step. With reduction of DPD activity, less 5-FU is catabolized and more 5-FU is available to be anabolized to 5-FU nucleotides (active metabolites), including, in particular, 5-fluoro-2′deoxyuridine monophosphate, which inhibits thymidylate synthase and is needed by cells for the synthesis of thymidylate necessary for DNA synthesis (98).

Clinical Presentation

Patients with DPD deficiency who receive a normal dose of 5-FU have a clinical presentation that is similar to that of patients who receive an accidental overdose of 5-FU. In both instances, an excess of 5-FU is present (8). As a result, the excess 5-FU can be anabolized to 5-FU nucleotides, which, in turn, can affect the primary 5-FU target sites (103,104) and produce increased side effects and toxicity (103).

Typical symptoms and signs include fever (secondary to neutropenia), mucositis, stomatitis, and diarrhea (8,105–107). Other symptoms and physical signs sometimes include nausea and vomiting, rectal bleeding, or skin changes (typically presenting as a maculopapular rash or increased pigmentation). Neurologic abnormalities are of particular interest because of their associated frequency with DPD deficiency. Many of these neurologic signs are subtle and unrecognized unless they are specifically sought during a complete neurologic examination. These signs may include cerebellar ataxia, presence of a broad-based gait, and subtle changes in cognitive function, including the inability to perform simple calculations (serial sevens). In cases of profound DPD deficiency in which there is complete or nearly-complete ab-

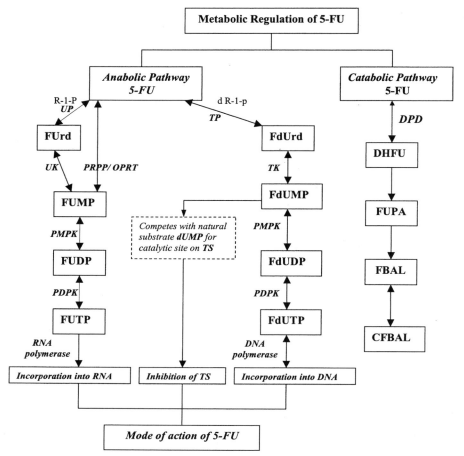

FIG. 25.2. Metabolic regulation of 5-fluorouracil (5-FU). Dihydropyrimidine dehydrogenase (DPD) plays an important role in regulating the bioavailability of 5-FU to exert its cytotoxic effect. The anabolic pathway results in incorporation of the active metabolites into RNA and DNA. In addition, 5-FU generates fluorodeoxyuridine monophosphate, which competes with deoxyuridine monophosphate (FUMP; the natural substrate of thymidylate synthase) for the active catalytic site. This prevents the formation of thymidylate, which is essential for DNA synthesis. In the catabolic pathway, DPD is essentially responsible for approximately 85% of 5-FU metabolism. CFBAL, carboxy-fluoro-β-alanine; DPD, dihydropyrimidine dehydrogenase; DHFU, dihydrofluorouracil; dR-1-P, deoxyribose-1-phosphate; FBAL, α-fluoro-β-alanine; FdUDP, fluorodeoxyuridine diphosphate; FdUMP, fluorodeoxyuridine monophosphate; FdUrd, fluorodeoxyuridine; FdUTP, fluorodeoxyuridine triphosphate; FUDP, fluorouridine diphosphate; FUMP, fluorouridine monophosphate; FUPA, fluoroureidopropionic acid; FUrd, fluorouridine; FUTP, fluorouridine triphosphate; OPRT, orotate phosphoribosyltransferase; PDPK, pyrimidine diphosphate kinase; PMPK, pyrimidine monophosphate kinase; PRPP, phosphoribosyl pyrophosphate; R-1-P, ribose-1-phosphate; TK, thymidine kinase; TP, thymidine phosphorylase; UP, uridine phosphorylase; UK, uridine kinase.

sence of enzyme activity, there may be an alteration in the level of consciousness, with coma (8,107).

Abnormalities may be observed in the initial routine laboratory tests at presentation (8,105–107). These include evidence of leukopenia, thrombocytopenia, and anemia on the initial complete blood count. Oftentimes this may be manifest as a decrease in the absolute neutrophil count (near 0). This is typically seen when 5-FU is administered as a bolus (with or without leucovorin). In contrast, results of routine chemistry tests and urinalysis typically are normal.

Diagnosing DPD Deficiency

Complete or profound DPD deficiency is relatively easy to diagnose. Elevated plasma or urine levels of uracil and/or thymine (the natural substrates for DPD) can be detected by various methods, including thin-layer chromatography, high-performance liquid chromatography, and mass spectrometry (mainly for confirmation) (8,108). Partial DPD deficiency is more difficult to diagnose. This typically requires a radioenzymatic assay of DPD activity to directly measure DPD enzyme activity (109). Although various cells or tissues have been assessed with this assay, PBM cells are particularly well suited because the cells are easy to obtain. Furthermore, the subsequent enzymes of the pyrimidine catabolic pathway are not present in these cells, making the assessment of DPD activity easier. An algorithm for the prediction of 5-FU toxicity and enzyme deficiency is given in Figure 25.3.

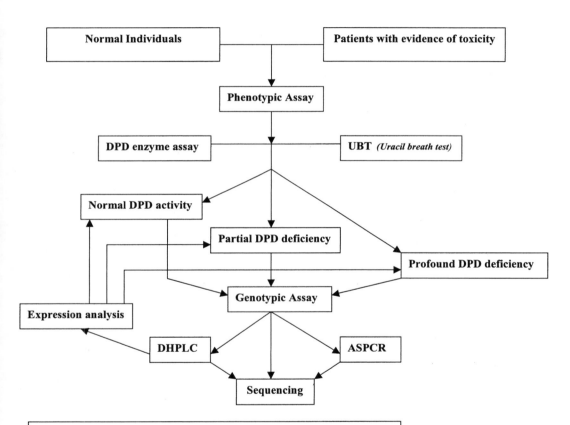

FIG. 25.3. Algorithm for the prediction of 5-fluorouracil (5-FU) toxicity in normal individuals and in cancer patients prior to initiation of treatment. The DPD enzyme assay remains the gold standard for the identification of individuals at risk for developing toxicity after the administration of 5-FU; however, the DPD enzyme assay is not always possible. Validation of a new and promising phenotypic test, the uracil breath test (UBT), currently is in progress. Preliminary results of this test indicate it is accurate in the differentiation of different enzyme phenotypes. The advance in genotypic tests offered by new techniques such as denaturing high-performance liquid chromatography (DHPLC) has allowed rapid and accurate screening of entire genes in considerably shorter periods of time. In addition, this technique allows the detection of known and unknown sequence variations, contrary to the allele-specific polymerase chain reaction (ASPCR) method, which allows the detection of previously known sequence variations only. Detected sequence variations should be confirmed by direct sequencing.

Pharmacologic Consequences of DPD Inhibition

The impact of complete deficiency of DPD on 5-FU metabolism, disposition, and pharmacokinetics was examined in one of the first reported DPD-deficient patients (8). The patient was given a "test" dose (1/20 of standard dose) of radiolabeled 5-FU (25 mg/m^2, 600 μCi [^{3}H-6]-5-FU) as an intravenous bolus, after which plasma, urine, and cerebrospinal fluid were sampled at specified times. The patient was observed to have a markedly altered pharmacokinetic pattern. 5-FU was detected in the plasma at unusually high levels for at least 8 hours, and more than 85% of the 5-FU was excreted unchanged in the urine over the 24-hour period after drug administration. The patient had an apparent 5-FU elimination half-life of 159 minutes, with a systemic clearance of 70 mL/min/M^2. This was in contrast to a group of "normal" patients given a standard bolus dose of 5-FU (450 mg/m^2) with the same radioactive tracer dose (600 μCi [^{3}H-6]-5-FU) (102). These patients had an apparent elimination half-life of 13 ± 7 minutes, with a systemic clearance of 594 ± 198 mL/min/M^2. The data imply that the increased 5-FU levels resulting from decreased catabolism secondary to DPD deficiency will lead to increased anabolism with formation of 5-FU nucleotides, leading to increased risk of toxicity.

Clinical Management

Because DPD deficiency currently is not easily diagnosed before 5-FU is administered, the consequences of most cases of DPD deficiency cannot be prevented. Unfortunately, the options for managing the resultant 5-FU toxicities are limited even when the possibility of DPD deficiency is considered soon after treatment (107). The initial and most obvious approach is to remove the source of any further 5-FU (or related drug), e.g., discontinue protracted intravenous infusion of 5-FU or stop further administration of an oral fluoropyrimidine drug (e.g., capecitabine). Obviously less can be done after administration of a standard intravenous bolus dose of 5-FU.

Although various other interventions (107) have been suggested (including hemoperfusion and hemodialysis, and administration of the nucleoside thymidine or granulocyte colony-stimulating factor in an attempt to rescue cells at risk), none has made much impact on reversing 5-FU toxicity. Perhaps the most useful approach for these patients has been aggressive supportive care with appropriate antibiotic coverage for infections (as well as antiinfectious coverage for potential nonbacterial infections, e.g., fungal infections) and appropriate fluid and electrolyte support with hospitalization in the intensive care unit if necessary (e.g., for sepsis with the additional need for hemodynamic support).

Molecular Basis for DPD Deficiency

As with TPMT deficiency and most other pharmacogenetic syndromes, it is useful to have a comprehensive understanding of the normal structure of the macromolecules involved, including protein, RNA, and DNA, as well as an understanding of the mechanisms controlling both the synthesis and degradation of these molecules prior to studying the molecular causes of the pharmacogenetic disorder.

When DPD deficiency was first reported or suspected in cancer patients in the late 1980s, little was known about the human enzyme (8,110). It was the recognition of the increasingly important role of DPD as a critical step in 5-FU metabolism and pharmacology that provided the impetus for undertaking the initial studies (111). Because results of animal studies and clinical experience with 5-FU administered intraperitoneally and by hepatic artery infusion suggested that this catabolic enzyme was abundant in the liver, initial approaches focused on human liver.

DPD protein has been purified from human liver to homogeneity and has permitted characterization of this protein, including analysis of substrate kinetics; location of functional domains, preparation of a polyclonal antibody, and determination of the N-terminal amino acid sequence that proved essential to elucidation of the cDNA sequence and the subsequent isolation and characterization of the DPD gene (known as *DPYD,* according to accepted genomics nomenclature) (100). These studies demonstrated that 5-FU was an excellent substrate for the human DPD enzyme, with a substrate affinity in the same range as that of the natural substrate uracil (100,112). This study also provided initial insight into the complexity of this enzyme, with multiple cofactors (NADPH, flavin) required for enzyme action.

Determination of the cDNA sequence provided further insight into the DPD protein because various functional domains within the translated amino acid sequence could be predicted (113,114). Thus, several potentially important regions within the linear sequence of amino acids were identified, including flavin-binding regions, NADPH-binding regions, two iron/sulfur domains, and the uracil-binding site. Awareness of these critical regions and of the conservation of the amino acid sequence during evolution of the DPD protein has helped in predicting the possible functional consequences of various mutations in the coding region of the gene on DPD activity (115).

The availability of pure protein in sufficient quantities has permitted initial studies of the three-dimensional structure. Porcine DPD, which shares greater than 99% homology with human DPD, has been crystallized with x-ray diffraction studies, permitting modeling of the DPD protein dimer with its two identical polypeptide chains (116,117). The availability of this structural analysis, together with identification of the location of the various functional domains such as the uracil binding site and of potentially important contact points, should prove useful for the assessment of various sequence variants that are determined.

Availability of the cDNA has permitted studies at the gene level. Initial studies using fluorescence in situ hybridization localized the gene for the DPD protein to chromosome 1p22 (118). The *DPYD* gene subsequently was shown to consist of 23 exons with exon length varying from 50 to over 1,550 base pairs (119,120) and several long introns (some greater than 10 kb), with the total gene size estimated at least 30 to 40 kb. These studies provided valuable information on the intron-exon junctions that has been useful in the identification of specific common mutations and has aided in the development of several of the newer genotyping tests (see later in text). More recently, the promoter for the *DPYD* gene has been cloned with initial characterization, which may prove valuable in future investigations of the regulation of expression of the *DPYD* gene (121).

With the availability of the cDNA initially and more importantly the DNA sequence of the *DPYD* gene, there was an effort to identify the structural changes that could account for the decrease in DPD activity. The initial mutation described in the *DPYD* gene was not in the cDNA but was a G-to-A mutation in the 5′ splicing recognition sequence of intron 14, resulting in a 165-bp deletion corresponding to exon 14 (121). This mutation is known by established nomenclature as DPYD*2A (122). This mutation not only was the first one described but subsequently was demonstrated to be the most frequently observed mutation accounting for decreased DPD activity (123–127). Today there are at least 30 known sequence variants, most of which have been reported in the literature (Table 25.3) (107,128–143). It should be noted that many of these are not actually mutations with functional consequences but are polymorphisms with little obvious functional significance.

As with the study of sequence variants with other genetic abnormalities, it has proved useful to evaluate these sequence variants to determine whether they have any effect on protein function (activity) after translation. Thus, after inserting or producing the de-sired sequence variant (e.g., by site directed mutagenesis) one can examine the protein produced in an expression system with an assay of protein function (e.g., assessment of DPD activity possibly with determination of K_m and V_{max}) (121). Additional insight into the potential functional consequence of the sequence variant can be obtained by determining whether the variant results in a conserved or nonconserved amino acid change, whether the locus is a highly conserved area, and whether the change occurs in potentially critical regions of the molecule (e.g., active site, critical binding regions) (114). Finally, family studies of both normal and deficient members can provide valuable insight into whether the particular sequence variant results in a functional change *in vivo* (131).

Pattern of Inheritance

Although initial family studies of a patient with complete DPD deficiency suggested an autosomal recessive pattern of inheritance (8), subsequent family studies of partially DPD-deficient patients who developed toxicity after receiving 5-FU demonstrated that the inheritance is best described as autosomal codominant (99,108). With the availability of genotypic tests for the various alleles, this has now been confirmed (108).

Population Studies

To better understand the extent of DPD variability, studies were undertaken in a population of 124 healthy individuals (45% males and 55% females) (144). DPD activity followed a normal distribution, with an approximate sixfold range in DPD enzyme activity. Although some initial study results (145) suggest that there is a preponderance of females with low DPD activity, no significant difference in DPD activity by gender was observed subsequently (146,147). In studies of healthy adult populations (145) and cancer patient populations (146,147) consisting of men and women from 20 to 70 years old, there was no obvious age-related variation in DPD activity.

DPD activity has been examined in different races. Studies from the United States suggest that there is no racial difference in DPD activity between Caucasians and African Americans. In the limited population studies of DPD activity in other racial groups, there is no suggestion of dramatic differences in the range of DPD activity in healthy populations; however, there are data suggesting that the frequency of DPD deficiency seems different across racial groups with DPD deficiency much less common in Japanese Americans

TABLE 25.3. *Reported sequence variations in the coding region of the* DPYD *gene*

DPYD*	Genotype	Amino acid change		DPD enzyme activity		
				Normal	Deficient	Uncertain
*12	62G>A	R21Q	2	[129]		
	74G>A	H25R	2			[130]
*9A	85T>C	C29R	2	[108, 131]	[132, 133]	
	257C>T	P86L	4		[134]	
*7	Del TCAT 295–298	Frameshift	4		[135]	
	496A>G	M166V	6	[108, 136]	[132]	
	545T>A	M182K	6			[152]
	601A>C	S201R	6		[134]	
	632A>G	Y211C	6		[134]	
*8	703C>T	R235W	7		[135]	
	812 del T	Frameshift	8			[130]
	775A>G	259E	8			
*11	1003G>A	V335L	10		[129]	
	1108A>G	370V	10		[134]	
	Del>TG 1039–1042	Frameshift	10		[134]	
*12	1156G>T	E386>stop	11		[129]	
	1217T>C	406T	11	[137]		
	1475C>T	S492L	12		[134]	
*4	1601G>A	S534D	13	[138]		[131, 139]
*5	1627A>G	I543V	13	[139]	[132]	
*13	1679T>G	I560S	13		[108, 131]	
	1714C>G	L572V	13			[130]
*2A	IVS14+1G>A	Del el4	14	[131]	[125, 132, 136, 140, 141]	
	T1896C	F632F				[130]
*3	1897delC	Frameshift	14		[142]	
*6	2194G>A	V7321	18	[131, 139]	[132]	
	2329G>A	A777S	19			[152]
	2657G>A	R886H	21			[133]
	2846A>T	D949V	22		[132]	
	2921A>T	D974V	23			[143]
	2933A>G	978R	23		[134]	
*10	2983G>T	V995F	23		[150]	
	3067C>T	1023S	23	[137]		

and Chinese Americans than in Caucasians and African Americans in the United States.

The initial population studies of healthy individuals permitted the establishment of a statistical "cutoff point" for the DPD radioassay described earlier, separating individuals with DPD activity in the normal range from individuals who are DPD deficient. Both fresh and frozen PBM cell samples were used in the studies of healthy individuals. A strong correlation was found between the cell samples, with a normal distribution pattern of DPD activity in both frozen and fresh samples (144). This has permitted the use of frozen samples from more distant locations for further DPD screening in cancer patients. A similar normal distribution was observed in human livers from cadaver donors (148).

A subsequent study examined DPD activity in PBM cells from 151 female breast cancer patients (149). The distribution pattern of DPD activity was similar (normal distribution) to that in PBM cells from a healthy population (144). Of interest, however, the mean DPD activity in the PBM cells from the breast cancer population was "shifted to the left" and statistically significantly lower than that from the healthy population. The difference also was shown after cross-analysis by age and race. Menopausal status, use of hormonal therapy or chemotherapy, or disease status did not appear to be related to this finding. The frequency of DPD deficiency in the population of breast cancer patients is similar (approximately 3.0%) to that of other reported pharmacogenetic syndromes (1,10).

Screening for DPD Deficiency

Over the past decade, the radioenzymatic assay has remained the gold standard for diagnosing DPD deficiency (108). This assay can detect not only individuals who are completely deficient in DPD activity but also those who are partially deficient. Unfortunately, the assay, while accurate and sensitive, is somewhat cumbersome, time consuming, and not well-suited for widespread use for screening patients before treatment with 5-FU.

Over the years there have been many attempts to develop more user-friendly assays. This initially included phenotypic assays, such as determining plasma (or urine) levels of uracil (or thymine) (8,10). More recently, antibody-based tests using polyclonal or monoclonal antibodies to DPD have been used (150,151). Although these assays could typically permit diagnosis of completely DPD-deficient individuals, they are somewhat less accurate in assessing partially deficient individuals (typically individuals with a heterozygous mutation) (152), which makes these assays of limited use because the vast majority of DPD-deficient individuals are partially deficient.

With sequencing of the cDNA (112,113) and subsequent characterization of the *DPYD* gene (118,119), it was hoped that it would be possible to develop a limited number of specific PCR-based tests. As shown in Table 25.3, many sequence variants with low DPD activity have been described. Furthermore, it now is recognized that complex compound heterozygote patterns exist with DPD deficiency (107,152); this makes these tests less valuable, with DPD activity levels lower than what a specific PCR test might suggest. For all of these reasons, simple genotypic assays alone are likely to be of limited value in screening for DPD deficiency.

New Phenotypic Assays

A recently developed assay permits rapid assessment of DPD activity and is sensitive enough to detect partially deficient individuals and to differentiate among individuals with normal-range DPD activity (low normal, mid normal, and high normal) (153). This assay uses a stable isotope (^{13}C) localized at the 2-carbon of

uracil. The uracil is administered as a tasteless (slightly alkaline) solution at a dose of 6 mg/kg in about 200 mL of water. Following the three-step catabolism of uracil (initially through the rate-limiting enzyme DPD), the 2-carbon of uracil is released as $^{13}CO_2$. At selected time points, expired air can be collected into specially designed self-sealing foil-lined breath bags. The $^{13}CO_2$ content in the bags can be assessed later with a specially designed infrared detector developed for this purpose (UBiT Infrared Detector, Meretek Inc., Nashville, TN, USA). This detector can distinguish between the levels of $^{13}CO_2$ and $^{12}CO_2$. The ratio of $^{13}CO_2$ to $^{12}CO_2$ can be shown to be proportional to DPD enzyme activity determined by the radioenzymatic assay. Of particular interest is that partially deficient individuals have a pattern very different from that of individuals with normal DPD activity. The UBiT detector can be used to identify DPD deficiency before the administration of 5-FU. This assay is rapid (90 minutes or less), noninvasive, cost effective, and suitable for use in a clinical laboratory.

New Genotypic Assays

Two new interesting approaches for genotyping sequence variants in the *DPYD* gene have recently been described. The first assay was developed to detect what appears to be the most common DPYD sequence variant, DPYD*2A, which results in defective protein. This defective DPD is rapidly degraded, resulting in decreased detectable DPD enzyme activity (below the normal range). Using specific primers and a fluorogenic probe, one can specifically use real-time PCR to detect this mutation (124).

Although this is thought to be the most common sequence variant, thus justifying the development of a specific assay, multiple sequence variants are associated with DPD deficiency, with additional complexity due to compound heterozygotes. Thus, it would be desirable to rapidly screen the entire coding region and, potentially, additional regions responsible for regulating the expression of DPD mRNA (e.g., promoter). Denaturing high-performance liquid chromatography is a relatively new method that permits relatively rapid examination of DNA fragments less than 1,000 bp by applying a temperature-modulated heteroduplex analysis gradient that can differentiate between mutant and wild-type sequences based on the differences in the melting temperatures and specific chromatogram patterns of the two fragments (154). The detected changes can be confirmed by direct sequencing (e.g., capillary gel electrophoresis). Using this method, the entire coding sequence and the promoter can be scanned within 12.5 hours.

Concluding Remarks

DPD deficiency provides an excellent example of how sequence variations in important regions of a gene coding for an enzyme with a critical role in drug metabolism can have pharmacologic and, in turn, clinical consequences. Most impressive with DPD deficiency is that in the most severe cases, death can occur essentially because of the presence of excessive drug, analogous to overdose through excess drug administration. The severity of adverse drug reactions with cancer chemotherapy is related to the typically narrow therapeutic window that characterizes many of the chemotherapeutic drugs. DPD deficiency is now one of several pharmacogenetic syndromes associated with cancer chemotherapy drugs. More recently, there has been an increased awareness of the role of altered expression of genes controlling drug-metabolizing enzymes in tumors (155). These genes may have a major role in determining the response to cancer chemotherapy agents. Genes coding for expression of critical enzymes that are involved in metabolism (both anabolism and catabolism) or are targets for drug action have been of particular interest. This is illustrated by recent studies examining the effectiveness of the cancer chemotherapy drug 5-FU, in which response was related to the expression of the target enzyme thymidylate synthase, the catabolic enzyme DPD, and the anabolic enzyme thymidylate phosphorylase (156).

URIDINE DIPHOSPHATE GLUCURONOSYLTRANSFERASE

Introduction

Uridine diphosphate glucuronosyltransferases (UGTs) are important drug-metabolizing enzymes that catalyze phase II reactions (157). Phase II reaction enzymes usually conjugate phase I reaction products, parent compounds, or other reactive intermediates to form more polar derivatives for renal and biliary elimination. Phase II reaction-metabolizing enzymes also include *N*-acetyltransferases (NAT1 and NAT2), glutathione *S*-transferases, and sulfotransferases.

UGTs constitute a superfamily of enzymes that exert their action through transfer of the glucuronic acid moiety uridine diphosphoglucuronate to the aglycone substrates (158). Conjugation with glucuronic acid (glucuronidation) is a major pathway for the detoxification and excretion of lipid-soluble endogenous substrates and xenobiotics (158). Glucuronides are inactive water-soluble conjugates (with the exception of a few examples, e.g., morphine-6-glucuronide)

(159), which are eliminated from the body via bile or urine (160). Most of the commonly administered drugs in medicine are targeted for glucuronidation, such as paracetamol (acetaminophen) (161), ibuprofen and amitriptyline (162,163), morphine (159), steroid hormones (synthesized as endobiotic substrates and administered as hormone therapy) (162,164–167), and the immunosuppressives cyclosporin and tacrolimus (168).

Irinotecan (CPT-11; 7-ethyl-10-[4-(1-piperidino)-1 piperidino]-carbonyl-oxycamptothecin), a camptothecin water-soluble chemical derivative, is a relatively new cancer chemotherapy drug currently used primarily in the first-line treatment of advanced metastatic colorectal cancer, with potential clinical activity in lung cancer and several other malignancies. This important cancer chemotherapy drug likely will find indications in several other tumor types in the future (169,170).

Metabolic Regulation

Irinotecan (CPT-11) is a prodrug that is converted by carboxylesterases in the liver to the active metabolite 7-ethyl-10-hydroxycamptothecin (SN-38) (169); its antitumor activity is mediated by the inhibition of topoisomerase I (170). In a normal drug metabolic pathway, SN-38 is glucuronidated by UGT1A1, the major UGT isoform, to the inactive SN-38 glucuronide SN-38G (169), which is excreted into bile and urine. Bacterial β-glucuronidase in the intestine can transform the inactive SN-38G to the active SN-38 (Fig. 25.4). Accumulation of large amounts of the active metabolite exceeding the capacity of the catabolic pathway, or in the presence of defective UGT1A1 gene, results in direct enteric injury that leads to severe, life-threatening diarrhea (171,172).

The variability in glucuronidation of SN-38 appeared to be a major determinant of the severity of diarrhea associated with the level of UGT1A enzyme isoform activity. UGT1A1 occupies a critical position in irinotecan metabolism because it has the major role in the disposition and hence detoxification of the active metabolite SN-38 (173). It was hypothesized that the presence of mutations in the UGT1A1 gene could produce a decrease in function or relative amount of UGT1A1 and in turn result in delayed clearance of SN-38 (3).

To date the genetic polymorphism of only six of the 16 functional UGT genes has been described and characterized (174). The most important and best studied of these isoforms is UGT1A1, the isoform that is known to have an important role in bilirubin dispo-

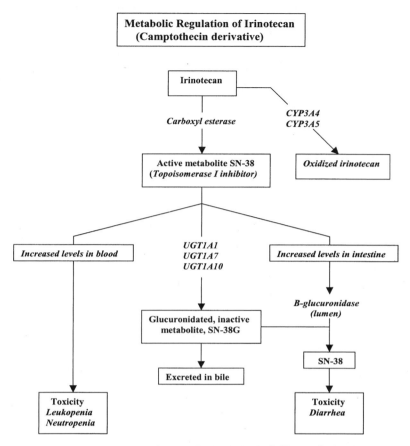

FIG. 25.4. Metabolic regulation of irinotecan (camptothecin derivative). The antileukemic drug irinotecan exerts its action through transformation into the active form SN-38 (7-ethyl-10-hydroxycamptothecin)via a reaction catalyzed by carboxylesterase. The enzyme uridine diphosphoglucuronyltransferase (UDPGT) regulates the bioavailability of the active metabolite SN-38 by transforming it into the inactive glucuronidated form SN-38G (10-*O*-glucuronyl-SN-38). SN-38 is primarily glucuronidated by UGT1A1, the main enzyme isoform of the UGT family of enzymes, responsible for glucuronidation of SN-38. The enzyme isoforms UGT1A7 and UGT1A10 have been implicated in the glucuronidation of SN-38. The cytochrome enzymes CYP3A4 and CYP3A5 also are involved in a minor pathway for the oxidation of irinotecan.

sition (175) and whose functional significance has been convincingly demonstrated (174). Polymorphism of this specific gene results in the well-characterized hyperbilirubin syndromes of the rare (1/1,000,000) type 1 and 2 Crigler-Najjar syndromes (CN-1 and CN-2, respectively) and the relatively common (estimated in up to 15% of general population) Gilbert syndrome (176).

Irinotecan is an excellent example of how a polymorphism in a drug-metabolizing enzyme can alter the metabolic pathway of the drug and consequently the therapeutic outcome in cancer chemotherapy.

Clinical Presentation

Clinical Presentation Associated with Inherited Disorders of Bilirubin Glucuronidation

Three grades of UGT1A1 deficiency occur in man and are associated with three forms of inherited unconjugated hyperbilirubinemia: CN-1, CN-2, and Gilbert syndrome (177). CN-1 was first described in 1952 (178). It is a genetic trait characterized by potentially lethal hyperbilirubinemia (serum bilirubin 20 to 50 mg/dL), with absent or very low UGT1A1 activity, and arises from mutant coding region alleles and promoter polymorphisms. The mechanism later was found to be a virtual absence of hepatic glucuronidation (UGT1A1 activity) (179). Untreated CN-1 invariably results in death from bilirubin encephalopathy. Liver transplantation is currently the only definitive therapy for CN-1 (180). Alternative therapeutic modalities, such as hepatocyte transplantation and gene therapy, currently are being examined (181,182).

CN-2 associated with intermediate levels of hyperbilirubinemia (approximately 7 to 20 mg/dL) and is due to partial deficiency of UGT1A1 activity (179). The bile contains significant amounts of bilirubin glucuronides, but the ratio of bilirubin diglucuronide to monoglucuronide is lower than normal (183).

Gilbert syndrome is a chronic mild hyperbilirubinemia inherited as an autosomal recessive trait. It is the mildest form of inherited unconjugated hyperbilirubinemia. Serum bilirubin levels range from normal to 5 mg/dL. Hemolyses, fasting, and stress may elevate serum unconjugated bilirubin levels (184). Hepatic UGT1A1 activity is reduced to about 30% of normal (185).

Clinical Presentation Associated with Irinotecan Toxicity

During the initial clinical evaluation of irinotecan, the deaths of 55 of 1,245 patients were attributed to severe toxicity including leukopenia and/or diarrhea (186–188). Several of the deaths occurred sporadically, even in patient with excellent performance status (186,189–191).

Pharmacodynamic studies have shown that patients with relatively lower glucuronidation rates had progressive accumulation of SN-38 leading to toxicity (171). The impaired glucuronidation of SN-38 in some patients with Gilbert syndrome was responsible for severe neutropenia and/or diarrhea (192). Using acetaminophen to phenotype patients proved to be a poor predictor of SN-38G conjugation in cancer patients (193), probably because acetoaminophen is mainly metabolized by UGT1A6 (194).

Diagnosing UGT1A1 Deficiency

Diagnosing UGT1A1 enzyme deficiency relies on two parameters directly related to UGT1A1 activity: serum bilirubin and UGT1A1 genotype. Although serum bilirubin is a function of many factors, including RBC lifespan and mass, the detection of unexplained serum hyperbilirubinemia warrants further investigation. Unconjugated serum bilirubin level was associated with syndromes that were directly cor-

related with varying grades of UGT1A1 deficiency. Gilbert syndrome (serum bilirubin level range from normal to less than 5 mg/dL) was associated with 30% reduction in enzyme activity (185), CN-2 syndrome (serum bilirubin level 7 to 20 mg/dL) with partial enzyme deficiency (179), and CN-1 syndrome (serum bilirubin level 20 to 50 mg/dL) with profound enzyme deficiency (179). Genotyping assays for UGT1A1 is currently an accepted procedure for the identification of normal individuals with inherited UGT1A1 deficiency or cancer patients at risk for developing life-threatening toxicity prior to the initiation of treatment with chemotherapeutic drugs (Fig. 25.5). Genotyping analysis proved that patients whose genotype exhibited a variant allele [VNTR, (TA)7] in the promoter region [T(TA)7TAA] are at lower risk than those with mutations in the coding region (CN-2) or those in (CN-1). These patients can experience lethal toxicity due to the presence of mutations in the promoter and coding regions, which result in profound enzyme deficiency.

Pharmacologic Consequences of UGT1A1 Deficiency

Genetic lesions resulting from more than 50 mutations in the UGT1A1 exons and promoter region have been reported to cause varying degrees of enzyme deficiency (195,196). UGT1A1 deficiency is associated with glucuronidation rates of irinotecan active metabolite (SN-38). The differences in bilirubin levels among the genotypes were found to be statistically significant but clinically a poor predictor of toxicity and UGT1A1 deficiency. Some cancer patients carrying genotypes associated with Gilbert syndrome may comply with irinotecan chemotherapy (197), based on the fact that genotypes detected in Gilbert syndrome also were reported in healthy individuals with normal bilirubin levels (198–201). UGT1A1*28 is associated with Gilbert syndrome but apparently is not solely responsible for the complete manifestation of the syndrome (176). However, patients who have the variant promoter genotype UGT1A1*28 are at increased risk for severe toxicity from irinotecan (197).

Interindividual differences in the pharmacokinetics of SN-38 and SN-38G are mostly associated with the UGT1A1 genotype; thus the excessive accumulation of the active metabolite SN-38 would increase the toxicity of irinotecan (202).

In vitro SN-38 glucuronidation rates in human liver microsomes were found to be significantly lower in homozygotes of the $(TA)_7$ allele (7/7) and heterozy-

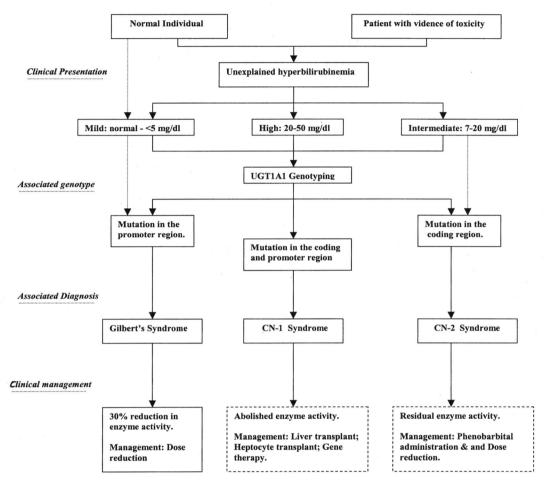

FIG. 25.5. Diagnosing UGT1A1 deficiency. Assessment of UGT1A1 deficiency depends on the measurement of enzyme level in the liver, which is an invasive procedure and should be avoided due to embedded risks. Fortunately, genotyping analysis for UGT1A1 gene polymorphisms and/or mutations proved to be a reliable predictor of enzyme activity in cancer patients and normal individuals. The genotypic pattern identified in cases with unexplained unconjugated hyperbilirubinemia correlated with enzyme activity in Gilbert syndrome and Crigler-Najjar type 1 and 2 (CN-1 and CN-2) syndromes.

gotes (6/7) than in homozygotes of the $(TA)_6$ allele (6/6) (155). Severe grades of neutropenia and diarrhea were observed after administration of irinotecan in some patients with Gilbert syndrome (155,192), and patients with solid tumors who received 300 mg/m^2 irinotecan every 3 weeks and were heterozygous or homozygous for the $(TA)_7$ allele displayed similar toxicity. Higher AUC SN-38 values were reported in

patients with genotypes 6/7 or 7/7 more than in patients with the 6/6 genotype and correlated significantly with absolute neutrophil count ($p < 0.0001$) (203). This genetic influence on irinotecan metabolism is critical in patients with reduced UGT1A1 activity.

In patients with the normal allele $(TA)_6/(TA)_6$, higher levels of SN-38 glucuronide were produced, which resulted in grade I diarrhea (204). Patients with the $(TA)_7$ mutation developed more severe diarrhea, without significant differences between homozygotes for $(TA)_7$ and heterozygotes $(TA)_6/(TA)_7$.

The relationship between the different grades of irinotecan toxicity and the multiple variant genotypes (UGT1A1*28 in the promoter and UGT1A1*6, UGT1A1*27, UGT1A1*29, and UGT1A1*7 in the coding region) suggest that the genotype for UGT1A1*28 (either heterozygous or homozygous) is a significant risk factor for severe toxicity by irinotecan ($p < 0.001$; odds ratio 7.23; 95% confidence interval 2.52 to 22.3) (197). Patients heterozygous for UGT1A1*27 also suffered severe toxicity. No statistical correlation was detected between the genotype UGT1A1*6 and the occurrence of severe toxicity (197).

Irinotecan has the tendency to cause diarrhea, usually of greater severity and clinical impact than its other major toxicity, myelosuppression. The severity of the diarrhea is generally unpredictable and inconsistently correlated to interindividual pharmacokinetic variability (205). It should be noted that clinical investigators were able to manage, but not prevent, diarrhea during phase II and III development of irinotecan (206,207).

Only a small fraction of administered irinotecan is converted to the active metabolite SN-38; the remaining drug is metabolized by CYP3A4 and/or CYP3A5 or excreted via hepatic or renal transport (208,209) via a number of transporters, including MDR1 (P-glycoprotein), MRP2 (cMOAT), and BCRP (210,211).

It is generally accepted that the late diarrhea ensuing from irinotecan administration is related to a direct effect of SN-38G on the intestinal mucosa, where the bacterial intestinal β-glucuronidase can convert SN-38G to the active metabolite SN-38 again. The genetic variability at the UGT1A1 promoter seems unlikely to be the sole element responsible for irinotecan pharmacokinetics and toxicity (212), although significant correlation was observed between UGT1A1 promoter polymorphism and both pharmacokinetics and toxicity of irinotecan (202,203).

Clinical Management

Dose reductions may be necessary in patients homozygous or heterozygous for the (TA)7 allele. Because the genetic polymorphism in UGT1A1 is not the sole determinant of irinotecan clearance and given the complex metabolism and elimination of irinotecan that involves carboxylesterase, CYP3A4, and transporters

(213), the possibility of reduced antitumor effect from altered irinotecan dosing is more likely to occur.

Although not directly related to irinotecan toxicity, study of other hyperbilirubinemias, such as CN-1 and CN-2, can provide insight into clinical management. It should be noted that CN-1 almost invariably results in death from bilirubin encephalopathy (180), and liver transplantation is currently the only definitive therapy for CN-1 (214,215). Alternative treatment modalities are currently under investigation. For example, hepatocyte transplantation in CN-1 has demonstrated that approximately 5% replacement of UGT1A1 function significantly reduces serum bilirubin levels (181,216). Low levels of UGT1A1 activity in CN-2 patients have provided significant protection (181,182). Another approach has been used to partially correct the genetic lesion (deletion of a single guanosine base in exon 4) (217) in Gunn rats (218). This approach uses the cell's own mismatch repair mechanism to correct point mutations or single-base deletions or insertions and requires information regarding the specific mutation in a given patient for the synthesis of an oligonucleotide directed at the site carrying the mutation.

Molecular Basis of UGT1 Deficiency

Based on structural homology (158,196,219), the human UGTs are classified into UGT1 and UGT2 families (196,219). The full-length UGT proteins are encoded by 16 genes (220,221). The UGT1A locus encodes eight genes (1a1, 1A3, 1A4, 1A6, 1A7, 1A8, 1A9, and 1A10) (222,223), and eight are encoded by UGT2 genes (2A1, 2B4, 2B7, 2B10, 2B11, 2B15, 2B17, and 2B28).

The UGT1 isoforms are derived from a single gene locus that spans more than 500 kb on chromosome 2q37 (196,219,224). The UGT1 gene consists of at least 13 unique isoforms with variable exon 1 and common exons 2 to 5. The four exons (exons 2–5) located at the 3′end of this locus encode the carboxy-terminal domain (which binds the common sugar donor substrate UDP-glucuronic acid) of all UGT isoforms (196,219,222,225,226). Each of the exons 1 is preceded by its own unique promoter, which is differentially spliced to the common exons, producing a unique mature mRNA that encodes the amino-terminal domain of these enzymes that confers aglycone substrate specificity (227). The UGT1 family is further classified into multiple isoforms named according to the unique exon (UGT1A1 through UGT1A12) (196,219). The UGT1A1 isoform is responsible for the glucuronidation of bilirubin (175,228) and is expressed from the UGT1A locus on human chromosome 2q37 (229). The human UGT2 enzyme isoforms are encoded by separate genes clustered on chromosome 4, each composed of six exons, and therefore exhibit differences in amino acid sequence throughout the entire polypeptide chain (196,219).

Even though most of the genetic polymorphisms in the numerous UGT isoforms have been reported, in most instances their functional significance remains unclear due to the undefined overlapping substrate specificities and yet undetermined substrate binding domains of the UGT protein isoforms.

Mutations in the Promoter Region of the UGT1A1 Gene

Mutations in the promoter region of the UGT1A1 gene have been implicated in interindividual variation in UGT1A1 expression due to the presence of VNTRs of TA in the TATA box sequence of the promoter region (176,198,230). The transcriptional activity of the UGT1A1 gene was found to be inversely related to the number of (TA) repeats in the TATA box (231).

Six TA repeats are found in the most common wild-type allele (UGT1A1*1). A variant allele containing seven TA repeats (UGT1A1*28) was found to be the most common among the variant alleles (219), whereas five and eight TA repeats were found almost exclusively in the African-American population: UGT1A1*33 [A(TA)5TAA] and UGT1A1*34 [A(TA)8TAA], respectively (232,233). The A(TA)7TAA and A(TA)8TAA UGT1A1 alleles were also reported to be associated with breast cancer demonstrating lower transcriptional activity in vitro (234) and a twofold increase in the risk of developing breast cancer in premenopausal African-American women.

Homozygosity for the variant promoter, with VNTR A(TA)$_7$TAA, is required for Gilbert syndrome, but it is not sufficient for the manifestation of hyperbilirubinemia, which is partly dependent on the level of bilirubin production (176). Individuals who are homozygous for the (TA)$_7$TAA allele [(TA)$_7$ TAA/(TA)$_7$TAA] have enzyme activity approximately 25% of normal, whereas individuals who are heterozygous [(TA)$_7$TAA/(TA)$_6$TAA] have approximately 50% of the homozygous wild-type [(TA)$_6$ TAA/(TA)$_6$TAA] activity (3).

In the Japanese population, variant alleles with VNTR (TA)7 were reported to be less frequent (homozygosity in 2% to 3%) (235–237), whereas a homozygous G71R mutation within the coding regions of UGT1A1 was found to be the common cause of the Gilbert phenotype (mild unconjugated hyperbilirubinemia) in this population.

Molecular Basis of UGT1A1 Deficiency Associated with Mutations in the Coding Region

To date, the genetic polymorphism of six of the 16 functional human UGT genes has been described and characterized, namely, UGT 1A1, 1A6, 1A7, 2B4, 2B7, and 2B15. The functional significance of only the UGT1A1 genetic polymorphism has been convincingly demonstrated (174). The catalytic activity of the mutants of UGT 1A6, 1A7, and 2B15 suggesting the toxicologic significance of these isoforms requires further investigation (174).

CN-1 results from genetic mutations, such as deletions or insertions (238), that cause a shift in the reading frame, which in turn abolishes UGT1A1 activity due to a truncated protein without one or more of its critical functional domains (238). Similarly, a point mutation can lead to the introduction of a premature termination codon or dramatically change the polarity, hydrophobicity, or charge of a single critical amino acid. In such cases, the phenotype cannot always be predicted from the mutation alone. Site-directed mutagenesis and expression studies have demonstrated that substitution of a single amino acid residue within certain microregions of UGT1A1 can lead to profound or partial loss of enzyme activity. In CN-1, enzyme activity was reported to be greatly reduced upon the deletion of critical amino acids or disruption of the polarity or hydrophobicity within a stretch of 20 aromatic/hydrophobic amino acids in the amino-terminal domain of UGT1A1 (encoded by exon 1) (239,240), or by a single amino acid substitution within a highly conserved region (amino acids 298–315) (241,242). Other mutations at a splice donor or splice acceptor site may cause partial or complete exon skipping during RNA processing (243).

In CN-2, amino acid changes resulting from an SNP in the coding region of the UGT1A1 gene usually reduce enzyme activity but do not abolish it (179). This explains the milder phenotype seen in CN-2 and the inducibility of residual enzyme activity by phenobarbital administration (244,245). Enzyme activity greatly varies in CN-2 patients carrying different mutations (246–248). Tables 25.4A and 25.4B list reported mutations in the UGT1A1 gene that are associated with enzyme activity in CN-1 and CN-2.

Intronic Sequence Variations

Intronic sequence variations occurring at a splice donor or splice acceptor site have been reported to cause frameshifts and/or premature stop codons due

TABLE 25.4A. *Sequence variations identified in UGT1A1 gene and associated syndromes*

Exon	Nucleotide change	Amino acid change	Activity	Associated syndrome	Reference
Exon 1	44T>G	L15R	Reduced activity	CN-2	247
	115C>G	H39D	Not detected	CN-1	213
	120-121delCT	(frame shift)	Inactive	CN-1	260
	145C>T	Q49X	Inactive	CN-1	249
	211G>A	G71R	Reduced activity	Gilbert's	236, 237, 273
	222C>A	Y74X	Inactive	CN-1	213
	395T>C	L132P	Reduced activity	CN-2	273
	474-475insT	Truncated (frame shift)	Inactive	CN-1	239, 266
	508-510delTTC	F170del	Inactive	CN-1	179, 239, 266
	517delC	Truncated (frame shift)	inactive	CN-1	213
	524T>A	L175Q	Reduced activity	CN-2	179
	529T>C	C177R	Inactive	CN-1	179
	625T>C	R209W	Reduced activity	CN-2	179, 246
	671T>G	V224G	Residual activity	CN-2	213
	686C>A	P229Q	Reduced activity	CN-2	236
	722-723delAG	Truncated (frame shift)	Truncated-inactive	CN-1/CN-2	213
	826G>T	G276R	Inactive	CN-1	179
	835A>T	B279Y	Not detected	CN-1	179, 226, 242
	840C>A	C280X	Truncated-inactive	CN-1	267
Intron 1	IVS1+1G>C]	Truncated protein	Inactive	CN-1	249
Exon 2	del Exon 2	Truncated	Inactive	CN-1	179
	872C>T	A291V	Inactive	CN-1	242
	879-892del	Truncated (frame shift)	Truncated-inactive	CN-1	179
	880T>A	Truncated (frame shift)	Inactive	CN-1	179, 268
	881-893del	Truncated (frame shift)	Inactive	CN-1	179, 268
	881T>C	1294T	Reduced activity	CN-2	269
	923G>A	G308E	Inactive	CN-1	241, 242
	973delG	Truncated (frame shift)	Truncated-inactive	CN-2	179
	991C>T	Q331X	Truncated-inactive	CN-1	243
Promoter	991C>T	Q331X	Reduced activity	CN-2	271
(TA)₆TAA/ *(TA)₇TAA*	992A>G	Q331R	Reduced activity	CN-2	248

to the interruption of cryptic sites within exons (249). A list of intronic sequence variations is given in Tables 25.4A and 25.4B.

Molecular Basis of UGT Activity Associated with Protein Dimerization

Dimerization of human UGT1A1 was suggested to be a functionally significant mechanism for the complementation or reconstitution of enzyme activity. Using gel permeation high-performance liquid chromatography of solubilized microsomal fractions and nearest-neighbor cross-linking analysis with disulfide cross-linking agents proved that intermolecular binding of UGT1A1 occurs within intact microsomal membranes and that human UGT1A1 molecules exist in a size class consistent with its dimer (250). Cysteine residues are required for cross-linking analysis with disulfide cross-linking agents. Human UGT1A1 contains 11 cysteine residues, one

of which lies within the signal peptide that is not present in the mature enzyme.

The primary structure of human UGT1A1 indicates that most of the molecule lies within the lumen of the endoplasmic reticulum, with only a 26-amino-acid fragment, including three cysteine residues, at the carboxy-terminus remaining in the cytoplasm (250). Complementation or reconstitution of activity was proven by interacting two inactive forms of rat liver UGT2B1 having two different mutations, which resulted in complementation of the enzyme activity toward testosterone upon coexpression in COS-7 cells (251).

Pattern of Inheritance

The pattern of inheritance for individuals who are likely to be affected with this pharmacogenetic syndrome is essentially the same as with Gilbert syndrome (252). Although previous studies of the various

TABLE 25.4B. *Sequence variations identified in UGT1A1 gene and associated syndromes*

Exon	Nucleotide change	Amino acid change	Activity	Associated syndrome	Reference
Exon 3	1005G>A	W335X	Inactive	CN-1	242
	1006C>T	R336W	Inactive	CN-1	269
Promoter	1021C>T	R341X	Truncated-inactive	CN-1	270
(TA)₆TAA/	1046delA	Truncated (frame shift)	Truncated-inactive	CN-1	213
(TA)₇TAA/	1069C>T	Q357X	Truncated-inactive	CN-1	179, 226, 242
	1070A>G	Q357R	Inactive	CN-1	242
	1081C>T	Q361X	Truncated-inactive	CN-1	260
Intron 3	IVS3-2A>G	Truncated protein	Inactive	CN-1	249
Exon 4	1102G>A	A368T	Inactive	CN-1	242
	1124C>T	S376F	Inactive	CN-1	179, 241, 243
	1130A>G	H377R	Not detected	CN-2	213
	1133G>T	G377V	Not detected	CN-2	213
	1143C>G	S381R	Inactive	CN-1	242
	1159C>G	P387R	Inactive	CN-1	260
	1201G>C	A401P	Inactive	CN-1	12, 41, 65
	1223delA	Truncated (frame shift)	Truncated-inactive	CN-1	213
	1223-1224 insT	Truncated (frame shift)	Inactive	CN-1	242
Exon 5	1308A>T	K437X	Inactive	CN-1	242
	1391A>C	Z464A	Residual activity	CN-2	272
	1451G>A	W484X	Truncated-inactive	CN-1	213
Promoter					
(TA)₇TAA/	1456T>G	Y486D	Reduced activity	Gilbert's	235, 236
(TA)₇TAA					
	1490T>A	L497X	Truncated-inactive	CN-1	213

hyperbilirubinemic syndromes, including Crigler-Najjar type 1 and 2 and Gilbert syndrome, were confusing as to the pattern of inheritance, it now is clear that an autosomal recessive pattern of inheritance is responsible for both Gilbert syndrome and the pharmacogenetic syndrome.

Population Studies

Based on serum bilirubin levels the incidence of Gilbert syndrome is 3% to 10% in Caucasians; however, based on genotyping the incidence is 7% to 19% (174). Among Europeans the most common mutation giving rise to Gilbert syndrome is $(TA)_7$ TAA (UGT1A1*28). The published frequency of UGT1A1*28 mutation among whites is extraordinarily high: 0.387(232), 0.4 (176), and 0.38 (198).

In most ethnic groups, Gilbert syndrome arises from a polymorphism in the UGT1A1 promoter, which contains a VNTR ranging from five to eight TA repeats, $(TA)_{5-8}TAA$, involved in the modulation of UGT1A1 transcriptional activity (176,177,232). In Caucasians, blacks, and Asians, homozygosity for the variant promoter UGT1A1*28, $(TA)_7TAA$, which occurs in 0.5% to 19% of these populations (198,254), is required for Gilbert syndrome, although it is not al-

ways sufficient for manifestation of hyperbilirubinemia. The $(TA)_6$ allele is the most common allele, and the frequency of VNTRs that differ from $(TA)_6$ was reported to be higher in blacks, intermediate in Caucasians, and lower in Asians (255).

Other promoter variant alleles having VNTR $(TA)_5$ and $(TA)_8$ were reported in the African population, with frequencies of 0.035 and 0.069, respectively (253). Accordingly, the high variability in SN-38 glucuronidation reported in liver samples from African populations (256) can be explained by the presence of five and eight TA repeats in the UGT1A1 promoter (232,257,258). The variant promoter allele having a VNTR of $(TA)_5$ has shown greater glucuronidation activity than that of the variant allele with $(TA)_8$ in liver samples (256).

In the Japanese population, a missense mutation leading to a heterozygous (sometimes homozygous) single nucleotide change in the UGT1A1 coding region (G71R, R367G, Y486D, P229Q) is a common cause of Gilbert syndrome. The Gly71Arg mutation in the coding region has been shown to result in 30% and 60% reduction in bilirubin glucuronidating activity in heterozygous and homozygous mutant alleles, respectively (257,259). Greater risk of toxicity from xenobiotics metabolized by UGT1A1 is anticipated in patients who exhibit promoter polymorphism and compound heterozygosity for mutations in the coding region.

UGT1A6*2 and the single mutation allele (Arg184Ser) demonstrated a frequency range from 17% to 29% and 0.5% to 2%, respectively (233). Rates of metabolism of a number of xenobiotic phenols by recombinant UGT1A6*2 were found to be lower than those of the wild-type enzyme UGT1A6 (260).

UGT2B4, the enzyme variant at locus Asp458, has shown an allele frequency that is threefold higher than that of the Glu458 variant in Caucasians. Apparently UGT2B4 substrate specificity was not altered by the Asp458Glu substitution. Moreover, genetic polymorphism of UGT2B4 was reported to unlikely be of any functional significance given the overlapping substrate specificity with the higher activity enzyme UGT2B7 (261).

The importance of UGT1A1 genotypes in irinotecan toxicity in the different ethnic and racial groups was demonstrated by the large differences in the distributions of UGT1A1 polymorphisms between Caucasians and Japanese populations; the frequency of UGT1A1*28 in Caucasians was higher than the frequency among the Japanese (199,232). This implies that Caucasians are at higher risk for irinotecan toxicity. The clinical significance of the variant alleles UGT1A1*6 and UGT1A1*27 in exon 1, which have been identified in the Japanese population only, remains unclear (176,200,201).

Screening for UGT1A1 Deficiency

Screening for UGT1A1 deficiency in cancer patients or even in normal individuals can follow three routes. The first is simple measurement of unconjugated serum bilirubin, which as previously mentioned is a poor predictor of enzyme deficiency or toxicity after the administration of chemotherapeutic drugs such as irinotecan. Second is measurement of enzyme activity in the liver; however, the liver is not easily accessible for assessment of enzyme activity. Third is the genotyping of UGT, where UGT1A1 has been demonstrated to be the most important UGT isoform. UGT1A1 is affected by several common mutations in the promoter region (Table 25.4) that have been associated with deficient enzyme activity (155,202, 262,263). In contrast to TPMT and DPD deficiency, where a combination of both phenotyping and genotyping usually is advised to confirm the existence of a pharmacogenetic syndrome, evaluation of UGT1A1 deficiency usually relies on genotyping tests for routine screening.

Concluding Remarks

Genetic polymorphisms in drug metabolism is gaining more clinical relevance with the better understanding of the pharmacogenetic properties of several drug-metabolizing enzymes. Metabolic polymorphism now is recognized as an important cause of interpatient variability after the administration of standard doses of a chemotherapeutic drug (264). With the administration of the maximal tolerated dose of a chemotherapeutic drug, it is anticipated that one third of patients will experience variable grades of toxicity. Elucidation of the pharmacogenetic basis underlying this variation has proved to be clinically relevant, where the pharmacokinetics of the drug and its metabolites correlates with drug activity and/or toxicity or when the drug has a narrow therapeutic index, but most importantly when the metabolic pathway is the main factor determining drug concentration and clearance.

Elucidation of a pharmacogenetic basis for variation in clinical toxicity is becoming increasingly important in cancer chemotherapy (262,265). Examples of genetic polymorphism in drug-metabolizing enzymes are increasingly being recognized as causing life-threatening toxicities, as in the case of irinotecan, where screening for genetic polymorphism in UGT1A1 has proved to be useful in identifying patients at risk for toxicity before the initiation of treatment.

IMPLICATIONS FOR OTHER CANCER CHEMOTHERAPY AGENTS

There is increasing evidence for the importance of pharmacogenetics and cancer chemotherapy. The three examples discussed involving TPMT, DPD, and UGT1A1 demonstrate how sequence variations in important regions of genes coding for enzymes having critical roles in drug metabolism or in a promoter region can have dramatic effects, producing an abnormal pattern of drug metabolism that in turn can lead to altered pharmacokinetics and severe often life-threatening toxicity.

It should be emphasized that genetic variations in other critical steps in drug action (e.g., drug transporters or drug targets) also may be responsible for pharmacogenetic syndromes, and one must remain vigilant that these sites may be the basis of an atypical response to a cancer chemotherapy agent. As noted in the introduction, one of the consequences of pharmacogenetic syndromes with cancer chemotherapy drugs is that severe toxicity, even death, may occur, particularly because these drugs are characterized by a narrow "therapeutic window," where the difference between the effective dose and the toxic dose is relatively small. An impressive example is DPD deficiency in the most severe cases, where death can occur essentially due to the presence of excessive drug, similar to what occurs when an overdose is mistakenly administered. The three examples discussed in detail (TPMT, DPD, and UGT1A1) remain the best characterized pharmacogenetic syndromes associated with cancer chemotherapy, but there is increasing evidence of the possible role of pharmacogenetics with other cancer chemotherapy drugs. These include effects on other classic cytotoxic drugs such as methotrexate and other antifolates (275–277). Investigations of other types of agents used in cancer management currently are underway, including agents as diverse as hormone receptor-based therapy (e.g., tamoxifen) and targeted therapies (e.g., agents that act on epidermal growth factor receptors).

Finally, there has been an increased awareness of the role of altered gene expression of genes that control drug-metabolizing enzymes in tumors (156). These genes may have a major role in determining the response to cancer chemotherapy agents. Genes coding for expression of critical enzymes that are involved in metabolism (both anabolism and catabolism) or are targets for drug action have been of particular interest. This is illustrated by recent studies examining the effectiveness of the cancer chemotherapy drug 5-FU, in which response was shown to be related to expression of the target enzymes thymidylate synthase, as well as the catabolic enzyme DPD and the anabolic enzyme thymidylate phosphorylase (278).

With the completion of sequencing of the human genome, the potential to rapidly screen individuals in the future, and the increasing understanding of the role of proteins (proteomics) coded for by newly identified genes, there is likely to be a new era in cancer chemotherapy. Although pharmacogenetics will remain important, there will be an increasing emphasis on pharmacogenomics, where the alteration in sequence or a difference in expression of a critical gene will provide the stimulus to investigate the pharmacologic consequences (4). This will include an increasing focus on the importance of SNPs and the role of these subtle nucleotide changes in drug response (279).

REFERENCES

1. Kalow W. Pharmacogenetics: its biological roots and the medical challenge. *Clin Pharmacol Ther* 1993;54: 235–241.
2. Weber WW. *Pharmacogenetics*. New York: Oxford University Press, 1997:–318.
3. Diasio RB. Pharmacogenetics. In: Chabner BA, Longo DL, eds. *Cancer chemotherapy & biotherapy,* 3rd ed. Philadelphia: Lippincott Williams & Wilkins, 2001:998–1011.
4. Evans WE, Relling MV. Pharmacogenomics: translating functional genomics into rational therapeutics. *Science* 1999;286:487–491.
5. Guttmacher AE, Collins FS. Genomic medicine—a primer. *N Engl J Med* 2002;347:1512–1520.
6. Pfost DR, Boyce-Jacino MT, Grant DM. A SNPshot: pharmacogenetics and the future of drug therapy. *Trends Biotechnol* 2000;18:334–338.
7. Lu Z, Diasio RB. Polymorphic drug-metabolizing enzymes. In: Schilsky RL, Milano GA, Ratain MJ, ed. *Principles of antineoplastic drug development and pharmacology*. New York: Marcel Dekker, 1996: 281–305.
8. Diasio RB, Beavers TL, Carpenter JT. Familial deficiency of dihydropyrimidine dehydrogenase: biochemical basis for familial pyrimidinemia and severe 5-fluorouracil-induced toxicity. *J Clin Invest* 1988;81: 47–51.
9. Sasvari-Szekely M, Gerstner A, Ronai Z, et al. Rapid genotyping of factor V Leiden mutation using single-tube bi-directional allele-specific amplification and automated ultrathin-layer agarose gel electrophoresis. *Electrophoresis* 2000;21:816–821.
10. Kalow W. Pharmacoanthropology and the genetics of drug metabolism. In: Kalow W, ed. *Pharmacogenetics of drug metabolism*. New York: Pergamon Press, 1992.
11. Relling MV, Dervieux T. Pharmacogenetics and cancer therapy. *Nat Rev Cancer* 2001;1:99–108.
12. Nagasubramanian R, Innocenti F, Ratain MJ. Pharmacogenetics in cancer treatment. *Annu Rev Med* 2003; 54:437–452.
13. Weinshilboum R. Methyltransferase pharmacogenetics. *Pharmacol Ther* 1989;43:77.
14. Paterson ARP, Tidd DM. 6-Thiopurines. In: Sartorelli AC, John DG, eds. *Antineoplastic and immunosuppressive agents II*. New York: Springer Verlag, 1975:384.
15. Lennard L. The clinical pharmacology of 6-mercaptopurine. *Eur J Clin Pharmacol* 1992;43:329.
16. Relling MV, Hancock ML, Boyett JM, et al. Prognostic importance of 6-mercaptopurine dose intensity in acute lymphoblastic leukemia. *Blood* 1999;93:2817.
17. Mcleod HL, Coulthard S, Thomas AE, et al. Analysis of thiopurine methyltransferase variant alleles in childhood acute lymphoblastic leukaemia. *Br J Haematol* 1999;105:696.
18. McLeod HL, Chokkalingam S. The thiopurine S-methyltransferase gene locus—implications for clinical pharmacogenomics. *Pharmacogenomics* 2002; 3:89.
19. Remy CN. Metabolism of thiopyrimidines and thiop-

urines: S-methylation with S-adenosylmethionine transmethylase and catabolism in mammalian tissue. *J Biol Chem* 1963;238:1078.

20. Woodson LC, Weinshilboum RM. Human kidney thiopurine methyltransferase: purification and biochemical properties. *Biochem Pharmacol* 1983;32: 819.

21. Krynetski EY, Evans WE. Pharmacogenetics as a molecular basis for individualized drug therapy: the thiopurine S-methyltransferase paradigm. *Pharm Res* 1999;16:342–349.

22. Krynetski EY, Tai HL, Yates CR, et al. Genetic polymorphism of thiopurine S-methyltransferase: clinical importance and molecular mechanisms. *Pharmacogenetics* 1996;6:279.

23. Lennard L, Maddocks J. Assay of 6-thioguanine nucleotide, a major metabolite of azathioprine, 6-mercaptopurine and 6-thioguanine, in human red blood cells. *J Pharm Pharmacol* 1983;35:15.

24. Weinshilboum RM, Sladek SL. Mercaptopurine pharmacogenetics: monogenic inheritance of erythrocyte thiopurine methyltransferase activity. *Am J Hum Genet* 1980;32:651.

25. McLeod HL, Relling MV, Liu Q, et al. Polymorphic thiopurine methyl-transferase in erythrocytes is indicative of activity in leukemic blasts from children with acute lymphoblastic leukemia. *Blood* 1995;85: 1897.

26. Dervieux T, Blanco JG, Krynetski EY, et al. Differing contribution of thiopurine methyltransferase to mercaptopurine versus thioguanine effects in human leukemic cells. *Cancer Res* 2001;61:5810.

27. McLeod HL, Evans W. Pharmacogenomics: unlocking the human genome for better drug therapy. *Annu Rev Pharmacol Toxicol* 2001;41:101.

28. Lennard L, Rees CA, Lilleyman JS, et al. Childhood leukemia: a relationship between intracellular 6-mercaptopurine metabolites and neutropenia. *Br J Clin Pharmacol* 1983;16:359.

29. Evans WE, Horner M, Chu YQ, et al. Altered mercaptopurine metabolism, toxic effects and dosage requirement in a thiopurine methyltransferase-deficient child with acute lymphocytic leukemia. *J Pediatr* 1991;119: 985–989.

30. Lennard L, Gibson BE, Nicole T, et al. Congenital thiopurine methyltransferase deficiency and 6-mercaptopurine toxicity during treatment for acute lymphocytic leukemia. *Arch Dis Child* 1993;69:577–579.

31. Lennard L, Van Loon JA, Weinshilboum RM. Pharmacogenetics of acute azathioprine toxicity; relationship to thiopurine methyltransferase genetic polymorphism. *Clin Pharmacol Ther* 1989;46:149–154.

32. Schutz E, Gummert J, Mohr F, et al. Azathioprine-induced myelosuppression in thiopurine methyltransferase deficient heart transplant recipient. *Lancet* 1993;341:436.

33. Relling MV, Hancock HL, Rivera GK, et al. Intolerance to mercaptopurine therapy related to heterozygosity at the thiopurine methyltransferase gene locus. *J Nat Cancer Inst* 1999;91:2001.

34. Relling MV, Yanishevski Y, Nemec J, et al. Etoposide and antimetabolite pharmacology in patients who develop secondary acute myeloid leukemia. *Leukemia* 1998;12:346.

35. Bo J, Schroder H, Kristinsson J, et al. Possible car-

cinogenic effect of 6-MP on bone marrow stem cells: relation to thiopurine metabolism. *Cancer* 1999;86: 1080.

36. Relling MV, Rubnitz JE, Rivera GK, et al. High incidence of secondary brain tumors after radiotherapy and antimetabolites. *Lancet* 1999;354:34.

37. Black AJ, Mcleod HL, Capell HA, et al. Thiopurine methyltransferase genotype predicts therapy-limiting severe toxicity from azathioprine. *Ann Intern Med* 1998;129:716.

38. Ishioka S, Hiyama K, Sato H, et al. Thiopurine methyltransferase genotype and the toxicity of azathioprine in Japanese. *Intern Med* 1999;38:944.

39. Naughton MA, Battaglia E, O'Brien S, et al. Identification of thiopurine methyltransferase (TPMT) polymorphisms cannot predict myelosuppression in systemic lupus erythematosus patients taking azathioprine. *Rheumatology (Oxford)* 1999;38:640.40.

40. Lennard L, Lilleyman JS, Van Loon J, et al. Genetic variation in response to 6-mercaptopurine for childhood acute lymphoblastic leukaemia. *Lancet* 1990; 336:225–229.

41. Elion GB. Biochemistry and pharmacology of purine analogues. *Fed Proc* 1967;26:898.42.

42. Weinshilboum RM, Raymond FA, Pazmino PA. Human erythrocyte thiopurine methyltransferase: radiochemical microassay and biochemical properties. *Clin Chim Acta* 1978;85:323.

43. Van Loon JA, Weinshilboum RM. Thiopurine methyltransferase biochemical genetics: human lymphocyte activity. *Biochem Genet* 1982;20:637.

44. Woodson LC, Dunnette JH, Weinshilboum RM. Pharmacogenetics of human thiopurine methyltransferase: kidney-erythrocyte correlation and immunotitration studies. *J Pharmacol Exp Ther* 1982;222:174.

45. Szumlanski CL, Honchel R, Scott MC, et al. Human liver thiopurine methyltransferase pharmacogenetics: biochemical properties, liver-erythrocyte correlation and presence of isozymes. *Pharmacogenetics* 1992; 2:148.

46. Weinshilboum RM, Otterness DM, Szumlanski CL. Methylation pharmacogenetics: catechol O-methyltransferase, thiopurine methyltransferase, and histamine N-methyltransferase. *Annu Rev Pharmacol Toxicol* 1999;39:19.

47. McLeod HL, Miller DR, Evans WE. Azathioprine induced myelosuppression in thiopurine methyltransferase deficient heart transplant recipient. *Lancet* 1993;341:1151.

48. Lennard L, Van Loon JA, Lilleyman JS, et al. Thiopurine pharmacogenetics in leukemia: correlation of erythrocyte thiopurine methyltransferase activity and 6-thioguanine nucleotide concentrations. *Clin Pharmacol Ther* 1987;41:18.

49. Thiopurine methyltransferase measurement. *Mayo Foundation Lab Med Bull* 1991;14:1.

50. Lennard L, Lilleyman JS. Individualizing therapy with 6-mercaptopurine and 6-t thioguanine related to the thiopurine methyltransferase genetic polymorphism. *Ther Drug Monit* 1996;18:328–334.

51. Lennard L, Keen D, Lilleyman JS. Oral 6-mercaptopurine in childhood leukemia: parent drug pharmacokinetics and active metabolite concentrations. *Clin Pharmacol Ther* 1986;40:287–292.

52. Woodson LC, Ames MM, Selassie CD, et al. Thiop-

urine methyltransferase: aromatic thiol substrates and inhibition by benzoic acid derivatives. *Mol Pharmacol* 1983;24:471.

53. Ames MM, Selassie CD, Woodson LC, et al. Thiopurine methyltransferase: structure-activity relationships for benzoic acid inhibitors and thiophenol substrates. *J Med Chem* 1986;29:354.

54. Lewis LD, Benin A, Szumlanski C, et al. Olsalazine and 6-mercaptopurine-related hematologic suppression: a possible drug-drug interaction. *Clin Pharmacol Ther* 1997;62:464.

55. Griffin MG, Miner PB. Conventional drug therapy in inflammatory bowel disease. *Gastroenterol Clin North Am* 1995;24:509.

56. Hanauer SB. Drug therapy: inflammatory bowel disease. *N Engl J Med* 1996;334:841.

57. Szumlanski C, Weinshilboum RM. Sulphasalazine inhibition of thiopurine methyltransferase: possible mechanism for interaction with 6-mercaptopurine and azathioprine. *Br J Clin Pharmacol* 1995;39:456.

58. Van Loon JA, Szumlanski CL, Weinshilboum RM. Human kidney thiopurine methyltransferase: photoaffinity labeling with S-adenosyl-L-methionine. *Biochem Pharmacol* 1992;44:775.

59. Honchel R, Aksoy I, Szumlanski C, et al. Human thiopurine methyltransferase: molecular cloning and expression of T84 colon carcinoma cell cDNA. *Mol Pharmacol* 1993;43:878.

60. Lee D, Szumlanski C, Houtman J, et al Thiopurine methyltransferase pharmacogenetics: cloning of human liver cDNA and presence of a processed pseudogene on human chromosome 18q21.1. *Drug Metab Dispos* 1995;23:398.

61. Weinshilboum RM. Thiopurine pharmacogenetics: clinical and molecular studies of thiopurine methyltransferase. *Drug Metab Dispos* 2001;29:601.

62. McLeod HL, Krynetski EY, Relling MV, et al. Genetic polymorphism of thiopurine methyltransferase and its clinical relevance for childhood acute lymphoblastic leukemia. *Leukemia* 2000;14:567.

63. Szumlanski C, Otterness D, Her C, et al. Thiopurine methyltransferase pharmacogenetics: human gene cloning and characterization of a common polymorphism. *DNA Cell Biol* 1996;15:17.

64. Tai H-L, Krynetski EY, Schuetz EG, et al. Enhanced proteolysis of thiopurine methyltransferase (TPMT) encoded by mutant alleles in humans (TPMT*3A, TPMT*2): mechanisms for the genetic polymorphism of TPMT activity. *Proc Natl Acad Sci USA* 1997; 94:6444.

65. Krynetski EY, Schuetz JD, Galpin AJ, et al. A single point mutation leading to loss of catalytic activity in human thiopurine methyltransferase. *Proc Natl Acad Sci USA* 1995;92:949.

66. Otterness D, Szumlanski C, Lennard L, et al. Human thiopurine methyl-transferase pharmacogenetics: gene sequence polymorphisms. *Clin Pharmacol Ther* 1997; 62:60.

67. Yates CR, Krynetski EY, Loennechen T, et al. Molecular diagnosis of thiopurine S-methyltransferase deficiency: genetic basis for azathioprine and mercaptopurine intolerance. *Ann Intern Med* 1997;126:608.

68. Tai HL, Krynetski EY, Yates CR, et al. Thiopurine S-methyltransferase deficiency: two nucleotide transitions define the most prevalent mutant allele associated with loss of catalytic activity in Caucasians. *Am J Hum Genet* 1993;58:694.

69. Delamoureyre CSV, Debuysere H, Sabbagh N, et al. Detection of known and new mutations in the thiopurine S-methyltransferase gene by single-strand conformation polymorphism analysis. *Hum Mutat* 1998; 12:177.

70. Otterness DM, Szumlanski CL, Wood TC, et al. Human thiopurine methyltransferase pharmacogenetics—kindred with a terminal exon splice junction mutation that results in loss of activity *J Clin Invest* 1998; 101:1036.

71. Tai HL, Fessing MY, Bonten EJ, et al. Enhanced proteasomal degradation of mutant human thiopurine S-methyltransferase (TPMT) in mammalian cells: mechanism for TPMT protein deficiency inherited by TPMT*2, TPMT*3A, TPMT*3B or TPMT*3C. *Pharmacogenetics* 1999;9:641.

72. Loennechen T, Yates CR, Fessing MY, et al. Isolation of a human thiopurine S-methyltransferase (TPMT) complementary DNA with a single nucleotide transition A719G (TPMT*3C) and its association with loss of TPMT protein and catalytic activity in humans. *Clin Pharmacol Ther* 1998;64:46.

73. Hon YY, Fessing MY, Pui CH, et al. Polymorphism of the thiopurine S-methyltransferase gene in African-Americans. *Hum Mol Genet* 1999;8:371.

74. Schaeffeler E, Lang T, Zanger UM, et al. M. High-throughput genotyping of thiopurine S-methyltransferase by denaturing HPLC. *Clin Chem* 2001;47:548.

75. Vuchetich JP, Weinshilboum RM, Price RA. Segregation analysis of human red blood cell (RBC) thiopurine methyltransferase (TPMT) activity. *Genet Epidemiol* 1995;12:1.

76. Spire VMC, Debuysere H, Mastain B, et al. Genotypic and phenotypic analysis of the polymorphic thiopurine S-methyl transferase (TPMT) gene in a European population. *Br J Pharmacol* 1998;125:879.

77. Fessing MY, Kreynetski EY, Zambetti GP, et al. Functional characterization of the human thiopurine S-methyltransferase gene promoter. *Pharmacogenetics* 1999;9:189.

78. Spire VMC, Debuysere H, Fizio F, et al. Characterization of a variable number tandem repeat region in the thiopurine S-methyltransferase gene promoter. *Pharmacogenetics* 1999;9:189.

79. Yan L, Zhang S, Eiff B, et al. Thiopurine methyltransferase (TPMT) promoter variable number tandem repeat (VNTR) polymorphism: genotype-phenotype correlation analysis for 1211 patients. *Clin Pharmacol Ther* 2000;68:210.

80. Alves S, Amorim A, Ferreira F, et al. Influence of the variable number of tandem repeats in the promoter region of the thiopurine methyltransferase gene on the enzymatic activity. *Clin Pharmacol Ther* 2001;70:165.

81. Kroplin T, Weyer N, Gutsche S, et al. Thiopurine S-methyltransferase activity in human erythrocytes: a new HPLC method using 6-thioguanine as substrate. *Eur J Clin Pharmacol* 1998;54:265.

82. Kroplin T, Fischer C, Iven H. Inhibition of thiopurine S-methyltransferase activity by impurities in commercially available substrates: a factor for differing results of TPMT measurements. *Eur J Clin Pharmacol* 1999; 55:285.

83. Lilleyman JS, Lennard L. Mercaptopurine metabolism

and risk of relapse in childhood lymphoblastic leukaemia. *Lancet* 1994;343:1188–1190.

84. Coulthard SA, Howell C, Robson J, et al. The relationship between thiopurine methyltransferase activity and genotype in blasts from patients with acute leukemia. *Blood* 1998;92:2856.

85. Collieduguid ESR, Prichard SC, Powrie RH, et al. The frequency and distribution of thiopurine methyltransferase alleles in Caucasian and Asian populations. *Pharmacogenetics* 1999;9:37.

86. McLeod HL, Pritchard SC, Githanga J, et al. Ethnic differences in thiopurine methyltransferase pharmacogenetics: evidence for allele specificity in Caucasian and Kenyan subjects. *Pharmacogenetics* 1999;9:773.

87. Delamoureyre CSV, Debuysere H, Mastain B, et al. Genotypic and phenotypic analysis of the polymorphic thiopurine S-methyltransferase gene (TPMT) in a European population. *Br J Pharmacol* 1998;125:879.

88. Ameyaw MM, Collieduguid ESR, Powrie RH, et al. Thiopurine methyltransferase alleles in British and Ghanaian populations. *Hum Mol Genet* 1999;8:367.

89. Collie-Duguid ESR, Pritchard SC, Powrie RH, et al. The frequency and distribution of thiopurine methyltransferase alleles in Caucasian and Asian populations. *Pharmacogenetics* 1998;9:37.

90. McLeod HL, Lin JS, Scott EP, et al. Thiopurine methyltransferase activity in American white subjects and black subjects. *Clin Pharmacol Ther* 1994;55:15.

91. Anstey A, Lennard L, Mayou SC, et al. Pancytopenia related to azathioprine—an enzyme deficiency caused by a common genetic polymorphism: a review. *J R Soc Med* 1992;85:752–756.

92. Kerstens PJSM, Stolk JN, De Abreu RA, et al. Azathioprine-related bone marrow toxicity and low activities of purine enzymes in patients with rheumatoid arthritis. *Arthritis Rheum* 1995;38:142.

93. Ari ZB, Mehta A, Lennard L, et al. Azathioprine-induced myelosuppression due to thiopurine methyltransferase deficiency in a patient with autoimmune hepatitis. *J Hepatol* 1995;23:351.

94. Escousse A, Mousson C, Santona L, et al. Azathioprine-induced pancytopenia in homozygous thiopurine methyltransferase-deficient renal transplant recipients: a family study. *Transplant Proc* 1995;27:1739.

95. Kumagai K, Hiyama K, Ishioka S, et al. Allelotype frequency of the thiopurine methyltransferase gene in Japanese. *Pharmacogenetics* 2001;11:275.

96. Hongeng S, Sasanakul W, Chuansumrit A, et al. Frequency of thiopurine S-methyltransferase genetic variation in Thai children with acute leukemia. *Med Pediatr Oncol* 2000;35:410.

97. Hall A, Hamilton P, Minto L, et al. The use of denaturing high-pressure liquid chromatography for the detection of mutations in thiopurine methyltransferase. *J Biochem Biophys Methods* 2001;47:65.

98. Scrip's cancer chemotherapy report. In: *Scrip World Pharmaceutical News*. London: PJB Publications, 2002.

99. Diasio RB, Lu Z, Zhang R, et al. Fluoropyrimidine catabolism. In: Muggia FM, ed. *Concepts, mechanisms, and new targets for chemotherapy*. Boston: Kluwer Academic Publishers, 1995:71–94.

100. Lu Z-H, Zhang R, Diasio RB. Purification and characterization of dihydropyrimidine dehydrogenase from human liver. *J Biol Chem* 1992;267:17102–17109.

101. Sommadossi JP, Gewirtz DA, Diasio Rbet, et al. Rapid catabolism of 5-fluorouracil in freshly isolated rat hepatocytes as analyzed by high performance liquid chromatography. *J Biol Chem* 1982;257:8171–8176.

102. Heggie GD, Sommadossi JP, Cross DS, et al. Clinical pharmacokinetics of 5-fluorouracil and its metabolites in plasma, urine, and bile. *Cancer Res* 1987;47: 2203–2206.

103. Sweeny DJ, Diasio RB. Toxicity of antimetabolites. In: Powis G, Hacker MP, eds. *Mechanisms of toxicity of anticancer drugs: a study in human toxicity*. New York: Macmillan, 1991.

104. Daher GC, Harris BE, Diasio RB. Metabolism of pyrimidine analogues and their nucleosides. In: *The international encyclopedia of pharmacology and therapeutics, vol. 1*. Oxford: Pergamon Press 1994.

105. Harris BE, Carpenter JT, Diasio RB. Severe 5-fluorouracil toxicity secondary to dihydropyrimidine dehydrogenase deficiency: a potentially more common pharmacogenetic syndrome. *Cancer* 1991;68: 499–501.

106. Takimoto CH, Lu Z-H, Zhang R, et al. Severe neurotoxicity following 5-fluorouracil-based chemotherapy in a patient with dihydropyrimidine dehydrogenase deficiency. *Clin Cancer Res* 1996;2:477–481.

107. Morrison GB, Bastian A, Dela Rosa T, et al. Dihydropyrimidine dehydrogenase (DPD) deficiency: a pharmacogenetic defect causing severe adverse reactions to 5-fluorouracil-based chemotherapy. *Oncol Nurs Forum* 1997;24:83–88.

108. Johnson MR, Wang K, Diasio RB. Profound dihydropyrimidine dehydrogenase (DPD) deficiency resulting from a novel compound heterozygote genotype. *Clin Cancer Res* 2002;8:768–774.

109. Johnson MR, Yan J, Shao L, et al. Semi-automated radioassay for determination of dihydropyrimidine dehydrogenase (DPD) activity. Screening cancer patients for DPD deficiency, a condition associated with 5-fluorouracil toxicity. *J Chromatogr B Biomed Sci Appl* 1997;696:183–191.

110. Tuchman M, Stoeckeler JS, Kiang DT, et al. Familial pyrimidinemia and pyrimidinuria associated with severe fluorouracil toxicity. *N Engl J Med* 1985;313: 245–249.

111. Diasio RB, Harris BE. Clinical pharmacology of 5-fluorouracil. *Clin Pharmacokinet* 1989;16:215–237.

112. Lu Z, Zhang R, Diasio RB. Comparison of dihydropyrimidine dehydrogenase from human, rat, pig and cow liver: biochemical and immunological properties. *Biochem Pharmacol* 1993;46:945–952.

113. Yokota H, Fernandez-Salguero P, Furuya H, et al. cDNA cloning and chromosome mapping of human dihydropyrimidine dehydrogenase, an enzyme associated with 5-fluorouracil toxicity and congenital thymine uraciluria. *J Biol Chem* 1994;269: 23192–23196.

114. Albin N, Johnson MR, Diasio RB. cDNA cloning of bovine liver dihydropyrimidine dehydrogenase. *DNA Sequence* 1996;6:231–238.

115. Mattison LK, Johnson MR, Diasio RB. A comparative analysis of translated dihydropyrimidine dehydrogenase (DPD) cDNA; conservation of functional domains and relevance to genetic polymorphisms. *Pharmacogenetics* 2002;12:133–144.

116. Dobritzsch D, Schneider G, Schnackerz KD, et al. Crystal structure of dihydropyrimidine dehydrogenase, a major determinant of the pharmacokinetics of the

anti-cancer drug 5-fluorouracil. *EMBO J* 2001;20: 650–660.

117. Dobritzsch D, Ricagno S, Schneider G, et al. Crystal structure of the productive ternary complex of dihydropyrimidine dehydrogenase with NADPH and 5-iodouracil. Implications for mechanism of inhibition and electron transfer. *J Biol Chem* 2002;277: 13155–13166.

118. Takai S, Fernandez-Salguero P, Kimura S, et al. Assignment of the human dihydropyrimidine dehydrogenase gene (DPYD) to chromosome region 1p22 by fluorescence in situ hybridization. *Genomics* 1994;24: 613–614.

119. Johnson MJ, Wang K, Tillmanns S, et al. Structural organization of the human dihydropyrimidine dehydrogenase gene. *Cancer Res* 1997;57:1660–1663.

120. Wei X, Elizondo G, Sapone A, et al. Characterization of the human dihydropyrimidine dehydrogenase gene. *Genomics* 1998;51:391–400.

121. Shestopol SA, Johnson MR, Diasio RB. Molecular cloning and characterization of the human dihydropyrimidine dehydrogenase promoter. *Biochim Biophys Acta* 2000;1494:162–169.

122. Wei X, McLeod HL, McMurrough J, et al. Molecular basis of the human dihydropyrimidine dehydrogenase deficiency and 5-fluorouracil toxicity. *J Clin Invest* 1996;98:610–615.

123. McLeod HL, Collie-Duguid ES, Vreken P, et al. Nomenclature for human DPYD alleles. *Pharmacogenetics* 1998;8:455–459.

124. Gardiner SJ, Begg EJ, Robinson BA. The effect of dihydropyrimidine dehydrogenase deficiency on outcomes with fluorouracil. *Adverse Drug React Toxicol Rev* 2002;21:1–16.

125. Johnson MJ, Hageboutros A, Wang K, et al. Life-threatening toxicity in a dihydropyrimidine dehydrogenase deficient patient following treatment with topical 5-fluorouracil. *Clin Cancer Res* 1999;5: 2006–2011.

126. Van Kuilenburg AB, Vreken P, Abeling NG, et al. Genotype and phenotype in patients with dihydropyrimidine dehydrogenase deficiency. *Hum Genet* 1999;104:1–9.

127. Johnson MR, Diasio RB. Importance of dihydropyrimidine dehydrogenase (DPD) deficiency in patients exhibiting toxicity following treatment with 5-fluorouracil. *Adv Enzyme Regul* 2001;41:151–157.

128. Raida M, Schwabe W, Häusler P, et al. Prevalence of a common point mutation in the dihydropyrimidine dehydrogenase (DPD) gene within the 5′-splice donor site of intron 14 in patients with severe 5-fluorouracil (5-FU)-related toxicity compared with controls. *Clin Cancer Res* 2001;7:2832–2839.

129. Kouwaki M, Hamajima N, Sumi S, et al. Identification of novel mutations in the dihydropyrimidine dehydrogenase gene in a Japanese patient with 5-fluorouracil toxicity. *Clin Cancer Res* 1998;4:2999–3004.

130. Yamaguchi K, Arai Y, Kanda Y, et al. Germline mutation of dihydropyrimidine dehydrogenase gene among a Japanese population in relation to toxicity to 5-fluorouracil. *Jpn J Cancer Res* 2001;92:337–342.

131. Collie-Duguid ES, Etienne MC, Milano G, McLeod HL. Known variant DPYD alleles do not explain DPD deficiency in cancer patients. *Pharmacogenetics* 2000; 10:217–223.

132. Van Kuilenburg ABP, Haasjes J, Richel DJ, et al.

Clinical implications of dihydropyrimidine dehydrogenase (DPD) deficiency in patients with severe 5-fluorouracil-associated toxicity: identification of new mutations in the DPD gene. *Clin Cancer Res* 2000;6: 4705–4712.

133. Vreken P, Van Kuilenburg A, Meinsma R, et al. Dihydropyrimidine dehydrogenase (DPD) deficiency: identification and expression of missense mutations C29R, R886H and R235W. *Hum Genet* 1997;101:333–338.

134. Van Kuilenburg ABP, Dobritzsch D, Meinsma R, et al. Novel disease-causing mutations in the dihydropyrimidine dehydrogenase gene interpreted by analysis of the three-dimensional protein structure. *Biochem J* 2002;364:157–163.

135. Vreken P, van Kuilenburg AB, Meinsma R, et al. Dihydropyrimidine dehydrogenase deficiency. Identification of two novel mutations and expression of missense mutations in E. coli. *Adv Exp Med Biol* 1998;431:341–346.

136. Meinsma R, Fernandez-Salguero P, Van Kuilenburg AB, et al. Human polymorphism in drug metabolism: mutation in the dihydropyrimidine dehydrogenase gene results in exon skipping and thymine uraciluria. *DNA Cell Biol* 1995;14:1–6.

137. Gross E, Neubauer S, Seck K, et al. High-throughput mutation screening of the DPYD gene by denaturing HPLC. *Proc Am Assoc Cancer Res* 2002;43:322A.

138. Ridge SA, Sludden J, Wei X, et al. Dihydropyrimidine dehydrogenase pharmacogenetics in patients with colorectal cancer. *Br J Cancer* 1998;77:497–500.

139. Ridge SA, Sludden J, Brown O, et al. Dihydropyrimidine dehydrogenase pharmacogenetics in Caucasian subjects. *Br J Clin Pharmacol* 1998;2:151–156.

140. van Kuilenburg AB, Vreken P, Beex LV, et al. Severe 5-fluorouracil toxicity caused by reduced dihydropyrimidine dehydrogenase activity due to heterozygosity for a G→A point mutation. *J Inherit Metab Dis* 1998;21:280–284.

141. Christensen E, Cezanne I, Kjaergaard S, et al. Clinical variability in three Danish patients with dihydropyrimidine dehydrogenase deficiency all homozygous for the same mutation. *J Inherit Metab Dis* 1998;21: 272–275.

142. Vreken P, Van Kuilenburg A, Meinsma R, et al. Identification of novel point mutations in the dihydropyrimidine dehydrogenase gene. *J Inherit Metab Dis* 1997;20:335–338.

143. Albin N, Johnson MR, Shahinian H, et al. Initial characterization of the molecular defect in human dihydropyrimidine dehydrogenase deficiency. *Proc Am Assoc Cancer Res* 1995;36:211A.

144. Lu Z, Zhang R, Diasio RB. Dihydropyrimidine dehydrogenase activity in human peripheral blood mononuclear cells and liver: population characteristics, newly identified patients, and clinical implication in 5-fluorouracil chemotherapy. *Cancer Res* 1993;53: 5433–5438.

145. Milano G, Etienne MC, Cassuto-Viguier E, et al. Influence of sex and age on fluorouracil clearance. *J Clin Oncol* 1992;10:1171–1175.

146. Fleming RA, Milano GA, Gaspard MH, et al. Dihydropyrimidine dehydrogenase activity in cancer patients. *Eur J Cancer* 1993;29A:740–744.

147. Fleming RA, Milano G, Thyss A, et al. Correlation between dihydropyrimidine dehydrogenase activity in peripheral mononuclear cells and systemic clearance

of fluorouracil in cancer patients. *Cancer Res* 1992;52: 2899–2902.

148. Lu Z, Zhang R, Diasio RB. Dihydropyrimidine dehydrogenase activity in human liver: population characteristics and clinical implication in 5-FU chemotherapy. *Clin Pharmacol Ther* 1995;58: 512–522.

149. Lu Z, Zhang R, Carpenter JT, et al. Decreased dihydropyrimidine dehydrogenase activity in population of patients with breast cancer: implications for 5-FU-based chemotherapy. *Clin Cancer Res* 1998;4: 325–329.

150. Vreken P, van Kuilenburg AB, Meinsma R, et al. Dihydropyrimidine dehydrogenase deficiency: a novel mutation and expression of missense mutations in E. coli. *J Inherit Metab Dis* 1998;21:276–279.

151. Diasio RB, Van Kuilenburg AB, Lu Z, et al. Determination of dihydropyrimidine dehydrogenase (DPD) in fibroblasts of a DPD deficient pediatric patient and family members using a polyclonal antibody to human DPD. *Adv Exp Med Biol* 1994;370:7–10.

152. Ezzeldin H, Johnson MR, Okamoto Y, et al. High performance liquid chromatography (DHPLC) analysis of the DPYD gene in patients with lethal 5-fluorouracil (5-FU) toxicity; multiple heterozygote sequence variations demonstrate a complicated DPYD genotype. *Clin Cancer Res* 2003 (in press).

153. Mattison LK, Carpenter M, Wang YH, et al. Rapid identification of dihydropyrimidine dehydrogenase (DPD) deficiency by a novel uracil breath test (UBT). ASCO 2003. In: Proceedings of the 39th Annual Meeting of the American Society of Clinical Oncology 2003 (A494).

154. Ezzeldin H, OkamotoY, Johnson MR, et al. A high-throughput denaturing high-performance liquid chromatography method for the identification of variant alleles associated with dihydropyrimidine dehydrogenase deficiency. *Ann Biochem* 2002;306: 63–73.

155. Iyer L, Hall D, Das S, et al. Phenotype-genotype correlation of in vitro SN-38 (active metabolite of irinotecan) and bilirubin glucuronidation in human liver tissue with UGT1A1 promoter polymorphism. *Clin Pharmacol Ther* 1999;65:576–582.

156. Diasio RB, Johnson MR. The importance of pharmacogenetics/ pharmacogenomics for the cancer chemotherapy drug 5-fluorouracil. *Pharmacology* 2000;61:199–203.

157. Dutton GJ, ed. *Glucuronidation of drugs and other compounds*. Boca Raton, FL: CRC Press, 1980.

158. Scriver RC, Beaudet AL, Valle D, et al., eds. *The metabolic and molecular bases of inherited disease*, 8th ed. New York: McGraw-Hill Book Company, 2001:3063–3101.

159. Coffman BL, Rios GR, King CD, et al. Human UGT2B7 catalyzes morphine glucuronidation. *Drug Metab Dispos* 1997;25:1–4.

160. Bock KW, Lilienblum W, von Bahr C. Studies of UDP-glucuronyltransferase activities in human liver microsomes. *Drug Metab Dispos* 1984;12:93–97.

161. de Wildt SN, Kearns GL, Leeder JS, et al. Glucuronidation in humans. Pharmacogenetic and developmental aspects. *Clin Pharmacokinet* 1999;36: 439–452.

162. Strassburg CP, Nguyen N, Manns MP, et al. UDP-glu-curonosyltransferase activity in human liver and colon. *Gastroenterology* 1999;116:149–160.

163. Green MD, King CD, Mojarrabi B, et al. Glucuronidation of amines and other xenobiotics catalyzed by expressed human UDP-glucuronosyltransferase 1A3. *Drug Metab Dispos* 1998;26:507–512.

164. Strassburg CP, Manns MP, Tukey RH. Expression of the UDP-glucuronosyltransferase 1A locus in human colon. Identification and characterization of the novel extrahepatic UGT1A8. *J Biol Chem* 1998;273:8719–8726.

165. Belanger A, Hum DW, Beaulieu M, et al. Characterization and regulation of UDP glucuronosyltransferases in steroid target tissues. *J Steroid Biochem Mol Biol* 1998;65:301–310.

166. Strassburg CP, Kneip S, Topp J, et al. Polymorphic gene expression and interindividual variation of UDP-glucuronosyltransferase activity in human small intestine. *J Biol Chem* 2000;275:36164–36171.

167. Hum DW, Belanger A, Levesque E, et al. Characterization of UDP-glucuronosyltransferases active on steroid hormones. *J Steroid Biochem Mol Biol* 1999;69:413–423.

168. Strassburg CP, Barut A, Obermayer-Straub P, et al. Identification of cyclosporine A and tacrolimus glucuronidation in human liver and the gastrointestinal tract by a differentially expressed UDP-glucuronosyltransferase: UGT2B7. *J Hepatol* 2001;34:865–872.

169. Humerickhouse R, Lohrbach K, Li L, et al. Characterization of CPT-11 hydrolysis by human liver carboxylesterase isoforms hCE-1 and hCE-2. *Cancer Res* 2000;60:1189–1192.

170. Iyer L, Ratain MJ. Clinical pharmacology of camptothecins. *Cancer Chemother Pharmacol* 1998; 42[Suppl]:S31–S43.

171. Gupta E, Lestingi TM, Mick R, et al. Metabolic fate of irinotecan in humans: correlation of glucuronidation with diarrhea. *Cancer Res* 1994;54:3723–3725.

172. Araki E, Ishikawa M, Iigo M, et al. Relationship between development of diarrhea and the concentration of SN-38, an active metabolite of CPT-11, in the intestine and the blood plasma of athymic mice following intraperitoneal administration of CPT-11. *Jpn J Cancer Res* 1993;84:697–702.

173. Gupta E, Lestingi TM, Mick R, et al. Metabolic fate of irinotecan in humans: correlation of glucuronidation with diarrhea. *Cancer Res* 1994;54:3723–3725.

174. Miners JO, Mckinnon RA, Mackenzie PI. Genetic Polymorphism of UDP-glucuronosyltransferase and their functional significance. *Toxicology* 2002;181–182.

175. Bosma PJ, Seppen J, Goldhoorn B, et al. Bilirubin UDP-glucuronosyltransferase 1 is the only relevant bilirubin glucuronidating isoform in man. *J Biol Chem* 1994;269:17960–17964.

176. Bosma PJ, Chowdhury JR, Bakker C, et al. The genetic basis of the reduced expression of bilirubin UDP-glucuronosyltransferase 1 in Gilbert's syndrome. *N Engl J Med* 1995;333:1171–1175.

177. Burchell B, Hume R. Molecular genetic basis of Gilbert syndrome. *J Gastroenterol Hepatol* 1999;14: 960–966.

178. Crigler JF, Najjar VA. Congenital familial non-hemolytic jaundice with kernicterus. *Pediatrics* 1952;10:169–180.

179. Seppen J, Bosma PJ, Goldhoorn BG, et al. Discrimina-

tion between Crigler-Najjar type I and II by expression of mutant bilirubin uridine diphosphate glucuronosyltransferase. *J Clin Invest* 1994;94:2385–2391.

180. Gourley GR. Bilirubin metabolism and kernicterus. *Adv Pediatr* 1997;44:173–229.

181. Fox IJ, Roy Chowdhury J, Kaufman SS, et al. Treatment of Crigler-Najjar syndrome type I with hepatocyte transplantation. *N Engl J Med* 1998;338:1422–1426.

182. Roy Chowdhury J. Prospects of liver cell transplantation and liver-directed gene therapy. *Semin Liver Dis* 1999;19:1–6.

183. Fevery J, Blanckaert N, Heirwegh KP, et al. Unconjugated bilirubin and an increased proportion of bilirubin monoconjugates in the bile of patients with Gilbert's syndrome and Crigler-Najjar syndrome. *J Clin Invest* 1977;60:970–979.

184. Felsher BF, Rickard D, Redeker AG. The reciprocal relation between caloric intake and the degree of hyperbilirubinemia in Gilbert's syndrome. *N Engl J Med* 1970;283:170–172.

185. Monaghan G, McLellan A, McGeehan A, et al. Gilbert syndrome is a contributory factor in prolonged unconjugated hyperbilirubinemia of the newborn. *J Pediatr* 1999;134:441–446.

186. Negoro S, Fukuoka M, Masuda N, et al. Phase I study of weekly intravenous infusion of CPT-11, a new derivative of camptothecin, in the treatment of advanced non-small-cell lung cancer. *J Natl Cancer Inst* 1991;83:1164–1168.

187. Akabayashi, A. Questions raised over release of side-effects data in Japan. *Lancet* 1997;350:124.

188. Pharmaceuticals and Cosmetics Division, Pharmaceutical Affairs Bureau, Ministry of Health, and Welfare. *Summary Basis of Approval (SBA) No. 1 (revised edition): irinotecan hydrochloride.* Tokyo: Yakuji Nippo, 1996.

189. Rougier P, Van Cutsem E, Bajetta E, et al. Randomised trial of irinotecan versus fluorouracil by continuous infusion after fluorouracil failure in patients with metastatic colorectal cancer. *Lancet* 1998;352: 1407–1412.

190. Kudoh S, Fujiwara Y, Takada Y, et al., for the West Japan Lung Cancer Group. Phase II study of irinotecan combined with cisplatin in patients with previously untreated small-cell lung cancer. *J Clin Oncol* 1998;16: 1068–1674.

191. Masuda N, Fukuoka M, Negoro S, et al., and The CPT-11 Lung Cancer Study Group West. Randomized trial comparing cisplatin (CDDP) and irinotecan (CPT-11) versus CDDP and vindesine (VDS) versus CPT-11 alone in advanced non-small cell lung cancer (NSCLC), a multicenter phase III study. *Proc Am Soc Clin Oncol* 1999;18:459a.

192. Wasserman E, Myara A, Lokiec F, et al. Severe CPT-11 toxicity in patients with Gilbert's syndrome: two case reports. *Ann Oncol* 1997;8:1049–1051.

193. Gupta E, Mick R, Ramirez J, et al. Pharmacokinetic and pharmacodynamic evaluation of the topoisomerase inhibitor irinotecan in cancer patients. *J Clin Oncol* 1997;15:1502–1510.

194. Bock KW, Forster A, Gschaidmeier H, et al. Paracetamol glucuronidation by recombinant rat and human phenol UDP glucuronosyltransferases. *Biochem Pharmacol* 1993;45:1809–1814.

195. Kadakol A, Ghosh SS, Sappal BS, et al. Genetic lesions of bilirubin uridine-diphosphoglucuronate-glucuronosyltransferase (UGT1A1) causing Crigler-Najjar and Gilbert syndromes: correlation of genotype to phenotype. *Mutat Update* 1993:16:297–306.

196. Mackenzie PI., Owens IS, Burchell B, Bock KW, et al. The UDP glycosyltransferase gene superfamily: recommended nomenclature update based on evolutionary divergence. *Pharmacogenetics* 1997;7:255–269.

197. Ando Y, Saka H, Ando M, et al. Polymorphisms of UDP-glucuronosyltransferase gene and irinotecan toxicity: a pharmacogenetic analysis. *Cancer Res* 2000; 60:6921–6926.

198. Monaghan G, Ryan M, Seddon R, et al. Genetic variation in bilirubin UDP-glucuronosyltransferase gene promoter and Gilbert's syndrome. *Lancet* 1996;347: 578–581.

199. Ando Y, Chida M, Nakayama K, et al. The UGT1A1*28 allele is relatively rare in a Japanese population. *Pharmacogenetics* 1998;8:357–360.

200. Akaba K, Kimura T, Sasaki A, et al. Neonatal hyperbilirubinemia and mutation of the bilirubin uridine diphosphate-glucuronosyltransferase gene: a common missense mutation among Japanese, Koreans and Chinese. *Biochem Mol Biol Int* 1998;46:21–26.

201. Maruo Y, Nishizawa K, Sato H, et al. Association of neonatal hyperbilirubinemia with bilirubin UDP-glucuronosyltransferase polymorphism. *Pediatrics* 1999;103:1224–1227.

202. Ando Y, Saka H, Asai G, et al. UGT1A1 genotypes and glucuronidation of SN-38, the active metabolite of irinotecan. *Ann Oncol* 1998;9:845–847.

203. Iyer L, Das S, Janish L, et al. UGT1A1*28 polymorphism as a determinant of irinotecan disposition and toxicity. *Pharmacogenom J* 2002;2:43–47.

204. Iyer L, Janisch L, Das S, et al. UGT1A1 promoter genotype correlates with pharmacokinetics of irinotecan (CPT-11). *Proc Am Soc Clin Oncol* 2000;19: 178A(abst).

205. Gupta E, Ratain MJ. Camptothecin analogues: topotecan and irinotecan. In: Grochow LB, Ames M, eds. *A clinician's guide to chemotherapy pharmacokinetics and pharmacodynamics.* Baltimore: Williams & Wilkins 1998:435–457.

206. Bleiberg H, Cvitkovic E. Characterisation and clinical management of CPT-11 (irinotecan)-induced adverse events: the European perspective. *Eur J Cancer* 1996; 32A:S18–S23.

207. Wadler S, Benson AB III, Engelking C, et al. Recommended guidelines for the treatment of chemotherapy-induced diarrhea. *J Clin Oncol* 1998;16:3169–3178.

208. Slatter JG, Schaaf LJ, Sams JP, et al. Pharmacokinetics, metabolism, and excretion of irinotecan (CPT-11) following I.V. infusion of [(14)C]CPT-11 in cancer patients. *Drug Metab Dispos* 2000;28:423–433.

209. Santos A, Zanetta S, Cresteil T, et al. Metabolism of irinotecan (CPT-11) by CYP3A4 and CYP3A5 in humans. *Clin Cancer Res* 2000;6:2012–2020.

210. Chu XY, Kato Y, Ueda K, et al. Biliary excretion mechanism of CPT-11 and its metabolites in humans: involvement of primary active transporters. *Cancer Res* 1998;58:5137–5143.

211. Schellens JH, Maliepaard M, Scheper RJ, et al. Transport of topoisomerase I inhibitors by the breast cancer resistance protein: potential clinical implications. *Ann N Y Acad Sci* 2000;922:188–194.

212. Mathijssen RHJ, Verweij J, de Jonge MJA, et al. Impact of body-size measures on irinotecan clearance: alternative dosing recommendations. *J Clin Oncol* 2002;20:81–87.

213. Kadakol A, Siddhartha S, Ghosh, et al. Genetic lesions of bilirubin uridine-diphosphoglucuronate glucuronosyltransferase (UGT1A1) causing Crigler-Najjar and Gilbert syndromes: correlation of genotype to phenotype. *Hum Mutat* 2000;16:297–306.

214. Sokal EM, Silva ES, Hermans D, et al. Orthotopic liver transplantation for Crigler-Najjar type I disease in six children. *Transplantation* 1995;60:1095–1098.

215. Van der Veere CN, Sinaasappel M, McDonagh AF, et al. Current therapy for Crigler-Najjar syndrome type 1: report of a world registry. *Hepatology* 1996;24: 311–315.

216. Roy Chowdhury J, Roy Chowdhury N, Strom SC, et al. Human hepatocyte transplantation: gene therapy and more? *Pediatrics* 1998;102:647–648.

217. Roy Chowdhury J, Huang TJ, Kasari K, et al. Molecular basis for the lack of bilirubin-specific and 3-methylcholanthrene-inducible UDP-glucuronosyltransferase activities in Gunn rats: the two isoforms are encoded by distinct mRNA species that share an identical single base deletion. *J Biol Chem* 1991;266:18294–18298.

218. Kren BT, Parashar B, Bandhopadhyaya B, et al. Correction of UDP glucuronosyltransferase gene defect in Gunn rat model of Crigler-Najjar syndrome type I with a chimeric oligonucleotide. *Proc Natl Acad Sci USA* 1999;96:10349–10354.

219. Clarke DJ, Burchell B. The uridine diphosphate glucuronosyltransferases multigene family: function and regulation. Conjugation-deconjugation reactions in drug metabolism and toxicity. *Handbook Exp Pharmacol* 1994;25:1–4.

220. Mackenzie PI. The UDP glucuronosyltransferase multigene family. In: Hodgson E, Bend JR, Philpot RM, eds. *Reviews in biochemical toxicology.* Raleigh, NC: Toxicology Communications, 1995:29–72.

221. Tukey RH, Strassburg CP. Human UDP-glucuronosyltransferases: metabolism, expression and disease. *Annu Rev Pharmacol Toxicol* 2000;40:581–616.

222. Ritter JK, Chen F, Sheen YY, et al. A novel complex locus UGT1 encodes human bilirubin, phenol and other UDP-glucuronosyltransferase isozymes with identical carboxyl termini. *J Biol Chem* 1992;267: 3257–3261.

223. Gong QH, Cho JW, Huang T, et al. Thirteen UDP glucuronosyl-transferase genes are encoded at the human UGT1 gene complex locus. *Pharmacogenetics* 2001; 11:357–368.

224. Owens IS, Ritter JK. Gene structure of the human UGT1 locus creates diversity in isozyme structure, substrate specificity and regulation. *Prog Nucleic Acid Res Mol Biol* 1995;51:305–338.

225. Ritter JK, Chen F, Sheen YY, et al. A novel complex locus UGT1 encodes human bilirubin, phenol, and other UDP-glucuronosyltransferase isoenzymes with identical carboxy termini. *J Biol Chem* 1992;267: 3257–3261.

226. Bosma PJ, Roy Chowdhury N, Goldhoorn BG, et al. Sequence of exons and flanking regions of human bilirubin UDP glucuronosyltransferase gene complex and identification of a genetic mutation in a patient with Crigler-Najjar syndrome, type I. *Hepatology* 1992;15:941–947.

227. Mackenzie PI. Expression of chimeric cDNAs in cell culture defines a region of UDP glucuronosyltransferase involved in substrate selection. *J Biol Chem* 1990;265:3432–3435.

228. Innocenti F, Iyer L, Ratain M. Pharmacogenetics of anticancer agents: lessons from amonafide and irinotecan. *Drug Metab Dispos* 2001;29:596–600.

229. van Es HH, Bout A, Liu J, et al. Assignment of the human UDP glucuronosyltransferase gene (UGT1A1) to chromosome region 2q37. *Cytogenet Cell Genet* 1993;63:114–116.

230. Bosma P, Chowdhury J, Jansen P. Genetic inheritance of Gilbert's syndrome. *Lancet* 1995;346:314–315.

231. Guillemette C, De Vivo I, Hankinson S, et al. Association of genetic polymorphisms in UGT1A1 with breast cancer and plasma hormone levels. *Cancer Epidemiol Biomarkers Prev* 2001;10:711–714.

232. Beutler E, Gelbart T, Demina A, et al. Racial variability in the Udglucuronosyltransferase 1 (UGT1A1) promoter: a balanced polymorphism for regulation of bilirubin metabolism? *Proc Natl Acad Sci USA* 1998;95:8170–8174.

233. Lampe JW, Bigler J, Horner NK, et al. UDP-glucuronosyltransferase (UGT1A1*28 and UGT1A6*2) polymorphisms in Caucasians and Asians: relationships to serum bilirubin concentrations. *Pharmacogenetics* 1999;9:341–349.

234. Guillemette C, Millikan R, Newman B, et al. Genetic polymorphisms in UGT1A1 and association with breast cancer among African Americans. *Cancer Res* 2000;60:950–956.

235. Maruo Y, Sato H, Yamano T, et al. Gilbert's syndrome caused by homozygous missense mutation (Tyr486Asp) of bilirubin-UDP glucuronosyl transferase. *J Pediatr* 1998;132:1045–1047.

236. Koiwai O, Nishizawa M, Hasada K, et al. Gilbert's syndrome is caused by a heterozygous missense mutation in the gene for bilirubin UDPglucuronosyltransferase. *Hum Mol Genet* 1995;4:1183–1186.

237. Soeda Y, Yamamoto K, Adachi Y, et al. Predicted homozygous mis-sense mutation in Gilbert's syndrome. *Lancet* 1995;346:1494.

238. Jansen PLM, Bosma PJ, Roy Chowdhury J. Molecular biology of bilirubin metabolism. In: Boyer JL, Ockner RK, eds. *Progress in liver diseases.* Philadelphia: WB Saunders, 1995:125–150.

239. Ritter JK, Yeatman MT, Kaiser C, et al. Phenylalanine codon deletion at the UGT1 gene complex locus of a Crigler-Najjar type I patient generates a pH-sensitive bilirubin UDP-glucuronosyltransferase. *J Biol Chem* 1993;268:23573–23579.

240. Ciotti M, Cho JW, George J, et al. Required buried-helical structure in the bilirubin UDP-glucuronosyl transferase, UGT1A1, contains a non-replaceable phenylalanine. *Biochemistry* 1998;37:11018–11025.

241. Erps LT, Ritter JK, Hersh JH, et al. Identification of two single base substitution in the UGT1 gene locus which abolish bilirubin uridine diphosphate glucuronosyltransferase activity in vitro. *J Clin Invest* 1994;93:564–570.

242. Labrune P, Myara A, Hadchouel M, et al. Genetic heterogeneity of Crigler-Najjar syndrome type I: a study of 14 cases. *Hum Genet* 1994;94:693–700.

243. Bosma PJ, Roy Chowdhury J, Huang T-J, et al. Mechanisms of inherited deficiencies of multiple UDP-glu-

curonosyltransferase isoforms in two patients with Crigler-Najjar syndrome, type I. *FASEB J* 1992;6: 2859–2863.

244. Arias IM. Chronic unconjugated hyperbilirubinemia without overt signs of hemolysis in adolescents and adults. *J Clin Invest* 1962;41:2233–2245.

245. Arias IM, Gartner LM, Cohen M, et al. Chronic non-hemolytic unconjugated hyperbilirubinemia with glucuronosyl transferase deficiency: clinical, biochemical, pharmacologic, and genetic evidence for heterogeneity. *Am J Med* 1969;47:395–409.

246. Bosma PJ, Goldhoorn B, Oude Elferink RPJ, et al. A mutation in bilirubin uridine 5′-diphosphate-glucuronosyltransferase isoform-1 causing Crigler-Najjar syndrome type-II. *Gastroenterology* 1993;105: 216–220.

247. Seppen J, Steenken E, Lindhout D, et al. A mutation which disrupts the hydrophobic core of the signal peptide of bilirubin UDP-glucuronosyltransferase, an endoplasmic reticulum membrane protein, causes Crigler-Najjar type II. *FEBS Lett* 1996;390:294–298.

248. Moghrabi N, Clarke DJ, Boxer M, et al. Identification of an A-to-G missense mutation in exon 2 of the UGT1 gene complex that causes Crigler-Najjar syndrome type 2. *Genomics* 1993;18:171–173.

249. Gantla S, Bakker CTM, Deocharan B, et al. Splice-site mutations: a novel genetic mechanism for Crigler-Najjar syndrome type 1. *Am J Hum Genet* 1998;62: 585–592.

250. Ghosh SS, Sappal BS, Kalpana GV, et al. Homodimerization of human bilirubin-uridine diphosphoglucuronate glucuronosyltransferase-1 (UGT1A1) and its functional implications. *J Biol Chem* 2001;45: 42108–42115.

251. Meech R, Mackenzie PI. UDP-glucuronosyltransferase, the role of the amino terminus in dimerization. *J Biol Chem* 1997;272:26913–26917.

252. Bosma P, Chowdhury JR, Jansen PH. Genetic inheritance of Gilbert's syndrome. *Lancet* 1995;346: 314–315.

253. Nakabayashi H, Taketa K, Miyano K, et al. Growth of human hepatoma cell lines with differentiated functions in chemically defined medium. *Cancer Res* 1982;42,3858–3863.

254. Monaghan G, Foster B, Jurima-Romet M, et al. UGT1A1 genotyping in a Canadian Inuit population. *Pharmacogenetics* 1997;7:153–156.

255. Beutler E, Gelbart T, Demina A. Racial variability in the UDP glucuronosyltransferase 1 (UGT1A1) promoter: a balanced polymorphism for regulation of bilirubin metabolism? *Proc Natl Acad Sci USA* 1998;95:8170–8174.

256. Iyer L, Bergseth AC, Ybazeta G, et al. High variability in SN-38 glucuronidation in liver samples from African population as predicted by UGT1A1 genotypes. *Clin Pharmacol Ther* 1999;65:197(abst).

257. Akaba K, Kimura T, Sasaki A, et al. Neonatal hyperbilirubinemia and mutation of the bilirubin uridine diphosphate-glucuronosyltransferase gene: a common missense mutation among Japanese, Koreans and Chinese. *Biochem Mol Biol Int* 1998:46:21–26.

258. DiRienzo A, Hall D, Iyer L. Two new alleles in the promoter of the bilirubin UDP-glucuronosyl transferase 1 (UGT1A1) gene. *Clin Pharmacol Ther* 1998: 63:207.

259. Akaba K, Kimura T, Sasaki A, et al. Neonatal hyperbilirubinemia and a common mutation of the bilirubin uridine diphosphate-glucuronosyltransferase gene in Japanese. *J Hum Genet* 1999;44:22–25.

260. Ciotti M, Obaray R, Martin M, et al. Genetic disease at the UGT1 locus associated with Crigler-Najjar syndrome type-1 disease, including a prenatal diagnosis. *Am J Med Genet* 1997;68:173–178.

261. Jin CJ, Miners JO, Lillywhite KJ, et al. cDNA cloning and expression of two new members of the human liver UDP-glucuronosyltransferase 2B subfamily. *Biochem Biophys Res Commun* 1993;194:496–503.

262. Iyer L, King CD, Whittington PF, et al. Genetic predisposition to the metabolism of irinotecan (CPT-11). Role of uridine diphosphate glucuronosyltransferase isoform 1A1 in the glucuronidation of its active metabolite (SN-38) in liver microsomes. *J Clin Invest* 1998;101:847–854.

263. Hall D, Ybazeta G, Destro-Bisol G, et al. Variability at the uridine diphosphate glucuronosyltransferase 1A1 promoter in human populations and primates. *Pharmacogenetics* 1999;9:591–599.

264. Ingelman-Sundberg M, Oscarson M, McLellan RA. Polymorphic human cytochrome P450 enzymes: an opportunity for individualized drug treatment. *Trends Pharmacol Sci* 1999;20:342–349.

265. Boddy AV, Ratain MJ. Pharmacogenetics in cancer etiology and chemotherapy. *Clin Cancer Res* 1997;3: 1025–1030.

266. Rosatelli MC, Meloni A, Faa V, et al. Molecular analysis of patients with Sardinian descent with Crigler-Najjar syndrome type 1. *J Med Genet* 1997;34: 122–125.

267. Aono S, Yamada Y, Keino H, et al. A new type of defect in the gene for bilirubin uridine 5-diphosphate-glucuronosyltransferase in a patient with Crigler-Najjar syndrome type I. *Pediatr Res* 1994;35:629–632.

268. Ritter JK, Yeatman MT, Ferreira P, et al. Identification of a genetic alteration in the code for bilirubin UDPglucuronosyltransferase in the UGT1 gene complex of a Crigler-Najjar type 1 patient. *J Clin Invest* 1992;9: 150–155.

269. Ciotti M, Chen F, Rubatelli FF, et al. Coding and a TATA Box mutation at the bilirubin UDP-glucuronosyl transferase gene cause Crigler-Najjar syndrome type 1 disease. *Biochem Biophys Acta* 1998;1407: 40–50.

270. Moghrabi N, Clarke DJ, Burchell B, et al. Cosegregation of intragenic markers with a novel mutation that cause Crigler-Najjar syndrome type I: implication in carrier detection and prenatal diagnosis. *Am J Hum Genet* 1993;53:722–729.

271. Koiwai O, Aono S, Adachi Y, et al. Crigler-Najjar syndrome type II is inherited both as a dominant and as a recessive trait. *Hum Mol Genet* 1996;5:645–647.

272. Chalasani N, Roy Chowdhury N, Roy Chowdhury J, et al. Kernicterus in an adult who is heterozygous for Crigler-Najjar syndrome and homozygous for Gilbert-type genetic defect. *Gastroenterology* 1997;112: 2099–2103.

273. Aono S, Adachi Y, Uyama E, et al. Analysis of genes for bilirubin UDPglucuronosyltransferase in Gilbert's syndrome. *Lancet* 1995;345:958–959.

274. Aono S, Yamada Y, Keino H, et al. Identification of a

defect in the gene for bilirubin UDP-glucuronosyl-transferase in a patient with Crigler-Najjar syndrome type II. *Biochem Biophys Res Commun* 1993;197: 1239–1244.

275. Ulrich CM, Robien K, Sparks R. Pharmacogenetics and folate metabolism—a promising direction. *Pharmacogenomics* 2002;3:299–313.

276. Ulrich CM, Yasui Y, Storb R, et al. Pharmacogenetics of methotrexate: toxicity among marrow transplantation patients varies with the methylenetetrahydrofolate reductase C677T polymorphism. *Blood* 2001;98: 231–234.

277. Stevenson JP, Redlinger M, Kluijtmans LA, et al. Phase I clinical and pharmacogenetic trial of irinotecan and raltitrexed administered every 21 days to patients with cancer. *J Clin Oncol* 2001;19: 4081–4087.

278. Salonga D, Danenberg KD, Johnson M, et al. Colorectal tumors responding to 5-fluorouracil have low gene expression levels of dihydropyrimidine dehydrogenase, thymidylate synthase, and thymidine phosphorylase. *Clin Cancer Res* 2000;6:1322–1327.

279. McCarthy JJ, Hilfiker R. The use of single-nucleotide polymorphism maps in pharmacogenomics. *Nat Biotech* 2000;18:505–508..

26

Designs for Phase II and Phase III Cancer Drug Studies

Gary L. Rosner and Donald A. Berry

Department of Biostatistics, M.D. Anderson Cancer Center,
Houston, Texas, 77030

In this chapter, we discuss statistical issues regarding the design and analysis of phase II and phase III clinical studies. Our focus is on anticancer therapy, although the issues we discuss arise in other areas of medicine as well. There are many good review discussions in books and journal articles (1–6). We include a review of the general issues, but our approach differs from that of other authors, namely, we focus on recent innovations in statistical methodology. We have used many of these innovations in the design and analysis of clinical trials, working with investigators at the Duke University Comprehensive Cancer Center, the University of Texas M.D. Anderson Cancer Center, the Cancer and Leukemia Group B, and in consultations with pharmaceutical companies. Although not a series of case studies, these examples illustrate the challenges of clinical study design and provide a foundation that allows us to propose additional novel solutions.

Many of the newer designs are based on the flexibility of Bayesian inference; therefore, we first introduce the basic concepts of Bayesian statistics. The approach is formally different from that of the more commonly used frequentist approach. There are a variety of reviews of Bayesian statistics and comparisons with frequentist methods (7–10).

In the frequentist paradigm, probability is defined as long-run frequency. One assumes a particular hypothesis and calculates probabilities of events conditionally on that hypothesis. An especially important hypothesis is that of no treatment effect. One identifies a set of outcomes that has a prespecified small probability (such as 0.05) under this assumption. If the actual outcome is in this set, then one "rejects the null hypothesis of no treatment effect."

In the frequentist approach, any particular statistical analysis plan has a calculable probability of rejecting the null hypothesis—the "small probability" indicated in the previous paragraph. This is its so-called type I error probability, the probability of wrongly concluding that an ineffective treatment is beneficial. A type II error probability is found by assuming some alternative hypothesis (that the treatment has a particular benefit) and calculating the probability of concluding that the treatment is ineffective. Both probabilities are interpreted as long-run relative frequencies, assuming many repetitions of the experiment. They are calculated under different assumptions of the true underlying hypothesis, however. At the start of the design process, one specifies null and alternative hypotheses and error probabilities. One then establishes rules to avoid exceeding these probabilities over the range of possible outcomes of the experiment.

The Bayesian paradigm, on the other hand, is based on calculating probabilities of unknowns. Because it is unknown whether the null or alternative hypothesis is correct, these hypotheses have probabilities. These probabilities are interpreted as "degrees of belief" [Berry (11), pp. 120–122] rather than long-run frequencies. The basis of the Bayesian approach is Bayes' rule, a basic property of conditional probability (11). It relates so-called inverse probabilities. A familiar example is finding the positive predictive value (PPV) for a diagnostic test. The probability of having disease given a positive test result is the inverse of the probability of a positive test result given disease (the latter being the test's sensitivity). PPV also is related to the test's specificity and the prevalence of disease in the population. The analog of PPV in the more general application of Bayes' rule to statistical inference is the "posterior probability" that a hypothesis is true given experimental results. The analog of disease prevalence is the "prior probability" that a hypothesis is true.

For a simple example, consider two very specific hypotheses: the null hypothesis H0 in which the proportion r of a population that responds (complete or partial, say) is 1/2 and the alternative hypothesis H1 in which r is 3/4. Viewing "response" as analogous to a positive test result, H1 as "disease," and H0 as "no disease," the sensitivity of the test is 3/4 (the probability of response under H1) and the test specificity is 1/2 (the probability of nonresponse under H0). Suppose the prior probabilities of H1 and H0 are both 50%: P(H1) = P(H0) = 0.5. After observing a response in one patient, the updated (posterior) probability of H1 is found using Bayes' rule:

P(H1 | response) =

$$P(\text{response} | \text{H1})P(\text{H1})/P(\text{response})$$

where

P(response) = P(response | H1)P(H1)

$$+ \ P(\text{response} | \text{H0})P(\text{H0}).$$

The probability of response r is 3/4 under H1 and r = 1/2 under H0. Therefore:

P(response) = (3/4)(0.5) + (1/2)(0.5) = 5/8,

and

P(H1 | response) = (3/4)(0.5)/(5/8) = 60%.

The new evidence increases the probability of H1 from 50% to 60% (and decreases the probability of H0 from 50% to 40%). If a second independent observation is a response, then a second use of Bayes' rule (with the prior probability to this observation being that posterior to the first observation) gives P(H1 | response, response) = 9/13 = 69%. If, however, the next patient does not respond, then P(H1 | response, nonresponse) = 3/7 = 43%. This process can continue indefinitely, updating either continually or all at once. The current probabilities of the various possible values of r can be found at any time. These probabilities depend on the original prior probability and on the intervening data.

These calculations were somewhat restrictive in that they considered only two possible hypotheses or values of r. More generally, r could be any value between 0 and 1. Consider a single-arm clinical study in which the tumors of three of the first ten patients responded and the other seven did not. Suppose that based on information prior to the trial, all possible values of response probability r between 0 and 1 are regarded to be equally likely. (This distribution has been variously called *uniform, flat, noninformative,* and *open minded.*) The probability of observing three responses in ten patients depends on r and is proportional to $r^3(1-r)^7$. This is called the *likelihood func-*

tion of r. Updating the distribution of r based on this information means, according to Bayes' rule, multiplying the prior distribution by the likelihood. For a flat prior, the current (or posterior) distribution of r is simply proportional to the likelihood. By applying Bayes' rule, our knowledge about possible values of r is no longer "flat" but now indicates that some values of r are more likely than other values. The updated distribution of r, shown in Figure 26.1, is called a *beta density* with parameters 4 (=3+1) and 8 (=7+1). [See Chapter 7 in Berry (11) for derivation of beta densities and further discussion of the uses of beta densities.]

A principal distinction between the Bayesian and frequentist approaches is that the latter considers probabilities of sets of data for particular parameter values (analogs of sensitivity and specificity), whereas the former also considers probabilities of parameter values (or hypotheses). Thus, for example, the Bayesian approach allows for finding the probability that one treatment is more effective than another.

An aspect of the Bayesian approach that is especially important in designing clinical trials is that it allows for calculating the probability of future data (for any given design) without having to condition on a particular value of parameter r. One effects such a calculation by averaging the conditional probabilities of the data (that is, the sampling distribution) over the various possible values of r. The distribution over

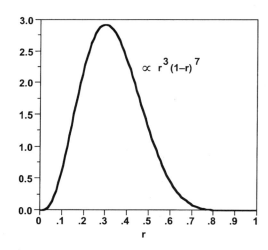

FIG. 26.1. Posterior distribution of response rate r after observing three responses among ten patients. This assumes a flat prior distribution, that each value of r has the same a priori probability. The symbol ∞ indicates "proportional to." The vertical axis is labeled so that the total area under the curve is 1.

which one averages is determined by the currently available information.

Consider again the clinical trial in which the tumors in three of the first ten patients responded and the other seven did not. If ten more patients are treated, how many will be responders? It is impossible to say for sure, of course, but there is some information available for predicting this number. Conditioning on information that currently is available allows one to calculate predictive probabilities for future results.

Bayesian predictive probabilities incorporate two types of variability. One is the usual sampling variability in the data that applies even if response rate are perfectly known. (You will not always observe the same number of responses in identical replicates of an experiment.) The other uncertainty is in the underlying response rate itself. The Bayesian approach comes in by ascribing to the response rate a distribution, namely, a prior distribution at the start of the trial and a current distribution at this point in the trial. This latter distribution is posterior to the previous results (three or ten responses) and prior to the subsequent part of the trial.

Figure 26.1 shows the distribution of r after three responses and seven nonresponses. Assuming that r is known, the probability of k responses is proportional to $r^k(1-r)^{10-k}$ for the next ten patients. For example, if r were known to be its current estimate of 3/10, then the probabilities of seeing k responses in the next ten patients is as shown in Figure 26.2. The parameter r is not known, however. The uncertainty associated with r is shown in Figure 26.1. Accounting for both the uncertainty in r (as in Fig. 26.1) and the sampling variability in the future experiment (as in Fig. 26.2) gives

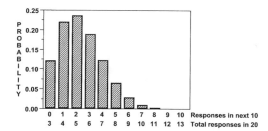

FIG. 26.3. Predictive probabilities of numbers of responses in the next ten patients when response rate r has the distribution shown in Fig. 26.1. These Bayesian predictive probabilities more accurately reflect the current uncertainty in predicting the future results than when assuming any particular value of r, such as in Fig. 26.2, where r was assumed to be 0.3. In particular, the probabilities of both zero responses and eight responses are greater in this figure, reflecting the possibilities that r may be less than 0.3 or greater than 0.3. Also shown in the figure are the total number of responses in the trial of 20 patients, adding the future number to the three observed so far.

the predictive probabilities in Figure 26.3. [For general calculations regarding Bayesian predictive distributions, see Berry (11) and Berry and Stangl (10).]

INTERIM ANALYSIS IN PHASE II STUDIES

The tradition in oncology drug development is to focus initially on toxicity. Initial studies, called *phase I,* are discussed in Chapters 21–23. Once the investigators decide on an appropriate dose from phase I, the agent undergoes evaluation for efficacy. This phase of the development process is called *phase II* and is the focus of this part of the chapter. One can think of phase II studies as screening studies in the sense that they seek to separate potentially active agents from agents that fail to show enough activity to warrant further evaluation. Some phase II studies evaluate combinations of agents, although most consider single-agent therapy. Treatments that are sufficiently promising undergo further evaluation in either follow-up phase II studies or large-scale randomized clinical trials, known as *phase III.*

Viewing phase II studies as means of screening new agents helps motivate the choice of short-term clinical endpoints for evaluating efficacy. In the tradition of cytotoxic drug development for solid tumors, the most common clinical endpoint in phase II studies has been tumor response: reduction in the size of a measurable tumor or in the extent of disease. Current response categories follow the Response Evaluation Criteria in Solid Tumors (RECIST) guidelines pro-

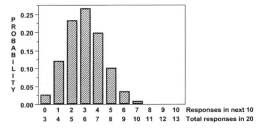

FIG. 26.2. Predictive probabilities of numbers of responses in the next ten patients assuming that r is exactly 0.3. This assumption is almost surely wrong, so this distribution of probabilities overestimates the precision in any predictions. The Bayesian probabilities shown in Figure 26.3 more accurately reflect the current uncertainty in predicting the future results. Also shown in the figure are the total number of responses among all 20 patients, adding the future number to the three observed so far.

posed by the European Organization for Research and Treatment of Cancer, National Cancer Institute of the United States, and the National Cancer Institute of Canada (12, Chapter 24). RECIST categories correspond to degrees of change in tumor size.

Most modern phase II studies incorporate interim analyses and early stopping rules. A popular design in phase II studies of anticancer agents is the two-stage optimal design of Simon (13). This design calls for analysis of the data part way through the study. The results of the interim analysis may lead the investigators to stop the study early and conclude that the therapy is not active enough to warrant further evaluation. Simon proposed an algorithm for calculating stopping boundaries that simultaneously minimize the expected sample size under the null hypothesis ("not active enough") and preserve type I and type II error probabilities. One may also set up a similar two-stage design that minimizes the maximum sample size (13).

Phase II studies that incorporate interim analyses have to deal with a time lag. Patients do not enter the study at the same time, and they do not usually respond to their therapy immediately. Clinical follow-up evaluations of tumor response follow a fixed schedule that typically allows 1 or 2 months between assessments. Thus, there is a time lag between when a patient begins therapy and when the patient's clinical assessment leads to a response determination. When initiating an interim analysis, the study investigators must decide whether to stop accruing patients into the study while waiting for full follow-up of the first n patients for the planned interim analysis. If accrual continues, should any outcomes among the new patients enter into the interim analysis? If the analysis should incorporate data—possibly incomplete—from these patients, then what is the best way to accomplish it?

Herndon (14) discusses options in a two-stage phase II study, allowing for continued accrual. He proposes what he calls a *hybrid design* in which the first interim analysis informs the decision on whether to stop accrual or continue to accrue patients while waiting for complete follow-up for the interim analysis. He develops his hybrid design using frequentist considerations (i.e., controlling the type I and type II error probabilities). In his design, the interim analysis uses only data from patients with complete follow-up. Treated patients under observation who have not yet responded but might still ("too soon to tell") are ignored.

Even though there are several RECIST categories, most phase II studies collapse them into a simple dichotomy for the primary endpoint: response (either complete or partial) and no response. Although possibly appropriate for trials involving cytotoxic agents, considering only two categories based on evidence of tumor shrinkage may not be appropriate for newer types of therapies.

CONSIDERATIONS FOR EVALUATING TARGETED THERAPY

Many new anticancer agents have specific molecular targets and seek to disrupt tumor growth and the cancer's potential to metastasize. An agent targeting the molecular signals involved in tumor growth and metastasis may delay disease progression rather than cause immediate tumor shrinkage, for example. Even if a new agent does not shrink the size of the tumor in the short term, the tumor may not appear to increase in size and evidence of new disease may not appear. Traditional measures of tumor growth, such as reduction in the size of the mass, may be desirable but may not be the most appropriate endpoints to consider when screening the targeted therapies in the search for agents with strong potential for clinical use (15,16). Thus, some investigators have chosen endpoints other than tumor shrinkage for evaluating potential new therapies (17–19).

A suitable endpoint for phase II evaluation may be progression-free survival (PFS) (17,18). PFS is the fraction of the patients who are alive and free of disease over time. Typically, one specifies a length of time from the initiation of therapy of interest, such as 6-month PFS, written as PFS(6). Thus, phase II studies of newer targeted anticancer therapies may choose to consider an agent as a potential winner if the estimated PFS (e.g., at 6 months) exceeds some threshold percentage, instead of basing decisions on the extent of tumor shrinkage. Suppose, for example, that one estimates the 6-month PFS associated with the study therapy to be 75% based on the study's data. If historical data indicate that around 50% of similar patients would survive 6 months without evidence of disease, then one might be inclined to consider the new agent a potential winner. The study's design should call for collecting enough data to impart reasonable precision to the estimate of 6-month PFS.

With newer therapies targeting molecular pathways involved in tumor growth, disease stabilization may be a useful endpoint to consider when deciding if the agent is active. For some cancers, such as metastatic renal cell carcinoma, there is great heterogeneity in tumor growth rates within the population of patients. This heterogeneity may make a cytostatic agent appear active simply by chance if a high percentage of patients enrolled in the study happen to have slow-growing tumors. Thus, stable disease may not be an appropriate endpoint in an uncontrolled study.

A potentially useful strategy for phase II evaluation of possibly cytostatic drugs is the randomized discontinuation design (20). Briefly, all patients receive the study drug for some fixed period of time specified ahead of time. At the end of this fixed follow-up period, patients are restaged. If there appears to be tumor shrinkage, either partial or complete, the patient would continue receiving the study drug. Patients who progress during the initial follow-up period go off the study. Patients with stable disease at the end of this open-label treatment period are randomized to continue receiving the study drug or to receive placebo in a blinded fashion. At the end of a second follow-up period following randomization fixed in the protocol, the two treatments are compared with respect to proportions of patients whose disease has progressed. Thus, the randomized discontinuation design identifies patients with apparently slow tumor growth while they are receiving the study drug, which one can compare to historical data. The design also incorporates a concurrent (randomized) control to determine if the drug or just naturally slow tumor growth is responsible for stable disease at the end of the first study follow-up period [for further details see Rosner et al. (21)].

Regardless of the chosen endpoint, the phase II study paradigm as practiced in cancer assumes that the earlier phase I studies had correctly determined the safety profile of the agent. Unfortunately, this assumption often is wrong. Patient populations enrolling in phase I studies in cancer typically are different from populations of patients who enroll in phase II studies. The former group of patients is sicker and less able to tolerate the adverse effects of many chemotherapeutic agents. Additionally, phase I studies generally have small sample sizes and are not designed to estimate the dose-toxicity curve efficiently, even within the range of doses around the targeted area of interest, such as the dose associated with a 25% risk of dose-limiting toxicity (22–26). Therefore, some have argued for inclusion of toxicity as a primary study endpoint in phase II. Bryant and Day (27) and Conaway and Petroni (28,29) discuss phase II study designs that consider safety and efficacy, with stopping rules determined to satisfy frequentist characteristics. Thall et al. (30) combined the two events into a single endpoint comprising several categories and then discussed study designs based on this composite outcome. These methods are more complicated than the more standard phase II designs, but the inclusion of safety monitoring seems to make them more appropriate.

As an example, Thall et al. (30) propose monitoring safety and toxicity in phase II studies of anticancer agents. Their design builds on already available data

by quantifying current knowledge about safety and efficacy through probability distributions, and Bayesian calculations update our knowledge about risks and benefits as data accrue. That is, one summarizes efficacy and safety as statistics (proportions) that are associated with some uncertainty. The experiment describes means for collecting data that can be combined with the numeric summaries already available for making inference about clinical endpoints, such as the proportions of patients one expects will respond to therapy, suffer adverse events, or both. The probabilities associated with the various outcomes are updated, integrating in some weighted manner the newly acquired data with the already available information. The investigators use this updated knowledge to inform decisions, such as whether to continue the study and treat more patients or to stop and declare the drug to be active, inactive, or too toxic.

An alternative approach to designing studies considers some optimization criterion to maximize (e.g., benefit) or minimize (e.g., cost). Such designs are called *decision-theoretic,* and several such proposals exist in the literature (31–46). As a simple example, one might want to consider designing a study that seeks to maximize the number of patients receiving beneficial therapy while simultaneously minimizing the number of patients experiencing toxicity. Additionally, one can imagine that there exists a tradeoff between toxicity and efficacy, whereby one might consider higher risks of toxicity if the therapy can deliver a much greater chance of cure.

With such a study, the design considerations include more than just the number of patients to enroll. Other considerations include rules for deciding to continue the study, as well as decision rules concerning choices one can make with respect to the agent under investigation. The decision rules incorporate losses and gains, such as the average number of patients receiving inferior treatment; the precision of the estimate of the treatment's effect, subject to some cost constraints; and the expected profit if the agent will receive regulatory approval, given the current treatment effect. Once the appropriate losses and gains are identified and included, one can compare various designs with respect to the expected risk (losses minus gains) associated with each design and identify the optimal one. Some examples of optimal designs have been described (37,41,43,46).

AUXILIARY VARIABLES

In addition to information about the target endpoint, a clinical study generates other valuable information that should be captured as it accumulates. Information about whether a tumor responds can be useful, but so can time to tumor response, even if time to tumor response is not the chosen endpoint. As stated earlier, newer agents are being designed for specific biologic targets or to interfere with the ability of cancer cells to grow and metastasize. Increasingly, biochemical markers of disease activity will serve as correlative measures of a treatment's effect. Similarly, information about a patient's current or changing status during the study can be valuable and can be incorporated prospectively into the clinical study's design. Such information, even if not the study's primary endpoint, may be useful in updating the probability distributions of a trial's parameters. Variables that correlate with a study's primary endpoint provide information that may be used to form early conclusions about the endpoint and to lend precision to final analyses of trial data. We call these *auxiliary variables.*

We distinguish auxiliary endpoints from surrogate endpoints. The surrogate endpoint stands in for the primary clinical outcome. Auxiliary endpoints, on the other hand, are helpful in making inferences about the primary endpoint because they may correlate with that endpoint. Auxiliary endpoints do not substitute for the primary endpoint, however; they provide information about it. In the end, one analyzes the primary endpoint to evaluate the treatment effect in the study. A possible way to distinguish the two types of outcomes is as follows. A variable is auxiliary if it is correlated with the ultimate endpoint—any correlation will do, including negative correlation—or the treatment in question. On the other hand, a variable can serve as a surrogate endpoint only if it is highly correlated with the primary endpoint.

Some have argued that surrogate measures of a treatment's activity will be useful endpoints only if certain criteria are met: the treatment is effective clinically; it alters these biochemical markers in a prescribed and reproducible manner; and the absence of a treatment effect on the markers corresponds to lack of clinical efficacy (47,48). These are demanding requirements, and not many endpoints will be good surrogates for the primary clinical outcome. Auxiliary variables serve a different purpose and do not have to meet such stringent criteria to be useful in clinical research.

Efficient designs incorporate information about auxiliary variables. These variables are tied to the target endpoint via mathematical models. Developing models that consider early trial information requires care. In particular, the models should allow for learning about the relationship between the auxiliary variables and the target endpoint based on the data they accumulate in the trial. One might even consider separate models for each possible auxiliary variable separately.

A model should be flexible and include the possibility that the auxiliary variable's correlation with the target endpoint depends upon the treatment under study. For example, measurable effects on some auxiliary variables may be more informative about one treatment than for another. If accumulating trial data indicate that the specific tumor response (the auxiliary variable) relates to survival in the control group but not in the experimental group, then the auxiliary variable is treatment dependent. In this case, a well-designed statistical model will disregard the auxiliary variable and rely only on overall survival.

Having information on auxiliary variables for patients before the long-term primary endpoints of a trial are available can allow for adaptation of a trial already underway. These variables give early information that can be used to modify a trial's conduct. Possibilities include stopping early for either futility or efficacy, dropping arms or doses, adding arms or doses, and ramping up accrual. Inclusion of auxiliary information into the design and analysis may contribute to the early approval of an experimental drug or to the early release of clinical trial findings.

Advantages of modeling with an auxiliary variable can be understood from the following example of a clinical trial. Suppose that a clinical trial has been designed to compare an experimental drug to a control therapy, with survival as the primary endpoint. Further, assume that tumor response—an auxiliary variable—also is considered in the study design, and response may correlate with survival. Reliable information about survival may not be available until long after all patients have entered the study and completed treatment. Some survival information is available, however, and full response information is available. Suppose it turns out that the experimental group has a higher tumor response than the control group and that all patients who respond (irrespective of treatment) survive substantially longer than those who do not respond. Analyzing the study data with a model that relates survival duration for all patients in the study to each patient's response information (and, perhaps, other clinical characteristics) may indicate that the drug prolongs survival. Notice that the comparison is on the basis of survival and not on the basis of tumor response. Such conclusions can be as strong statistically as those for a comparable clinical trial with much longer follow-up, if the analysis of the latter trial focuses only on survival and ignores auxiliary variables. Of course, the model must be flexible enough to allow discounting of the influence of the auxiliary variable on the inference if it should turn out that the auxiliary variable is related to the primary endpoint in only one treatment group but not the other.

An agent with a measurable target can be evaluated as a biomarker within the setting of an actual clinical trial. Biomarkers are distinct types of auxiliary variables. A possible use of a biomarker is measuring it over time and incorporating the data in a longitudinal model. The longitudinal model relates the level or change in level of the biomarker with the primary endpoint, which commonly is time to progression or overall survival. Methodologic developments have appeared in disease settings, such as acquired immunodeficiency syndrome (49,50) and stroke (51). The increasing interest in, and development of, agents that target specific biologic processes in medical oncology requires new strategies in clinical trial design. Changes in measurable biomarkers, such as gene expression or even imaging studies, may turn out to be useful auxiliary variables for use in clinical studies. Such information is gathered during early phase I and phase II studies, which allows the development of models for incorporating the auxiliary variables into clinical studies.

Agents that have a measurable target are fundamentally different from those that do not. Certain oncoproteins are examples of biologic agents without measurable targets. A biologic agent is not effective if it does not affect its target. Some agents may have more than one target, however, and some targets may be unknown. If no measurable target can be identified, one still may be able to determine auxiliary variables that could correlate with the primary endpoint. In this case, one models the possibility of a relationship between the auxiliary variables and the primary endpoint. Clearly, there are demands to learn as much as possible about the drugs in development in order to come up with efficient clinical trial designs. Again, the goal in designing the study is efficient learning: learning if and how the targeted therapy is beneficial in treating the disease as demonstrated by its effect on the primary endpoint.

SAMPLE SIZE

The most common method for calculating the number of patients is based on the frequentist paradigm. The structure depends on a so-called *null hypothesis* that corresponds to the proposition that the new agent is not any better than what is already available and an alternative hypothesis that the new agent improves on what is currently available with respect to the study endpoint(s). Coming up with these null and alternative hypotheses may be less than straightforward, especially for single-arm studies. The usual way of

thinking of the hypothesized response rates, however, is as the level of activity one expects from current therapies (p_0 in the null hypothesis) and the target level of activity one would hope to see with the new therapy (p_1 in the alternative hypothesis). The typical study is designed to maintain a low probability of incorrectly favoring the alternative hypothesis over the null hypothesis (type I error). The sample size, on the other hand, must be large enough to allow a high probability of *correctly* favoring the alternative hypothesis (i.e., power, which equals one minus the type II error). Several books develop the formulas for computing sample sizes for phase II and phase III clinical trials according to frequentist considerations (1,2).

Type I and II error probabilities have frequentist interpretations. One evaluates the study design in terms of the relative frequencies of key study characteristics, such as how often the study will decide in favor of the null or alternative hypothesis. The operating characteristics of a design summarize relative frequencies of key measures, such as the error probabilities and average sample size (if there is sequential monitoring of study data). Bayesian designs, however, are built on considerations of decision making rather than on achieving prespecified error probabilities. It still is possible to evaluate any given design's operating characteristics—however it was constructed—using computer simulation. Additionally, the decision-theoretic designs generally require numeric methods to determine the desired sample size (or upper limit sample size, in the case of sequential monitoring).

ADAPTIVE DESIGNS OF CLINICAL TRIALS

Many phase II studies have inefficient designs. Dose recommendations resulting from phase I studies are commonly based on the maximally tolerated dose (MTD). Targeted therapy favors a dose that achieves optimal biologic effect rather than the maximum dose that can be tolerated. Information needed to determine the dose that will provide optimal biologic effect often is gained during phase I and early phase II studies. In practice, however, neither the MTD nor the dose associated with optimal biologic effect is known exactly. If the phase II study restricts attention solely to the phase I MTD or putative optimal biologic dose, then the study will likely be inefficient. Instead, it would seem that one should continue refining one's knowledge as the treatment undergoes further development. This imprecise knowledge about what dose is "the right dose" calls for adaptive trial designs for phase II studies. Adaptive trial designs will allow for learning by dynamically changing certain design parameters as the study data accrue. For example, adaptive phase II study designs can allow for dose adjustments as patients enter the study, based on findings of biologic effect among patients already enrolled and treated. This flexibility enables the study to determine the most effective dose prior to the initiation of the phase III clinical trials. Thus, adaptive designs are more efficient because the "established" MTD or optimal biologic dose may well be wrong, and further investigation of dose toxicity and dose efficacy would be wise.

Carrying the idea of dose-finding phase II study designs further, consider a study that assigns a predetermined number of patients to each of a prespecified set of doses. Such phase II studies are common in clinical trials outside of oncology, and they are becoming increasingly utilized in cancer research. It is not uncommon to find at the end of such a trial that many patients were assigned to doses that provided little benefit and gave little or no information about the important aspects of the dose-response curve. In the case of an effective agent, some of the patients could have been treated more effectively had they been assigned doses where the drug produced more responses. In the case of an ineffective agent, the trial should have stopped sooner, thus saving patient resources and not exposing patients to ineffective therapy. Additionally, if during the course of the study it appears that the underlying statistical assumptions were incorrect, such as when the standard deviation of the target response (e.g., change in some marker level) is larger or smaller than expected, the sample size should have been different. The study will have enrolled more patients than necessary or not enrolled enough patients to address the study's questions. Patient resources could have been used more effectively.

An alternative approach is adaptive dose finding (52,53). This sort of study design proceeds sequentially, assigning patients with higher probability to the dose currently considered best. Here, we mean "best" in the sense of efficacy or in the sense of providing information about relative efficacy among the set of doses under consideration. One does not predetermine the number of patients to assign to each dose. Instead, as the study data inform us of the relative benefits of the different doses or treatments, the allocation ratios change to reflect the evolving knowledge. That is, the data help determine how the study allocates patients to the doses under consideration.

This method will use a large sample size when the dose-response curve has a gentle slope over the range of doses studied or in settings where there is relatively great heterogeneity in patient responses to therapy. When the available data suggest only a moderate effect of the experimental treatment, then there are two possibilities to consider. One is that the trial can be abandoned because the effect is too modest to be clinically meaningful. Alternatively, if the benefit is real and important but not big relative to the variation in the study population, then the study would need a larger sample size to show the benefit. An advantage of adaptive designs is that one can learn about the effect and variation and decide whether, given that information, it is worth further exploration.

Adaptive designs may lead to smaller sample sizes, such as when there is little variation among patient responses, a lack of benefit or substantial benefit from the experimental drug, or a dose-response curve that rises steeply over a short dose range. Moreover, as more data accrue, more information accumulates about which doses appear more effective. A new patient is then assigned to the dose that is best for the patient, given the available information. Compared to a design that is not adaptive, adaptive dosing will treat more patients with the better performing doses and fewer patients will receive the apparently less effective doses.

Adaptive dosing provides a more efficient method for identifying an optimal dose and requires a smaller number of patients to do so, on average, compared to a phase II trial design that uses only predetermined dose assignments. Even though adaptive dose finding may not assign patients to every dose within the range under study, this methodology allows the investigator to consider more doses at the start of the study and to approximate better the dose-response curve than a static study design that focuses on just one or two doses.

We illustrate these ideas by describing the clinical trial design of Berry et al. (53). This study used adaptive dose finding in the investigation of a biologic neuroprotective agent for patients who experienced a stroke. As part of the design, there were two stages to the study. The first stage, a dose-ranging stage, continued until a decision was made either to stop the drug from further evaluation or to move onto the second stage, a randomized clinical trial. Because the dose-ranging part of the study included randomization to placebo, the second-stage randomized trial would commence only if the data indicated the existence of an optimal dose that might prove better than placebo in a confirmatory phase III trial. In fact, as we discuss later in this chapter, the switch to phase III can be seamless and accrual need not stop. Furthermore, even though the study of Berry et al. (53) enrolled stroke patients in an acute setting, the key aspects of the study's design apply equally well to cancer studies.

The dose-ranging stage considered 16 doses, including placebo. The randomization algorithm assigned to each entering patient the dose that would provide maximum information about the relationship of dose to response, given the currently available data. Thus, the assigned dose might be the dose in the range of the steepest part of the dose-response curve, or the placebo, or even one of the highest doses. With accumulating data, the study learned about the dose-response relationship and, therefore, could avoid assigning doses in the flat part of the dose-response curve, unless some of the doses were at a plateau of the curve.

Although the study consisted of two stages, the number of patients in each stage was not fixed before the study started. Additionally, in keeping with the adaptive nature of the study's design, the number of patients assigned to each of the 16 doses was not prespecified; instead, the number of patients in the first stage depended on the accumulating data. If there appeared to be only a shallow dose-response curve, or the drug's benefit appeared to be only moderate, or the variation of the responses at the doses was relatively large, then the study would end up putting more patients in the dose-finding stage. On the other hand, the sample size in the dose-finding stage would tend to be smaller if the drug appeared to provide substantial benefit, no benefit, or there was relatively little variation in the responses. Somewhat paradoxically, the design also would tend to have a small sample size if there were great heterogeneity in responses, because a very large variance would necessitate a very large sample size, a sample size so large that one would not wish to continue the study.

The study's primary endpoint was the change from baseline to the assessment at 13 weeks. The assessments were measured by a scale that quantified the severity and disability caused by the stroke. The design incorporated further efficiencies by incorporating weekly assessments via the stroke scale. A longitudinal model characterized these weekly measures for each patient. With this model, interim analyses could incorporate data from all patients, including patients with fewer than 13 weeks of follow-up, that is, the model accounted for within-patient correlation and allowed for Bayesian prediction of the 13-week assessment for patients taking into account currently available information on each patient. Bayesian calculations allowed continual updating of the relevant probability distributions of the effect of therapy.

The sequential dose-finding part of the study (phase II) proceeded until the resulting data either identified an optimal dose for use in the next part of the study (i.e., phase III) or indicated an inadequate therapeutic effect, warranting discontinuation of the trial. In general, the transition from a phase II study to a phase III clinical trial can be accomplished while maintaining patient accrual. The idea of a "seamless" phase II to phase III design is described in a subsequent section.

We have incorporated adaptive allocation methods into more than 12 clinical trial designs that are underway at the M.D. Anderson Cancer Center. These designs randomly assign patient to each treatment arm, weighting the assignment probabilities to favor the more beneficial treatment arms as the study data accumulate. In some of these adaptive studies, the treatment arms represent distinctly different therapies, whereas in other studies two treatment arms represent similar therapies.

One ongoing study incorporates an adaptive design to determine the optimally effective dose of a particular drug. In this study, the different treatment arms represent the varying dose levels. For this study, we initially use a slow and graduated increase in assigned doses. This strategy allows for the possibility of a steep dose-toxicity relationship or for increasing benefit with dose until some threshold beyond which toxicity leads to lower overall benefit. Having gathered some information about the relationship between dose and clinical benefit over a range of doses, we preferentially assign patients to the doses that show treatment benefit. The study continues using a degree of randomization, however, to account for remaining uncertainty and to allow for continued learning. For a patient newly enrolled in the study, we use all information from patients treated to date to calculate the current Bayesian probabilities that each admissible dose would be better than placebo. The study allocates doses randomly, with weights proportional to these probabilities.

When designing a study that includes adaptive randomization, we evaluate different allocation algorithms, including assigning patients to treatment arms in proportion to powers of the probabilities that the treatment is superior to placebo or some control therapy. (Using powers of the probabilities can hasten or slow the progression to the best performing treatment, according to the desires of the investigators.) We use computer simulation to evaluate each design's frequentist operating characteristics, such as the average sample size, the average proportion of patients ultimately receiving the best treatment, and the type I and type II errors. An important part of the design process includes modifying the parameters of the algorithm the study will use for making treatment assignments. These changes sometimes are necessary in order for the study to have the desired characteristics.

Using adaptive allocation in a clinical study, new patients are more likely to receive the better performing treatments and are less likely to be assigned treatments that are performing poorly in the study. The study is designed to stop when we learn that the treatment is either ineffective or effective. Patients in the trial benefit, because more of them will have received more effective treatments during the course of the trial than if the randomization were fixed throughout the course of the study. The investigators benefit from a more efficient method of learning. Providing more beneficial treatment to greater numbers of study participants can increase enrollment while it also increases the efficiency of the trial.

Finding the optimal dose is an issue in the development of all drug therapies, including cancer therapy. Many clinical studies involve design elements similar to those just described for the stroke study. These elements of drug development allow the study statistician to incorporate adaptive dose-finding methods using early information about the expected target endpoint.

Historically, clinical study designs have evaluated each new therapy one at a time. Evaluating each new therapy in sequence results in an inefficient expenditure of enormous patient and financial resources. The number of potentially beneficial therapies in research and development is increasing at an extremely rapid pace, however, and the static trial design remains a rate-limiting factor in the process. The high cost of drug development and of medical treatment, in general, requires the drug development/experimental trial system to focus on controlling the cost of developing new drugs by more efficiently using patient resources. With the large number of experimental therapies in the development queue, drug development must be able to evaluate a larger number of experimental therapies over a given period of time than is possible with the one-at-a-time approach. Study designs for clinical research must now allow researchers to investigate many drugs at the same time in trials requiring smaller sample sizes. Furthermore, these studies will gain efficiency if they assess dose response while screening for activity and evaluating the best way to deliver the new therapy. Accomplishing all of these goals requires trial designs that are flexible and adaptive. With adaptive treatment allocation as we have discussed, the studies will gravitate toward assigning the better performing therapies and away from the poorer drugs.

There are other aspects of many study designs that lead to inefficiency. Sample sizes, patient randomization methods, and stopping criteria for clinical studies usually are determined and fixed in advance of the start of the trial. In this sense, most trial designs are static or inflexible. The static character of traditional clinical trials allows for simplicity in quantifying the uncertainty of one treatment arm's benefit compared to that of the other, namely, everything is conditional on a particular value for the treatment effect. These so-called null and alternative hypotheses, so pervasive in clinical trial designs, are almost certainly wrong, yet the sample size is chosen assuming that a specific and fixed (alternative) treatment effect is at work and that we know what it is. Sample sizes are relatively large, and a direct comparison usually is made between the results of two treatment arms within the same study. Common exceptions to this static design are phase II protocols that stop the study after the first stage if the drug treatment is not adequately beneficial and phase III protocols that stop the trial if one treatment is shown to be highly advantageous over another. In practice, however, early stopping criteria are very cautious, resulting in clinical studies that rarely stop early, except for administrative reasons, such as when accrual is very slow.

In summary, adaptive designs use results obtained during the study to direct the study's continuing course. This periodic decision making involves intermittent, or even ongoing, evaluation of the study data as they are gathered, in order to adapt the study's design. The goals of adapting the design are to provide the most beneficial treatment to the largest number of patients and to extract the most valuable information that can be gleaned from the trial. The information learned from the accumulating data will determine what adaptations are made to the trial design. Adaptations to the study include modifying eligibility criteria, adding or dropping a treatment arm, adding or dropping a dose level, expanding enrollment to additional sites, early stopping, or increasing accrual beyond the original sample size to reach a clear conclusion. The accumulating data are used to effect each of these possible trial adaptations. Dynamically changing randomization proportions of patients based on the accumulating data, as discussed previously, is also considered in adaptive designs. Patient randomization to treatment arms that are performing better or that provide more information about the study's hypotheses can be more heavily weighted as the study continues (55). Through the use of Bayesian hierarchical modeling, adaptive study design can also incorporate information learned from other ongoing or completing studies.

DECISION ANALYSIS AND CHOOSING SAMPLE SIZE

Choosing a design for a clinical study involves making decisions; in particular, choosing a sample size is making a decision. There is an extensive literature that deals with decision analysis (52–57). Consider all the components of a particular design, including the sample size. Typically there will be a well-defined set of outcomes that will result from the study. A critical aspect of decision analysis is to assign a worth or value (called a *utility*) to each possible outcome. Each outcome also has a probability of occurring. Averaging each outcome's utility with respect to these probabilities gives an overall expected utility for the design itself. The expected utility for each design provides a basis for choosing one design over another. Designs with the highest utilities are preferred in much the same way that one would prefer the design that is expected to yield the greatest return on one's investment.

Decision-theoretic concepts can enter into calculations for determining sample sizes for clinical studies. We carry out randomized clinical trials to learn how one therapeutic regimen compares to another. The ultimate beneficiaries of this knowledge are the patients with the disease under study, and the ultimate utility of the trial is the net benefit gained by patients who receive the therapy, patients within and beyond the clinical trial. We call the size of this group of patients the "patient horizon," symbolically N. This patient horizon includes all patients participating in the study and those patients outside of the trial who stand to benefit from the information generated by the trial.

The size of N depends on the particular cancer and the treatments that are available to treat individuals with the disease. Many more people will benefit from improvements in the treatment of a relatively more common form of cancer, such as colorectal cancer, than would benefit from better treatments for much rarer cancers, such as cancer of the larynx. Comparing these two situations illustrates opposite extreme values of N. If the ultimate intent of running clinical trials is to treat as many patients as effectively as possible, then one would expect that the sample sizes would be different in these two extreme situations. Typically, however, with sample size calculations based on traditional power calculations, both the more prevalent and the rarer disease situations are managed in the same way. That is, the number of patients in the clinical study is the same, regardless of whether a relatively large number or small number of patients stand to benefit from a treatment, assuming the goal of the study is to detect treatment effects of the same magnitude. From the standpoint of wanting to carry out clinical research to benefit as many people as possible, though, it does not seem right that these two extreme situations would be treated in exactly the same way when determining sample size. For example, a much higher percentage of patients with the rarer cancer will participate in the clinical trial than of the more prevalent cancer. If, for example, almost all of the patients with cancer of the larynx at some time participate in the study, there will be relatively few patients outside the trial who stand to benefit from the knowledge. On the other hand, the number of patients in the clinical trial of a new agent for treating colorectal cancer may be too small to allow definitive statements about which treatment is better for everyone and anyone with the disease. As a result, the large group of patients outside of the study may receive inferior therapy that happened to look good in the clinical trial. In summary, one should approach sample size calculation differently depending on whether one is studying a relatively rare or prevalent disease.

Of course, one does not typically know the number of patients who are outside of the trial but stand to benefit from any improvements in treating their cancer as a result of the trial. One also does not typically know just how effective the treatment will be and how extensive the side effects of the treatment will be. All of these factor into the determination of the patient horizon N. The investigator could estimate the annual number of patients with the disease under study and consider the potential therapies expected to become available over a set number of years. The number of patients who would present in the future can be discounted by the probability that other treatments will become available. Luckily, precision is not essential and only the order of magnitude of N matters. In practice, if N is not known, one would estimate its mean and use this estimate in the calculations.

The optimal trial sample size is one that maximizes the expected overall beneficial treatment in the patient horizon N. Consider clinical trials evaluating therapies with respect to a dichotomous outcome, with subsequent clinical practice picking up the better performing therapy. It turns out that the order of magnitude of the optimal sample size for one clinical trial is on the order of the square root of N (58). When designing two trials to compare treatments in sequence for the same form of cancer, the sample size of the first trial will be on the order of the cube root of N. A single trial addressing effective treatment for a cancer with a patient horizon of 1 million would have size of order 1,000; if it is the first of two trials, the optimal sample size is 170. By comparison, if the horizon is smaller, such as on the order of 1,000, then the optimal sample size for a single trial is 32 (and 17 for the first of two trials). Comparing these two scenarios illustrates how decision-theoretic considerations lead to different clinical trial sample sizes, depending on the size of the population likely to benefit from improvements in therapy under investigation. The theory is discussed by Cheng et al. (58).

This discussion assumed a fixed sample size within each trial. Interim monitoring with the possibility of expanding or curtailing accrual has the potential to improve considerably the overall treatment benefit of patients with the disease under study.

SEAMLESS PHASES II AND III

Investigators move into a new clinical trial phase when they presume to have learned something from the study. Estimating an MTD prompts them to move into the second phase, and estimating that a drug will have a beneficial effect based upon a given endpoint prompts them to initiate a phase III clinical trial. Unfortunately, this division of the drug evaluation process into phases invites delays in drug development. These delays are not beneficial to the patients. The Bayesian view of clinical drug development, on the other hand, is that of a continuous process. Bayesian methods do not presume that a quantity is precisely known. Investigators following the Bayesian paradigm assess and reassess uncertainty of any predicted outcomes or treatment effects as additional information accrues throughout the study process. It seems to us that a preferred method of drug development, therefore, is to design and effect each clinical trial as a continuous process, applying Bayesian methods of analysis along the way.

Such a continuous process involves the repeated analyses of accruing study data and the use of a statistical algorithm that employs decision analysis to direct decisions regarding the conduct of the study. On a periodic basis (e.g., weekly, monthly, after every "event"), the decision analysis selects among three possible choices for the trial: (i) continuing the study, (ii) stopping the study for insufficient evidence of a meaningful treatment effect, or (ii) moving forward into a validating phase of the trial. If data support the selection of the third choice, then a move into the validating phase can be made without stopping patient accrual.

We designed a trial effecting a continuous or seamless transition from phase II to phase III at the M.D. Anderson Cancer Center (59). The anticipated treatment effect was on local control. Survival was the main endpoint, however, with local control as an auxiliary endpoint, the utility of which we needed to demonstrate based on the accumulating study data. Therefore, we incorporated into a mathematical model of survival associations with local control and with treatment. Our model also allowed for the possi-

bility that any treatment-related increase in survival is not accompanied by improved local control.

Repeating interim analyses inform decisions to change the study as data accumulate. If the observed data result in a strong prediction that the treatment has no effect on survival or on local control, then the study will stop. If our prediction from the accumulating data suggests that the treatment might improve local control and that this improvement may result in a survival benefit, then we would enlist the participation of other treatment centers and increase accrual to the study. Of course, enrollment of patients at M.D. Anderson to the study continues while new centers join the study, because stopping enrollment would be an inefficient use of patient resources. The absence of a break in patient accrual at the initial study site provides a larger patient base having longer follow-up, thus providing more information for analysis of the treatment's effect on survival.

The expanded trial will continue until one of three outcomes occurs: (i) the predictive probability of eventually reaching statistical significance becomes sufficiently large (in which case the research company would apply for regulatory approval to market the treatment); (ii) predictive probabilities indicate that continuing the trial would be futile; or (iii) the maximum sample size is reached. The maximum sample size for a randomized phase III study of the treatments in the M.D. Anderson study would be 900 patients. In the seamless design, the maximum sample size also is 900 patients. Based on simulations, we determined that the actual patient accrual to the seamless study will be much less than 900—more likely about half that size. The reduction in sample size occurs as a result of frequent determinations of the predictive probability of achieving statistical significance and modeling the specific relationship between local control and survival. The criteria for decision making at the interim analyses are set to ensure adequate control of frequentist error probabilities (i.e., of type I and type II errors).

The application of this design can result in decreased drug development time and more efficient use of patient and financial resources. The seamless design will enroll relatively more patients when the treatment effect is relatively smaller or less clear than originally anticipated, precisely when one would want to have a larger study to sort out the treatment effect.

An additional benefit of a Bayesian design is the ability to continue accruing patients to a trial that has reached maximum sample size if conclusions are still unclear, in order to achieve clarification of the conclusions. The reduced expected sample size and efficient use of patient resources in a seamless trial design are not as likely to occur in a traditional trial design, where the stopping boundaries generally allow for only a modest reduction in required sample size.

PROCESS OR TRIAL?: SUMMARY

With the large number of drugs under development, there is great demand for more rapid evaluation of experimental drugs. This demand will result in increased use of adaptive allocation in order to evaluate many drugs simultaneously. The benefits of adaptive designs can lead to single studies having multiple treatment arms with the ability to add or drop treatment arms or to considering a collection of experiments for which information is updated frequently and shared. The order in which drugs enter clinical studies and the degree to which patients in a study receive treatment with a particular drug will be determined by the data that become available. A drug suggesting treatment benefit will move through clinical evaluation and development more quickly, whereas drugs without apparent benefit will not progress. Furthermore, sample sizes will be sufficiently large to clarify uncertainties about the benefits and toxicities of each drug.

At M.D. Anderson we are creating a process to replace the discrete sequence of phase II studies followed by phase III clinical trials. This process begins with a number of experimental treatment arms plus a control, with the latter possibly the standard treatment. The process includes randomly assigning patients to the different treatments, with learning about their relative effectiveness as the study progresses. The better performing treatment arms will receive more patients as we gather data. Treatment arms that do not perform well will be dropped. A treatment that shows a sufficiently effective level will move into the next phase of the process (i.e., the traditional phase III clinical trial). This successful treatment might even replace the current control in the phase II portion of the process once the superiority of its effectiveness is demonstrated. As a new drug therapy becomes available, we will add it to the process as a new treatment arm. The overall benefits of this process are more effective treatment for patients enrolled in the process, rapid discontinuation of poor treatments, faster dissemination of study results, and shorter delays in granting accessibility to better treatments for patients outside the trial. For drug developers, a benefit of this process is a shortening of the length of time spent developing a drug and potentially quicker approval than that seen by following the traditional path.

Bayesian methods are particularly suited to adaptive trial design. The investigator considers the available information regarding the hypothesis and parameters to be studied. Then he or she characterizes this information and associated uncertainty quantitatively in a prior distribution or incorporates it in a hierarchical model along with the trial's results. While designing the trial, the investigator anticipates the possible implications and consequences of each trial outcome. The investigator calculates the predictive probability of each possible outcome, which may require simulation. These calculations will facilitate determining other characteristics of the trial important to trial design, such as the probability of reaching a statistically significant benefit from one treatment over another, the anticipated number of patients needed for the trial, and the anticipated number of patients who will realize a beneficial treatment effect. Adaptive trial designs do not specifically consider utilities of the possible outcomes; however, they are directed toward efficient learning and effective patient treatment.

REFERENCES

1. Friedman LM, Furberg CD, DeMets DL. *Fundamentals of clinical trials,* 3rd ed. New York: Springer Verlag, 1998.
2. Piantadosi S. *Clinical trials: a methodologic perspective.* New York: John Wiley & Sons, 1997.
3. Altman DG. *Practical statistics for medical research.* London: Chapman and Hall, 1990.
4. Rosner B. *Fundamentals of biostatistics,* 5th ed. Florence, KY: Duxbury Press, 1999.
5. Bast RC, Gansler TS, Holland JF, et al. *Cancer medicine,* 5th ed. Hamilton, Ontario: Decker, 2000.
6. DeVita VT, Rosenberg SA, Hellman S. *Cancer: principles & practice of oncology,* 6th ed. Philadelphia: Lippincott Williams & Wilkins, 2001.
7. Berger JO, Berry DA. Statistical analysis and the illusion of objectivity. *Am Sci* 1988;76:159–165.
8. Goodman SN. Toward evidence-based medical statistics. 1: the P value fallacy. *Ann Intern Med* 1999;130:995–1004.
9. Goodman SN. Toward evidence-based medical statistics. 2: the Bayes factor. *Ann Intern Med* 1999;130:1005–1013.
10. Berry DA, Stangl DK. *Bayesian biostatistics.* New York: Marcel Dekker, 1996.
11. Berry DA. *Statistics: a Bayesian perspective.* Belmont, CA: Duxbury Press, 1996.
12. Therasse P, Arbuck SG, Eisenhauer EA, et al. New guidelines to evaluate the response to treatment in solid tumors. European Organization for Research and Treatment of Cancer, National Cancer Institute of the United States, National Cancer Institute of Canada. *J Natl Cancer Inst* 2000;92:205–216.
13. Simon R. Optimal two-stage designs for phase II clinical trials. *Control Clin Trials* 1989;10:1–10.
14. Herndon JE 2nd. A design alternative for two-stage, phase II, multicenter cancer clinical trials. *Control Clin Trials* 1998;19:440–450.

15. Stadler WM, Ratain MJ. Development of target-based antineoplastic agents. *Invest New Drugs* 2000;18:7–16.
16. Korn EL, Arbuck SG, Pluda JM, et al. Clinical trial designs for cytostatic agents: are new approaches needed? *J Clin Oncol* 2001;19:265–272.
17. Von Hoff DD. There are no bad anticancer agents, only bad clinical trial designs—twenty-first Richard and Hinda Rosenthal Foundation Award Lecture. *Clin Cancer Res* 1998;4:1079–1086.
18. Mick R, Crowley JJ, Carroll RJ. Phase II clinical trial design for noncytotoxic anticancer agents for which time to disease progression is the primary endpoint. *Control Clin Trials* 2000;21:343–359.
19. Ratain MJ, Stadler WM. Clinical trial designs for cytostatic agents. *J Clin Oncol* 2001;19:3154–3155.
20. Kopec JA, Abrahamowicz M, Esdaile JM. Randomized discontinuation trials: utility and efficiency. *J Clin Epidemiol* 1993;46:959–971.
21. Rosner GL, Stadler W, Ratain MJ. Randomized discontinuation design: application to cytostatic antineoplastic agents. *J Clin Oncol* 2002;20:4478–4484.
22. Geller NL. Design of phase I and II clinical trials in cancer: a statistician's view. *Cancer Invest* 1984;2:483–491.
23. O'Quigley J, Pepe M, Fisher L. Continual reassessment method: a practical design for phase I clinical trials in cancer. *Biometrics* 1990;46:33–48.
24. Piantadosi S, Fisher JD, Grossman S. Practical implementation of a modified continual reassessment method for dose-finding trials. *Cancer Chemother Pharmacol* 1998;41:429–436.
25. Storer BE. Design and analysis of phase I clinical trials. *Biometrics* 1989;45:925–937.
26. Faries D. Practical modifications of the continual reassessment method for phase I cancer clinical trials. *J Biopharm Stat* 1994;4:147–164.
27. Bryant J, Day R. Incorporating toxicity considerations into the design of two-stage phase II clinical trials. *Biometrics* 1995;51:1372–1383.
28. Conaway MR, Petroni GR. Bivariate sequential designs for phase II trials. *Biometrics* 1995;51:656–664.
29. Conaway MR, Petroni GR. Designs for phase II trials allowing for a trade-off between response and toxicity. *Biometrics* 1996;52:1375–1386.
30. Thall PF, Simon RM, Estey EH. New statistical strategy for monitoring safety and efficacy in single-arm clinical trials. *J Clin Oncol* 1996;14:296–303.
31. Chang MN, Therneau TM, Wieand HS, et al. Designs for group sequential Phase II clinical trials. *Biometrics* 1987;43:865–874.
32. Weiss GB, Hokanson JA. Optimal phase II trials. *Biometrics* 1988;44:910–911.
33. Storer BE. A class of phase II designs with three possible outcomes. *Biometrics* 1992;48:55–60.
34. Berry DA, Wolff MC, Sack D. Decision making during a phase III randomized controlled trial. *Control Clin Trials* 1994;15:360–378.
35. Ensign LG, Gehan EA, Kamen DS, et al. An optimal three-stage design for phase II clinical trials. *Stat Med* 1994;13:1727–1736.
36. Chen TT. Optimal three-stage designs for phase II cancer clinical trials. *Stat Med* 1997;16:2701–2711.
37. Stallard N. Approximately optimal designs for phase II clinical studies. *J Biopharm Stat* 1998;8:469–487.
38. Stallard N. Sample size determination for phase II clinical trials based on Bayesian decision theory. *Biometrics* 1998;54:279–294.
39. Erkanli A, Soyer R, Angold A. Optimal Bayesian two-phase designs. *J Stat Plan Inference* 1998;66:175–191.
40. Wang YG, Leung DH. An optimal design for screening trials. *Biometrics* 1998;54:243–250.
41. Yao TJ, Venkatraman ES. Optimal two-stage design for a series of pilot trials of new agents. *Biometrics* 1998;54:1183–1189.
42. Hanfelt JJ. Optimal multi-stage designs for a phase II trial that permits one dose escalation. *Stat Med* 1999;18:1323–1339.
43. Stallard N, Thall PF, Whitehead J. Decision theoretic designs for phase II clinical trials with multiple outcomes. *Biometrics* 1999;55:971–977.
44. Leung DH, Wang YG. A Bayesian decision approach for sample size determination in phase II trials. *Biometrics* 2001;57:309–312.
45. Leung DH, Wang YG. Optimal designs for evaluating a series of treatments. *Biometrics* 2001;57:168–171.
46. Stallard N, Thall PF. Decision-theoretic designs for pre-phase II screening trials in oncology. *Biometrics* 2001;57:1089–1095.
47. George SL. Statistical considerations and modeling of clinical utility of tumor markers. *Hematol Oncol Clin North Am* 1994;8:457–470.
48. Fleming TR, DeMets DL. Surrogate end points in clinical trials: are we being misled? *Ann Intern Med* 1996;125:605–613.
49. Tsiatis AA, DeGruttola V, Wulfsohn MS. Modeling the relationship of survival to longitudinal data measured with error. Applications to survival and CD4 counts in patients with AIDS. *J Am Stat Assoc* 1995;90:27–37.
50. Wang Y, Taylor JMG. Jointly modeling longitudinal and event time data with application to acquired immunodeficiency syndrome. *J Am Stat Assoc* 2001;96:895–905.
51. Stallard N, Whitehead J, Todd S, et al. Stopping rules for phase II studies. *Br J Clin Pharmacol* 2001;51:523–529.
52. Malakoff D. Bayes offers a "new" way to make sense of numbers. *Science* 1999;286:1460–1464.
53. Berry DA, Müller P, Grieve AP, et al. Adaptive Bayesian designs for dose-ranging drug trials. In: Gatsonis C, Carlin B, Carriquiry A, eds. *Case studies in Bayesian statistics V.* New York: Springer Verlag, 2001:99–181.
54. Sox HC, Blatt MA, Higgins MC, et al. *Medical decision making.* Boston: Butterworth-Heinemann, 1980.
55. Clemen RT. *Making hard decisions,* 2nd ed. Belmont, CA: Duxbury Press, 1996.
56. Berry DA. Decision analysis and Bayesian methods. In: Thall PF, ed. *Recent advances in clinical trial design and analysis.* Boston: Kluwer Academic Publishers, 1995:Chapter 7.
57. Lewis RJ, Berry DA. Decision theory. In: Armitage P, Colton T, eds. *Encyclopedia of biostatistics.* New York: John Wiley & Sons, 1998.
58. Cheng Y, Su F, Berry DA. Choosing sample size for a clinical trial using decision analysis. *Biometrika* 2003 *(in press).*
59. Inoue LYT, Thall PF, Berry DA. Seamlessly expanding a randomized phase II trial to phase III. *Biometrics* 2002;58:823–831.

PART 7

Specific Issues in Drug Development

27

Data Verification and Scientific Auditing

Raymond B. Weiss

Lombardi Cancer Center, Georgetown University Medical Center, Washington, DC 20007

WHY DO DATA AUDITS?

No clinical trial for any disease is worthwhile unless the data are trustworthy and reliable. Whenever any scientific observation is made (whether in the laboratory or the clinic), the usual scientific process involves attempted duplication by peers to validate the observations and conclusions. Such duplication and verification are relatively simple with laboratory experiments and clinical trials involving small numbers of patients (e.g., fewer than 50). However, large randomized trials comparing two to four treatments may involve hundreds or even several thousand patients to provide adequate statistical power for testing whatever hypothesis is being evaluated and drawing valid conclusions. Such large studies commonly involve several stratification categories, which add further complexity to the trials, and they may take 5 or more years to complete. They also involve expenditures of large amounts of money to collect the data and perform analyses. Whatever conclusions are drawn from such studies are going to be quoted extensively and used by many physicians as the basis for clinical care of many future patients. They also involve multiple institutions spread all over the country or even the world to obtain the necessary numbers of patient entries, with a resultant high degree of variability in the skills of the participating investigators and their dedication to excellence. Although duplication of such studies by other investigators would be the ideal means of verifying the data and the conclusions drawn, the complexity, cost, and time involved make it impractical to attempt such reproduction. It would be better to be certain in the first place that the data are as reliable as possible.

The conduct of scientific experiments and the presentation of results is a process based on trust. Peer review of a manuscript before publication is one means of assessing the validity of data, but no peer reviewer can be certain the actual data collection has been reliable. Although some bias may be present in any presentation of scientific data, the peer assumes the investigator is at least honest; unfortunately, investigator honesty is not always the case. The following episode well illustrates this unfortunate situation.

In 1990s, no scientific issue in the field of oncology engendered more debate, both orally at meetings and in print, than whether or not high-dose chemotherapy (HDC), with progenitor cell support, provided a greater benefit than conventional-dose chemotherapy for patients with any stage of breast cancer. Uncontrolled phase II trials involving groups of highly selected patients suggested that HDC improved both disease-free and overall survival for patients with stage II, III, or IV disease. Randomized prospective trials comparing HDC and conventional chemotherapy for breast cancer were initiated in the early 1990s in the United States and Europe, but it would take time to accrue sufficient patients with the necessary follow-up interval after treatment completion. In the meantime, many women and their oncologists clamored for this new aggressive therapy based on both the limited data and the simple and intuitive concept that more chemotherapy must be better. Entwined in this scientific debate was the financial issue regarding how such therapy would be funded for women with breast cancer. HDC with transplant support is costly, and this new demand for an expensive therapy for a common malignancy hit medical insurance companies in the same decade as efforts were being initiated to restrain medical care costs in the United States. When insurance coverage for a proposed transplant was denied, litigation involving multimillion-dollar suits was inevitable. The scientific arguments always came down to the fact that uncontrolled studies suggested a benefit from HDC, but randomized controlled studies are the gold standard for assessing the value of a therapy. At the height of this scientific debate amid much litigation in 1995, a prominent investigator from South Africa reported a randomized trial purporting to show

HDC was superior in efficacy to conventional chemotherapy for the treatment of metastatic breast cancer (1). Now there could no longer be argument about the benefit of such therapy, because the gold standard randomized trial had been published, and it was published in the most prominent journal in the field of oncology. An editorial praising the study, written by a respected transplant oncologist, was printed in the same journal issue (2). Although there were scientific criticisms of the trial (3), as is often the case with any scientific study, oncologists trusted the results and quoted the report widely, both in other journal articles and for care of individual patients. As of February 2001, the article (1) had been referenced in other publications at least 354 times (Institute for Scientific Information, *personal communication,* March 2001).

The article (1) achieved a great deal of prominence and brought international preeminence to the investigator, resulting in invitations to scientific meetings to recapitulate the results of this trial (4). When the investigator submitted to the May 1999 meeting of the American Society of Clinical Oncology (ASCO) an abstract reporting a second purported randomized trial (5), this time in early-stage, high-risk breast cancer, he was invited to present his paper at the Plenary Session of this large meeting with an international audience of thousands, the most prestigious segment of this annual event. He again reported a favorable effect of HDC over a conventional-dose regimen. However, other randomized studies reported by US and European investigators at this same meeting did not show such a favorable effect. Thus, US investigators involved in breast cancer research and transplant were planning to launch a similar randomized trial to see if the South African study results could be duplicated, using the same HDC regimen reported by the investigator (5). However, before such an expensive and time-consuming study was initiated, an on-site audit of the primary patient records was requested. When this audit was conducted, it was discovered that much of the data were totally unreliable and that no randomized study had been conducted, as reported at the ASCO meeting (6). Based on suspicion that the fully published trial (1) reported similarly unverifiable results, a second on-site audit of patient records was done (7) and the suspicions fulfilled. The whole reported clinical trial and the results (1) had been made up. Many patients could not be verified as being eligible for the study, there was no randomization, the conventional-dose treatments given were inconsistent with the published report, patient follow-up was inadequate, and no records for 29 of the patients alleged to have been entered on the study could be located despite a supreme effort to find them at several institutions in Johannesburg. The final

chicanery was the fact the protocols for these two alleged studies were written 9 years after the studies were supposed to have been started and just before an audit team arrived. Not only did this investigator commit scientific fraud (which he admitted in a letter (8) to his South African colleagues) in a published paper and an oral presentation at the most prestigious session of an international meeting with a peer audience of thousands, but nine other of his publications contained at least one statement that could be established as being false (7). The actions of this oncologist were monumental scientific misconduct, and the most unfortunate aspect of this whole affair is that the original publication (1) directly influenced the use of HDC for thousands of women with breast cancer around the world, costing untold amounts of money. Another, more carefully conducted, randomized study did not demonstrate any benefit for HDC in metastatic breast cancer, and few women now receive this sort of therapy for this cancer (9). Incidentally, this study (9) was conducted by one of the National Cancer Institute (NCI)-funded cooperative groups (the Eastern Cooperative Oncology Group) that has an on-site auditing program in place, as discussed later.

This example of scientific misconduct unfortunately is not the only instance of such dishonesty, and it is not limited to the field of oncology, one country, or clinical trials. A number of known examples of similar dishonesty, although certainly not exhaustive, can be cited (10–18). It is not unique to medicine or a new phenomenon (19). The authors (20) of a publication by investigators in the European Organization for Research in the Treatment of Cancer (EORTC) asked the rhetorical question, "Chemotherapy administration and data collection in an EORTC collaborative group—can we trust the results?" The answer to this question is, "Not always," as is well illustrated by the examples of scientific fraud described earlier (10–18). Such misconduct fortunately is rare, but what is not rare is plain human error, produced by the human frailties of sloppiness, inattention to detail, procrastination, attempting shortcuts, forgetfulness, and sloth. All of these human deficiencies can result in errors in a trial that may bias or invalidate the results. In order to minimize errors it is necessary to verify the raw data, and there is no more reliable means of data verification than on-site peer review of the medical records of the patients entered on the clinical trial. If such on-site review of a trial has been accomplished in a large fraction of the patients entered, a reader of the final scientific publication can be more confident of the results. An example is a study that has been cited in the medical literature at least 332 times (Institute for Scientific Information, personal *communication,* December 2002) since its publication in 1994 (21). There were 1,529 patients who were treated in this study, and a large fraction (24%) had on-site review and validation of the medical records (21). Although it was not feasible, or even necessary, to audit all 1,529 patients, a sufficient fraction, involving entries at all the participating institutions, were reviewed. Results from a study validated with this sort of scientific audit presumably can be trusted more than one without such quality assurance.

WHO DOES AUDITS?

Since 1981 the cooperative groups funded by the NCI have performed on-site audits of a sample of patients entered in all clinical trials conducted by these groups. A component of the NCI designated as the Clinical Trials Monitoring Branch (CTMB), with a staff of seven, oversees these audits and monitors the results provided in reports for every institution audited. A 40-page set of "Guidelines for Monitoring of Clinical Trials" (22) is the document that is the basis for conducting these audits, and each cooperative group funded by NCI has a committee of data managers and physicians who spend part of their professional time doing them. Other entities that perform audits (Table 27.1) are NCI contractors outside the cooperative groups, the US Food and Drug Administration (FDA) (18,23), and pharmaceutical companies sponsoring trials with their new agents. In very unusual circumstances the investigative arm of the US Congress, the General Accounting Office, may conduct audits (24). Cancer centers funded by the NCI are also charged with the responsibility of auditing the trials conducted within their purview. In the United States there are no trials funded by either the federal government or a drug company that do not have some sort of auditing process in place.

One of the NCI-funded large cooperative groups is the Cancer and Leukemia Group B (CALGB). This group of collaborating institutions has some 300 members consisting of large academic institutions, community hospitals, veterans hospitals, and private practices. At any one time approximately 100 studies are open, and the annual patient entries number approximately 3,500, with more than half of these patients also being entered in one or more "companion" studies involving assessment of some aspect of tumor biology. This adds another 2,000 annual study accruals. One of the standing CALGB administrative committees is the Data Audit Committee (DAC). This committee consists of approximately 20 CALGB investigators, half of whom are physicians and half are clinical research associates (CRAs). The DAC chair provides audit manager services as a contractor to CALGB and is the only committee member paid separately for this particular work. The other committee members are all active investigators at CALGB member institutions and give their time auditing as part of their contribution to the research activities of CALGB. They are compensated by the salary already being paid by their home institutions. A separate budget for travel costs for auditing is maintained in the NCI grant that supports the work of the CALGB central office.

The DAC members are self-selected for interest in doing this sort of work, skill in performing the task, willingness to travel for several days four to six times annually, and good knowledge of the various CALGB studies. An audit usually is accomplished in at most 2.5 days, because the volunteers in CALGB who do auditing are unable to spare any more time away from their regular work at their home institutions. In addition, the tedium of scrutinizing extensive medical records and verifying data is tolerable for only so long. Because the 20 DAC members cannot do all the audit work for 300 institutions, ad hoc auditors who also are active CALGB investigators (but not DAC members) are invited on many of the larger audits as a means of distributing the workload and as an educational experience valuable for all concerned.

HOW TO DO DATA AUDITS

Once it is established that on-site review of patient records is valuable for quality assurance purposes, the next question is how such audits should be done. What first must be done before a clinical trial is even initiated is to be certain permission is given by the

TABLE 27.1. *Entities involved in audits of cancer clinical trials*

- Cooperative groups funded by the National Cancer Institute (NCI)
- Pharmaceutical companies
- Food and Drug Administration (FDA)
- Contractors to the NCI
- European Organization for Research in the Treatment of Cancer (EORTC)
- Cancer centers
- Clinical Center at the National Institutes of Health, Bethesda, Maryland
- General Accounting Office

patients for such review of their medical records by professionals outside the institution involved. Such permission should be a standard component of the consent form signed by the patient for entry in the trial. In US studies this granting of permission is standard for all consents for studies at institutions funded by the NCI. For example, the consent contains phrasing that the patients authorize review of their medical records by representatives of the FDA, the NCI, and the cooperative group conducting the study. When relevant, permission also is granted to representatives of the drug company involved in the study. With the implementation of the Health Insurance Portability and Accountability Act (HIPAA) in the United States in 2003, written granting of permission for review of medical records will become even more important.

Audit Procedures

The CTMB guidelines for audits of NCI-funded institutions direct that each institution entering at least one patient in an NCI-sponsored trial will be audited at least every 36 months, with every institution being subject to audit during any 1 year (22). A minimum of 10% of the annual patient entries at each institution are audited, but in CALGB the fraction is usually at least 15% and may be as high as 100%, or nearly so, for institutions entering only small numbers of patients yearly. When a pharmaceutical company is the sponsor of a study, on-site audits may be done much more frequently by company representatives (as often as every other month), and all patients are reviewed. In addition, the audit process may differ from that of entities under the jurisdiction of the CTMB guidelines and is likely to vary with each company conducting audits. The remainder of this discussion focuses on the audit methods of CALGB. Its sister cooperative groups under CTMB oversight have similar audit methods.

For CALGB audits the team leader is always a member of the DAC and is an experienced auditor, usually a physician. The team leader heads the exit interview at the end of every audit, is the final arbiter of any deviations and deficiencies cited at the audit, and writes the final report that is submitted to the CTMB at NCI. A CRA and a physician almost always work as a pair, with the physician reviewing the on-site medical records and the CRA handling all the case report forms (CRFs) submitted. The audit process is one of matching whatever is reported in the CRFs with source documents in the local records. If deviations from the protocol are noted, a decision is made between the two auditors whether it is trivial, minor (lesser), or major. A trivial deviation is one so minor that it is not even worth comment. An example would be a patient who

received the day 8 dose of one therapy cycle on day 10 because of clinic scheduling issues. A minor or lesser deviation would be one where the data from that patient are still usable and valid even though the protocol was not followed exactly. An example would be the failure to do the required baseline electrocardiogram on a patient with no history of any heart disease. A major deviation would be any deficiency where the data from that patient are questionable and may cause the patient to be disallowed from the final analysis. An example would be a patient who does not meet all the eligibility requirements of the study.

Depending on the number of patients to be audited, the number of auditors visiting any one institution may vary from two to ten. Some major institutions with up to 70 patients to be audited in 2 days would require four pairs of auditors (one pair consists of one physician and one CRA) to accomplish the workload. Experience in CALGB has shown that one audit team can review approximately ten patient records in one workday, plus accomplish the required administrative reviews. Teams reviewing complex studies, such as those for treating acute myelogenous leukemia, may be able to handle only seven or eight records in one workday.

The patient lists are provided to the institution staff 3 or 4 weeks prior to the audit date and involve a cross-section of the protocols to which patients have been entered at the institution and usually a sample of patients from each study, with the number varying according to the accruals to particular studies. In CALGB an attempt is also made to review at least one patient entered by each participating physician-investigator. The institution staff assembles all inpatient and outpatient records, all relevant radiographs when evaluable tumor is being assessed for study purposes, and all relevant administrative records. The staff then tags important study items in the local records so that they may be readily located at the audit. Searching for particular items through unfamiliar medical records without tagging would waste considerable amounts of auditor time. Institution staff stay with the auditors at all times to assist with locating items or explaining questions the auditors raise regarding why some particular action was, or was not, taken.

At the same time the institution is preparing for the audit, the Data Operations Unit of the CALGB Statistical Center copies all CRFs submitted for the patients being audited. These documents are then used for comparison with the on-site medical records. Instead of copying CRFs, some of the NCI-funded groups provide printouts of the computerized data submitted on the patients to be audited, again to be compared with the on-site medical records.

Administrative Reviews

The first item for review in data audits conducted in the United States is to verify that the institutional review board (IRB; also known as the ethics committee in other countries) has initially reviewed and approved the study protocol and the consent form and has provided the required oversight in the form of annual reviews and renewals of the study, review of substantive revisions in the protocol, and timely reporting and review of unexpected serious adverse events. Failure to accomplish any of these required components of IRB oversight are considered "major deviations" in the administrative aspects of the trial conduct.

Another administrative aspect subject to outside audit is the content of the consent form and its signing. The contents of a sample of consents are reviewed for compliance with all information required by both the federal government and the local IRB, and then all consents signed by the audited patients are checked for a patient signature and date (with the date being prior to official entry onto the trial) and any other required items such as a witness signature. Such review of the consent and IRB oversight assures compliance with important aspects of patient protection and adherence to the tenets of clinical research in the Declaration of Helsinki (25).

In the United States another administrative function performed at audits is review of the handling and dispensing of investigational agents. The NCI has a number of requirements for record keeping and handling of the drugs it provides for clinical trials (26). The auditors verify that all drug supplies provided by the NCI were administered to a patient properly entered in the particular clinical trial, are in stock in the institution pharmacy, or, when no longer needed, have been returned to the NCI.

Patient Case Reviews

The bulk of audit work involves review of patient records, which is, of course, the main purpose of a scientific audit. As described earlier, the patient charts have been assembled prior to the audit and tagged to identify salient items regarding the clinical trial, such as all the preentry items that verify the patient met the eligibility criteria of the study, the treatment cycles, the radiology reports or pathology information that support the claimed tumor outcome (response or lack thereof and degree of response), and follow-up.

The first step is to verify that the patient met all the eligibility criteria of the study, that all required baseline blood tests and radiographs were performed, and that the tests were performed within the time limits specified in the protocol. This assessment will include review of the pathology reports, operative reports, and notes written by physicians and other health personnel. Once the patient is confirmed as being eligible, stratification in the proper category at the time of randomization (if applicable) is verified.

Treatment doses and schedule are reviewed for all treatment cycles, be it four cycles of adjuvant chemotherapy after surgery or ten cycles of therapy, for example, for metastatic disease. Physician notes and chemotherapy administration records are reviewed and compared with the CRFs for accuracy and compliance with the protocol. Toxicity information is evaluated for accuracy in reporting and grading on the CRFs. Drug dose modifications, if made, are assessed for compliance with protocol directives for such dose changes.

If the study involves monitoring evaluable tumor for changes in response to therapy, the physicians on the audit team will review the relevant radiographs to confirm the claimed responses. Although the oncologists performing audits are not radiologists, they can, for example, generally assess the difference between a partial and a complete response or concur with an assessment of progressive disease. Compliance with the protocol requirements for frequency of patient follow-up and long-term outcome is reviewed.

Finally, the auditors verify that all required CRFs have been submitted, and submitted on time. If relevant to the particular study, special blood or marrow sample submissions and pathology submissions for central review are verified. For patients who received protocol-directed irradiation, there are quality assurance centers funded by the NCI for assessing treatment compliance. For example, one such center is the Quality Assurance Review Center (QARC), which acts as the central reviewer of radiation therapy for a number of NCI-funded studies being conducted by the cooperative groups. A radiation oncologist and a dosimetrist at QARC review all radiation therapy records and the relevant radiographs to verify compliance with the protocol. Most protocols require this central review of radiation treatment planning data within a few days of initiating therapy so that any errors detected can be corrected early in the treatment.

AUDIT REPORTS

Results for audits conducted by the cooperative groups and NCI contractors are reported to the CTMB at NCI. If a pharmaceutical company is sponsoring the trial and conducting the audit, a report is made to the company; the report eventually may be subject to review by the FDA if marketing approval is sought for the new drug. CTMB has a Web-based program in a special format that is used for all audit reports to the NCI. It is divided into three sections (IRB/consent content, pharmacy, and patient cases) of the review. The patient case review section has six categories for assessment: consent signing; eligibility; treatment; toxicity; outcome and follow-up; and data quality and special sample submissions. Each of these six categories is rated as being "OK," a lesser deviation, or a major deviation. A summary rating of acceptable, acceptable needs follow-up, or unacceptable is given for each of the three major report segments. Too many major deviations or deficiencies in any of these three categories requires at least a response by the principal investigator (PI) regarding how the work quality can be improved and may trigger the need for a re-audit within 12 months. The work of some institutions is so egregiously poor that the institution may be dropped from the group.

DATA MODIFICATIONS

There is little point in performing scientific audits if the information from the audit is not utilized to improve data quality and protocol adherence. CALGB has a system of providing feedback to the database with audit information. The data coordinators at the Data Operations Unit of the CALGB Statistical Center go over every audit report and take note of any deviations for each patient that may require a change in the database. For example, if the patient were found ineligible at the audit, this information would be entered. If a toxicity were graded incorrectly or not reported at all, a correction would be made. If, for example, the auditors believed the patient had only stable disease instead of the reported partial response of the evaluable tumor, a request would be made of the institution staff to reassess the radiographs with their radiologists to take another look at the issue of response. If certain data are delinquent, the PI at the institution would have to provide a plan on how such delinquencies are going to be corrected. If the audit result rating was "unacceptable," the PI would have to provide a detailed plan on how work at that institution is going to be improved and accomplished by the time of a re-audit, which usually is done 10 to 12 months later.

AUDIT RESULTS

The results of CALGB audits conducted in the years 1982 to 1992 have been reported (27). The CALGB DAC has existed for 22 years and has acted as a constant prod to institution staff to adhere to protocols when entering and treating a patient and reporting accurately on the involved CRFs. The percentage of patients ineligible for the protocol on which they were entered stays at a rate of approximately 4%, which probably is the best it will ever be keeping in mind the human error factor. Accuracy in rating responses (or lack thereof) stays at a level of approximately 96%, with the 4% error rate reflecting an approximately equal rate of inaccurately upgrading and downgrading response assessments (27). Audits also serve as an educational tool because while auditors are reviewing data there is ample opportunity to teach CRAs the proper procedures for various data entries and protocol adherence and to point out errors. In addition, the auditors themselves gain valuable experience to carry back to their own institutions after observing how others perform protocol and data tasks better, or worse, than they do.

Reports of audit results are rare in the medical literature, but several examples of problems revealed by audits reiterate their value. When an outside audit of a phase I study was performed, some of the tumor responses were found to have been "overstated" (28) A CALGB audit uncovered scientific fraud committed by a physician involved in its clinical trials (29). This physician subsequently was prosecuted by the US Department of Justice for submitting false information to the government. Another anecdote illustrates the problems that can occur when the rate of ineligible patients in a study exceeds what would be considered reasonable. An ineligibility rate of 26% occurred in a study that was used as the basis for a fast-track approval application to the FDA for a new antitumor antibody (30). When the FDA staff reviewed the data from this study, they rejected the approval application as being inadequate, and the drug company involved has had to initiate new studies to meet the FDA requirements for marketing approval, which has considerably increased the time to eventual marketing of this drug, if approval is ever granted.

CONCLUSION

Each cooperative group funded by the NCI has an audit program in place that provides constant oversight for protocol compliance and data collection accuracy in all studies conducted by each group. In addition, pharmaceutical firms audit their funded institutions conducting company-sponsored trials. Of course, on-site data audits are not the only means for assuring data accuracy (Table 27.2). For example, eligibility checks are done on *all* patients in the central data management facilities of the cooperative groups, whereas this is done only for a sample of patients at an audit. However, audits sometimes find information in

TABLE 27.2. *Quality assurance mechanisms for clinical trials*

- Good training of the physician-investigators and the clinical research associates (CRAs) regarding all required responsibilities
- Statistical expertise involvement and oversight
- Close oversight by a principal investigator
- Close oversight by the institutional review board (ethics committee)
- Oversight by an independent Data Safety and Monitoring Board
- Continuous monitoring of case report forms (CRFs) and protocol compliance at a central data management facility
- Periodic on-site audits of medical records for a meaningful sample of patients
- Correction of errors detected by either audits or review of CRFs
- Periodic assessment of investigator performance and removal of poorly performing individuals and institutions

the medical record that makes the patient ineligible and was never transmitted to the data center. A basic tenet is that all participating investigators and CRAs should have good training in the clinical trial process before beginning to accrue patients. The PI should be directly involved in the study and review of CRFs and should not just be a figurehead. The IRB should be aware what investigators are doing in their institutions. Some IRBs even conduct their own internal audits to verify compliance with all required patient safety procedures. Periodic and comprehensive performance monitoring of all institution participants in a trial is another valuable prod for good work (31). All of these measures provide the observer of the results of reported trials with assurance that the studies have been conducted with as much accuracy as possible, given the number of patients and centers involved and variability in the capabilities of the professionals entering their patients in the study. When studies have various mechanisms in place to assure data accuracy (Table 27.2) and are reported to have, for example, 24% of the patients entered (21) subject to audit, the study can be reasonably assumed to be reporting accurate results. When studies not subject to such on-site peer review of medical records are reported, one may have some degree of skepticism about the results. The data are not always as reliable as they might be. These programs of continuous trial monitoring with on-site audits in the NCI-funded cooperative groups can serve as models for others to emulate, thus providing assurance in the accuracy of data reporting for all published clinical trials.

Supported by grants U10 CA 31946 and U10 CA 77597 from the National Cancer Institute, Bethesda, MD, USA.

REFERENCES

1. Bezwoda WR, Seymour L, Dansey RD. High dose chemotherapy with hematopoietic rescue as primary treatment for metastatic breast cancer: a randomized trial. *J Clin Oncol* 1995;13:2483–2489.
2. Kennedy MJ. High-dose chemotherapy of breast cancer: is the question answered? [Editorial] *J Clin Oncol* 1995;13:2477–2479.
3. Weiss RB. The randomized trials of dose-intensive therapy for breast cancer: what do they mean for patient care and where do we go from here? *Oncologist* 1999;4: 450–458.
4. Bezwoda WR. High-dose chemotherapy with hematopoietic rescue in breast cancer: from theory to practice. *Cancer Chemother Pharmacol* 1997;40: S79–S87.
5. Bezwoda WR. Randomised, controlled trial of high dose chemotherapy (HD-CNVp) versus standard dose (CAF) chemotherapy for high risk, surgically treated, primary breast cancer. *Proc Am Soc Clin Oncol* 1999; 18:2(abst).
6. Weiss RB, Rifkin RM, Stewart FM, et al. High-dose chemotherapy for high-risk primary breast cancer: an on-site review of the Bezwoda study. *Lancet* 2000; 355:999–1003.
7. Weiss RB, Gill GG, Hudis CA. An on-site audit of the South African trial of high-dose chemotherapy for metastatic breast cancer and associated publications. *J Clin Oncol* 2001;19:2771–2777.
8. Anonymous. South African investigator Bezwoda admits falsifying data in high-dose chemo study. *Cancer Lett* 2000;26:1–4.
9. Stadtmauer EA, O'Neill A, Goldstein LJ, et al. Conventional-dose chemotherapy compared with high-dose chemotherapy plus autologous hematopoietic stem-cell transplantation for metastatic breast cancer. *N Engl J Med* 2000;342:1069–1076.
10. Ferriman A. Consultant suspended for research fraud. *BMJ* 2000;321:1429.
11. Birmingham K. Misconduct trouble brewing in Göttingen. *Nature Med* 2001;7:875.
12. Anonymous. ORI misconduct findings announced in two cases. *Cancer Lett* 1996;22:4–6.
13. Weber W. Freiburg oncologist found guilty of scientific misconduct. *Lancet* 2001;357:780.
14. Greenberg DS. US genome chief withdraws five papers over fraud. *Lancet* 1996;348:1303.
15. Culliton BJ. Harvard researchers retract data in immunology paper. *Science* 1986;234:1069.
16. McCarthy M. US government suspends clinical research at another university. *Lancet* 2000;356: 320.

17. Neaton JD, Bartsch GE, Broste SK, et al. A case of data alteration in the Multiple Risk Factor Intervention Trial (MRFIT). The MRFIT Reseach Group. *Control Clin Trials* 1991;12:731–740.
18. Shapiro MF, Charrow RP. Scientific misconduct in investigational drug trials. *N Engl J Med* 1985;321: 731–736.
19. Weiss MP. Falsifying priority of species names: a fraud of 1892. *Earth Sci History* 1997;16:21–32.
20. Steward WP, Vantongelen K, Verweij J, et al. Chemotherapy administration and data collection in an EORTC collaborative group—can we trust the results? *Eur J Cancer* 1993;29A:943–947.
21. Wood WC, Budman DR, Korzun AH, et al. Dose and dose intensity of adjuvant chemotherapy for stage II, node-positive breast carcinoma. *N Engl J Med* 1994; 330:1253–1259.
22. Anonymous. Guidelines for monitoring of clinical trials for cooperative groups, CCOP research bases, and the Cancer Trials Support Unit (CTSU). Available at: *http://ctep.cancer.gov/monitoring/guidelines.html.*
23. Shapiro MF, Charrow RP. The role of data audits in detecting scientific misconduct. Results of the FDA program. *JAMA* 1989;261:2505–2511.
24. Kosty MP, Herndon JE, Green MR, et al. Placebo-controlled randomized study of hydrazine sulfate in lung cancer. *J Clin Oncol* 1995;13:1529–1530.
25. Declaration of Helsinki. Recommendations guiding medical doctors in biomedical research involving human subjects. *Med J Aust* 1976;1:206–207 (an updated version is also available at: *http://www.wma.net).*
26. Anonymous. Requisition of agents. Available at: *http://ctep.cancer.gov/requisition.*
27. Weiss RB, Vogelzang NJ, Peterson, BA, et al. A successful system of scientific data audits for clinical trial. A report from the Cancer and Leukemia Group B. *JAMA* 1993;270:459–464.
28. Cheung N-KV, Lazarus H, Miraldi FD, et al. Reassessment of patient response to monoclonal antibody 3F8. *J Clin Oncol* 1992;10:671–672.
29. Anonymous. Physician indicted for mail fraud after allegedly falsifying data of patients on ECOG, CALGB trials. *Cancer Lett* 1984;10:1–2.
30. Anonymous. Expert Raymond Weiss finds "incredible" protocol violations. *Cancer Lett* 2002;28:4–7.
31. Knatterud GL, Rockhold FW, George SL, et al. Guidelines for quality assurance in multicenter trials: a position paper. *Control Clin Trials* 1998;19:477–493.

28

Role of the Cooperative Groups in Drug Development

Christopher W. Ryan and Richard L. Schilsky*

*Biological Sciences Division, University of Chicago, Chicago, Illinois 60637

The United States cancer cooperative groups comprise a large network of physicians, nurses, clinical research associates, and other affiliated investigators who voluntarily work together to conduct cancer clinical trials. The cooperative group system plays a critical role in anticancer drug development and is considered the major vehicle for conducting publicly supported large-scale, multiinstitutional, randomized studies. The scope of research activities performed through the cooperative group system has expanded greatly since its inception and includes studies that encompass all phases of anticancer drug development, all modalities of treatment, as well as correlative science and translational research studies.

The Clinical Trials Cooperative Groups were originally organized by the National Cancer Institute (NCI) with the mission to conduct clinical trials of new cancer therapies. The cooperative group program began in 1955 when Dr. Sidney Farber, Mary Lasker, and others appealed to Congress for increased support of chemotherapy research. The Chemotherapy National Service Center was established within the NCI with $5 million in congressional support. By 1958, 17 groups were receiving NCI funding to perform cancer clinical trials using new agents from the NCI's drug development program. Out of this initiative, the groups evolved to become the NCI Clinical Trials Cooperative Group Program. Currently, more than 2,200 institutions and 16,000 investigators participate in the program, which encompasses comprehensive cancer centers, medical schools, and large public hospitals. The NCI's Community Clinical Oncology Program (CCOP) allows community physicians to participate in cooperative group studies, expanding the availability of clinical trials for patients who are unable to travel to a major medical center. Nearly 30,000 patients participate yearly in cooperative group studies, comprising approximately 60% of all patients participating in cancer clinical trials nationwide. Since their inception, the groups have enrolled more than 500,000 patients in more than 4,000 clinical trials (1). Approximately $180 million in annual funding currently is provided to the cooperative groups by the NCI.

The US cooperative groups have evolved and coalesced over the years to emerge as distinct focused entities that are vital to clinical cancer research. The ten current NCI-sponsored cooperative groups are listed in Table 28.1. Certain cooperative groups focus on limited types of cancer, others focus on specific modalities of treatment, and others are broadly multidisciplinary.

COOPERATIVE GROUP PROCESS

Each cooperative group is funded by the NCI to continually develop new studies in its particular areas of interest. Funding is not linked to any specific clinical trial, as is the format for most National Institutes of Health (NIH)-sponsored initiatives. Because the mechanism for generating new studies is always in place, this allows considerable flexibility and potential for rapid testing of new cancer therapies.

The Cancer Therapy Evaluation Program (CTEP) is the program within the Division of Cancer Treatment and Diagnosis (DCTD) of the NCI that oversees the research activities of the cooperative groups. Cooperative groups obtain new anticancer agents via CTEP, as well as directly from industry. CTEP sponsors Investigational New Drug applications (INDs) for more than 175 agents that are supplied by numerous pharmaceutical companies. Several branches within CTEP are responsible for the development of agents and work closely with the cooperative groups, as summarized in Table 28.2.

TABLE 28.1. *United States Cancer Cooperative Groups*

American College of Radiology Imaging Network (ACRIN)
American College of Surgeons Oncology Group (ACOSOG)
Cancer and Leukemia Group B (CALGB)
Children's Oncology Group (COG)
Eastern Cooperative Oncology Group (ECOG)
Gynecologic Oncology Group (GOG)
National Surgical Adjuvant Breast and Bowel Project (NSABP)
North Central Cancer Treatment Group (NCCTG)
Radiation Therapy Oncology Group (RTOG)
Southwest Oncology Group (SWOG)

The general structure of each cooperative group includes an operations center and a statistical center, which are overseen by the group chair and the group statistician, respectively. Groups are composed of institutions that are main members, affiliates of a main institution, or members of a participating CCOP. Each institution is represented by a principal or senior investigator who is responsible for overseeing and managing the cooperative group activities within the institution. A minimum level of accrual is required to maintain membership, as well as consistent quality in the conduct of research protocols as appraised by periodic on-site audits and other quality control measures. The audit program serves to verify study data through independent verification with source documentation (2). The audit program of each cooperative group is overseen by the Clinical Trials Monitoring Branch of CTEP.

Each cooperative group includes multiple disease or modality committees, each charged with developing research initiatives within their respective areas of expertise. Investigators typically present study con-

TABLE 28.2. *Structure of the Cancer Therapy Evaluation Program (CTEP) at the National Cancer Institute (NCI)*

Investigational Drug Branch: oversees and monitors studies using CTEP-sponsored agents
Pharmaceutical Management Branch: provides for distribution of investigational agents
Regulatory Affairs Branch: liaison between industry and the Food and Drug Administration (FDA)
Clinical Investigations Branch: supports comparative clinical trials
Biometric Research Branch: assesses clinical trial design
Clinical Trials Monitoring Branch: oversees cooperative group audits and quality assurance

cepts at semiannual group meetings, where discussions within the committees may lead to acceptance of the concept. If the concept is approved, then a complete protocol is written by the study chair. The protocol undergoes several levels of internal review, including peer review by the committee membership and the group statistical center.

Protocols subsequently undergo additional review by CTEP, and if applicable, the Food and Drug Administration (FDA). Following such approval, the study is distributed to individual institutions for activation. Activating a trial is at the discretion of the local institution and requires approval by the local institutional review board (IRB). IRB approval is mandated by federal regulations and assures that the trial meets local standards for the conduct of clinical research. The recent establishment of a Central IRB by the NCI provides a further level of ethical review for phase III studies.

Patients are enrolled in studies only if they meet the inclusion criteria; have been adequately informed regarding the potential risks, benefits, and alternatives; and have signed an IRB-approved consent form. Upon enrollment, patients are registered centrally with the group's statistical center, and data are submitted at regular intervals to the statistical center. Phase III treatment studies are subject to monitoring by a data and safety monitoring board (DSMB) at predefined points during study accrual. Unexpected toxicities or results can lead the DSMB to modify or close a study or release results early. The multiple levels of peer, federal, and local review ensure that cooperative group trials are exemplary models of clinical research.

UNIQUE CAPABILITIES OF THE COOPERATIVE GROUPS

The emphasis of the cooperative group program traditionally has been to conduct definitive, prospective randomized studies of new cancer treatments. Although the majority of patients treated in cooperative group studies are enrolled in phase III trials, the scope of research performed by the groups encompasses a far greater spectrum. Phase I and phase II studies comprise a large portion of the research portfolio of the groups and can be completed rapidly because of the large patient population available at hundreds of sites. Multicenter phase II studies are likely to provide more objective and generalizable results than single-center trials and provide data that reflect treatment outcomes more likely to be obtained in phase III trials. Multicenter phase II trials are the only efficient mechanism for evaluating new agents in rare tumor types and in special populations, such as those with organ dysfunction, minority populations, and the elderly. Studies involving pathologic and basic science correlates also are an important component of the groups' work. Indeed, the introduction of molecularly targeted therapies that may be appropriate for only a small segment of a patient population (e.g., Her2/neu + breast cancer) requires the conduct of multicenter trials to enable completion of accrual in a timely fashion.

Studies shared between the cooperative groups (the so-called Intergroup) allow rapid accrual to large phase III trials and make feasible studies of rare diseases or rare subpopulations. Intergroup cooperation promotes sharing of resources and expertise from the respective groups. The Intergroup process was pioneered within the breast cancer committees and now includes meetings between leaders of all the major disease sites. Advances in adjuvant therapies often are made through Intergroup collaboration, due to the large numbers of patients required to answer such questions.

The cooperative group mechanism facilitates research in special populations. For example, the Cancer and Leukemia Group B (CALGB) Cancer in the Elderly Committee is addressing questions relevant to cancer care in older patients. Initiatives in this population have included pharmacokinetic analyses of commonly used chemotherapeutic agents, such as paclitaxel and irinotecan, to detect age-related variability in toxicity and pharmacokinetics and investigation of less toxic treatment regimens in breast cancer and leukemia. Pharmacologic studies in patients with hepatic or renal dysfunction have answered questions regarding dosing and safety that could not be answered with the limited number of patients available in single institutions. These studies are particularly important because early clinical trials of new agents virtually always exclude patients with organ dysfunction, yet such patients are commonly seen in oncology practices and no dosing guidelines exist for the safe administration of chemotherapy in these circumstances. The CALGB has completed studies of paclitaxel, gemcitabine, and irinotecan in patients with organ dysfunction that have led to specific dosing recommendations in these special populations (3,4).

The cooperative groups also have an important mission to make clinical trials available to minorities and other underserved populations. CTEP developed an initiative to increase minority accrual to clinical trials that has been met with enthusiasm by the groups. Some groups have minority-based CCOPs or have designated individual institutions with access to large minority populations to increase minority accrual.

The cooperative groups have served as a forum to test novel clinical trial designs that might not be feasible in single institutions. For example, the CALGB successfully accrued 374 patients to a randomized discontinuation study of carboxyaminoimidazole for metastatic renal cell carcinoma. In this study, patients who had stable disease after a prolonged run-in with this potential cytostatic agent were randomized to continue the agent or to receive placebo until progression. Randomized phase II studies and other designs that screen agents for activity can be performed rapidly through the cooperative groups. Novel trial designs will be increasingly important as the development of molecularly targeted anticancer agents changes our concept of clinical benefit.

As anticancer drug therapies evolve from nonspecific cytotoxic treatments to therapies directed against molecular targets, the nature of clinical research will continue to evolve. Selection of appropriate patients for directed therapies will be increasingly based on tumor expression of specific cellular and genetic targets. Such selective therapy will require a concerted effort among clinical oncologists, pathologists, and basic scientists. The cooperative groups are ideally poised to face this challenge, with access to specialized experts within each network of academic and community centers.

ACHIEVEMENTS OF THE COOPERATIVE GROUPS

The contribution of the cooperative groups to development of anticancer drug therapies has been significant. Seminal cooperative group studies have led to approval of new agents by the FDA and new indications for approved agents; they also have led to refined treatment approaches in all major malignancies. Given the high level of peer review associated with cooperative group studies and the quality of the institutions that participate, these studies are held in high regard by the oncology community and are considered to define the standard of care in cancer treatment.

The achievements of the cooperative groups in cancer drug development during the past 5 decades constitute an exhaustive list. The following is a selection of some of the major accomplishments and represents the scope and importance of cooperative group research in bringing therapeutic advances to the public.

Breast Cancer Adjuvant Chemotherapy

The National Surgical Adjuvant Breast and Bowel Project (NSABP) has performed numerous studies that have refined the optimal adjuvant treatment for women with localized breast cancer. Selected studies in patients with node-negative disease include NSABP B-13 and B-19, which demonstrated that systemic chemotherapy increased disease-free survival in women with estrogen receptor-negative tumors and overall survival in women 50 years or older (5). NSABP B-14 established the benefit of tamoxifen for node-negative, estrogen receptor-positive tumors, whereas the B-20 trial demonstrated increased benefit with the addition of chemotherapy to tamoxifen (6,7).

Recent advances in the adjuvant treatment of node-positive breast cancer include CALGB 9344, an Intergroup study that demonstrated that sequential addition of paclitaxel to doxorubicin/cyclophosphamide improved disease-free and overall survival for women with node-positive breast cancer (8). These results led to FDA approval of paclitaxel following doxorubicin/cyclophosphamide for the adjuvant treatment of node-positive breast cancer.

Negative studies have had equal importance in refining the approach to adjuvant therapy. The lack of utility of adjuvant high-dose chemotherapy with autologous bone marrow transplantation was demonstrated clearly by an Intergroup study (9).

Ovarian Cancer

The Gynecologic Oncology Group (GOG) has been instrumental in defining the most active chemotherapeutic agents for treatment of ovarian cancer. Two studies performed by the GOG (GOG-22 and GOG-47) established the value of cisplatin in the treatment of advanced ovarian cancer (10,11). The activity of paclitaxel was established by GOG-111, which randomized women with advanced ovarian carcinoma to cyclophosphamide and cisplatin versus paclitaxel and cisplatin and demonstrated improved progression-free and overall survival for women receiving paclitaxel (12). This was the first phase III trial of paclitaxel in the primary treatment of patients with cancer and was the primary study that led to FDA approval of paclitaxel for this indication.

Colorectal Cancer

A series of cooperative group studies established the long-term survival benefit of adjuvant chemotherapy for colorectal cancer. INT-0035 was a collaborative effort among the North Central Cancer Treatment Group (NCCTG), Eastern Cooperative Oncology Group (ECOG), and the Southwest Oncology Group (SWOG) that demonstrated a survival advantage for patients with Dukes stage C colon cancer who received 1 year of postoperative 5-fluorouracil (5-FU) in combination with levamisole (13). The early results of this study served as the basis for the NIH Consensus Panel recommendation of 5-FU/levamisole as standard adjuvant treatment. Further studies involving NCCTG, ECOG, CALGB, NSABP, and SWOG have refined the adjuvant treatment regimen, with 6 months of 5-FU and leucovorin emerging as standard of care for treatment of stage C disease (14–16). Recently completed Intergroup trials have examined whether addition of either irinotecan or oxaliplatin to 5-FU/leucovorin results in further improvement in survival of patients with node-positive colon cancer.

Adjuvant Treatment of Melanoma

A series of randomized trials demonstrated the benefit of adjuvant interferon therapy for patients with node-positive malignant melanoma and led to an FDA indication for use of interferon in this disease. ECOG 1684 randomized patients with deep primary or regionally metastatic melanoma to observation or to maximally tolerated doses of interferon alfa 2b. Both relapse-free and overall survival were prolonged with interferon treatment, with median survival increasing from 2.8 years to 3.8 years (17). ECOG 1690 confirmed a relapse-free but not overall survival advantage for interferon alfa in a three-arm trial randomizing patients to high-dose interferon, lower-dose interferon, or observation (18). ECOG 1694 tested a vaccine therapy in comparison to high-dose interferon and found the vaccine arm to be inferior, establishing interferon as the standard to which all other adjuvant therapies should be compared in future studies for high-risk patients (19). All of these studies were completed through Intergroup collaboration.

Adult Leukemia and Lymphoma

The approval of fludarabine for second-line treatment of chronic lymphocytic leukemia was partly based on SWOG 8378, a phase I/II study that demonstrated unequivocal activity of this agent (20). CALGB 9011 demonstrated a significantly higher complete response rate and progression-free survival for fludarabine over chlorambucil in first-line treatment of chronic lymphocytic leukemia (21). High-dose cytarabine was established by CALGB 8525 as standard consolidation therapy for patients younger than 60 years old with acute myeloid leukemia (22). For Hodgkin disease, a CALGB study established the ABVD (doxorubicin, bleomycin, vincristine, and dacarbazine) regimen as standard therapy for patients with advanced disease, based on less toxicity, fewer second malignancies, and no difference in outcome compared to the MOPP (mechlorethamine, vincristine, procarbazine, and prednisone)/ABV hybrid regimen (23). In INT-0067, the standard regimen of CHOP (cyclophosphamide, doxorubicin, vincristine, and prednisone) was found to be the best available treatment for advanced non-Hodgkin lymphoma, demonstrating no difference in 3-year survival and a lower incidence of treatment-related mortality compared to three third-generation regimens (24).

Lung Cancer

Data collected over the years from cooperative group studies can yield valuable information following retrospective analysis. A SWOG analysis of 2,531 patients with advanced non–small cell lung cancer (NSCLC) treated in clinical trials from 1974 to 1988 identified treatment with cisplatin as an independent predictor of improved outcome (25). These data, along with later studies of cisplatin combination therapy, led to platinum-based regimens becoming standard of care for NSCLC. The superiority of paclitaxel plus cisplatin over etoposide plus cisplatin was demonstrated by an ECOG study (26). The improved time to tumor progression observed with the paclitaxel combination led to an FDA indication and adoption of paclitaxel plus platinum as a common treatment for advanced NSCLC.

Cooperative group trials can serve as a mechanism to test controversial cancer therapies that may not be of interest to the pharmaceutical industry. Despite positive reports from small studies and anecdotes from vocal supporters, several randomized cooperative group studies failed to demonstrate any anticancer activity of hydrazine sulfate, a component of jet fuel with purported nutrition-enhancing properties. Two definitive studies were performed in advanced NSCLC and a third in advanced colorectal cancer by the NCCTG and the CALGB, each of which failed to show any benefit from the use of hydrazine sulfate (27–29).

Genitourinary Cancer

Cooperative group studies have led to approvals and new indications of drugs for prostate cancer. A Radiation Therapy Oncology Group (RTOG) study comparing radiation with or without combined androgen blockade in men with locally confined prostate cancer demonstrated improved disease-free survival and decreased local failure rates for patients receiving the hormone therapy. This study led to an FDA indication for the use of goserelin in combination with flutamide for men undergoing radiotherapy for localized disease (30). An FDA indication for the use of mitoxantrone in patients with hormone-refractory prostate cancer was partially based on results from a CALGB study that randomized such patients to hydrocortisone with or without mitoxantrone (31). The mitoxantrone arm had a delay in time to treatment failure and disease progression, as well as a possible benefit in pain control. A randomized study of mitoxantrone plus prednisone versus the newer docetaxel/estramustine combination is completing accrual through SWOG with Intergroup participation.

The groups have contributed to refining the chemotherapy regimens used to cure testicular cancer. A SWOG study demonstrated the necessity of using high-dose cisplatin in treatment of this disease (32). The importance of including bleomycin with platinum and etoposide when limiting chemotherapy to three cycles was shown by an ECOG study (33). The Testicular Cancer Intergroup study established the effectiveness of adjuvant, cisplatin-based chemotherapy for stage II disease in preventing relapse (34).

Pediatric Cancers

The Children's Oncology Group was formed recently by the merger of four pediatric cancer cooperative groups: the Children's Cancer Group, the Intergroup Rhabdomyosarcoma Study Group, the National Wilms' Tumor Study Group, and the Pediatric Oncology Group. The research achievements of these groups have set the standard of care for pediatric cancer over the past 30 years and have led directly to the cure of the majority of childhood cancer patients.

Step-by-step refinements in treatment regimens have improved the outcome of children with leukemia and lymphoma. Recent studies by the Children's Cancer Group that have adjusted chemotherapy regimens for acute lymphoblastic leukemia based on prognostic factors have improved outcome for all risk groups (35,36). The four Intergroup Rhabdomyosarcoma Study Group studies (IRSG-I to IRSG-IV) have contributed greatly to the cure rate of childhood rhabdomyosarcoma, which has increased from 20% to over 70% during the last 25 years, and were used to develop a clinical prognostic schema that is the standard for choosing appropriate treatment based on risk category (37,38). Treatment of Wilms tumor has likewise been refined, and over 90% of patients are currently cured with combination therapy developed by the National Wilms' Tumor Study Group (39).

Cancer Prevention

Cooperative group studies have proved important in the area of cancer prevention. The National Surgical Adjuvant Breast and Bowel Project Breast Cancer Prevention Trial (NSABP P-1) successfully randomized 13,000 women at high risk for developing breast cancer to either placebo or 5 years of tamoxifen (40). After a median follow-up of 4.2 years, the incidence of invasive breast cancer was reduced by 44% among women assigned to tamoxifen, leading to an FDA-approved indication for use of tamoxifen to reduce the risk of developing breast cancer in high-risk women. The Study of Tamoxifen and Raloxifene (STAR) is designed to determine whether raloxifene is as effective as tamoxifen in reducing the risk of developing breast cancer. This ongoing NSABP study plans to enroll 22,000 women.

The Prostate Cancer Prevention Trial (PCPT) was an Intergroup randomized, phase III, double-blind study of finasteride or placebo for the prevention of prostate cancer involving nearly 19,000 participants that completed accrual in 1996 (41). The subsequent Selenium and Vitamin E Cancer Prevention Trial (SELECT) is investigating whether selenium and vitamin E can prevent prostate cancer (42). This ambitious study is coordinated by SWOG and plans to enroll more than 32,000 men.

FUTURE DIRECTIONS

Since the 1950s the cooperative groups have contributed greatly to anticancer drug development. Although the accomplishments of the past are obvious, less clear is the future role of the cooperative groups in the changing landscape of clinical cancer research. Whereas the NCI was once the near-exclusive force in drug development and clinical research, industry now plays a much greater role. The growing pipeline of agents being developed by industry will necessitate an increasing number of studies and more expeditious completion of trials. This will lead to increasing competition for the limited pool of patients available to enroll in studies.

A trend by pharmaceutical companies to work directly with contract research organizations (CROs) could have a negative impact on the cooperative groups. The ability of these for-profit organizations to efficiently conduct clinical studies is attractive to the pharmaceutical industry. Industry-sponsored studies often focus on regulatory issues directed toward drug approval. Although the scientific premise of such studies may not be particularly interesting, the financial incentives for enrolling patients may lure physicians away from participating in cooperative group studies. CROs provide an efficient mechanism for recruiting patients to trials, but they generally lack the expertise in cancer care and research that is the hallmark of the cooperative groups. Although the quality of research and the rigor of the peer review process will remain a forte of the groups, new strategies will be needed to maintain a leadership role in cancer investigation. This may require more direct relationships with industry and development of new management strategies to ensure efficient conduct of studies. As an example, the Coalition of National Cancer Cooperative Groups was formed by the leaders of six cooperative groups to develop and implement strategies to ensure the success of the groups in the future, including plans for interaction with industry and other private foundations.

In conclusion, the cooperative group program has played a major role in the evolution of anticancer therapies for nearly half a century and remains a vital mechanism for drug development. Comprised of thought leaders in clinical oncology and basic science, the cooperative groups are well positioned to meet the challenges of cancer research in the twenty-first century.

REFERENCES

1. Kelahan AM, Catalano R, Marinucci D. The history, structure, and achievements of the cancer cooperative groups. *Managed Care Cancer* 2001;May/June:28–33.
2. Weiss RB, Vogelzang NJ, Peterson BA, et al. A successful system of scientific data audits for clinical trials: a report from the Cancer and Leukemia Group B. *JAMA* 1993;270:459–464.
3. Venook AP, Egorin MJ, Rosner GL, et al. Phase I and pharmacokinetic trial of paclitaxel in patients with hepatic dysfunction: Cancer and Leukemia Group B 9264. *J Clin Oncol* 1998;16:1811–1819.
4. Venook AP, Egorin MJ, Rosner GL, et al. Phase I and pharmacokinetic trial of gemcitabine in patients with hepatic or renal dysfunction: Cancer and Leukemia Group B 9565. *J Clin Oncol* 2000;18:2780–2787.
5. Fisher B, Dignam J, Mamounas EP, et al. Sequential methotrexate and fluorouracil for the treatment of node-negative breast cancer patients with estrogen receptor-negative tumors: eight-year results from National Surgical Adjuvant Breast and Bowel Project (NSABP) B-13 and first report of findings from NSABP B-19 comparing methotrexate and fluorouracil with conventional cyclophosphamide, methotrexate, and fluorouracil. *J Clin Oncol* 1996;14:1982–1992.
6. Fisher B, Costantino J, Redmond C, et al. A randomized clinical trial evaluating tamoxifen in the treatment of

patients with node-negative breast cancer who have estrogen-receptor-positive tumors. *N Engl J Med* 1989;320:479–484.

7. Fisher B, Dignam J, Wolmark N, et al. Tamoxifen and chemotherapy for lymph node-negative, estrogen receptor-positive breast cancer. *J Natl Cancer Inst* 1997;89:1673–1682.

8. Henderson IC, Berry D, Demetri G, et al. Improved outcomes from adding paclitaxel but not from escalating doxorubicin dose in an adjuvant chemotherapy regimen for patients with node positive primary breast cancer. *J Clin Oncol* 2003;21:976–983.

9. Peters WP, Rosner G, Vredenburgh J, et al. Updated results of a prospective, randomized comparison of two doses of combination alkylating agents (AA) as consolidation after CAF in high-risk primary breast cancer involving ten or more axillary lymph nodes (LN): CALGB 9082/SWOG 9114/NCIC Ma-13. *Proc Am Soc Clin Oncol* 2001:A81.

10. Omura G, Blessing J, Ehrlich C, et al. A randomized trial of cyclophosphamide and doxorubicin with or without cisplatin in advanced ovarian carcinoma. *Cancer* 1986;57:1725–1730.

11. Omura G, Morrow P, Blessing J, et al. A randomized comparison of melphalan versus melphalan plus hexamethylmelamine versus Adriamycin plus cyclophosphamide in ovarian carcinoma. *Cancer* 1983;51:783–789.

12. McGuire WP, Hoskins WJ, Brady MF, et al. Cyclophosphamide and cisplatin compared with paclitaxel and cisplatin in patients with stage III and stage IV ovarian cancer. *N Engl J Med* 1996;334:1–6.

13. Moertel CG, Fleming TR, MacDonald JS, et al. Fluorouracil plus levamisole as effective adjuvant therapy after resection of stage III colon carcinoma: a final report. *Ann Intern Med* 1995;122:321–326.

14. O'Connell MJ, Laurie JA, Kahn M, et al. Prospectively randomized trial of postoperative adjuvant chemotherapy in patients with high-risk colon cancer. *J Clin Oncol* 1998;16:295–300.

15. Haller DG, Catalano PJ, Macdonald JS, et al. Fluorouracil (FU), leucovorin (LV) and levamisole (LEV) adjuvant therapy for colon cancer: four-year results of INT-0089. *Proc Am Soc Clin Oncol* 1997;16:A940.

16. Wolmark N, Rockette H, Mamounas E, et al. Clinical trial to assess the relative efficacy of fluorouracil and leucovorin, fluorouracil and levamisole, and fluorouracil, leucovorin, and levamisole in patients with Dukes' B and C carcinoma of the colon: results from National Surgical Adjuvant Breast and Bowel Project C-04. *J Clin Oncol* 1999;17:3553–3559.

17. Kirkwood JM, Strawderman MH, Ernstoff MS, et al. Interferon alfa-2b adjuvant therapy of high-risk resected cutaneous melanoma: the Eastern Cooperative Group EST 1684. *J Clin Oncol* 1996;14:7–17.

18. Kirkwood JM, Ibrahim JG, Sondak VK, et al. High- and low-dose interferon alfa-2b in high-risk melanoma: first analysis of intergroup trial E1690/S9111/C9190. *J Clin Oncol* 2000;18:2444–2458.

19. Kirkwood JM, Ibrahim JG, Sosman JA, et al. High-dose interferon alfa-2b significantly prolongs relapse-free and overall survival compared with the GM2-KLH/QS-21 vaccine in patients with resected stage IIB-III melanoma: results of intergroup trial E1694/S9512/C509801. *J Clin Oncol* 2001;19:2370–2380.

20. Grever MR, Kopecky KJ, Coltman CA, et al. Fludarabine monophosphate: a potentially useful agent in chronic lymphocytic leukemia. *Nouv Rev Fr Hematol* 1988;30:457–459.

21. Rai KR, Peterson B, Elias L, et al. A randomized comparison of fludarabine and chlorambucil for patients with previously untreated chronic lymphocytic leukemia. A CALGB, SWOG, CTG/NCI-C and ECOG intergroup study. *Blood* 1996;88:141a(abst 552).

22. Mayer RJ, Davis RB, Schiffer CA, et al. Intensive postremission chemotherapy in adults with acute myeloid leukemia. Cancer and Leukemia Group B. *N Engl J Med* 1994;331:896–903.

23. Duggan D, Petroni G, Johnson J, et al. MOPP/ABV versus ABVD for advanced Hodgkin's disease—a preliminary report of CALGB 8952 (with SWOG, ECOG, NCIC). *Proc Am Soc Clin Oncol* 1997;16:A43.

24. Fisher RI, Gaynor ER, Dahlberg S, et al. Comparison of a standard regimen (CHOP) with three intensive chemotherapy regimens for advanced non-Hodgkin's lymphoma. *N Engl J Med* 1993;328:1002–1006.

25. Albain KS, Crowley JJ, LeBlanc M, et al. Survival determinants in extensive-stage non-small-cell lung cancer: the Southwest Oncology Group experience. *J Clin Oncol* 1991;9:1618–1626.

26. Bonomi P, Kim K, Fairclough D, et al. Comparison of survival and quality of life in advanced non-small-cell lung cancer patients treated with two dose levels of paclitaxel combined with cisplatin versus etoposide with cisplatin: results of an Eastern Cooperative Oncology Group trial. *J Clin Oncol* 2000;18:623–631.

27. Loprinzi CL, Goldberg RM, Su JQ, et al. Placebo-controlled trial of hydrazine sulfate in patients with newly diagnosed non-small-cell lung cancer. *J Clin Oncol* 1994;12:1126–1129.

28. Loprinzi CL, Kuross SA, O'Fallon JR, et al. Randomized placebo-controlled evaluation of hydrazine sulfate in patients with advanced colorectal cancer. *J Clin Oncol* 1994;12:1121–1125.

29. Kosty MP, Fleishman SB, Herndon JE 2nd, et al. Cisplatin, vinblastine, and hydrazine sulfate in advanced, non-small-cell lung cancer: a randomized placebo-controlled, double-blind phase III study of the Cancer and Leukemia Group B. *J Clin Oncol* 1994;12:1113–1120.

30. Pilepich MV, Winter K, John MJ, et al. Phase III Radiation Therapy Oncology Group (RTOG) Trial 86-10 of androgen deprivation adjuvant to definitive radiotherapy in locally advanced carcinoma of the prostate. *Int J Radiat Oncol Biol Phys* 2001;50:1243–1252.

31. Kantoff PW, Halabi S, Conaway M, et al. Hydrocortisone with or without mitoxantrone in men with hormone-refractory prostate cancer: results of the cancer and leukemia group B 9182 study. *J Clin Oncol* 1999;17:2506–2513.

32. Samson MK, Rivkin SE, Jones SE, et al. Dose-response and dose-survival advantage for high versus low-dose cisplatin combined with vinblastine and bleomycin in disseminated testicular cancer. A Southwest Oncology Group study. *Cancer* 1984;53:1029–1035.

33. Loehrer PJ Sr, Johnson D, Elson P, et al. Importance of bleomycin in favorable-prognosis disseminated germ cell tumors: an Eastern Cooperative Oncology Group trial. *J Clin Oncol* 1995;13:470–476.

34. Williams SD, Stablein DM, Einhorn LH, et al. Immediate adjuvant chemotherapy versus observation with treatment at relapse in pathological stage II testicular cancer. *N Engl J Med* 1987;317:1433–1438.

35. Nachman J, Sather HN, Gaynon PS, et al. Augmented Berlin-Frankfurt-Munster therapy abrogates the adverse prognostic significance of slow early response to induction chemotherapy for children and adolescents with acute lymphoblastic leukemia and unfavorable presenting features: a report from the Children's Cancer Group. *J Clin Oncol* 1997;15:2222–2230.

36. Lange B, Sather H, et al. Double delayed intensification improves outcome in moderate risk pediatric acute lymphoblastic leukemia: a Children's Cancer Group Study. *Blood* 1997;90:A2489.

37. Crist W, Gehan EA, Ragab AH, et al. The third intergroup rhabdomyosarcoma study. *J Clin Oncol* 1995;13:610–630.

38. Crist WM, Anderson JR, Meza JL, et al. Intergroup rhabdomyosarcoma study-IV: results for patients with nonmetastatic disease. *J Clin Oncol* 2001;19:3091–3102.

39. Neville HL, Ritchey ML. Wilms' tumor: overview of National Wilms' Tumor Study Group results. *Urol Clin North Am* 2000;27:435–442.

40. Fisher B, Constantino JP, Wickerham DL, et al. Tamoxifen for prevention of breast cancer: report of the National Surgical Adjuvant Breast and Bowel Project PI Study. *J Natl Cancer Inst* 1998;90:1371–1388.

41. Thompson IM, Coltman CA Jr, Crowley J. Chemoprevention of prostate cancer: the Prostate Cancer Prevention Trial. *Prostate* 1997;33:217–221.

42. Klein EA, Thompson IM, Lippman SM, et al. SELECT: the next prostate cancer prevention trial. Selenium and Vitamin E Cancer Prevention Trial. *J Urol* 2001;166:1311–1315.

29

Drug Development in the Elderly

Stuart M. Lichtman

Section of Geriatric Oncology, Don Monti Division of Medical Oncology, North Shore University Hospital, New York University School of Medicine, Manhasset, New York 11030

This chapter discusses drug development in elderly patients. These patients traditionally have not been the subject of clinical drug development; however, they are the largest consumers of chemotherapy and their numbers are rising dramatically. This points to the increased need to develop information in this patient group. The complexity of this development is due to the specific characteristics of older patients: physiologic changes that occur with aging, comorbidity leading to end-organ dysfunction, and functional decline.

BACKGROUND

Epidemiology

Persons older than 65 years are the fastest growing segment of the United States population and will account for an estimated 20% of Americans by the year 2030. Increasing age is directly associated with increasing rates of cancer, corresponding to an 11-fold greater incidence in persons older than 65 years versus those younger than 65 years. Consequently, the older population comprises a majority of cancer patients. The over-75-year-old group will triple by 2030, and the over-85-year-old will double in the same period (1). The average life expectancy of a 75-year-old-person currently is 10 years and that of an 85-year-old is 6 years (2–6). Together, these statistics outline an increasingly elderly cancer population that will require specific management for various cancers (1,5).

Despite the increasing incidence of cancer with aging and the aging of the population, only a minority of elderly patients have been entered into clinical trials. Limited information on single-agent chemotherapy and combinations is available (7,8). The European Organization for Research and Treatment of Cancer (EORTC) conducted an analysis of European trials (9). Twenty-two percent of the patients were 65 years or older, and 8% were 70 years or older. Older patients underwent surgery, radiotherapy, and chemotherapy less often. More elderly patients experienced a delay in dose administration or dose reduction compared with younger patients. There was no difference in toxicity in the older patients compared with the younger patients, except for oral toxicity. Increased dose reductions and delays may explain the lack of toxicity differences. There also may have been a bias toward positive selection, which may increase with age. The EORTC investigators, as well as others, advocate that the elderly should be candidates for all phases of clinical trials and that they should not be excluded on an age basis. The Cancer and Leukemia Group B (CALGB) has reviewed their experience with non–small cell lung cancer (10). Despite the absence of a specified upper age limit entry criterion, no patients older than 80 years were accrued. Traditionally, patient selection has been based on good clinical practice, clinical judgment with performance status, and organ function parameters. There seems to be a need for a more comprehensive tool of pretreatment assessment so that the potential problems in treating elderly patients can be predicted and avoided (9). As in any clinical investigation, patient selection is always crucial for adequate completion of the program. An increased rate of discontinuance, patient refusal or loss to follow-up, or excessive toxicity may lead to a decreased number of evaluable patients, which would jeopardize the study (11).

A number of barriers that limit the participation of elderly patients in clinical trials have been identified (Table 29.1) (12). Physicians involved in a study of potential breast cancer trials participants were questioned. Physicians' perceptions of the most important barriers to accrual of older patients were as follows: elderly patients have significant comorbid conditions that are not excluded by the protocol but may affect

TABLE 29.1. *Barriers to participation*

1. Focus on aggressive therapy, which can be unacceptably toxic in the elderly
2. Comorbidity
3. Fewer trials available
4. Limited expectation of benefit from patient, physicians, and family
5. Lack of financial and social supports
6. Trials have not specifically addressed this group
7. Patient and physician reluctance to include older patients; physicians not recommending therapy, particularly clinical trials
8. Social supports
9. Insurance
10. Futility of therapy
11. Mistrust of clinical trials, i.e., guinea pig syndrome
12. Competition of alternative and complementary therapy

how they would respond to treatment (16%); elderly patients have difficulty understanding what is required in a complicated treatment trial, which results in poor compliance (16%); treatment toxicity (14%); and elderly patients often do not meet the eligibility criteria (15%). Cognitive dysfunction is particularly important in understanding the complicated informed consent documents. Cognitive impairments can be as high as 36% in adults aged 85 years and older (13). In 1998 the National Bioethics Advisory Commission published guidelines delineating specific recommendations about research that includes subjects with limitations in decision-making capacity.

Oncologists most frequently suggested that the most effective interventions for improving the accrual of elderly patients to trials included making personnel available in the clinic to explain clinical trials to older patients and their families (25%) and providing physicians with educational materials concerning treatment toxicity in the elderly (18%). Physicians viewed barriers to accruing older patients with breast carcinoma to clinical trials as multidimensional, with the most important involving protocol requirements, treatment specific issues, and older patients' medical and cognitive characteristics. Thus, a variety of interventions would be needed to improve accrual of older patients to clinical trials, including increasing physicians' knowledge concerning treatment toxicity in the elderly, simplifying protocol requirements, and reducing treatment toxicity (12). In another part of this study, after controlling for other conditions, age was significantly associated with whether or not a patient was offered participation in a clinical trial. Among the 60 patients who were offered participation, there was no evidence that age was associated with whether or not a patient agreed to participate. Older patients were just as likely as younger patients to agree to participate. Failure of clinicians to offer a clinical trial to eligible older patients is a significant barrier to enrollment (14).

Aging and Cancer Chemotherapy

Aging is a multidimensional process and is highly individualized. Chronologic age does not always predict the physiologic decline in an individual. These effects are due in part to the interaction of comorbidity on aging. It has been suggested that the process of aging is a functional continuum with frailty at the midpoint of independence and predeath (15). In the primary health stage, there are no significant limitations in activity and minimally reduced functional reserve. Many individuals then become somewhat more vulnerable, with critically reduced functional reserve causing some functional limitations. Reversibility of some conditions is possible. The stage of frailty is characterized by severe limitations with no significant recovery of functional reserve. Cancer chemotherapy needs to be tailored to the individual and needs to take into consideration these phases of aging. Truly frail patients probably are not optimal candidates for new drug development. Their ability to tolerate even minimal toxicity is greatly impaired. After drugs have been approved at doses applicable to patients with an adequate performance status, studies should be performed in frail and vulnerable populations to determine whether lower doses can be given safely and possibly used in a palliative setting.

CLINICAL PHARMACOLOGY

Elderly patients are the largest users of pharmaceuticals and incur 30% of the total drug cost. Fifty percent of all drugs marketed will have some use in treating problems of the elderly (16,17), yet most studies are conducted in healthy patients younger than 55 years (18). This divergence can make decision making, particularly with regard to dosing, quite difficult. This effect also may contribute to some degree to the increased incidence of drug toxicity with age. These toxicity differences also can be the result of age-related changes in pharmacokinetics and pharmacodynamics. A number of physiologic changes accompany human aging. These include increase in body fat, decrease in lean body mass, and decrease in total body water (19–22). Elderly cancer patients have a number of significant comorbid illnesses that also may affect the disposition and effect of the drug (23,24).

Pharmacokinetics

Pharmacokinetics can be defined as the characteristic interaction between the drug and the body in terms of its absorption, distribution, metabolism, and excretion. We will discuss each entity separately and highlight the age-related variation and its influence on cancer chemotherapy. These issues must be taken into account when planning drug studies in the elderly (Table 29.2).

Absorption

A number of changes in the digestive system can affect drug absorption. These parameters include decreased gastrointestinal motility, decreased splanchnic blood flow, decreased secretion of digestive enzymes, and mucosal atrophy (18,25). All of these factors can result in reduced absorption rate (i.e., in the amount of drug absorbed in the unit of time). Of special concern is the oldest patient in whom the sum effect of these changes can significantly impair the intestinal absorption of drugs. Because most of the chemotherapy drugs are administered parenterally, absorption abnormalities do not usually affect chemotherapy. Drug compliance is an important issue with oral therapy (26).

Distribution

The volume of distribution of drugs is a function of body composition and the concentration of circulating plasma proteins, such as serum albumin and red blood cells (25,27,28). Fat content doubles from 15% to 30% of body weight in the elderly, and intracellular water decreases from 42% to 33% in the average 25-year-old compared to the average 75-year-old. These findings emphasize that obesity is a significant problem in the elderly and should be considered in trials (29). In one study, 24% of men and 29.7% of women (mean age 73.1 years) were considered obese (30). This change leads to a decreased volume of distribution of more polar drugs that primarily distribute to body water while that of the lipid-soluble drugs increases. This effect can lead to a lower peak concentration and prolonged terminal half-life (25,27). The CALGB evaluated the effect of obesity in patients receiving adjuvant treatment for breast cancer. They found that patients treated within 5% of their actual weight did not experience excessive toxicity; therefore, they recommended that initial doses be computed according to actual body weight (31). As an individual ages there is a decrease of 15% to 20% in plasma albumin and a reduction of red blood cell concentration. Hypoalbuminemia and anemia are known adverse prognostic factors in the elderly with regard to functional ability and survival (32–35). Serum albumin can explain some of the pharmacokinetic and pharmacodynamic variability seen with chemotherapy, such as with etoposide (36,37). Hypoalbuminemia is associated with low protein binding, which results in more free drug being available for renal elimination (38). Anemia also can be particularly relevant for treatment with anthracyclines, taxanes, and epipodophyllotoxins, which are heavily bound to red blood cells. The correction of anemia with erythropoietin may be particularly beneficial to older individuals, given that anemia is the only component of volume of distribution that can be manipulated. One retrospective study showed changes in response to chemotherapy related to anemia (39–41).

TABLE 29.2. *Specific features of absorption and distribution of drugs in the elderly*

Factors that may affect absorption
  Reduced gastric secretion
  Reduced gastric emptying time
  Reduced gastrointestinal motility
  Diminished splanchnic blood flow
  Decreased absorption surface
  Concomitant medication, i.e., H2 blockers, antacids
Factors that affect distribution
  Changes in body composition
    Fat content doubles
    Decreased intracellular water
    Albumin concentrations reduced (etoposide, taxanes are highly protein bound)
    Anemia
  Increase in volume of distribution
  Lower peak concentration and prolonged terminal $t_{1/2}$

Metabolism

The liver is the main site of drug metabolism. There is lack of agreement regarding age-related changes in hepatic drug-metabolizing capacity; however, there is consensus that liver size decreases with age (27). Liver blood flow is reduced at a rate of 0.3% to 1.5% per year after age 25 years. This may lead to lower clearances of drugs that are highly dependent on blood flow for elimination. Phase 1 metabolism occurs primarily via the cytochrome P-450 microsomal system, which consists of a number of isoenzymes. Phase 2 reactions are primarily conjugation reactions.

Cytochrome P-450

These heme-based enzymes are grouped into various classes based on various types of metabolic processes and genetic homology. In addition to hepatic locations, these enzymes are located in the small bowel, kidneys, lungs, and brain to a much lesser extent. The nomenclature of the various cytochrome (CYP) enzymes (e.g., CYP2D6, CYP1A2) is based on the family, subfamily, and specific gene for each enzyme. Despite large numbers of various enzymes, genetic variability accounts for differing levels of enzyme activity through various pathways that may lead to clinically important pharmacodynamic differences among individuals (42–44).

For a drug to be susceptible to pharmacokinetic drug interactions from enzyme substrates or induction, it generally must have at least 30% of its metabolism through that one enzyme substrate. The potential for drug interactions is relatively high, particularly with the CYP3A4 enzyme. This enzyme is inhibited by a variety of commonly prescribed medications and is involved in the metabolism of a variety of anticancer agents. Cyclophosphamide, ifosfamide, paclitaxel, etoposide, teniposide, vincristine, vinblastine, busulfan, and tamoxifen all are substrates of CYP3A4 and may be significantly affected by common enzyme inhibitors of this enzyme (45).

Age-related declines in these systems have been demonstrated in animal studies and some human trials. It has been demonstrated that cytochrome P-450 (CYP) 1A2 shows a 20% to 25% decrease in clearance in healthy elderly men and women compared with younger subjects (46,47). This effect may result in decreased first-pass metabolism of drugs that are highly extracted by the liver such as morphine. The predominant P-450 isoform, CYP3A4, also is present in the intestinal mucosa. Other variables be considered are the effect of age, diet, genetic polymorphisms, and stereoselective drug metabolism (47). Many alterations of enzyme activity involve either drug-induced increases or decreases in metabolism. Phase 2 reactions appear to be unaffected by age (48). The biliary excretion of drugs has been studied, but no age-related alterations have been noted (48).

Excretion

Age-related changes in excretory function occur. There is a gradual loss in renal mass and decline in function with age. The combined weight of the kidneys declines by 30% by age 90 years. This loss is due primarily to loss of cortical mass with relative preservation of the renal medulla. Glomerular sclerosis produces loss of capacity to perform ultrafiltration of plasma, which leads to a decreased glomerular filtration (GFR) rate by approximately 1 mL/min for every year over age 40 years (49–51). The im-

portance of this decline was first emphasized in a study of doses based on renal function leading to a higher therapeutic index (52). The reduction in GFR is not reflected by an increase in serum creatinine levels because of the simultaneous loss of muscle mass that occurs with age. Estimations of creatinine clearance in the elderly may lead to errors in dosing (53).

Traditionally, serum creatinine has been used to estimate the glomerular filtration function of the kidney because it is primarily filtered through the glomerulus; however, a small portion undergoes tubular secretion. In order to facilitate the estimation of glomerular clearance, various equations have been evaluated to calculate creatinine clearance based on serum creatinine and other factors. Two common equations used clinically are the Cockcroft-Gault and Jelliffe equations (54,55). The equations are less accurate in populations such as patients with severe renal failure, patients with decreased muscle mass, and the elderly. Many individuals lose muscle mass with age. Many elderly individuals with a low serum creatinine of less than 1 mg/dL may actually have diminished muscle mass and diminished production of creatinine rather than exceptional renal function. A comparison of the accuracy of various formulas was performed recently (56).

The decline in GFR with age translates into pharmacokinetic alterations of drugs or their active metabolites, which are excreted by the kidneys. Due to the physiologic decline in renal function with age, chemotherapy agents, which are primarily renally excreted, must be used with extreme care in the elderly. Standard doses may be too toxic. This is particularly true of the frail elderly. Dosing modifications for these physiologic declines have been suggested (57,58).

A study by Gelman and Taylor (52) highlighted the importance of GFR impairment in the management of older persons with cancer. In a retrospective analysis, the authors demonstrated that the toxicity of CMF (cyclophosphamide, methotrexate, and fluorouracil) was reduced without compromising efficacy when the doses of cyclophosphamide and methotrexate were adjusted to the GFR in women aged 65 and over (52). The Calvert and Chatelut formulas can be used to calculate the dose of carboplatin for the desired area under the curve based on age and serum creatinine (59,60). Other drugs can be dose adjusted per Kintzel and Dorr (61), who provide general guidelines to adjust doses of renally excreted or nephrotoxic anticancer drugs in patients who present with altered renal function. The dosage adjustments for renal impairment were calculated using a formula to determine the fraction of the normal dose (61). The formula is as follows:

Fraction of normal dose = (normal dose)

$$\times\ f(kf - 1) + 1$$

where f is the fraction of the original dose excreted as active or toxic moiety, and kf is the patient's creatinine clearance (mL/min)/(120 mL/min).

However, one must realize that the pharmacokinetics of drugs is not a sole function of the GFR. For example, Borkowski et al. (62) studied the pharmacokinetics of nine drugs in patients younger than 65 years or 65 years and over. Of particular interest is the drug dichloromethotrexate. Although the renal clearance of the drug decreased with age, the plasma clearance did not suggest that compensatory mechanisms, such as hepatic clearance, exist. This finding was especially interesting because dichloromethotrexate is completely excreted via the kidneys (62).

COMORBIDITY AND FUNCTIONAL STATUS

Comorbidity is a key factor in the overall survival of patients and therefore of the benefits and toxicity of therapy. The role of comorbidity and survival was evaluated by Charlson et al. (63), who determined that the severity of comorbid illness can predict survival in general medical patients admitted to an inpatient unit. With each increased level of the comorbidity index there were stepwise increases in the cumulative mortality attributable to comorbid disease. In follow-up, age was also a predictor of mortality (63). The affect of comorbidity on survival of patients with colorectal cancer was evaluated by Yancik et al. (64). A retrospective analysis of 1,610 patients showed that hypertension, significant heart disease, gastrointestinal problems, arthritis, and chronic obstructive pulmonary disease were the most prominent conditions. Forty percent of patients older than 75 years had at least five conditions. Within 2 years of diagnosis, 28% of the patients had died. The number of comorbid conditions was significant in predicting early mortality in a model, including age, gender, and disease stage. Certain conditions significantly increased the risk of mortality (e.g., heart problems, alcohol abuse, liver disease, and deep vein thrombosis). Although disease stage is a crucial determinant of survival, comorbidity increases the complexity of management and affects survival duration (64). Satariano and Ragland (24) assessed the effect of comorbidity and stage of disease on 3-year survival in women with primary breast cancer. Patients who had three or more of seven selected comorbid conditions had a 20-fold higher rate of mortality from causes other than breast cancer and a fourfold higher rate of all-cause mortality compared with patients who had no comorbid conditions. The effects of comorbidity were independent of age, disease stage, tumor size, histologic type, type of treatment, race, and social and behavioral factors. Comorbidity in patients with breast cancer appears to be a strong predictor of 3-year survival, independent of the effects of breast cancer stage.

Functional status is also a significant issue in the elderly (65). Comorbidity and functional status are independent in older cancer patients and therefore need to be assessed independently. The traditional oncology measures, such as the Karnofsky score and European Cooperative Oncology Group (ECOG) performance scale, are not good predictors in the elderly. The degree of dependency and geriatric functional scores can predict survival in older patients (23,65–67). Future drug development will require new and easy-to-administer functional scales for the oncologist. These scales must aid the oncologist in predicting toxicity and outcome.

END-ORGAN DYSFUNCTION

Patients with end-organ dysfunction usually are excluded from clinical trials, particularly for new drugs. Comorbidity is common, as previously mentioned in elderly patients both with and without cancer (68). Forty-five of sixty-four nursing home residents had four or more comorbid diseases (68). Repetto et al. (68) evaluated patients older than 70 years and younger than 70 years, with and without cancer. The most common comorbid diseases for cancer patients were arthrosis, arthritis, and bone diseases and for noncancer patients were cardiovascular disorders. Compared with younger cancer patients, older cancer patients had a higher prevalence of psychiatric disorders, cardiovascular diseases, stroke and central nervous system diseases, bone disorders, and cataracts. Compared with noncancer patients, older cancer patients had a lower prevalence of most conditions. The prevalence of comorbid conditions was higher among the noncancer patients than the cancer patients. The older noncancer patients presented with at least one comorbid disease in addition to the condition prompting the initial clinic visit and more than four comorbid conditions were present in 57.6% of the patients. The majority of the other patients presented with two or fewer conditions in addition to the cancer.

The assessment of patients with end-organ dysfunction is critical to guide physicians in dosing. A number of clinical trials have used this study design (69–72).

The Pharmacology and Experimental Therapeutics committee of the CALGB has completed a series of trials. Although not specifically geared for the elderly, this approach is a good example of what is possible in a cooperative group setting. The data have broad applicability. The first trial was with paclitaxel. The authors demonstrated that for patients with elevated levels of aspartate transaminase (AST) or bilirubin, dose reductions are necessary and an increase in toxicity can be anticipated. Increased myelosuppression, partially due to altered paclitaxel pharmacokinetics, is observed in such patients (70). The second trial was with gemcitabine. Patients with elevated AST levels tolerated gemcitabine without increased toxicity, but patients with elevated bilirubin levels had significant deterioration in liver function after gemcitabine therapy. Patients with elevated creatinine levels had significant toxicity even at reduced doses of gemcitabine, including two instances of severe skin toxicity. Patients with elevated bilirubin levels have an increased risk of hepatic toxicity, and a dose reduction is recommended. Patients with elevated creatinine levels seem to have increased sensitivity to gemcitabine, but the data are not adequate to support a specific dosing recommendation (71). Patients in the irinotecan trial were treated in one of four cohorts: (i) AST twice the upper limit of normal; (ii) direct bilirubin 1.6 to 7.0 mg/dL with any AST; (iii) creatinine 1.6 to 5.0 mg/dL with normal AST and bilirubin; or (iv) normal liver function tests and creatinine but prior pelvic radiation therapy. CPT-11, SN-38, and SN-38G were measured in blood and urine. Pharmacokinetic results showed that the median CPT-11 clearance was 12.5 L/hour. Cohort II patients had 28%, 40%, and 53% decreases in clearance estimates for CPT-11, SN-38 and SN-38G, respectively, compared to cohorts III and IV. This reduced clearance is consistent with the clinical observation that patients with increased bilirubin require dose modification to avoid dose-limiting toxicity (DLT). Accrual has continued in an attempt to define optimal doses (69). Studies of organ dysfunction with chemotherapy and the epithelial growth factor receptor inhibitor OSI-774 are ongoing.

DESIGN ISSUES

Issues of clinical trial design are given in Table 29.3.

Endpoint

Cause of Death

When new therapies are being developed for older patients, it is important to determine the appropriate

TABLE 29.3. *Clinical trial design*

Clinical trials specific for elderly patients
Some form of geriatric assessment should be performed
Comorbidity should be assessed
Studies should emphasize particular aspects of aging, i.e., frailty, vulnerable elderly, well elderly
Polypharmacy and concomitant medications should be evaluated, particularly those drugs that interact with the cytochrome P-450 system
Limited sampling strategies should be used when appropriate
Limit office visits and testing to facilitate compliance to the protocol
Quality-of-life assessment should be included

endpoint. Particular care must be taken when overall survival is a study endpoint. A number of studies determined that cause of death may differ in older versus younger patient populations. Vose et al. (73) studied cause of death in a lymphoma trial. The deaths attributed to tumor or treatment-related toxicity were similar in patients older and younger than age 60 years. The differences in survival were due to other causes of death not obviously related to the lymphoma or its therapy, occurring in 22% of patients 60 years or older but in only 2% of patients younger than 60 years ($p = 0.005$). These data supported the position that aggressive non-Hodgkin lymphoma in elderly patients is not significantly less responsive than in younger patients. However, the inclusion of older patients in clinical trials will decrease the overall survival secondary to deaths due to apparently unrelated causes (73). As mentioned earlier, Satariano and Ragland (24) showed that there was a fourfold higher rate of all-cause mortality in patients with comorbid conditions compared with patients who had no comorbid conditions. The effects of comorbidity were independent of age, disease stage, tumor size, histologic type, type of treatment, race, and social and behavioral factors (24). This phenomenon is particularly important in cancers, which can have a relatively indolent course. It has been shown in prostate cancer studies that competing causes of death are substantive contributors to mortality. In one cohort of patients with local-stage disease who were followed for 15 years, nearly 90% of the observed deaths were believed to be from causes other than prostate cancer (74,75).

Quality of Life

Quality of life has emerged as an important endpoint in clinical trials. In elderly patients in whom treatment often is palliative, this is a particularly significant concern. Patient quality of life is affected by a number of factors related to the disease and treatment characteristics. Quality of life should be as important an objective as survival. There are different priorities and problems for different cancers or different stages of disease (76). In advanced disease, issues about quality of life are focused on palliation of cancer-related symptoms and treatment-induced toxicity. A number of elements thought to determine quality of life, such as symptom status and physical, emotional, role, and social functioning should be measured. A number of measures of quality of life have been established (77). Geriatric assessment also has become an integral part of evaluating elderly patients (78). There are many parallels between geriatric assessment and quality-of-life assessment in that they are multidimensional and broad. They share many dimensions and focus on issues that are among the most important to older persons, particularly the ability to function fully in social roles and participate in various activities. Differences in quality of life are best measured by the patient, but functional status and other dimensions of geriatric assessment are better assessed by clinicians or family members (77). Therefore, drug development should include quality-of-life and functional assessments.

Oral Cancer Therapy

There are a number of issues that are specific to oral anticancer therapy and should be considered in the development of oral agents (Table 29.4). An increasing trend over the past 20 years has been the increased use of oral chemotherapy for the treatment of a variety of malignancies (79). Cost has been a significant impetus for this development. Oral therapy can eliminate charges for items such as administration and nursing, central intravenous catheters, and infusion pump costs, and costs related to adverse effects of intravenous administration such as line sepsis (80). Patient

TABLE 29.4. *Factors often associated with nonadherence to prescribed oral medication regimens*

Complex treatment regimen
Substantial behavioral change required
Inconvenient or inefficient clinics
Inadequate supervision
Poor communication with health care providers
Patient dissatisfaction with care
Patient health beliefs in favor of nonadherence
Inadequate social support
History of nonadherence
History of mental illness

preferences and quality-of-life issues are important factors for the development of oral chemotherapy. More than 90% of patients prefer an oral agent, provided efficacy is maintained. Reasons include convenience, concerns or difficulties with intravenous access lines, and ability to control the chemotherapy administration environment (81). In addition, oral agents may be preferable for elderly patients with limited means to travel to and from the medical caregiver.

Compliance

Patient noncompliance is a potential major obstacle for orally formulated chemotherapy (Table 29.4). Dose reductions, such as occurs with poor compliance, in the adjuvant treatment of breast cancer can lead to a markedly inferior disease-free survival (82). Factors associated with higher rates of noncompliance include lower socioeconomic status, treatment in a community-based setting, and the number of doses administered per day (83). In elderly patients, noncompliance can lead to a higher risk of hospitalization. Factors statistically associated with this risk include poor recall of medication regimen, seeing numerous physicians, female gender, medium income category, use of numerous medications, and having the opinion that medications are expensive (84). Pharmacokinetic analysis showed actual compliance was less than half that suggested by patient self-report. Measures designed to increase compliance, including patient education, home psychologic support, and exercises in pill taking, were shown to increase compliance nearly threefold (26,85). There are data indicating that compliance with oral chemotherapy may influence survival (86). A number of studies have evaluated compliance with regard to oral chemotherapy regimens (87–91). A number of risk factors have been identified with regard to adherence to prescribed oral mediation regimens (Table 29.4) (91).

To overcome problems of compliance in the elderly, providers should prescribe a simple dosage regimen for all medications to be taken (preferably one or two doses daily), help the patient select cues that will assist him or her in remembering to take doses (time of day, mealtime, or other daily rituals), provide devices to simplify remembering doses (medication boxes), and regularly monitor compliance.

Dose-Limiting Toxicity

Phase I drug development involves the determination of the dose of chemotherapy to use in subsequent phase II studies. Various well-defined phases of clinical investigation have been established to provide an organized approach to the drug evaluation process (92). At each step in the process, the toxicity profile is more accurately defined. In the phase I clinical trial, the ultimate goal is to determine the toxicity and pharmacology of a new agent. The DLT(s) and the maximal tolerated dose (MTD) of a particular dose and schedule are established. The DLT is the adverse effect that limits further escalation of the dose. The MTD is defined differently in various phase I trials, but in general it is the dose that results in either serious (i.e., life-threatening) or irreversible toxicity in a predetermined percentage of patients. The procedure for demonstrating the MTD involves careful escalation of doses from an initial starting dose until the DLT is achieved. The phase I investigation is considered to be successfully completed when both the DLT and the MTD on a specific schedule have been identified. The recommendation of a dose and schedule for further phase II testing should result from data derived from the phase I trial (92). Phase I trials of chemotherapy specifically in elderly patients have not been performed. This limits the applicability of these studies to the older patient population. Studies of new agents in predetermined stages of aging (i.e., frail, vulnerable) or in patients with specific common comorbidities or functional impairments would be invaluable.

Alteration of Dose-Limiting Toxicity

In certain cases, the DLT may be ameliorated with various interventions. For example, administration of 2-mercaptoethane sulfonate (MESNA) has dramatically reduced bladder toxicity associated with high doses of either cyclophosphamide or ifosfamide (93,94). Several agents, including amifostine, have demonstrated chemoprotection from cisplatin toxicity, and use of dexrazoxane may ameliorate cardiotoxicity associated with doxorubicin (95). The current effective antiemetic therapies has been important, allowing the use of more antiemetic drugs. This approach has been particularly important in elderly patients in whom highly emetogenic drugs such as cisplatin and high-dose cyclophosphamide would have been prohibitive (96,97). Likewise, the use of colony-stimulating factors may markedly reduce the period of myelosuppression associated with high doses of cytotoxic chemotherapy and has increased the therapeutic ratio of standard doses of chemotherapy for elderly patients (98–100). These supportive drugs need further study in the elderly and should be strongly considered in dose-finding studies in elderly patients.

Alternating the schedule of drug administration may affect the potential for producing a toxic event. For example, administration of doxorubicin as a continuous intravenous infusion or a weekly, lower-dose intravenous bolus appears to be effective in reducing the observed cardiac toxicity compared with that from a higher dose given as an intravenous bolus on a 3-week schedule. Different formulations of the same drug may alter toxicity, such as been seen with liposomal preparations (101). This schedule and formulation may allow potentially toxic agents to be used in the elderly population. Although a change in the schedule of administration may lessen toxicity, it is important to ensure that the change also does not alter therapeutic efficacy.

Traditionally during the phase I investigation, acute toxicities are identified and the potential duration and reversibility of the toxicities are defined. Patients with malignancy who have limited therapeutic options may be offered an opportunity to participate in these trials, but selection of appropriate patients to accurately evaluate toxicity in a phase I clinical investigation is extremely important (92). In general, patients should have reasonably good performance status and basically normal organ function. As a result, entry criteria may exclude elderly patients from dose-finding trials. Because the major objective of this phase of clinical investigation is to define organ toxicity, patients with significant pretreatment organ dysfunction will be unevaluable when assessing certain toxic events. In addition, abnormal organ function may increase the risk of participation in this early phase. Studies in the elderly can be defined differently than what has been historically done. Variations in performance and functional status can be defined in the eligibility criteria. If such a study is performed, the final dose that is determined will be applicable to that particular group of patients. The heterogeneity of the elderly limits the value of drug studies performed in fit younger patients. Endpoints may be different because of age-related changes in organ function, as previously discussed, or secondary to comorbid conditions. Organ dysfunction studies can be performed in both younger and older patients to define the dose in each population.

Polypharmacy

Polypharmacy is frequent in the older population. The number and type of concomitant medications need to be carefully assessed when patients are entered into clinical trials. If this requirement is too rigid, it may limit the number of older patients accrued. Older ambulatory patients use threefold more medications than younger patients (47). At least 90% of the older patients use at least one medication, and the average is at least four medications per patient. Self-medication with herbal remedies and other alternative therapies are becoming increasingly common. The large number of drugs also leads to a number of inappropriate medications and increased toxicity (102). Significant drug interactions, particularly those involved in the cytochrome P-450 system, are of major concern (103,104). In an analysis of comorbidity, the number of medications taken was assessed (68). Sixty percent of cancer patients older than 70 years took medications compared with 73% of younger cancer patients. Fifty-four percent of older noncancer patients received four or more different daily medications. The increased number of medications and the physiologic changes of the older patients often lead to serious adverse sequela. Adverse drug reactions cause 3% to 5% of all hospital admissions (105–107). An Italian study demonstrated that 3.4% of admissions were due to adverse drug reactions. Gastrointestinal complaints (19%) represented the most common events, followed by metabolic and hemorrhagic complications (9%). The drugs most frequently responsible for these events were diuretics, calcium channel blockers, nonsteroidal antiinflammatory drugs, and digoxin. Female gender, alcohol use, and number of drugs were independent predictors of hospital admissions. For severe adverse events, age, comorbidity, and number of drugs were the only predisposing factors (105). Drug doses often must be decreased because of age-related losses in weight and decreases in renal and hepatic function. When writing prescriptions for patients or designing trials, the potential problems of the use of concomitant medications that use the P-450 system should be considered (108).

Sampling

There is a clear need for the involvement of elderly patients early in the development of anticancer agents. Pharmacokinetic drug sampling is an integral part of the process. Accuracy of specimen acquisition is critical. To help ensure accurate pharmacologic results, the schedule of blood sampling must be carefully considered. In one study, a limited sampling strategy was utilized in which the patient was only required to be at the center for 4 additional hours and not required to have a 24-hour sample. Patients and families are reluctant to participate in studies if there is the burden of frequent office visits. This strategy was utilized successfully in a trial evaluating the effect of aging on the pharmacokinetics and pharmacodynamics of paclitaxel (109–111). Limiting sampling has been applied to many agents (112–121). A few data points can be used in the approach of population pharmacokinetics (122).

Complementary and Alternative Medicine

The use of complementary and alternative medicine (CAM) is common in the general population (123). Data show that at least one third of cancer patients use some form of CAM (124,125). A significant knowledge gaps exists regarding alternative therapies in cancer patients and how alternative therapies may interact with more conventional therapy. Increasing evidence indicates that CAM treatments are biologically active, and research is needed to define the potential interactions with drug metabolism and therapeutic outcomes. For example, St. John's wort *(Hypericum perforatum)* has been reported to induce CYP P-450 metabolism, thus affecting drug concentrations in some patients (126,127). St. John's wort lowers the area under the curve of digoxin by induction of the P glycoprotein drug transporter (128). Induction of cytochrome P-450 CYP3A4 isoenzymes decreases indinavir and cyclosporine levels, which could significantly affect patient outcomes (129–131). Irinotecan metabolism also can be altered. During therapy, St. John's wort was found to reduce the plasma levels of the metabolite SN-38 (126,127). Additional potential drug interactions due to cytochrome P-450 include the ability of various foods to alter the drug-metabolizing potential. Grapefruit juice is a potent inhibitor of cytochrome P-450 (132). Cruciferous vegetables, charcoal-grilled beef, red wine, ethanol, and cigarette smoke also can induce the cytochrome P-450 system and have the potential to alter the rate at which many drugs are metabolized (133). The use of complementary therapy has been studied in prostate cancer. Of the patients presenting to urology clinics and the support group, 27.4% and 38.9% with prostate cancer and 25.8% and 80% at high risk for prostate cancer, respectively, used some form of complementary therapy. The use significantly differed according to disease status ($p = 0.001$), and was highest among men who were clinically disease free after radical therapy. Of the patients, 24% did not inform the urologist of alternative therapy use. Urologists and other physicians need to be aware of this of use and consider the potential effects when assessing patients for and with prostate cancer (134). In another study, patients with progressive disease or those primarily treated with hormones were most likely to use complementary therapy. Among the patients using complementary therapy, 90% believed that it would help them live longer and improve quality of life, 60% believed it would relieve symptoms, and 47% expected it to cure disease. Among patients who use complementary therapy, the perception of benefit is much greater than that supported by scientific data

(135). The herbal supplement PC-SPES has been used by many patients with prostate cancer. It is known to have significant estrogenic activity. In a phase II study, PC-SPES seems to have activity in the treatment of both androgen-dependent and androgen-independent prostate cancer with acceptable toxicity (136). The surreptitious use of this herbal substance by patients may alter the effect of clinical trials.

CONCLUSION

There is an increasing recognition of the importance of geriatric oncology. The elderly are the largest group of patients for the medical oncologist. Many of the drugs that have been approved recently have an improved therapeutic index for the elderly, as well as a broad range of activity. This result has particularly affected the treatment of solid tumors such as lung, bladder, prostate, and breast cancers.

The introduction of oral medications will allow a broader spectrum of patients to derive benefit from chemotherapy, particularly those with a poorer performance status. The elderly are still underrepresented in clinical trials (137). More studies on toxicity, drug metabolism, and drug effect are required. We will need improved methods to guide our decision making as to the appropriate therapy for this group, taking into account comorbidity, performance status, and geriatric functional assessment (65). Appropriate clinical trial design is mandatory if the results of these studies will be applicable to what is the majority of cancer patients (Table 29.3). Future studies will need to incorporate more older patients to yield meaningful data to make evidence-based decisions. Given the projected increase in the number of elderly cancer patients, research and educational initiatives targeted to this population need to be a priority (138,139).

REFERENCES

1. Yancik R. Cancer burden in the aged: an epidemiologic and demographic overview. *Cancer* 1997;80:1273–1283.
2. Barry P, Katz PR. On cancer screening in the elderly [Editorial]. *J Am Geriatr Soc* 1989;37:913–914.
3. Black JS, Kapoor W. Health promotion and disease prevention in older people. Our current state of ignorance. *J Am Geriatr Soc* 1990;38:168–172.
4. Robie PW. Cancer screening in the elderly. *J Am Geriatr Soc* 1989;37:888–893.
5. Yancik R, Yates JW. *Cancer in the elderly. Approaches to diagnosis and treatment.* New York: Springer, 1989.
6. Yancik R, Ries LG. Caring for elderly cancer patients. Quality assurance considerations. *Cancer* 1989;64[1 Suppl]:335–341.
7. Begg CB, Carbone PP. Clinical trials and drug toxicity in the elderly: the experience of the Eastern Cooperative Oncology Group. *Cancer* 1983;52:1986–1992.
8. Begg CB, Elson PJ, Carbone PP. A study of excess hematologic toxicity in elderly patients treated on cancer chemotherapy protocols. In: Yancik R, Yates JW, eds. *Cancer in the elderly. A approach to early detection and treatment.* New York: Springer, 1989:149–163.
9. Monfardini S, Sorio R, Boes GH, et al. Entry and evaluation of elderly patients in European Organization for Research and Treatment of Cancer (EORTC) new-drug-development studies. *Cancer* 1995;76:333–338.
10. Rocha Lima C, Herndon J, Kosty M, et al. Therapy choices among older patients with lung carcinoma: an evaluation of two trials of the Cancer and Leukemia Group B. *Cancer* 2002;94:181–187.
11. Yancik R. Integration of aging and cancer research in geriatric medicine [Editorial]. *J Gerontol A Biol Sci Med Sci* 1997;52:M329–M332.
12. Kornblith AB, Kemeny M, Peterson BL, et al. Survey of oncologists' perceptions of barriers to accrual of older patients with breast carcinoma to clinical trials. *Cancer* 2002;95:989–996.
13. Black SA, Rush RD. Cognitive and functional decline in adults aged 75 and older. *J Am Geriatr Soc* 2002;50:1978–1986.
14. Kemeny MM, Muss H, Kornblith A, et al. Barriers to participation of older women with breast cancer in clinical trials. *Proc Annu Meet Am Soc Clin Oncol* 2000;19:2371a.
15. Hamerman D. Toward an understanding of frailty. *Ann Intern Med* 1999;130:945–950.
16. Morris LA, Grossman R, Barkdoll G, et al. Information search activities among elderly prescription drug users. *J Health Care Mark* 1987;7:5–15.
17. Schmucker DL. Drug disposition in the elderly: a review of the critical factors. *J Am Geriatr Soc* 1984;32:144–149.
18. Yuen GJ. Altered pharmacokinetics in the elderly. *Clin Geriatr Med* 1990;6:257–267.
19. Tumer N, Scarpace PJ, Lowenthal DT. Geriatric pharmacology: basic and clinical considerations. *Annu Rev Pharmacol Toxicol* 1992;32:271–302.
20. Shock NW, Watkin DM, Yiengst BS, et al. Age differences in water content of the body as related to basal oxygen consumption in males. *J Gerontol* 1963;18:1–8.
21. Forbes GB, Reina JC. Adult lean body mass declines with age: some longitudinal observations. *Metabolism* 1978;19:653–663.
22. Adelman LS, Liebman J. Anatomy of body water and electrolytes. *Am J Med* 1959;27:256–277.
23. Repetto L, Vercelli M, Simoni C, et al. Comorbidity among elderly patients with and without cancer. *Proc Am Soc Clin Oncol* 1994;13:1625a.
24. Satariano WA, Ragland DA. The effect of comorbidity on 3-year survival of women with primary breast cancer. *Ann Intern Med* 1994;120:104–110.
25. Baker SD, Grochow LB. Pharmacology of cancer chemotherapy in the older person. *Clin Geriatr Med* 1997;13:169–183.

26. Kastrissios H, Blaschke TF. Medication compliance as a feature in drug development. *Annu Rev Pharmacol Toxicol* 1997;37:451–475.

27. Egorin MJ. Cancer pharmacology in the elderly. *Semin Oncol* 1993;20:43–49.

28. Rossman I. *Clinical geriatrics,* 2nd ed. Philadelphia: Lippincott, 1979.

29. Kotz CM, Billington CJ, Levine AS. Obesity and aging. *Clin Geriatr Med* 1999;15:391–412.

30. Lin CC, Li TC, Lai SW, et al. Epidemiology of obesity in elderly people. *Yale J Biol Med* 1999;72:385–391.

31. Rosner GL, Hargis JB, Hollis DR, et al. Relationship between toxicity and obesity in women receiving adjuvant chemotherapy for breast cancer: results from cancer and leukemia group B study 8541. *J Clin Oncol* 1996;14:3000–3008.

32. Ania BJ, Suman VJ, Fairbanks VF, et al. Incidence of anemia in older people: an epidemiologic study in a well defined population. *J Am Geriatr Soc* 1997;45:825–831.

33. Corti MC, Guralnik JM, Salive ME, et al. Serum albumin level and physical disability as predictors of mortality in older persons. *JAMA* 1994;272:1036–1042.

34. Hazzard WR. Depressed albumin and high-density lipoprotein cholesterol: signposts along the final common pathway of frailty. *J Am Geriatr Soc* 2001;49:1253–1254.

35. Volpato S, Leveille SG, Corti MC, et al. The value of serum albumin and high-density lipoprotein cholesterol in defining mortality risk in older persons with low serum cholesterol. *J Am Geriatr Soc* 2001;49:1142–1147.

36. Schwinghammer TL, Fleming RA, Rosenfeld CS, et al. Disposition of total and unbound etoposide following high-dose therapy. *Cancer Chemother Pharmacol* 1993;32:273–278.

37. Arbuck SG, Douglass HO, Crom WR, et al. Etoposide pharmacokinetics in patients with normal and abnormal organ function. *J Clin Oncol* 1986;4:1690–1695.

38. Stewart CF. Use of etoposide in patients with organ dysfunction: pharmacokinetic and pharmacodynamic considerations. *Cancer Chemother Pharmacol* 1994;34:S76–S83.

39. Eisenhauer EA, Vermorken JB, van Glabbeke M. Predictors of response to subsequent chemotherapy in platinum pretreated ovarian cancer: a multivariate analysis of 704 patients. *Ann Oncol* 1997;8:963–968.

40. Teicher BA, Ara G, Herbst R, et al. PEG-hemoglobin: effects on tumor oxygenation and response to chemotherapy. *In Vivo* 1997;11:301–311.

41. Schrijvers D, Highley M, De Bruyn E, et al. Role of red blood cells in pharmacokinetics of chemotherapeutic agents. *Anticancer Drugs* 1999;10:147–153.

42. Rieseman C. Antidepressant drug interactions and the cytochrome P450 system: a critical appraisal. *Pharmacotherapy* 1995;15[6 Pt 2]:84S–99S.

43. Michalets EL. Update: clinically significant cytochrome P-450 drug interactions. *Pharmacotherapy* 1998;18:84–112.

44. Evans W, Schentag J, Jusko W. *Applied pharmacokinetics, principles of therapeutic drug monitoring,* 3rd ed. Vancouver, WA: Applied Therapeutics, 1994.

45. Flockhart D. Cytochrome P450 drug interaction table (online). Available at: *http://medicine.iupui.edu/flockhart/* (accessed September 18, 2002).

46. Sotaniemi EA, Arranto AJ, Pelkonen O, et al. Age and cytochrome P450-linked drug metabolism in humans: an analysis of 226 subjects with equal histopathologic conditions. *Clin Pharmacol Ther* 1997;61:331–339.

47. Vestal RE. Aging and pharmacology. *Cancer* 1997;80:1302–1310.

48. Balducci L, Corcoran MB. Antineoplastic chemotherapy of the older cancer patient. *Hematol Oncol Clin North Am* 2000;14:193–212.

49. Brenner BM, Meyer GW, Hostetter TH. Dietary protein intake and the progressive nature of kidney disease: the role of hemodynamically mediated glomerular injury in the pathogenesis of progressive glomerular sclerosis in aging, renal ablation, and intrinsic renal disease. *N Engl J Med* 1982;307:652–659.

50. Tauchi H, Tsuboi K, Okutoni J. Age changes in the human kidney of the different races. *Gerontology* 1971;17:87–97.

51. Evers BM, Townsend CMJ, Thompson JC. Organ physiology of aging. *Surg Clin North Am* 1994;74:23–39.

52. Gelman RS, Taylor SGt. Cyclophosphamide, methotrexate, and 5-fluorouracil chemotherapy in women more than 65 years old with advanced breast cancer: the elimination of age trends in toxicity by using doses based on creatinine clearance. *J Clin Oncol* 1984;2:1404–1413.

53. Smythe M, Hoffman J, Kizy K, et al. Estimating creatinine clearance in elderly patients with low serum creatinine concentrations. *Am J Hosp Pharm* 1994;51:198–204.

54. Cockcroft DW, Gault MH. Prediction of creatinine clearance from serum creatinine. *Nephron* 1976;16:31–41.

55. Jelliffe RW. Estimation of creatinine clearance when urine cannot be collected. *Lancet* 1971;1:975–976.

56. Marx GM, Steer CB, Galani E, et al. Evaluation of the Cockroft Gault, Jelliffe and Wright formulae in estimating renal function in elderly patients. *Proc Annu Meet Am Soc Clin Oncol* 2002;21:1486a.

57. Balducci L, Extermann M. Cancer chemotherapy in the older patient: what the medical oncologist needs to know. *Cancer* 1997;80:1317–1322.

58. Skirvin JA, Lichtman SM. Pharmacokinetic considerations of oral chemotherapy in elderly patients with cancer. *Drugs Aging* 2002;19:25–42.

59. Calvert AH, Newell DR, Gumbrell LA, et al. Carboplatin dosage: prospective evaluation of a simple formula based on renal function. *J Clin Oncol* 1989; 7:1748–1756.

60. Chatelut E, Canal P, Brunner V, et al. Prediction of carboplatin clearance from standard morphological and biological patient characteristics. *J Natl Cancer Inst* 1995;87:573–580.

61. Kintzel PE, Dorr RT. Anticancer drug renal toxicity and elimination: dosing guidelines for altered renal function. *Cancer Treat Rev* 1995;21:33–64.

62. Borkowski JM, Duerr M, Donehower RC, et al. Relation between age and clearance rate of nine investigational anticancer drugs from phase I pharmacokinetic data. *Cancer Chemother Pharmacol* 1994;33:493–496.

63. Charlson ME, Pompei P, Ales KL, et al. A new method of classifying prognostic comorbidity in longitudinal studies: development and validation. *J Chronic Dis* 1987;40:373–383.

64. Yancik R, Wesley MN, Ries LA, et al. Comorbidity and age as predictors of risk for early mortality of male and female colon carcinoma patients: a population-based study. *Cancer* 1998;82:2123–2134.

65. Extermann M, Overcash J, Lyman GH, et al. Comorbidity and functional status are independent in older cancer patients. *J Clin Oncol* 1998;16:1582–1587.

66. Rockwood K, Stadnyk K, MacKnight C, et al. A brief clinical instrument to classify frailty in elderly people. *Lancet* 1999;353:205–206.

67. Reuben DB, Rubenstein LV, Hirsch SH, et al. Value of functional status as a predictor of mortality: results of a prospective study. *Am J Med* 1992;93:663–669.

68. Repetto L, Venturino A, Vercelli M, et al. Performance status and comorbidity in elderly cancer patients compared with young patients with neoplasia and elderly patients without neoplastic conditions. *Cancer* 1998;82:760–765.

69. Venook A, Klein C, Kastrissios H, et al. Phase I study of irinotecan (CPT-11) in patients with abnormal liver or renal function or with prior pelvic radiation therapy. *Proc Annu Meet Am Soc Clin Oncol* 2001;20:293a.

70. Venook AP, Egorin MJ, Rosner GL, et al. Phase I and pharmacokinetic trial of paclitaxel in patients with hepatic dysfunction: Cancer and Leukemia Group B 9264. *J Clin Oncol* 1998;16:1811–1819.

71. Venook AP, Egorin MJ, Rosner GL, et al. Phase I and pharmacokinetic trial of gemcitabine in patients with hepatic or renal dysfunction: Cancer and Leukemia Group B 9565. *J Clin Oncol* 2000;18:2780–2787.

72. Lichtman SM, Etcubanas E, Budman DR, et al. The pharmacokinetics and pharmacodynamics of fludarabine phosphate in patients with renal impairment: a prospective dose adjustment study. *Cancer Invest* 2002;20:904–913.

73. Vose JM, Armitage JO, Weisenburger DD, et al. The importance of age in survival of patients treated with chemotherapy for aggressive non-Hodgkin's lymphoma. *J Clin Oncol* 1988;6:1838–1844.

74. Johansson JE, Adami HO, Andersson SO, et al. High 10-year survival rate in patients with early, untreated prostatic cancer. *JAMA* 1992;267:2191–2196.

75. Newschaffer CJ, Otani K, McDonald MK, et al. Causes of death in elderly prostate cancer patients and in a comparison nonprostate cancer cohort. *J Natl Cancer Inst* 2000;92:613–621.

76. Gridelli C, Cortesi E, Roila F. Survival and quality of life: comparing end points in oncology. *Ann Oncol* 2001;12[Suppl]:S1.

77. Ganz PA, Reuben DB. Assessment of health status and outcomes: quality of life and geriatric assessment. In: Hunter CP, Johnson KA, Muss HB, eds. *Cancer in the elderly.* New York: Marcel Dekker, 2000:521–542.

78. Cohen HJ, Feussner JR, Weinberger M, et al. A controlled trial of inpatient and outpatient geriatric evaluation and management. *N Engl J Med* 2002;346:905–912.

79. Greco FA. Evolving role of oral chemotherapy for the treatment of patients with neoplasms. *Oncology* 1998; 12:43–50.

80. DeMario MD, Ratain MJ. Oral chemotherapy: rationale and future directions. *J Clin Oncol* 1998;16: 2557–2567.

81. Liu G, Franssen E, Fitch MI, et al. Patient preferences for oral versus intravenous palliative chemotherapy. *J Clin Oncol* 1997;15:110–115.

82. Bonadonna G, Valagussa P. Dose-response effect of adjuvant chemotherapy in breast cancer. *N Engl J Med* 1981;304:101–105.

83. Lebovits AH, Strain JJ, Schleifer SJ, et al. Patient noncompliance with self-administered chemotherapy. *Cancer* 1990;65:17–22.

84. Col N, Fanale JE, Kronholm P. The role of medication noncompliance and adverse drug reactions in hospitalizations of the elderly. *Arch Intern Med* 1990;150: 841–845.

85. Cramer JA. Enhancing patient compliance in the elderly. Role of packaging aids and monitoring. *Drugs Aging* 1998;12:7–15.

86. Richardson JL, Shelton DR, Krailo M, et al. The effect of compliance with treatment on survival among patients with hematologic malignancies. *J Clin Oncol* 1990;8:356–364.

87. Levine AM, Richardson JL, Marks G, et al. Compliance with oral drug therapy in patients with hematologic malignancy. *J Clin Oncol* 1987;5:1469–1476.

88. Richardson JL, Marks G, Levine A. The influence of symptoms of disease and side effects of treatment on compliance with cancer therapy. *J Clin Oncol* 1988;6:1746–1752.

89. Lee CR, Nicholson PW, Souhami RL, et al. Patient compliance with prolonged low-dose oral etoposide for small cell lung cancer. *Br J Cancer* 1993;67:630–634.

90. Urquhart J. Patient compliance with crucial drug regimens: implications for prostate cancer. *Eur Urol* 1996; 29:124–131.

91. Partridge AH, Avorn J, Wang PS, et al. Adherence to therapy with oral antineoplastic agents. *J Natl Cancer Inst* 2002;94:652–661.

92. Grever MR, Grieshaber CK. Toxicology by organ system. In: Holland JF, Frei E, eds. *Cancer medicine,* 5th ed. Hamilton, Ontario: BC Decker, 2000:602–611.

93. Lichtman SM, Ratain MJ, Van Echo DA, et al. Phase I trial of granulocyte-macrophage colony-stimulating factor plus high-dose cyclophosphamide given every 2 weeks: a Cancer and Leukemia Group B study. *J Natl Cancer Inst* 1993;85:1319–1326.

94. Tew KD, Colvin OM, Chabner BA. Alkylating agents. In: Chabner BA, Longo DL, eds. *Cancer chemotherapy and biotherapy: principles and practice,* 3rd ed. Philadelphia: Lippincott-Raven, 2001:373–414.

95. Hensley ML, Schuchter LM, Lindley C, et al. American Society of Clinical Oncology clinical practice guidelines for the use of chemotherapy and radiotherapy protectants. *J Clin Oncol* 1999;17:3333–3355.

96. Koeller JM, Aapro MS, Gralla RJ, et al. Antiemetic guidelines: creating a more practical treatment approach. *Support Care Cancer* 2002;10:519–522.

97. Hesketh PJ, Kris MG, Grunberg SM, et al. Proposal for classifying the acute emetogenicity of cancer chemotherapy. *J Clin Oncol* 1997;15:103–109.

98. Crawford J. Pegfilgrastim: the promise of pegylation fulfilled. *Ann Oncol* 2003;14:6–7.

99. Crawford J, Ozer H, Stoller R, et al. Reduction by granulocyte colony-stimulating factor of fever and neutropenia induced by chemotherapy in patients with small-cell lung cancer. *N Engl J Med* 1991; 325: 164–170.

100. Balducci L, Lyman GH. Patients aged > or = 70 are at high risk for neutropenic infection and should receive hemopoietic growth factors when treated with moder-

ately toxic chemotherapy. *J Clin Oncol* 2001;19: 1583–1585.

101. Safra T, Muggia F, Jeffers S, et al. Pegylated liposomal doxorubicin (Doxil): reduced clinical cardiotoxicity in patients reaching or exceeding cumulative doses of 500 mg/m². *Ann Oncol* 2000;11:1029–1033.

102. Corcoran ME. Polypharmacy in the older patient with cancer. *Cancer Control* 1997;4:419–428.

103. Kivisto KT, Kroemer HK, Eichelbaum M. The role of human cytochrome P450 enzymes in the metabolism of anticancer agents: implications for drug interactions. *Br J Clin Pharmacol* 1995;40:523–530.

104. King RS. Drug interactions with cancer chemotherapy. *Cancer Pract* 1995;3:57–59.

105. Onder G, Pedone C, Landi F, et al. Adverse drug reactions as cause of hospital admissions: results from the Italian Group of Pharmacoepidemiology in the Elderly (GIFA). *J Am Geriatr Soc* 2002;50:1962–1968.

106. Lazarou J, Pomeranz BH, Corey PN. Incidence of adverse drug reactions in hospitalized patients: a meta-analysis of prospective studies. *JAMA* 1998;279: 1200–1205.

107. Einarson TR. Drug-related hospital admissions. *Ann Pharmacother* 1993;27:832–840.

108. Flockhart DA, Tanus-Santos JE. Implications of cytochrome P450 interactions when prescribing medication for hypertension. *Arch Intern Med* 2002;162: 405–412.

109. Huizing MT, Keung AC, Rosing H, et al. Pharmacokinetics of paclitaxel and metabolites in a randomized comparative study in platinum-pretreated ovarian cancer patients. *J Clin Oncol* 1993;11:2127–2135.

110. Kearns C, Gianni L, Vigano L, et al. Validation of paclitaxel limited sampling strategies. *Proc Annu Meet Am Soc Clin Oncol* 1997;16.

111. Lichtman SM, Egorin M, Rosner G, et al. Clinical pharmacology of paclitaxel in relation to patient age: CALGB 9762. *Proc Annu Meet Am Soc Clin Oncol* 2001;19:265a.

112. Ratain MJ, Staubus AE, Schilsky RL, et al. Limited sampling models for amonafide pharmacokinetics. *Proc AACR* 1988;29:766a.

113. Mick R, Gupta E, Vokes EE, et al. Limited-sampling models for irinotecan pharmacokinetics-pharmacodynamics: prediction of biliary index and intestinal toxicity. *J Clin Oncol* 1996;14:2012–2019.

114. Minami H, Beijnen JH, Verweij J, et al. Limited sampling model for area under the concentration time curve of total topotecan. *Clin Cancer Res* 1996;2: 43–46.

115. Ratain MJ, Robert J, van der Vijgh WJ. Limited sampling models for doxorubicin pharmacokinetics. *J Clin Oncol* 1991;9:871–876.

116. Egorin MJ, Forrest A, Belani CP, et al. A limited sampling strategy for cyclophosphamide pharmacokinetics. *Cancer Res* 1989;49:3129–3133.

117. Ratain MJ, Staubus AE, Schilsky RL, et al. Limited sampling models for amonafide (NSC 308847) pharmacokinetics. *Cancer Res* 1988;48:4127–4130.

118. Ratain MJ, Vogelzang NJ. Limited sampling model for vinblastine pharmacokinetics. *Cancer Treat Rep* 1987; 71:935–939.

119. van Warmerdam LJ, ten Bokkel Huinink WW, Maes RA, et al. Limited-sampling models for anticancer agents. *J Cancer Res Clin Oncol* 1994;120: 427–433.

120. Tranchand B, Amsellem C, Chatelut E, et al. A limited-sampling strategy for estimation of etoposide pharmacokinetics in cancer patients. *Cancer Chemother Pharmacol* 1999;43:316–322.

121. van Warmerdam LJ, Verweij J, Rosing H, et al. Limited sampling models for topotecan pharmacokinetics. *Ann Oncol* 1994;5:259–264.

122. Aarons L. Population pharmacokinetics: theory and practice. *Br J Clin Pharmacol* 1991;32:669–670.

123. Eisenberg DM, Kessler RC, Foster C, et al. Unconventional medicine in the United States—prevalence, costs, and patterns of use. *N Engl J Med* 1993;328: 246–252.

124. Jacobson JS, Workman SB, Kronenberg F. Research on complementary and alternative therapies for cancer: issues and methodological considerations. *J Am Med Womens Assoc* 1999;54:177–180,183.

125. Ernst E, Cassileth BR. The prevalence of complementary/alternative medicine in cancer: a systematic review. *Cancer* 1998;83:777–782.

126. Mathijssen RHJ, Verweij J, de Bruijn P, et al. Effects of St. John's wort on irinotecan metabolism. *JNCI Cancer Spectrum* 2002;94:1247–1249.

127. Mansky PJ, Straus SE. St. John's wort: more implications for cancer patients. *JNCI Cancer Spectrum* 2002; 94:1187–1188.

128. Johne A, Brockmoller J, Bauer S, et al. Pharmacokinetic interaction of digoxin with an herbal extract from St. John's wort (Hypericum perforatum). *Clin Pharmacol Ther* 1999;66:338–345.

129. Ernst E. Second thoughts about safety of St. John's wort. *Lancet* 1999;354:2014–2016.

130. Piscitelli SC, Burstein AH, Chaitt D, et al. Indinavir concentrations and St. John's wort [Letter]. *Lancet* 2000;355:547–548.

131. Ruschitzka F, Meier PJ, Turina M, et al. Acute heart transplant rejection due to Saint John's wort [Letter]. *Lancet* 2000;355:548–549.

132. Dresser GK, Spence JD, Bailey DG. Pharmacokinetic-pharmacodynamic consequences and clinical relevance of cytochrome P450 3A4 inhibition. *Clin Pharmacokinet* 2000;38:41–57.

133. Yue QY, Bergquist C, Gerden B. Safety of St. John's wort (Hypericum perforatum) [Letter]. *Lancet* 2000; 355:576–577.

134. Nam RK, Fleshner N, Rakovitch E, et al. Prevalence and patterns of the use of complementary therapies among prostate cancer patients: an epidemiological analysis. *J Urol* 1999;161:1521–1524.

135. Wilkinson S, Gomella LG, Smith JA, et al. Attitudes and use of complementary medicine in men with prostate cancer. *J Urol* 2002;168:2505–2509.

136. Small EJ, Frohlich MW, Bok R, et al. Prospective trial of the herbal supplement PC-SPES in patients with progressive prostate cancer. *J Clin Oncol* 2000;18: 3595–3603.

137. Trimble EL, Carter CL, Cain D, et al. Representation of older patients in cancer treatment trials. *Cancer* 1994;74:2208–2214.

138. Lichtman SM. Integration of geriatrics in oncology training—the relationship between the academic center and the community. *Crit Rev Oncol Hematol* 2000;33:57–59.

139. Muss HB, Cohen HJ, Lichtman SM. Clinical research in the older cancer patient. *Hematol Oncol Clin North Am* 2000;14:283–291.

30

Quality-of-Life Measurement

Kelly Dineen, David Cella, and Kimberly Davis

Center on Outcomes, Research and Education (CORE), Evanston, Illinois 60201

Although quality of life has always been an important consideration in the care of people with cancer, the past 20 years have witnessed the emergence of more formal attention to this issue. The development and validation of several health-related quality-of-life (HRQOL) instruments (questionnaires) defined the quality-of-life issues important to patients. Research findings and information gained from clinical practice also contributed to the inclusion of quality-of-life assessment with other important components of the treatment decision-making process, such as toxicity, length of treatment, and survival advantage. As people live longer with cancer, assessing and maintaining quality of life becomes a priority.

Extended survival, often with long disease-free periods, is a reality for many forms of cancer. However, for many patients, extended survival comes with significant short-term and sometimes long-term costs. Some new treatments that offer increased survival benefits have high side-effect profiles. These side effects can severely affect quality of life. Understanding the impact of symptoms such as fatigue, pain, and nausea on a patient's daily life can help tailor interventions to minimize impact on quality of life. Therefore, finding a balance between treatment toxicity and efficacy is a prevailing concern in clinical care (1).

Today's new cancer treatments often are a refinement of the structure or delivery of existing agents or of new drugs with favorable side effect profiles to equally effective existing therapy. "Cytostatic" treatment (e.g., "targeted" or "small-molecule" therapy) offers promise of disease control with minimal toxicity. In cases where the outlook for survival is limited (e.g., advanced lung cancer), there has been a shift in emphasis from aggressive cytotoxic therapy to palliative treatment to maximize quality of life. Increasingly for physicians and patients, HRQOL is carrying a greater weight in the treatment decision-making process, along with treatment efficacy, treatment burden, and side effects.

In this chapter we first provide a brief overview of the development of the HRQOL concept and its measurement. We highlight some important measurement issues and discuss choosing appropriate instruments. Finally, we review new applications of HRQOL instruments pertinent to those working in clinical and research settings.

DEFINING HEALTH-RELATED QUALITY OF LIFE

Until recently, health care providers were generally considered reliable informants of a patient's HRQOL, so HRQOL was assessed primarily by proxy raters. Numerous studies have demonstrated that agreement between patient and proxy is limited; thus, it is best to ask patients directly (2–4). The importance of understanding the subjective nature of the quality-of-life appraisal process is further highlighted by research that compares the treatment choices of advanced cancer patients with those made by proxy's reading clinical case scenarios. Patients with advanced disease more often choose aggressive treatments, despite toxic side effects and "minimal" survival benefits (5). Given comparable scenarios, proxy raters often state that they would refuse such treatment (6). For example, some drugs may have a palliative intent, thereby offering no survival benefit, but in the patient's mind, symptom relief may outweigh objectively comparable toxicity. Stephens et al. (4) found a similar discrepancy in the reporting of symptoms between patients and physicians. The symptom scores diverge most significantly at the extreme end, with patients reporting more severe symptoms than their physicians. Knowledge of the discrepancies in health ratings and treatment preferences between patients and proxies serves as a reminder that patients should ideally be given HRQOL information and support to participate in ongoing treatment decisions.

In the past, the assessment of HRQOL was dominated by unidimensional instruments weighted heavily toward the measurement of physical and functional abilities (7). For example, the Karnofsky Performance Status Rating, a single global rating of physical function, has been used to infer overall quality of life, despite evidence that HRQOL is multidimensional (3). This and other supportive research findings helped to expand the conceptualization of HRQOL to include other important dimensions.

Early definitions of HRQOL focused upon one's subjective appraisal of current level of functioning compared to one's perception of an ideal level of functioning (8). The gap between where one currently is and where one wants to be was considered important (1). The definition became further enhanced as the dimensionality of the overall construct of HRQOL was defined and expanded to encompass physical, emotional, and social well-being. The present consensus is that HRQOL is a *subjective* and *multidimensional* construct (1,8–12). This revised definition establishes the important parameters for QOL measurement: using the *patient's* perspective, and assessing *physical, mental,* and *social well-being.*

Many have expanded upon this basic conceptualization and include other factors in HRQOL measurement. For example, a review of the many available questionnaires revealed that more than 30 different names for QOL dimensions were listed by various authors (13). Review of these dimensions and available factor analytic studies suggest up to *seven* distinct dimensions: (i) physical concerns (symptoms; pain); (ii) functional ability (activity); (iii) family well-being; (iv) mental well-being; (v) treatment satisfaction (including financial concerns); (vi) sexuality/intimacy (including body image); and (vii) social functioning (Table 30.1). In addition, there are two relevant summary dimensions that are available using some QOL questionnaires. Global evaluation of QOL (i.e., a single question rating the patient's global or overall perception of QOL or health status) can provide important information about a patient's overall perspective of their HRQOL. Likewise, having a total score (i.e., the summation of dimension scores into an aggregate index of QOL) can allow for comparison across instruments if standard scores are available (13,14).

CHOOSING AN INSTRUMENT

Although there is no accepted gold standard for measurement of HRQOL, many questionnaires are available for use with cancer patients. These questionnaires have been described and discussed elsewhere (13,15,16). Questionnaires can be either disease specific or more generic. Disease-specific measures of HRQOL assess symptoms and side effects specific to a disease and/or treatment, such as lymphedema in breast cancer patients, along with other dimensions of quality of life. Table 30.2 provides a brief description of several well-known and often-used instruments.

No single instrument is best for *all* studies. A questionnaire that performs well in one setting may be ineffective in another. The researcher or clinician must find a balance between psychometric concerns such as reliability, validity, and breadth of coverage and clinical concerns that call for brevity, understandability, and ease of administration. When evaluating instruments for use in clinical or research settings, several questions must be considered: (i) How was the instrument developed? (ii) Which populations were used in the initial validation process? (ii) How was HRQOL defined? (iv) Has there been further validation of the instrument in clinical populations? To summarize, typically the best strategy is to select a questionnaire that comes closest to asking the most clinically appropriate questions, confirm its reliability and validity, and supplement with a *few* additional disease-specific/treatment-specific questions.

General and disease-specific instruments have advantages and disadvantages. General instruments can provide a more comprehensive measure of HRQOL, and disease-specific instruments can provide impor-

TABLE 30.1. *Dimensions of quality of life*

Physical concerns	General physical functioning, disruption in functioning from disease and symptoms such as pain, fatigue, nausea/vomiting
Functional ability	Ability to care for oneself, ability to work and maintain one's usual roles and activities
Family well-being	Family role functioning, support, family role responsibilities
Mental well-being	Emotional distress, impact of illness, cognitive functioning
Treatment satisfaction	Satisfaction with treatment, financial concerns
Sexuality intimacy	Includes body image concerns
Social functioning and well-being	Perceived level of support, social activity

TABLE 30.2. *Health-related quality-of-life instruments commonly used in oncology*

Instrument	Items	Scales	Validity/reliability
FACT Measurement System	27 items; Likert scaling	4 subscales; total scores; disease-specific additional concerns	Good reliability and validity; sensitive to clinical change; used in clinical trials
Medical Outcomes Study 36 Item Short-Form Health Survey (SF-36)	36 items; Likert scaling	8 subscales; 2 indices (Physical Component Summary and Mental Component Summary)	Good reliability; ample supportive validity data; used extensively with cancer patients
EORTC Quality-of-Life Questionnaire (EORTC QLQ-C30)	30 items; Likert scaling	7 scales; global quality-of-life score	Good reliability for individual scales; extensive validity data available
Functional Living Index-Cancer (FLIC)	22 items; combined visual analog/Likert scaling	Global score; optional use of 5 subscale scores	Good reliability and validity; total score most commonly used
Cancer Rehabilitation Evaluation System (CARES)	59 items; Likert scaling	5 summary scale scores; total score	Adequate test-retest reliability; internal consistency and concurrent validity

tant information about disease-specific and treatment-specific concerns. Instruments that strike a balance between these two approaches have tended to become most popular in oncology. Disease-specific and treatment-specific questions usually are of benefit when they are added to a general measure of quality of life. Together they can provide comparability across diseases and sensitivity to specific issues or symptoms relevant to a given disease or treatment. Ultimately, researchers or clinicians can select an instrument to suit their specific needs.

Quality-of-life measurement in oncology has advanced to the desirable point where we have become less concerned with creating reliable and valid instruments and more concerned with the acceptance of the importance of the concept in research and clinical care (14). We now are faced with the tasks of fine-tuning the important details, such as optimal symptom assessment, determining clinically meaningful change in scores, and developing responsive short forms for clinical trials. New applications for the administration of HRQOL assessments, such as computerized adaptive testing (CAT) for use in clinical settings, are also coming into play. Each of these issues will be discussed later in this chapter.

SYMPTOM ASSESSMENT

Intuitively, most people understand that the experience of many and/or severe symptoms from disease and/or treatment can diminish quality of life. Interest in formalized symptom assessment has evolved from two sources: clinicians wishing to plan treatments

based on a sound evaluation; and investigators wishing to accurately determine the efficacy of interventions targeted at specific symptoms (17). In clinical settings, symptom assessment measures often are used in conjunction with either general or disease-specific QOL measures to provide a detailed look at the patient's experience. Clinicians can track the improvement or worsening of symptoms across time and assess the effectiveness of palliative treatments (e.g., pain management).

In research settings there is a growing interest in understanding the complex relationship among symptom intensity, symptom duration, and HRQOL (18–21). Symptom assessments are used in clinical trial work as key patient-related endpoints, especially when evaluating disease or symptom focused therapies. Most exciting is the growing body of work showing that patient-reported QOL, including report of physical symptoms, is predictive of length of survival and tumor response, independent of other disease-related factors. The predictive value of symptom assessment has been demonstrated in a variety of patient samples, including heterogeneous (mixed cancer) samples, and site-specific samples such as advanced breast cancer, malignant melanoma, and colorectal, head and neck, lung, and esophageal cancer (21–28). The physical symptoms of pain and fatigue have been the best predictors of survival.

There are problems inherent in the measurement of symptoms. Symptoms may be episodic and of varying duration (29). Some symptoms may develop slowly, whereas others may have a more acute onset. There are questions as to whether one should measure intensity or frequency of the symptoms or the level of distress/bother to the patient (18,19,29,30). Finally, how does one weigh the suffering caused by the symptom(s) and the relative contribution of this suffering to a diminished HRQOL (17)? In addition to these more methodologically based concerns are the concerns of patient burden and time constraints. Comprehensive symptom assessment often is time consuming and difficult for patients to complete (18). To address these concerns, work is being done on the development and validation of shorter and more user-friendly forms (18,19,30).

More work needs to be done to integrate formalized symptom assessment into the routine care of cancer patients (7). Some researchers have demonstrated that ongoing monitoring of symptoms and HRQOL can improve quality of care and in turn improve quality of life (32,33). This is important because there is a good likelihood that many potentially treatable symptoms are missed due to failure to report (18).

SHORT FORMS

In a clinical trial, the measurement of HRQOL in the testing of new treatments with modest survival benefit may provide pivotal information in determining treatment value (14). However, existing instruments often are perceived as too long for some settings, particularly the assessment of symptomatic patients in declining health. Although short forms of the longer "parent" questionnaire often provide less precision than full-length counterparts, they can provide sufficient information about HRQOL for group comparisons, thereby reducing patient and administrative burden (34). Group comparisons, which benefit from large sample size, can overcome the problem of lower precision found in short forms.

Short forms typically are derived from existing instruments and are composed of selected items, usually picked because they maximize accurate estimation of the full-length score. Typically, their reliability and validity are confirmed through further research studies. Many well-known instruments now have short forms available, such as the Profile of Mood States (35), the Medical Outcomes Study (SF-20) (12), the Hospital Anxiety and Depression Scale (HADS) (9), and the MOS 36-Item Short Form Health Survey (SF-36) (36,37).

COMPUTER-BASED ASSESSMENT

Computer technology is being used to facilitate the use of QOL data in clinical practice and research. Computer-based testing (CBT), an innovative and alternate methodology for data collection, affords improved accuracy, precision, and interpretation that may make QOL assessment more "user friendly" (38). Computer-based assessments have been used recently in several medical setting applications (39–41), including oncology patients (33,34,38, 42–44). Interviews with patients have demonstrated a high level of acceptability (45).

CAT is a specific type of CBT that provides a platform for the administration of HRQOL assessments, only asking questions that will provide a maximum amount of information. Using probabilistic measurement models [Rasch or Item Response Theory (IRT)], item selection is guided by an individual's response to previously administered questions from a large item bank (46–51). Therefore, each patient need only answer a small number of items to obtain a measure that accurately estimates what would have been obtained had the entire set of items been administered. The result is an individually tailored HRQOL/symptom assessment.

Compared to traditional paper-and-pencil administration, CAT offers several advantages, including (i) speed of assessment; (ii) fewer items for the same level of precision; (iii) mechanism for completing routine assessments; (iv) immediate data entry; (v) easier scoring and interpretation; (vi) comparison of scores across time; and (vii) immediate presentation of results in "real time."

The use of CAT to administer HRQOL and symptom assessments has particular relevance for routine administration in the outpatient oncology setting. Although it has been the expectation that health care providers would gradually incorporate formal HRQOL assessments into clinical practice, this has been slow to materialize (32,52–57). Integration into clinical practice appears to be an essential factor in obtaining HRQOL assessments seen as viable clinical tools for guiding treatment planning and decision making. In a recent review of the use of HRQOL in the oncology setting, Davis and Cella (58) presented a list of barriers to assessing HRQOL and critical success factors for overcoming these barriers.

Logistic barriers that inhibit feasibility of clinical implementation were cited as one of three broad categories of barriers. Within this category were concerns about administrative burden on staff and patients, delayed presentation of results, perceived time constraints of conducting assessments, and the lack of universally accepted instruments. CAT specifically addresses each of those logistic barriers, therefore reducing several factors that impede clinical feasibility.

With respect to the critical success factors, Davis and Cella (58) also proposed three broad categories:

(i) the need for an acceptable set of core measures; (ii) clinical relevance and ease of use; and (iii) buy-in from staff and patients. Again, CAT addresses many of the suggested success factors included in the first two categories (59,60).

Having addressed both barriers and success factors, CAT and CBT offer opportunity for integrating HRQOL assessments into clinical practice. It is the belief of many in the field of HRQOL that ongoing improvements in technology can continue to offer solutions to the concerns that have historically interfered with the use of HRQOL assessments, particularly in busy outpatient clinics. It is the hope that collaborative efforts between researchers and clinicians will result in HRQOL becoming a more routine component of clinical care and research protocols, ultimately providing benefits for patients and providers.

DETERMINING CLINICALLY MEANINGFUL CHANGE

Until fairly recently there has been a tendency for statistical significance testing to dominate our decisions regarding the relevance of findings, especially in clinical trials. However, there is an important distinction to be made between statistically significant change and clinically significant or meaningful change. If a sample is large enough, statistically significant changes are more likely to be found (61). For example, a large clinical trial might obtain statistically significant differences between treatment arms, and these differences may reflect measurement of a true effect (i.e., the instrument was valid). Still, because of the large sample size (and perhaps the small score difference), we might question the clinical meaning of the difference score (62). Is the difference clinically significant? What is the meaningful pattern of change that deserves clinical attention? Does a significant difference between arms transfer to single case interpretation? What is the meaning of a 5-, 10-, or 15-point difference score? Unfortunately, a finding of statistically significant change gives us little to no sense of how the patient perceives the change.

Clinically meaningful change, or *minimally important difference,* refers to the smallest measure of change in quality of life that the patient perceives as an important or meaningful change (63). Lydick and Epstein (64) provide a summary of the various methods used to assess minimally important differences. Some approaches that have been used include the statistical examination of effect size across different thresholds of quality of life (61), calibration of change/difference scores to an external criterion (10,34,65), direct longitudinal assessment of patients

(63,66), determination of population weights or valuations (67,68), and utility/tradeoff/willingness to pay interviewing. For seven-point Likert scaling of symptoms, Jaeschke et al. (63) have suggested a difference of approximately 0.5 units per item as a minimal clinically important difference. Jacobson and Truax (69) recommend a Reliable Change Index that estimates whether a measured change can be considered real with confidence.

More recently, it has been suggested that there may be asymmetry in the magnitude of a meaningful change, depending upon whether the change is an improvement or worsening. Recent research suggests that patients will tolerate a greater degree of worsening in their quality of life before reporting a negative change, whereas smaller degrees of change in the positive direction are noted as meaningful (70). This may be due to the dispositional optimism of some people or an adaptation to one's illness and symptoms resulting in a modification of one's internal sense of ideal HRQOL. Further research is needed to confirm and explain this observation.

CROSS-CULTURALLY VALID ASSESSMENT

Culture influences health behavior and perceptions by shaping explanations of sickness, social position, and meaning of life (71,72). In any multicultural context, people with medical conditions possess attributes that create barriers to standard QOL evaluation, such as different language and low literacy. The most commonly used QOL instruments were originally developed in English. Exceptions include the World Health Organization QOL questionnaire (WHOQOL) (73), EuroQoL (74,75), and the Rotterdam Symptom Checklist (31,76).

There is increasing need for QOL instruments that are reliable and valid across cultures and languages. Thus, many groups have conducted translation and validation studies of various questionnaires originally written in the English language. Translation of an existing single-language document ideally involves an iterative forward-backward-forward sequencing and review of difficulties on an item-by-item basis. *Decentering,* or selective modification of the source document based upon problems encountered in this process, is ideal when possible. The final translated document should be pretested for acceptability and content validity and then implemented in multilingual clinical trials, where the derived data can be tested statistically for cross-cultural equivalence or bias. Translations are available for the Cancer Rehabilitation Evaluation System (CARES) (77,78), the European Organization for the Research and Treatment of

Cancer (EORTC) QLQ-C30 (10,19), the Functional Assessment of Cancer Therapy (FACT) Measurement System (16,34,79), the Functional Living Index-Cancer (FLIC) (11), the Medical Outcomes Study 36-Item Short-Form Health Survey (MOS SF-36) (36,37,80), the Sickness Impact Profile (SIP) (81–83), the Nottingham Health Profile (NHP) (84,85), the Mc-Master Health Index (86), and the Southwest Oncology Group (SWOG) questionnaire (87). Information about the current status of translations for any questionnaire is best obtained from the scale developer; however, a good review can be found in Spilker (88).

SUMMARY AND CONCLUSION

Treatment, evaluation, and planning of quality-of-life assessment in oncology have come a long way over the past 10 years. Quality of life is a multidimensional, subjective, and fluid endpoint, so its measurement must be comprehensive, include the patient's perspective, and be sensitive to meaningful change. Given the challenges and burdens of providing quality care in busy oncology practices, QOL measurement also must be brief. Because there is no "gold standard" or "best" quality-of-life measure, it is important to be aware of the strengths and weaknesses of available questionnaires when deciding upon instruments for use in either research or clinical practice. There are many exciting new areas of research of QOL measurement in oncology: establishing cross-cultural validity; enhancing interpretability of scores; standardizing scores across questionnaires; and implementing computerized practical assessment. Social, statistical, and measurement scientists have a tremendous opportunity to contribute meaningfully to the future health and well-being of our society by immersing themselves in these new challenges of measuring and evaluating QOL in people with cancer.

REFERENCES

1. Cella DF. Quality of life: concepts and definition. *J Pain Symptom Manage* 1994;9:186–192.
2. Presant CA. Quality of life in cancer patients. Who measures what? *Am J Clin Oncol* 1984;7:571–573.
3. Spitzer WO, Dobson AJ, Hall J, et al. Measuring the quality of life of cancer patients: a concise QL-index for use by physicians. *J Chronic Dis* 1981;34: 585–597.
4. Stephens RJ, Hopwood P, Girling DJ, et al. Randomized trials with quality of life endpoints: are doctors' ratings of patients' physical symptoms interchangeable with patients' self-ratings? *Qual Life Res* 1997;6: 225–236.
5. Yellen SB, Cella D. Someone to live for: social well-being, parenthood status, and decision-making in oncology. *J Clin Oncol* 1995;13:1255–1264.
6. Mischel MH. Reconceptualization of the uncertainty in illness theory. Image. *J Nurs School* 1990;22: 256–262.
7. Osoba D. Lessons learned from measuring health-related quality of life in oncology. *J Clin Oncol* 1994; 12(3), 608–616.
8. Cella DF, Cherin EA. Quality of life during and after cancer treatment. *Compr Ther* 1988;4:69–75.
9. Aaronson NK. Quality of life: what is it? How should it be measured? *Oncology* 1988;2:69–74.
10. Aaronson NK, Ahmedzai S, Bergman B, et al. The European Organization for the Research and Treatment of Cancer QLQ-C30: a quality of life instrument for use in international clinical trials in oncology. *J Natl Cancer Inst* 1993;85:365–376.
11. Schipper H, Clinch J, McMurray A, et al. Measuring the quality of life of cancer patients: the Functional Living Index-Cancer: development and validation. *J Clin Oncol* 1984;2:472–483.
12. Stewart AL, Hays RD, Ware JE. The MOS Short Form General Health Survey. Reliability and validity in a patient population. *Med Care* 1988;26:724–735.
13. Kornblith AB, Holland JC. *Handbook of measures for psychological, social and physical function in cancer. Volume 1: quality of life.* New York: Memorial Sloan-Kettering Cancer Center, 1994.
14. Cella DF. Quality of life. In: Holland JC, Breitbart W, Jacobson PB, et al., eds. *Research methods in psycho-oncology.* New York: Oxford University Press, 1998:1135–1146.
15. Cella DF. Measuring quality of life in palliative care. *Semin Oncol* 1995;22[Suppl 3]:73–81.
16. Cella DF, Bonomi AE. Measuring quality of life: 1995 update. *Oncology* 1995;9[Suppl 11]:47–60.
17. Ingham JM, Portenoy RK. Symptom assessment. *Hematol Oncol Clin North Am* 1996;10:21–39.
18. Chang VT, Thaler HT, Polyak T. Quality of life and survival: the role of multidimensional symptom assessment. *Am Cancer Soc* 1998;83:173–179.
19. Chang VT, Hwang SS, Feuerman M, et al. The Memorial Symptom Assessment Scale Short Form (MSAS-SF). *Cancer* 2000;89:1162–1171.
20. Osoba D, Zee B, Pater J, et al. Psychometric properties and responsiveness of the EORTC quality of life questionnaire (QLQ-30) in patients with breast, ovarian and lung cancer. *Qual Life Res* 1994;3:353–364.
21. Portenoy RK, Thaler HT, Kornblith AB, et al. Symptom prevalence, characteristics, and distress in a cancer population. *Qual Life Res* 1994;3:183–189.
22. Dancey J, Zee B, Osoba D, et al. Quality of life scores: an independent prognostic variable in a general population of cancer patients receiving chemotherapy. *Qual Life Res* 1997;6:151–158.
23. Kramer JA, Curran D, Piccart M, et al. Identification and interpretation of clinical and quality of life prognostic factors for survival and response to treatment in first-line chemotherapy in advanced breast cancer. *Eur J Cancer* 2000;36:1498–1506.
24. Butow PN, Coates A, Dunn SM. Psychosocial predictors of survival in metastatic melanoma. *J Clin Oncol* 1999;17:2256–2263.

25. Earlam S, Glover C, Fordy C, et al. Relation between tumor size, quality of life, and survival in patients with colorectal liver metastases. *J Clin Oncol* 1996;14: 171–175.

26. de Graeff A, de Leeuw JRJ, Ros WJG, et al. Sociodemographic factors and quality of life as prognostic indicators in head and neck cancer. *Eur J Cancer* 2001;37: 332–339.

27. Eton D, Fairclough DL, Yount S, et al. Quality of life during chemotherapy predicts clinical outcome in lung cancer: results from Eastern Cooperative Oncology Group Study 5592. *J Clin Oncol* 2003;21:1536–1543.

28. Blazeby JM, Brookes ST, Alderson D. The prognostic value of quality of life scores during treatment for oesophageal cancer. *Gut* 2001;49:227–230.

29. Kroenke K. Studying symptoms: sampling and measurement issues. *Ann Intern Med* 2001;134[9 Pt 2]: 844–853.

30. Osoba D. Self-rating symptom checklists: a simple method for recording and evaluating symptom control in oncology. *Cancer Treat Rev* 1993;19:43–51.

31. de Haes JC, van Knippenberg FC, Neijt JP. Measuring psychological and physical distress in cancer patients: structure and application of the Rotterdam Symptom Checklist. *Br J Cancer* 1990;62:1034–1038.

32. Detmar S, Aaronson N. Quality of life assessment in daily clinical oncology practice: a feasibility study. *Eur J Cancer* 1998;34:1181–1186.

33. Velikova G, Brown J, Smith A, et al. Computer-based quality of life questionnaires may contribute to doctor-patient interactions in oncology. *Br J Oncol* 2002;86: 51–59.

34. Cella DF, Tulsky DS, Gray G, et al. The Functional Assessment of Cancer Therapy (FACT) Scale: development and validation of the general version. *J Clin Oncol* 1993;11:570–579.

35. Cella DF, Jacobsen PB, Orav EJ, et al. A brief POMS measure of distress for cancer patients. *J Chronic Dis* 1987;40:939–942.

36. McHorney CA, Ware JE, Raczek AE. The MOS 36-item short form health survey (SF–36): II. Psychometric and clinical test of validity in measuring physical and mental health constructs. *Med Care* 1993;31:247–263.

37. McHorney CA, Ware JE, Lu J, et al. The MOS 36-Item Short Form Health Survey (SF-36). III. Tests of data quality, scaling assumptions and reliability across diverse patient groups. *Med Care* 1994;32:40–66.

38. Cella D, Lloyd S. Data collection strategies for patient-reported information. *Qual Manage Health Care* 1994; 2:28–35.

39. Swanston M, Abraham C, Macrar W, et al. Pain assessment with interactive computer animation. *Pain* 1993; 53:347–351.

40. Roizen M, Coalson C, Hayward R, et al. A patients use an automated questionnaire to define their current health status? *Med Care* 1992;30:74–84.

41. Lenart L, Horberger J. Computer-assisted quality of life assessment for clinical trials. Division of Clinical Pharmacology, Stanford University School of Medicine, CA. *Proceedings/AMA Annual Fall Symposium* 1996: 992–996.

42. Buxton J, White M, Osoba D. Patients' experiences using a computerized program with a touch-sensitive video monitor for the assessment of health-related quality of life. *Qual Life Res* 1998;7:513–519.

43. Sigle J, Porzolt F. Practical aspects of quality of life measurement, design, and feasibility: study of the qual-ity of life recorder and the standardization measurement of quality of life in an outpatient clinic. *Cancer Treat Rev* 1996;22[Suppl A]:75–89.

44. Taenzer P, Speca M, Atkinson M, et al. Computerized quality of life screening in an oncology clinic. *Clin Pract* 1997;5:168–175.

45. Velikova G, Wright E, Smith A, et al. Automated collection of quality of life data: comparison of paper and computer touch screen questionnaires. *J Clin Oncol* 1999;7:998–1007.

46. Weiss D, Kingsbury G. Application of computerized adaptive testing to educational problems. *J Educ Measure* 1984;21:361–375.

47. Green B, Brock R, Humphreys L, et al. Technical guidelines for assessing computerized adaptive tests. *J Educ Measure* 1984;21:347–360.

48. McKinely R, Reckase M. Implementing an adaptive testing program in an instructional program environment. Paper presented at the meeting of the American Educational Research Association, New Orleans, Louisiana, March 1984.

49. Urry V. Tailored testing: a successful application of latent trait theory. *J Educ Measure* 1997;14:181–196.

50. Olson J, Maynes D, Slawson D, et al. Comparison and equating of paper-administered, computer-administered and computerized adaptive tests of achievement. Paper presented at the meeting of the American Educational research Association. San Francisco, California, April 1986.

51. Weiss D. *New horizons in testing: latent trait test theory and computerized adaptive testing.* New York: Academic Press, 1983.

52. Till J, Osoba D, Pater J, et al. Research on health-related quality of life: dissemination into practical applications. *Qual Life Res* 1994;3:279–283.

53. Lohr K. Applications of health status assessment measures in clinical practice. Overview of the third conference on advances in health status assessment. *Med Care* 1992;30:MS1–MS14.

54. Bezjak A, Ng P, Taylor K, et al. A preliminary survey of oncologists' perceptions of quality of life information. *Psycho-Oncology* 1997;6:107–113.

55. Tanaka T, Gotay C. Physicians' and medical students' perspectives on patient's quality of life. *Acad Med* 1998;73:1003–1005.

56. Morris J, Perez D, McNoe B. The use of quality of life data in clinical practice. *Qual Life Res* 1998;7:85–91.

57. Bezjak A, Ng P, Skeel R, et al. Oncologists' use of quality of life information: results of a survey of Eastern Cooperative Oncology Group Physicians. *Qual Life Res* 2001;10:1–13.

58. Davis K, Cella D. Assessing quality of life in oncology clinical practice: a review of barriers and critical success factors. *J Clin Outcomes Measure* 2002;9:327–332.

59. Higginson I, Carr A. Using quality of life measures in the clinical setting. *BMJ* 2001;322:1297–1300.

60. Chang C, Cella D. Equating health-related quality of life instruments in applied oncology settings. *Phys Med Rehabil State Art Rev* 1997;11:397–406.

61. Kraemer H. Reporting the size of effects in research studies to facilitate assessments of practical or clinical significance. *Psychoneuroendocrinology* 1992;17: 527–536.

62. Braitman L. Statistical, clinical, and experimental evidence in randomized controlled trials. *Ann Intern Med* 1983;98:407–408.

63. Jaeschke R, Singer J, Guyatt G. Measurement of health status: ascertaining the minimal clinically important difference. *Control Clin Trials* 1989;10:407–415.

64. Lydick E, Epstein R. Interpretation of quality of life changes. *Qual Life Res* 1993;2:221–226.

65. Brady MJ, Cella DF, Mo F, et al. Reliability and validity of the Functional Assessment of Cancer Therapy-Breast (FACT-B) quality of life instrument. *J Clin Oncol* 1997;15:974–986.

66. Guyatt G, Walter S, Norman G. Measuring change over time: assessing the usefulness of evaluative instruments. *J Chronic Dis* 1987;40:171.

67. Torrance GW. Measurement of health state utilities for economic appraisal: a review article. *J Health Econ* 1986;5:1–30.

68. Torrance G, Feeny D. Utilities and quality-adjusted life years. *Int J Technol Assess Health Care* 1989;5:559–575.

69. Jacobson N, Truax P. Clinical Significance: a statistical approach to defining meaningful change in psychotherapy research. *J Consult Clin Psychol* 1991;59:12–19.

70. Cella D, Hahn E, Dineen K. Meaningful change in cancer-specific quality of life scores: differences between improvement and worsening. *Qual Life Res* 2002;11:207–221.

71. Harwood A, Kleinmann A. Ethnicity and clinical care: selected issues in treating Puerto Rican patients. *Hosp Physician* 1981;17:113–118.

72. Pennebaker J, Epstein D. Implicit psychophysiology: effects of common beliefs and idiosyncratic physiological responses on symptom reporting. *J Pers* 1983;51:468–496.

73. Sartorius N. WHO's working on the epidemiology of mental disorders. *Soc Psychiatry Psychiatr Epidemiol* 1993;28:147–155.

74. Brooks R, Jendteg S, Lindgren B, et al. EuroQol: health related quality of life measurement. Results form the Swedish questionnaire exercise. *Health Policy* 1991;18:37–48.

75. Nord E. EuroQol. Health-related quality of life measurement. Valuations of health states by the general public in Norway. *Health Policy* 1991;18:25–36.

76. Watson M, Law M, Maguire GP, et al. Further development of a quality of life measure for cancer patients: the Rotterdam Symptom Checklist (revised). *Psycho-Oncology* 1992;1:35–44.

77. Schag CA, Ganz PA, Heinrich RL. Cancer Rehabilitation Evaluation System-Short Form (CARES-SF): a cancer specific rehabilitation and quality of life instrument. *Cancer* 1991;68:1406–1413.

78. Ganz P, Coscarelli A. Quality of life after breast cancer: a decade of research. In: Dimsdale JE, Baum A, eds. *Quality of life in behavioral medicine research.* Hillsdale, NJ: Erlbaum, 1995:97–113.

79. Bonomi AE, Cella DF, Bjordal K, et al. Multilingual translation of the Functional Assessment of Cancer Therapy (FACT) quality of life measurement system. *Qual Life Res* 1996;5:309–320.

80. Ware JE, Kosinski MA, Bayliss MS, et al. Comparison of methods for scoring and statistical analysis of SF-36 health profile and summary measures: summary results from the Medical Outcomes Study. *Med Care* 1995;33:AS264–AS279.

81. Bergner M, Bobbitt RA, Carter WB, et al. The Sickness Impact Profile: development and final revision of a health status measure. *Med Care* 1981;19:787–806.

82. Chwalow AJ, Luire A, Bean K, et al. A French version of the Sickness Impact profile (SIP): stages in the cross validation of a generic quality of life scale. *Fund Clin Pharmacol* 1992;6:319–326.

83. De Bruin AF, De Witte LP, Diedeeriks JP. Sickness Impact Profile: the state of the art of a generic functional status measure. *Soc Sci Med* 1992;8:1003–1014.

84. Hunt S, McKenna SP, McEwen J, et al. The Nottingham Health Profile: subjective health status and medical consultations. *Soc Sci Med* 1981;15A:221–229.

85. Wiklund I. The Nottingham Health Profile—a measure of health-related quality of life. *Scand J Prim Health Care* 1990;1:15–18.

86. Chambers LW. The McMaster Health Index Questionnaire: an update. In: Walker SR, Rosser RM, eds. *Quality of life assessment: key issues in the 1990's.* London: Kluwer Press, 1993:131–149.

87. Moinpour CM. Quality of life assessment in Southwest Oncology Group clinical trials: translating and validating a Spanish questionnaire. In: Orley J, Kuyken W, eds. *Quality of life assessment: international perspectives.* Berlin: Springer-Verlag, 1994:83–97.

88. Spilker B, Cramer J, ed. *Quality of life and pharmacoeconomics in clinical trials,* 2nd ed. Philadelphia: Lippincott-Raven 1997.

31

Development of Supportive Care Agents in Oncology

Scott Z. Fields and *Alessandra Cesano

*EISAI Medical Research Inc., Teaneck, New Jersey 07666; and *Amgen Inc., Thousand Oaks, California 91320*

Patients with cancer experience morbidity from both the underlying disease and the toxicity of the antineoplastic agents used in the treatment of the cancer itself.

In general, a *supportive care drug* can be defined as an agent not intended to target the underlying cancer but to ameliorate cancer or chemotherapy-related symptoms. Supportive care agents define a broad range of products with varying mechanisms of action; as a consequence, development varies from product to product. These agents do, however, share a number of features that allow some general principles of development to be defined and contrasted to chemotherapeutics.

In this chapter we review issues related specifically to the development of cancer-related supportive care products.

PRECLINICAL STUDIES

Prior to entering the clinic, all drugs undergo considerable preclinical evaluation. For a variety of supportive care agents, including growth factors (hematopoietic or epithelial), bisphosphonates, and antiemetics, preclinical studies share a number of key factors.

Typically, *healthy* animals are used for these studies, because the effect being targeted is on *normal* cells. Because normal cells are targeted, the *variability* in the results tend to be relatively low, the *"response rate"* usually is high, and a *reproducible pharmacokinetic/pharmacodynamic (PK/PD) relationship* usually can be obtained using a relatively *small* number of animals. In addition, it is more likely to be *reproducible across species,* including human. These concepts are illustrated by the following examples.:

Hematopoietic growth factors: Hematopoietic growth factors are glycoproteins that stimulate the proliferation of bone marrow progenitor cells and their maturation into fully differentiated circulating blood cells. Two of these factors [granulocyte colony-stimulating-factor (G-CSF) and erythropoietin] are used for the prevention/treatment of myelosuppression following cytotoxic cancer therapy.

A. *Recombinant human G-CSF (rhG-CSF; Filgrastim, Neupogen):* Human G-CSF is a hematopoietic growth factor that promotes the proliferation and differentiation of neutrophils both *in vitro* (1) and *in vivo* (2). When administered to healthy animals (e.g., mice, rats, hamsters, dogs, and nonhuman primates), rhG-CSF induced a dose-dependent, rapid increase in neutrophil number in the vast majority of treated animals (3–5). In these experiments, normal animals were injected [intravenously (IV) or subcutaneously (SC)] with increasing doses of rhG-CSF or appropriate control solution and white blood cells were assessed on blood samples taken at different time points after drug administration (to determine the kinetics of the response). Virtually all animals treated with rhG-CSF showed a dose-dependent/time-dependent increase in the neutrophil counts with very similar kinetics (6). The use of a placebo *control* in these experiments is particularly important because a nonspecific increase in white blood cells often is observed in animals due to stress from manipulation. In view of the ability of rhG-CSF to elevate blood neutrophil numbers, the follow-up studies addressed its potential benefit in the prevention/treatment of neutropenia associated with myelosuppressive therapy for malignancy. In animal models pretreated with chemotherapeutic drugs (e.g., 5-fluorouracil, cyclophosphamide), administration of rhG-CSF was shown to decrease the neutrophil nadir and enhance neutrophil recovery in the majority of the treated animals compared to animals treated with control solution (7,8).

B. *Recombinant human erythropoietin (Epogen, Procrit):* Erythropoietin is a glycoprotein that stimulates the division and differentiation of committed erythroid progenitors in the bone marrow (9,10). When administered to healthy animals (rodents, dogs, monkeys), rh-erythropoietin resulted in a dose-dependent increase in red blood cells (RBCs) in virtually all the treated animals (11). In these experiments, healthy animals received an increasing dose of rh-erythropoietin or control solution, and determination of RBCs, hemoglobin, and hematocrit was performed on blood samples taken at varying time points after drug administration. Virtually all treated animals receiving rh-erythropoietin showed a dose-related increase in RBCs, hemoglobin, and hematocrit with highly reproducible kinetic curves (11).

Noteworthy, when the second-generation products for both agents were developed as longer-acting versions (Neulasta-pegylated G-CSF or pegfilgrastim and Aranesp-hyperglycosylated erythropoietin or darbepoietin alfa), animal models once were again predictive of the longer duration of action of these two new molecules (12,13). This was confirmed in the human clinical studies that followed (14,15).

Keratinocyte growth factor: Keratinocyte growth factors (KGF-1 and KGF-2) are members of the fibroblast growth factor family of protein that under physiologic conditions exert their activity on epithelial cell proliferation and differentiation. When administered in pharmacologic doses to healthy animals (mice, dogs, monkeys), KGFs resulted in a dose-dependent thickening of the gastrointestinal mucosa, including tongue epithelium, oral mucosa (cheek), nasal passages, and intestinal tract (mucosal epithelium and goblet cells), as determined by pathologic analysis of these organs (16–18). In animal models of chemotherapy/radiotherapy-induced mucosal injury (19,20), KGF given at various doses and schedules before, during, or after fractionated radiotherapy or chemotherapy resulted in a pronounced increase in oral mucosal chemotolerance/radiotolerance, as measured by the dose of chemotherapy/radiotherapy after which ulceration of the tongue (in case of locally applied radiotherapy) or significant weight loss/ death (for chemotherapy) is expected in 50% of the mice (EC_{50}).

These examples of preclinical development of supportive care agents can be contrasted with the preclinical development of antitumor agents. Generally speaking, cytotoxic anticancer agents typically undergo in vitro screening for lytic activity against a standard panel of tumor cell lines. *In vitro* assays are standard tests that measure the number of viable cells after exposure to the experimental agent (which represents either *overt cell killing* or *decreased rate of cell proliferation*). For the emerging anticancer "targeted" therapeutics [e.g., anti-epidermal growth factor receptor agents, anti-vascular endothelial growth factor (VEGF) agents], *in vitro* tests require tumor cells expressing the target of interest. This can be done by using human tumor cell lines naturally expressing the target (e.g., human breast cancer cell line expressing estrogen receptors) or by transfecting tumor cell lines that do not naturally express the molecule of interest with cDNA coding for it. The *in vitro* prescreening usually leads to selection of the most promising candidates for *in vivo* testing based on the ability to kill or inhibit the growth of the tumor cell lines at very low concentrations. *In vivo* testing of the lead compounds typically requires the use of SCID or nude rodents (immunocompromised mice who cannot reject xenografts) in which human tumor/cell lines can be transplanted and grow and, in some cases, transgenic animals [in particular for testing of targeted therapy in syngeneic animal models, e.g., transgenic mice expressing *herB2/neu* for *in vivo* testing of trastuzumab (Herceptin) and vaccine approaches] (21). These animal models are more costly and, especially for the latter, difficult and lengthy to develop. More importantly, the results observed in these animal models have not yet been very predictive of the results observed in cancer patients. For example, in the field of antiangiogenesis, very promising results have been observed preclinically with different inhibitors targeting various pathways (21). In these models, a high percentage of animals bearing tumor experienced tumor growth delay and/or regression after administration of the antiangiogenic agent, and these results led to extensive clinical investigations of these agents in a wide array of cancers. To date, clinical responses to antiangiogenic therapy have not paralleled what was observed in preclinical studies. The same has been true for chemotherapeutic drugs for which animal models have generally been poor predictors of antitumor activity and tumor type sensitivity in humans. For some targeted therapy, such as antibodies, for which cross-species reactivity may be lacking, specific reagents may need to be generated (e.g., an antibody directed against the animal version of the antigen), which adds time and cost to the development process. Finally, an additional consideration with some supportive care agents is that they might have a direct and/or indirect anticancer benefit. For instance, preclinical studies have suggested that animals (23) may have better outcomes if hemoglobin is kept in the normal range, perhaps due to enhancement of cell killing from chemotherapy or radiotherapy due to better tumor oxygenation, and/or possibly by decreasing the secretion of tumor growth factors such as VEGF. Alternatively, Mittleman et al. (24) have suggested a possible immune-mediated benefit on tumor cell control through T-cell activation from administration of rh-erythropoietin. In the case of bisphosphonates, some antitumor effect has also been postulated. Clinical data seem to suggest there might be some benefit in terms of time to first tumor lesion in bone when prophylactic administration of these compounds is given to patients at high risk for bone metastasis (25–27). However, if a supportive care agent is developed for a therapeutic indication instead of a supportive care indication (e.g., erythropoietin as an agent that may increase cancer survival), preclinical models become less reliable and more typical of a cancer-targeting agent.

In conclusion, preclinical models of supportive care agents target normal cells, generally are simpler to perform and less costly, and in most cases appear to be better predictors of success in clinical trials than their therapeutic counterparts.

TOXICOLOGY

Preclinical toxicity studies vary between oncology supportive care agents and cytotoxic therapy. Because supportive care in oncology is aimed at decreasing morbidity and does not treat the underlying disease, significant acute toxicity from such an agent would generally be clinically unacceptable. This is in contrast to antitumor agents where considerable toxicity may be acceptable and such agents often are used at their maximum tolerated dose (MTD).

In addition to acute toxicity, other safety concerns are important for supportive care agents.

A. *Antigenicity:* If an agent is intended to support a function supplied by an endogenous compound (e.g., a platelet or RBC growth factor), consideration must be given to the potential effect of an immune response against the agent cross-reacting with either the endogenous factor or its receptor. Unfortunately, animal models are of no use in terms of predicting the antigenicity of a human protein in humans (i.e., all human proteins are antigenic in animal models). However, experiments in mice genetically "knocked out" for the agent/pathway being tested are very useful and typically are required by the Food and Drug Administra-

tion (FDA) in order to evaluate the potential *effects* of a neutralizing antibody cross-reacting with endogenous agents/receptors. It should be noted, however, that not all antibodies are neutralizing, and the major effect of nonneutralizing antibodies usually is limited to the PK of the agent, that is, increase clearance with loss or decrease pharmacologic activity.

B. *Effects on tumor growth/response to therapy:* Another issue to be considered when dealing with supportive care agents is the potential effects of these drugs on the underlying tumor growth and/or response to treatment. When growth factors are used as supportive agents in cancer patients, they should not stimulate tumor growth *in vivo* or *in vitro*. This consideration is particularly important when the tumor originates from cells that express the receptor for the supportive agent and whose growth could, at least in theory, be stimulated by it, for example, hematopoietic factors in leukemia. In these cases, *in vitro* testing of the growth factor on the proliferative activity of numerous tumor cell lines and, where possible, fresh tumor samples expressing the growth factor receptor, together with some *in vivo* testing of the activity of the growth factor on the *in vivo* growth and response to antitumor treatment(s), usually are required by the FDA before proceeding to human studies.

These issues are generally not relevant to antitumor agents.

PHASE I STUDIES

Initial human studies for supportive care agents may be done in healthy volunteers because of the benign toxicity profile generally expected from these agents. This is advantageous in that enrollment is rapid, and the safety and PK profile can be determined without potential interference from the underlying disease. In many cases, an adequate PK/PD relationship can be established, thus allowing a rapid narrowing of the dose range most likely to be safe and effective. For example, the clinical PK and PD of filgrastim (Neupogen) have been studied in healthy volunteers after IV and SC dosing (28). In a dose-ranging study in healthy male volunteers, filgrastim was administered daily in escalating doses for 10 consecutive days. Serum concentration profiles were collected after the first and tenth dose. Elevations of the absolute neutrophil counts (ANC) above 10×10^9/L within 5 hours of filgrastim administration were observed after either a single IV or SC injection at doses above 1.15

μg/kg. Dose-dependent autoinduction of filgrastim clearance was evident: the ratios of the first dose area under the curve to the tenth dose area under the curve were 2.5, 3.3, 5.9, and 7.2 after 75, 150, 300 and 600 μg/day, respectively. The magnitude of autoinduction appeared closely related to the degree of neutrophilia in the recipients, which is consistent with increased receptor-mediated clearance by the expanded neutrophil pool (28).

When the agent being developed is a protein and "knocked out" animal studies suggest that a nonredundant pathway may be impaired if a neutralizing antibody against the growth factor is formed, single-dose studies in healthy volunteers are preferred to multidose studies because they may limit the risk of a potentially serious immune response against the agent. For small molecules, multidose studies may be more acceptable because antigenicity usually is not an issue. Because of this potential for antibody formation, when biologics/proteins enter development, a satisfactory test(s) for measuring and characterizing antibody formation must be available, for example, an enzyme-linked immunosorbent assay for antibody screening followed by a cell-based test on positive samples to test for neutralizing activity of the antibody.

When the second-generation product Neulasta (pegfilgrastim, a long-lasting version of filgrastim) was developed to improve the dosing schedule from daily to once per chemotherapy cycle, phase I studies in healthy volunteers showed not only that the drug was effective in increasing neutrophils but also that the duration of action and the $t_{1/2}$ of the drug were longer than those of filgrastim (29). In such healthy volunteer studies, a (placebo or active) control group typically is included in the study design to provide greater reliability to the results. Therefore, a phase I program with supportive care agents frequently results in PK/PD, safety, and some evidence of activity, thus providing valuable dose/schedule information before moving into phase II. This is in contrast to traditional cytotoxic development where phase I studies are done in cancer patients with heterogeneous tumor types and advanced disease that usually has been heavily pretreated. In these studies, PK data usually are limited because dose level cohorts are generally small (e.g., three patients per cohort, and in some rapid dose escalation schemes only a single patient is treated at the lower doses). In addition, responses in this patient population tend to be infrequent even with agents that eventually prove to be clinically active. Therefore, a true PK/PD relation is difficult to establish, the dose chosen is generally the MTD (which may not be the optimal dose), and the schedule of

administration selected for further development is chosen somewhat empirically. Perhaps more problematic is designing a phase I study for the new "targeted" anticancer agents, which are beyond the scope of this discussion. Because these agents may have a good safety profile and are mainly cytostatic in their antitumor activity, the determination of dose/schedule can be quite challenging unless appropriate surrogate markers of biologic activity are available (e.g., blood flow reduction for antiangiogenic agents). Although these products may be similar to supportive care agents because a relationship between PK/PD usually is sought to determine dose when the MTD is not expected to be the optimal dose, it is generally less informative because the PD markers presently available are less validated/predictive in terms of clinical benefit.

In conclusion, phase I trials for supportive care agents usually can be performed more rapidly and provide considerably more information than studies of therapeutic agents.

PHASE II TRIALS

After completion of the phase I program, supportive care agents typically enter phase II trials. Phase II trials for supportive care agents typically are *randomized controlled* (placebo or active control) studies. They *may or may not be tumor specific* (e.g., antiemetic), and they usually evaluate the *same endpoints* that will be used in phase III trials. In these studies, the control groups are critical, especially when the endpoints of the trial are subjective (e.g., pain, quality of life). For instance, in the phase II program of KGF for the treatment and prevention of chemotherapy/radiotherapy-induced mucositis, pain reduction was used as one measure of evaluating reduction in duration of mucositis. In patients undergoing chemotherapy/radiotherapy as a conditioning regimen before Peripheral Blood Stem Cell Transplantation (PBSCT), the duration of grade 3 to 4 mucositis was reduced from 7.7 to 4 days by administration of KGF before and after the transplant conditioning regimen (30). Without a placebo control group the 3.4-day reduction in grade 3 to 4 mucositis would be difficult to interpret (in contrast to objective reduction in tumor size used for therapeutics). Knowing the number of days of mucositis for the control group provided a more meaningful comparison than a historical control could provide. A potential clinical benefit could be postulated, and this difference allowed for powering the phase III study appropriately. In addition, secondary endpoints, such as reduction in pain medication (secondary to reduction in days of mucositis), would be difficult to evaluate without the control group. By contrast, in the case of Aranesp, some phase II studies used erythropoietin as an active control because in this case a standard treatment for anemia was available and it was important to evaluate how Aranesp compared to already available treatment (31).

In some circumstances, sufficient information is available from the phase I/II trials to allow proceeding directly to phase III. For instance, once the dose and schedule and PK/PD of Neulasta was determined in phase I/II studies (32), there was reasonable expectation of success in phase III. This was because early studies suggested that a once-per-cycle dosing regimen of Neulasta was adequate due to the mechanism of clearance, in which the agent is cleared only as the level of neutrophils recovers, and the level of neutrophil increase appeared to be as good as with Neupogen in volunteer studies (15,33).

In contrast to the supportive care phase II studies described earlier, studies of new cytotoxic agents traditionally have used a *single-arm design,* are *tumor specific,* and usually are designed to detect evidence of *tumor size reduction* (response rate) because such reduction would not be expected spontaneously and hence would provide evidence of drug activity. Unfortunately, response rate does not necessarily translate into survival or quality of life advantages, which are generally believed to provide evidence of patient benefit and therefore are the required endpoints for most phase III registration trials. A number of studies have shown that partial responses are not necessarily good predictors of survival in cancer patients receiving chemotherapy and in some cases are no better than disease stabilization (34,35). Therefore, traditional phase II studies for cytotoxic agents provide far less predictive information than typical controlled trials for supportive care agents, and the risk of failure in phase III for these agents is greater (36). It should be noted, however, that safety issues are far less likely to halt development of cancer therapeutic trials in which agents are frequently used at their MTDs while supportive care agents generally require benign safety profiles.

PHASE III TRIALS

Phase III trials of supportive care agents may be similar to phase II trials in that both typically are randomized and controlled, but phase III trials are larger and their design is based on phase II findings. For instance, in the case of Aranesp, multiple phase II trials suggested that this agent was superior to placebo in increasing hemoglobin levels and improving ane-

mia-related symptoms in cancer patients receiving chemotherapy (31). The phase III study of Aranesp to reduce RBC transfusions in patients undergoing chemotherapy was designed as randomized, placebo-controlled, double-blinded, multinational study conducted in anemic patients with advanced lung cancer, small cell lung cancer, or non–small cell lung cancer who underwent a platinum-containing chemotherapy regimen (36). The study was powered based on phase II data that used the same chemotherapy and endpoints. This maximized study efficiency because the number of patients was very likely to be adequate to detect the hypothesized difference versus placebo given that the phase II and III studies were similar but not so large as to unnecessarily enter patients into the study. Alternatively, Neulasta was compared to Neupogen, and not to placebo, in the phase III registration trials to show that once-per-cycle dosing of Neulasta was comparable to daily dosing of Neupogen using febrile neutropenia as the primary endpoint, which previously had been accepted by the FDA as evidence for patient benefit (15,32,33). Based on data obtained prior to phase III, the likelihood of success of both products in phase III trials was very high and the powering of the studies was far more reliable than for typical therapeutic trials. This is in contrast to phase III trials of therapeutic agents, which have a greater risk of failing because they typically enter this stage with only a single arm or occasionally underpowered phase II randomized data, use different endpoints in phase II and III (e.g., response rate vs survival), and generally are trying to detect smaller differences in benefit than seen with supportive care agents.

A critical issue for some supportive care agents is assuring that the drug does not have a negative effect on patient outcome. For instance, because the tumor cells in acute myeloid leukemia have the G-CSF receptor, it was crucial in the development of filgrastim to show that there was no evidence of increased proliferation with a worse outcome when Neupogen was administered to patients with acute myeloid leukemia undergoing induction and/or consolidation therapy. This was accomplished by a phase III randomized trial in which filgrastim administration was compared to placebo in patients undergoing induction and consolidation chemotherapy (37). In this study, important differences in remission rate between arms were excluded, and disease-free survival and overall survival were comparable, although the study was not designed to detect important differences in these endpoints (37). In the Aranesp pivotal registration trial, because Aranesp is a hematopoietic growth factor an analysis was done to evaluate long-term patient outcome (36). The data provided no evidence of inferior outcome, and a subset of patients with small cell lung cancer in the arm receiving Aranesp appeared to have improved survival (36). Similarly, amifostine, which generically protects cells against the side effects of chemotherapy/radiotherapy and has been approved for reduction of cumulative renal toxicity associated with repeated administration of cisplatin in patients with advanced ovarian cancer or non–small cell lung cancer and for prevention of radiotherapy-induced xerostomia in patients with Head and Neck Cancer (HNC) undergoing localized radiotherapy (38), required proof that it did not protect tumor cells from the effects of cytotoxic therapy. Phase III randomized trials evaluating this endpoint did not suggest that the effectiveness of the primary therapy was altered by the administration of amifostine (38). However, due to limited data on the effects of amifostine on the efficacy of chemotherapy in other settings, amifostine is not indicated in some settings where chemotherapy can produce significant survival benefit or cure (e.g., certain malignancies of germ cell origin) (38).

In summary, phase III trials of supportive care agents typically use a randomized, double-blinded, controlled design with active or placebo control as comparator. This is crucial because endpoints can be subjective and safety issues (both acute and chronic) are critical. However, being based on far more informative phase II trials, phase III trials in supportive care have a greater chance of success. Importantly, safety issues are of greater concern because these agents do not treat the underlying disease and phase III trials must be designed to conclusively define safety as well as efficacy so that the risk-to-benefit ratio can be adequately determined.

CONCLUSION

Although therapeutic and supportive care agents in oncology both are aimed at improving treatment for cancer patients, their development is very different. This is true starting from the preclinical program where *in vitro/in vivo* testing differs significantly and throughout the pivotal phase III trials. Because supportive care agents target normal cells, smaller studies usually can define the efficacy of these agents, and the PK/PD relationship usually is better defined and more reproducible across species. In addition, supportive care agents are generally active across a heterogeneous group of malignancies because the cells being targeted are not tumor cells. For this reason their development time tends to be shorter than that for therapeutics. Because supportive care agents differ, each will need a unique development program. However, the basic principle described in this chapter should provide a good framework for issues to be considered in designing such a program.

REFERENCES

1. Souza LM, Boone TC, Gabrilove J, et al. Recombinant human granulocyte colony-stimulating factor: effects on normal and leukemic myeloid cells. *Science* 1986; 232:61–65.
2. Cohen AM, Zsebo KM, Inoue H, et al. In vivo stimulation of granulopoiesis by recombinant human granulocyte colony-stimulating factor. *Proc Natl Acad Sci USA* 1987;84:2484–2488.
3. Metcalf D. The colony stimulating factors. Discovery, development, and clinical applications. *Cancer* 1990; 65:2185–2195.
4. Groopman JE, Molina JM, Scadden DT. Hematopoietic growth factors. Biology and clinical applications. *N Engl J Med* 1989;321:1449–1459.
5. Cohen AM, Zsebo KM, Inoue H, et al. In vivo stimulation of granulopoiesis by recombinant human granulocyte colony-stimulating factor. *Proc Natl Acad Sci USA* 1987;84:2484–2488.
6. Tamura M, Hattori K, Nomura H, et al. Induction of neutrophilic granulocytosis in mice by administration of purified human native granulocyte colony-stimulating factor (G-CSF). *Biochem Biophys Res Commun* 1987; 142:454–460.
7. Hattori K, Shimizu K, Takahashi M, et al. Quantitative in vivo assay of human granulocyte colony-stimulating factor using cyclophosphamide-induced neutropenia in mice. *Blood* 1990;75:1228–1233.
8. Welte K, Bonilla MA, Gillio AP, et al. Recombinant human granulocyte colony stimulating factor. Effects on hematopoiesis in normal and cyclophosphamide treated primates. *J Exp Med* 1987;165:941–948.
9. D'Andrea AD, Lodish HF, Wong GG. Expression cloning of the murine erythropoietin receptor. *Cell* 1989;57:277–285.
10. Lodish HF, Hilton DJ, Klingmuller U, et al. The erythropoietin receptor: biogenesis, dimerization, and intracellular signal transduction. *Cold Spring Harbor Symp Quant Biol* 1995;60:93–104.
11. Egrie JC, Browne JK. Development and characterization of novel erythropoiesis stimulating protein (NESP). *Br J Cancer* 2001;84[Suppl 1]:3–10.
12. Molineux G. Pegylation: engineering improved pharmaceuticals for enhanced therapy. *Cancer Treat Rev* 2002; 28[Suppl A]:13–16.
13. Aranesp label, Amgen Inc., Thousand Oaks, CA.
14. Neulasta label, Amgen Inc., Thousand Oaks, CA.
15. Finch PW, Rubin JS, Miki T, et al. Human KGF is FGF-related with properties of a paracrine effector of epithelial cell growth. *Science* 1989;245:752–755.
16. Igarashi M, Finch PW, Aaronson SA. Characterization of recombinant human fibroblast growth factor (FGF)-10 reveals functional similarities with keratinocyte growth factor (FGF-7). *J Biol Chem* 1998;273: 13230–13235.

17. Farrell CL, Rex KL, Kaufman SA, et al. Effects of keratinocyte growth factor in the squamous epithelium of the upper aerodigestive tract of normal and irradiated mice. *Int J Radiat Biol* 1999;75:609–620.

18. Dorr W, Spekl K, Farrell CL. Amelioration of acute oral mucositis by keratinocyte growth factor: fractionated irradiation. *Int J Radiat Oncol Biol Phys* 2002;54:245–251.

19. Farrell CL, Rex KL, Chen JN, et al. The effects of keratinocyte growth factor in preclinical models of mucositis. *Cell Prolif* 2002;35[Suppl 1]:78–85.

20. Amici A, Venanzi FM, Concetti A. Genetic immunization against neu/erbB2 transgenic breast cancer. *Cancer Immunol Immunother* 1998;47:183–190.

21. Boehm T, Folkman J, Browder T, et al. Antiangiogenic therapy of experimental cancer does not induce acquired drug resistance. *Nature* 1997;390:404–407.

22. Joy MS. Darbepoietin alfa: a novel erythropoiesis-stimulating protein. *Ann Pharmacother* 2002;36:1183–1192.

24. Mittleman M, Neumann D, Peled A, et al. Erythropoietin induces tumor regressions and antitumor immune responses in murine myeloma models. *Proc Natl Acad Sci USA* 2001;98:5181–5186.

25. Fontana A, Herrmann Z, Menssen HD, et al. Effects of intravenous ibandronate therapy on skeletal related events (SRE) and survival in patients with advanced multiple myeloma. *Blood* 1998;92[10 Suppl 1–2]:106A.

26. Berenson JR, Lipton A. Bisphosphonates in the treatment of malignant bone disease. *Annu Rev Med* 1999; 50:237–248.

27. Major PP, Lipton A, Berenson J, et al. Oral bisphosphonates: a review of clinical use in patients with bone metastases. *Cancer* 2000;88:6–14.

28. Roskos LK, Cheung EN, Vincent M, et al. Pharmacology of Filgrastim (r-metHuG-CSF). Filgrastim (r-metHuG-CSF). *Clin Pract* 1998;51–71.

29. Curran MP, Goa KI. Pegfilgrastim. *Drugs* 2002;62: 1207–1213.

30. Spielberger RT, Stiff PT, Emmanoullides C, et al. ASH 2001. *J Clin Oncol* 2001;20:7A abstract 25.

31. Glaspy JA, Tchekmedyian NS. Darbepoietin alfa administered every two weeks alleviates anemia in cancer patients receiving chemotherapy. *Oncology* 2002;16:23–29.

32. Holmes FA, Jones SE, O'Shaughnessy J, et al. Comparable efficacy and safety profiles of once-per-cycle pegfilgrastim and daily injection filgrastim in chemotherapy-induced neutropenia: a multicenter dose-finding study in woman with breast cancer. *Ann Oncol* 2002;13:903–909.

33. Holmes FA, O'Shaughnessy JA, Vukeljia S, et al. Blinded, randomized, multicenter study to evaluate single administration pegfilgrastim once per cycle versus daily filgrastim as an adjunct to chemotherapy in patients with high-risk stage II or stage III/IV breast cancer. *J Clin Oncol* 2002;20:727–731.

34. Cesano A, Lane S, Poulin R, et al. Stabilization of disease as a useful predictor of survival following second-line chemotherapy in small cell lung cancer and ovarian cancer patients. *Int J Oncol* 1999;15:1233–1238.

35. Cesano A, Lane S, Ross G, et al. Stabilization of disease as an indicator of clinical benefit associated with chemotherapy in non-small cell lung cancer. *Int J Oncol* 2000;17:587–590.

36. Pirker R, Vansteenkiste J, Gateley J, et al., NESP 980297 Study Group. A phase III, double-blind, placebo-controlled, randomized study of novel erythropoiesis stimulating protein (NESP) in patients undergoing platinum-treatment for lung cancer. *Eur J Cancer* 2001;37[Suppl 6]:S264–S265.

37. Heil G, Hoelzer D, Sanz MA, et al. A randomized, double-blind, placebo-controlled, phase III study of filgrastim in remission induction and consolidation therapy or adults with de novo acute myeloid leukemia. The International Acute Myeloid Leukemia Study Group. *Blood* 1997;90:4710–4718.

38. Ethyol label, Med Immune Oncology, Gaithersberg, MD.

32

Cancer Vaccines

Howard Z. Streicher, *Adriana A. Byrnes, and Jay J. Greenblatt

*Division of Cancer Treatment and Diagnosis, National Cancer Institute, Bethesda, Maryland 20892;
and *Technical Resources International, Inc., Bethesda, Maryland 20817*

The past decade has seen the emergence of detailed experimental data that are beginning to form the basis for a science of human tumor immunology. Immunology, which developed during a century of intense research into protection against infectious disease, provides a detailed molecular picture that suggests immunity can be understood as a cluster of inherited interacting biologic systems responding to external "danger" signals and which are highly modulated to avoid autoimmune or bystander damage (1). For most infections the outcome is that the host eliminates the infection, the infection eliminates the host, or in some cases the host and infecting organism exist together. Tumors present the immune system with an "infection" that is largely "self." Traditional vaccines are intended to prevent infection. Vaccines for tumors, as well as infections such as human immunodeficiency virus (HIV), tuberculosis, and malaria, will require better understanding of how chronic or recurrent infections can be controlled (2).

More than 100 years ago, after the discovery of microbial infection as a cause of disease, Hericourt and Richert attempted passive immunization with antisera produced in animals injected with human tumors [cited in Anderson (3)]. Perhaps the first reports of tumor regression in response to immunotherapy using nonspecific stimulation with bacteria were made by the surgeon William Coley (4). He is reported to have had the good fortune of seeing a remarkable regression of a sarcoma in his very first case, but he was unable to establish this treatment with consistently convincing responses, reflecting a pattern of ups and downs that has persisted into the modern era. Much of the enthusiasm for this approach seems to have diminished, replaced by radiation treatment and undermined by the characterization of malignancy as noninfectious and nonimmunogenic. Ludwig Gross (5), who was the first to demonstrate virally transmissible tumors in mammals, reintroduced the concept of tumor-specific immunity within a single strain. Understanding that the underlying mechanism of tumor rejection in mice across strains may be based on rejection of foreign antigens led to the unifying hypothesis of "cancer immunosurveillance." Burnet suggested that new antigenic potentials appearing on a tumor may allow the immune system to destroy a tumor even before it becomes clinically detectable [cited in Dunn et al. (6)]. About the same time, Thomas proposed that the primary function of cellular immunity was not to promote graft rejection but to protect from neoplastic disease [cited in Dunn et al. (6)]. However, the lack of strong evidence that immunodeficient patients had a markedly increased frequency of tumors, except for virally associated tumors such as lymphoma, and the inability to detect an underlying immunologic defect in patients who developed cancer challenged the hypothesis that immune surveillance played a major role in protection from neoplasias.

A resurgence of interest in cancer immunotherapy was triggered by the discovery that tumor cells contain antigens recognized by the immune system that are not found on most normal cells of adults (7). Interest has been sustained not only by the demonstration of immunologic effector cells capable of attacking tumors, occasionally with dramatic responses, but also with the discovery of a rapidly increasing number of potential antigenic targets. The current era of tumor vaccine development rests on three concepts: reactivity to tumor antigens can be demonstrated; endogenous antitumor reactivity may be limited by the nature of the antigens and by the milieu, which selects tumor variants that evade immune control; and the immune system is capable of controlling or eliminating even large tumor masses if a sufficient number of potent cells can be actively stimulated or provided by passive adoptive cellular transfer.

ROLE OF IMMUNITY IN PROTECTION FROM TUMORS

In a sense, cancer vaccines already exist for some of the viruses that are causally associated with cancer. The widespread use of hepatitis B virus vaccine prevents cancers that are associated with chronic hepatitis B infection, and a vaccine that could prevent hepatitis C infection is expected to have a similar role. New and striking evidence of the effectiveness of type-specific human papilloma virus vaccine is emerging that could lead to prevention of the most prevalent global gynecologic tumor, cervical cancer (8).

Evidence that the human immune system and immunotherapy may control or even eradicate tumors at all stages is abundant if inconsistent. Perhaps the most intriguing suggestion of an antitumor response is evidence that tumors are selected during their growth to avoid immune elimination. It has been proposed that tumor–host interaction may evolve through three stages: elimination, equilibration, and escape. The process of immune selection of tumor cells is itself a demonstration of the importance of effects exerted by the immune system on the tumor (6,9). There also is evidence that T-cell responses, tumor infiltrating lymphocytes, antibody responses, and even autoimmune phenomena presenting as paraneoplastic syndromes are associated with better prognosis (10,11).

Monoclonal antibodies, such as rituximab (Rituxan) and trastuzumab (Herceptin), have entered clinical practice 25 years after their discovery. Although these antibodies target surface signaling molecules, they may require intact Fc function and are likely to use immunologic effector mechanisms for their antitumor activity (12).

Systemic interleukin-2 therapy at high doses induced long-lasting complete remissions in 8% of patients with melanoma. The antitumor effect is thought to be immunologically mediated because interleukin-2 has no direct effects on tumor cells (13).

RECENT ADVANCES IN TUMOR VACCINES

Progress in the rational development of vaccine strategies to augment antigen-specific immunity raises the possibility that currently available vaccines may be clinically effective. For example, Grosenbach et al. (14) pioneered the use of viral vectors containing genes coding for costimulatory molecules and granulocyte-macrophage colony-stimulating factor to induce immune responses to carcinoembryonic antigen and prostate-specific antigen, among others. These vectors, as well as many other approaches, are beginning to show clear if modest antitumor responses that indicate both immunologic and clinical activity. Perhaps the strongest evidence for immune-mediated tumor activity comes from bone marrow and stem cell grafts. Allogeneic hematopoietic stem cell transplantation, a principal therapy for hematopoietic malignancy, may work through a single immunodominant minor H antigen to mediate graft versus leukemia effects (15). Using the ability to recreate part of an immune system from matched histocompatible donors for solid tumors, nonmyeloablative allogeneic peripheral blood stem cell transplant has resulted in antitumor responses in patients with renal cell cancer (16).

Antitumor activity and complete regression of bulky metastatic melanoma after nonmyeloablative adoptive cell transfer demonstrates the potential of large numbers of potent effector cells in selected patients (17). After nonmyeloablative adoptive transfer, this effect may be mediated by the expansion of adoptively transferred tumor infiltrating lymphocytes taken from a patient's own tumor. Several of the responding patients also developed autoimmunity, including vitiligo and uveitis, demonstrating that an antitumor response also may involve a response to normal tissues.

TUMOR ANTIGENS

T-cell receptors bind specifically to small peptides held in a groove of the major histocompatibility complex (MHC) molecules, on the surface of either the target or antigen-presenting cells. Class I MHC molecules holding 9-amino-acid sequences bind to receptors on CD8[+] T cells, which may have cytolytic effector function. Class II MHC–peptide complexes bind to CD4[+] helper T cells. These epitopes, peptides recognized by T cells, are created by proteolysis either in proteosomes or lysosomes. Of the estimated 10^5 to 10^6 MHC–peptide complexes on the surface of a typical cell, the number of peptides made from genes active in a tumor cell that are actually presented on the surface has been estimated to be about 10^4 (18). Because this number may represent only a small fraction (perhaps 1%) of the total number of possible peptides that can be generated from a protein and because the average representation of these peptides may be just 10 to 100 molecules of each per cell, any given tumor antigen cannot be assumed to be present on the cell surface at an effective density. The demonstration for any candidate vaccine that the proposed target is a T-cell epitope that is, in fact, presented on a tumor cell is essential.

At least in theory, these peptides, which represent self-antigens, are poorly immunogenic. For example, estimating one epitope for each ten amino acids, there are more than 60 potential HLA-A201 binding sequences in the open reading frame of the 661-amino-acid gp100 peptide of melanoma tumor cells and at least ten have been shown to be physically processed and presented by MHC molecules. Yet, one peptide, which was modified to enhance MHC binding, has been shown to be clinically active as a vaccine (19). A colon tumor may express 11,000 genomic alterations, and such genomic instability should provide multiple opportunities for the development of cancer antigens either by the overexpression of individual proteins or the expression of mutated proteins that can be targeted by vaccines (20). More knowledge about how a protein is processed for presentation and the rules that govern which proteins and epitopes become immunodominant would be extremely helpful in designing vaccines. The discovery of predictable, as well as unique and unusual, tumor antigens has been in itself a fascinating story (21,22). An extensive listing of human tumor antigens is provided in a recent review (23).

TUMOR–HOST IMMUNE SYSTEM

The reasons that tumors continue to grow in humans, despite the expression of highly immunogenic proteins or carbohydrates and even despite strong immune responses following vaccination, is not well understood. In a murine model of fibrosarcoma, eradication by adoptive transfer of tumor-specific cells was dose and time dependent, suggesting that there is an ongoing battle between tumor growth and immune effector cells (24).

It is easy to think of the immune system as being too weak to control cancer. In spite of this assumption, most cancer patients are not immune deficient and can be vaccinated. However, prior treatment may reduce or abrogate a patient's ability to mount an immune response, and immune responses to vaccines are significantly diminished after several rounds of chemotherapy (25,26). Almost invariably the subgroup of patients that makes a tumor-specific immune response to vaccine has better outcome compared to the subgroup that does not, and this observation is not explained by any independent measure of immune competence such as skin tests for anergy or response to control antigens.

Selective immune dysfunction appears to be a common feature that may allow cancers to survive and grow even in the face of a strong antitumor immune response. Many mechanisms have been proposed to account for the ability of tumors to evade immune control. A lack of T-cell precursors may be associated with thymic or "central" anergy that deletes T cells re-

active to self-proteins. Even where T cells can be detected, "peripheral" anergy or antigen-specific unresponsiveness may be based on altered signaling capability and function. Because this involves a failure to recognize or respond to antigen, this process has been called *selective blindness, immune ignorance,* or *escape by hiding.* T cells may make the wrong kind of responses by shifting Th1- to Th2-like responses, sometimes called *immune deviation.* Finally, tumors may be resistant to immune attack or death signals and alter strength of immune effectors by multiple mechanisms. Immune evasion may occur early in the growth of a tumor and persist even in minimal disease states. In mice defective interferon production may be an early event in tumor progression (27). Increasing tumor vulnerability by countering these mechanisms may be an essential element of a successful therapeutic vaccine strategy. As a hypothetical example, down-regulation of interferon-gamma (IFN-γ) receptors may decrease vulnerability to T-cell control but also may decrease expression of class I antigens. This may make the tumor cell more vulnerable to natural killer (NK) cell killing. It would be reasonable then, under these circumstances, to use a strategy to stimulate NK cell killing (28–31).

IMMUNE RESPONSE TO VACCINES

Immune assays in vaccine trials serve three important functions: (i) demonstration of immune activity as a biologic endpoint; (ii) demonstration of the mechanism of immune effectors; and (iii) as an intermediate endpoint to guide clinical development, or as a possible surrogate endpoint if an immune correlate to clinical benefit were established. Almost all traditional vaccines have used antibody responses as a measure of effectiveness. Although improved methods to measure antigen-specific T-cell subsets are providing consistent data for human immune responses to tumors, at present there are no consistently convincing data demonstrating a relationship between individual immune responses and tumor response in a specific patient (32). The combination of a functional assay, such as Elispot or cytokine flow, with a quantitative tetramer assay may provide the kind of data that could be correlated with clinical benefit in large trials. Validated standardized assays are essential to allow reliable comparisons among trials. Delayed-type hypersensitivity, the classic biologic assay for T-cell responses, if carefully standardized, may predict a measurable systemic response (33). Issues relevant to the manufacture of tumor vaccines, including lot release specifications for identity, purity, and potency, require assays that are validated. Standards for credentialing an assay include accuracy, precision, detection limits, specificity, linearity and range, and robustness (30).

Multiple elements of the immune system may play a role in antitumor responses. Recent technologic advances have begun to shed light on human CD4[+] and CD8[+] T-cell dynamics in chronic viral infections such as HIV and Epstein-Barr virus (34). Tumor-reactive cells with a broad range of antitumor activity may be found in peripheral blood, lymph nodes, and tumors of patients with cancer. There is no clear explanation for their coexistence with continuing tumor growth (35). It is possible that these cells are not functional or are turned off by factors such as the population of CD4[+]CD25[+] cells that express CTLA-4, which plays a critical role in blocking stimulation of both autoimmune and antitumor effectors cells (36,37). In HIV infections the initial immunologic response to infection may play a crucial role in early clearance of virus and subsequent disease progression by establishing a virologic set point. Such early immunologic responses may go unobserved in cancer patients but could influence responses to vaccines that stimulate antitumor activity. Later immune response to vaccine may be quite different from this initial response. Even in a patient with minimal residual disease, tumor resistance mechanisms may be maintained by the remaining tumor, and the antitumor response has evolved through several, presumably nonreversible, stages (38). Even though there is limited expression of HLA class II molecules on most tumor cells, inducing both CD4[+] and CD8[+] T-cell responses is likely to be critical to developing an effective response. The inherent ability of tumor to stimulate an immune response may play a crucial role in survival. For example, a dramatic difference in survival for patients with B-cell lymphoma may be associated with HLA class II gene expression (39,40). An additional and unexpected role of CD4[+] T-cell help in overcoming immune suppression opens new therapeutic possibilities for human trials (41).

The induction of effective T-cell responses usually requires stimulation by activated dendritic cells (DCs), sometimes called the *professional antigen-presenting cells* (42). Immunologic immaturity or neonatal tolerance may be associated with the relative absence of these cells. Tumor growth is associated with the accumulation of immature myeloid cells capable of inhibiting T-cell responses (43). Although DCs have been called nature's adjuvant, multiple factors control the strength and expression of immune responses. Effective T-cell responses require initial stimulation of naïve cells, proliferation and survival factors to avoid activation-induced apoptosis, localization, and targeting of potent effector cells to the tu-

mor. The fact that different vaccines may require augmentation in different aspects of this sequence may explain why it is difficult to draw a general conclusion based on empiric assessment of which adjuvant is the "best" for any given vaccine (44–47).

NK cells may play a functionally important role in linking the innate and adaptive systems. Several subsets identified by surface markers may have diverse functions. Recent evidence suggests that mismatched NK receptors and ligands are associated with prevention of leukemia relapse after allogeneic bone marrow transplantation (48).

Searching for antibodies that can distinguish cancer cells led to the discovery of lymphocyte surface antigens but required the development of humanized monoclonal antibodies for therapeutic success (49). Attempts to induce antibodies against traditional protein and carbohydrate tumor surface antigens has had limited success as a vaccine strategy, in contrast to the functionally targeted antibodies such as rituximab and Herceptin. However, the development of antitumor antibodies plays a role in monitoring immune responses and identifying targets, and may yet be shown to have importance in antitumor effector function.

VACCINE DESIGN

The lack of naturally occurring immunity to tumors, such as that following measles or small pox infection, makes it difficult to find a model for designing cancer vaccines. Methodologically, vaccines may be formulated from defined antigens or largely unidentified components in whole tumor cells. Both stimulate antigen-specific immunity, possibly to the same antigens, and so both ultimately may lead to similar results (50,51). Defined or targeted antigens may be formulated as peptides (52), proteins, viruses (53), deoxyribonucleic acid (DNA) plasmids, and pulsed DCs. There are numerous strategies for producing more potent vaccines, but there are sparse data comparing one strategy to another (54,55).

CLINICAL DESIGNS AND ENDPOINTS

Standard Trial Designs Might Not Be Suitable for Phase I and II Studies

Although the traditional structure of clinical trials progressing through phase I, II, and III may be difficult to alter, within this framework the objectives for each trial should be appropriate to vaccine development (56,57).

Any trial is predicated on the manufacture of a sufficient quantity of stable clinical grade agent, characterization of the agent including a measure of potency, stability, and the demonstration of safety in an appropriate animal model. For most vaccines, little direct toxicity is expected. Immune-mediated toxicity requires that an immune response be generated and that an appropriate target is present. In addition, vaccine potency and immune responses may be difficult to measure, toxicity may not be dose related, and both may take time to develop. Animal models, including transgenic mice expressing tumor antigens, oncogenes that produce spontaneous tumors, or HLA molecules that bind human epitopes may be most useful for understanding biologic mechanisms of immune effector responses to tumors. Biotechnology has made some types of reagents readily accessible in pharmacologic quantities, and recombinant DNA technology may make designer vaccines ever more feasible. However, the ability to make a product should depend on a clear rationale for development and testing of a candidate vaccine.

Phase I Considerations

The traditional phase I trial designed for cytotoxic agents in patients with refractory metastatic disease may not be appropriate for tumor vaccines. Most preventative vaccines rely on producing a threshold level of immunity rather than the highest possible immune response. Most tumor vaccines trials are not designed to reach the highest tolerated dose but to choose a dose and schedule aimed at generating the best antitumor effect, which may not be linear with dose. Patients with advanced disease may not have a vigorous immune response, so immune-mediated toxicity may be missed. The initial trial should be designed to determine immune activity and safety at the proposed dose. In addition, development of validated immune assays to standardize the potency of the vaccine, measure the specific immune response, and determine biologic activity are urgently needed. Estimating the magnitude of any beneficial clinical effects even in early studies may be very helpful in planning further studies. Based on the National Cancer Institute experience and a review of the literature, direct toxicity of most agents has been relatively mild. Autoimmunity may be the most important safety factor to evaluate.

Phase II Development

The challenge of choosing an appropriate endpoint for vaccine clinical trials is made more complex by the fact that vaccines do not kill tumor cells directly or inhibit tumor cell growth. Antitumor responses must depend on both the vaccine generating an immune response and the tumor being a susceptible target. In addition, depending on the strength of the response, vaccines may need to be evaluated more like drugs that are expected not to result in reduction of tumor masses but which interfere with tumor growth.

Four types of endpoints for phase II trials may be available: (i) tumor response, (ii) time to progression or survival, (iii) surrogate endpoints, and (iv) immunologic response. Objective tumor responses, which occur with some regularity in 5% to 10% of patients in vaccine phase II trials, may dramatically illustrate the activity of the agent but often are limited to individual patients and may be difficult to reproduce and use to reliably select a regimen for a larger trial. There is a reasonable supposition that the evaluation of such agents would best be done in patients with no detectable disease or minimal tumor burden, little prior treatment, and a high risk for disease progression (58). However, there is also reason to believe that even uncontrolled observations of disease stabilization may indicate benefit in more advanced disease. Given the great variability in the immunologic responses to vaccine and individual localized tumor sensitivity, achieving success may depend on choosing objectives appropriate to each vaccine as well as a measure of good fortune. One difficulty in demonstrating activity based on overall survival or time to progression endpoints lies in the fact that historical controls for small trials are unreliable and controlled trials in the adjuvant setting may be large and lengthy. Developing prognostic and predictive stratification and the use of valid and reliable laboratory endpoints, including immunologic assays, would provide more efficient trials. Choosing an appropriate study population, vaccine schedule, and observation period may be crucial to a successful trial. A successful phase II trial using a biologic agent for renal cell cancer demonstrated a hazard ratio of 2.3 but only three partial responses in 110 randomized patients (59).

A reliable approach to testing for immunologic competence that predicts vaccine response would be very useful but requires development. For example, skin test response to common antigens does not reliably predict an inability to respond to vaccine, and hematologic recovery from prior treatment may not reflect immunologic recovery. Vaccine responses take time to develop and, in the therapeutic setting, require continued boosting to maintain an effective level of sustained response. Both immune and subsequent clinical responses may take time to develop, so patients must remain in a trial long enough to finish the protocol treatment and to be observed for responses. Therefore, those patients who can successfully complete the vaccine regimen and be available for observation are a selected group because they must be immunocompetent to enter the trial and have survived long enough to complete the vaccination regimen. Using toxicity to determine the highest dose that can be given safely is not usually appropriate as an endpoint to determine a recommended dose. The selection of the patient population may have a significant impact on response to vaccine. For example, a population with advanced disease often is not the group of patients most likely to have a strong immunologic response. This weakens the power of a study to evaluate both efficacy and toxicity. Most vaccines have a threshold dose for triggering a response so that higher doses do not necessarily produce a better response. The ability to determine an effective dose and vaccine regimen to achieve the desired endpoint is the principal challenge to phase II development. This may be difficult to accomplish in the traditional phase II trial design where tumor response is the objective endpoint. The ability to adapt current information from basic and clinical science to ongoing trials of these agents, while maintaining the integrity of the study, would enhance the efficiency of vaccine development.

Phase III Trials

Based on encouraging results from phase I/II trials, more than 50 phase III trials on cancer vaccines have been conducted in the past 20 years. Although there are several very promising trials in progress, none to date has been successful enough to lead to a Food and Drug Administration (FDA)-licensed product.

Table 32.1 summarizes the results of selected ongoing phase III trials, along with the supporting phase I/II trials. A brief analysis of selected completed studies may be instructive in understanding the role of study design in the outcome for clinical trial. Autologous tumor cell bacillus Calmette-Guérin (BCG) vaccine in resected colon cancer significantly improved both survival and disease-free survival in phase II (60,61). However, in two phase III trials there were no significant differences in clinical outcomes (62,63), except for a retrospective subgroup analysis (63). Differences in disease stage, patient population, change in vaccine regimen, and possibly immune responses among the studies were not accounted for in the design of the phase III trials.

Some studies have used standard therapy to compare with less toxic vaccines. For example, ganglioside GM2 conjugated to KLH with QS-21 was compared to high-dose interferon-alpha (IFN-α) (64),

after first demonstrating that GM2-KLH/QS-21 treatment induced antibodies in most melanoma patients (65). High-dose IFN-α was significantly superior in the phase III trial (64). In this case, the phase II trial compared adjuvants and selected one on the basis of antibody response but did not evaluate whether antibody response to vaccination had any impact on patient survival. Other surrogate markers could have been studied to try to estimate the magnitude of the potential effect to be tested in a phase III trial.

Patient selection may play a role in certain vaccine strategies, most obvious with the many HLA class I restricted peptide epitopes. Melacine, a vaccine prepared from lysed cells of two human melanoma cell lines combined with detox adjuvant, showed antitumor and immunologic responses (66–68). In the phase III trial, no significant overall improvement in survival was observed. Only when survival was analyzed in the context of HLA class I expression was a highly significant benefit found among a subgroup of patients expressing two or more of five HLA class I antigens, particularly the A2 and C3 phenotypes (69,70). Another study suggests that preexisting responses to a class II ESO-1 peptide occur with DRw3 (71).

It is important to consider whether these selected examples illustrate product or clinical trial design failures (72). Larger trials usually are designed based on data from phase II efficacy trials. The types of study design issues that should be taken into account include the following:

- Drawing conclusion from trials that are underpowered to detect small differences between treatment groups
- Data from small studies that, even if statistically significant, may not readily reproduce and speculation from small sample sizes that may produce biased assumptions
- Comparison of clinical data with historical controls that frequently is misleading, especially with respect to survival data
- Retrospective subgroup analysis that may provide useful clues but invites data selection
- Sporadic individual responses that may not be consistently reproduced in larger trials
- Failure to demonstrate the biologic effect of the vaccine in a sufficient number of patients, lack of an appropriate target, or changing the vaccine regimen from earlier studies without an understanding of the consequences to biologic activity
- Choosing a patient population, disease stage, or endpoints for the study that may not be appropriate for the vaccine strategy

TABLE 32.1. *Selected ongoing phase III trials of cancer vaccines*

Vaccine/adjuvant	Disease/stage	Phase I and II trial results leading to phase III trial (reference)
MART-1:27-35; gp100:209-217(210M); tyrosinase:368-376(370D) + GM-CSF vs GM-CSF alone	Locally advanced or metastatic melanoma	GM-CSF prolonged survival in resected patients with high risk for recurrence as single agent (73); GM-CSF enhanced DTH responses to melanoma peptides in 3 of 3 patients, all had objective responses (74)
gp100:209-217(210M) + high-dose IL-2 vs high-dose IL-2 alone	Locally advanced or metastatic melanoma	High-dose IL-2 treatment resulted in ~17% response rate (75); high-dose IL-2 + gp100:209-127(210M) resulted in 42% response rate (19)
Polyvalent melanoma vaccine (CancerVax) + BCG vs BCG + placebo	Resected stage III melanoma (one trial)	47% 10-year overall survival rate with CancerVax + BCG vs 33% in historical controls with resected stage III melanoma (76)
	Resected stage IV melanoma (one trial)	31% 5-year overall survival rate vs 10% in historical controls w/ resected stage IV, M1b melanoma (76)
Id-KLH + GM-CSF vs KLH-KLH control + GM-CSF following chemotherapy	Stage II with bulky adenopathy, stage III and IV follicular lymphoma	Of 20 patients studied, tumor-specific CD8$^+$ T-cell responses seen in 85% of patients; 90% of patients in clinical CR after median follow-up of 36+ months; 73% of sampled patients converted to PCR negative for t(14;18) translocations (77).
Id-KLH + GM-CSF vs KLH-KLH control + GM-CSF following chemotherapy	Stage III or IV follicular NHL	Amplified genes cloned into plasmid vectors as source of Id protein coupled to KLH + GM-CSF generated cellular and/or humor Id-specific responses in ~70% of vaccinated patients (78)
Provenge (autologous DC loaded ex vivo with rec. fusion protein PAP linked to GM-CSF	Patients with rising PSA after radical prostatectomy with no evidence of metastases (one trial) Hormone-refractory prostate cancer (one trial)	Of 31 patients with hormone-refractory prostate cancer treated with Provenge, all developed immune responses to the PAP-GM-CSF construct after vaccination and 38% developed immune responses to PAP (79). Three patients had >50% decline in serum PSA and 3 other patients had 25%–49% decline. Time to disease progression correlated with an immune response to PAP and with the dose of DC received.
THERATOPE vaccine [which contains a synthetic form of a cancer-associated carbohydrate antigen sialyl Tn (STn)] vs placebo	Patients with metastatic breast cancer who completed first-line chemotherapy	Patients with stage II–IV breast cancer received THERATOPE vaccine following high-dose chemotherapy and autologous stem cell transplant (80), compared to unvaccinated historical controls, a trend toward decreased risk for relapse and death was found.

BCG, bacillus Calmette-Guérin; CR, complete response; GM-CSF, granulocyte-macrophage colony-stimulating factor; IL-2; interleukin-2; NHL, non-Hodgkin's lymphoma; PAP, prostatic acid phosphatase; PCR, polymerase chain reaction; PSA, prostate-specific antigen.

CONCLUSION—FUTURE DIRECTIONS

After a century of research there are no FDA-licensed cancer vaccines that can be used for treatment. The ability to develop a more detailed molecular analysis of the tumor to predict biologic behavior and identify appropriate targets for each patient will enable clinical trials to be done more efficiently and effectively in the near future. It is likely that no single group can do this alone. Although cytotoxic and immune-modulating treatment may either inhibit or enhance immune responses, vaccine strategies should take advantage of the ability to combine with other modes of therapy. Development of these combinations will require cooperation among investigators and sponsors of trials in order to share phase II data that will be essential to planning larger efficacy trials.

The sustained efforts of a few groups have made tumor immunology a science. The conception of a trial should start by advancing the best science-based vaccines and applying the best molecular technology to vaccine design and production. However, at the clinical level, in order to put these advances into practice, the ability to coordinate and compare studies in order to answer commonly occurring questions would be a

significant advantage. This will require not only communication among investigators but also the development of standardized clinical and laboratory methodologies, access to standardized reagents, and some additional flexibility in combining agents from multiple sources.

REFERENCES

1. Zinkernagel RM. What is missing in immunology to understand immunity? *Nat Immunol* 2000;1:181–185.
2. Abbas AK, Janeway CA Jr. Immunology: improving on nature in the twenty-first century. *Cell* 2000;100: 129–138.
3. Anderson JM. Immunotherapy of cancer. In: Halnan KE, ed. *Recent advances in cancer and radiotherapeutics: clinical oncology.* Baltimore: Williams & Wilkins, 1972:193–215.
4. Hall S. *A commotion in the blood.* New York: Henry Holt, 1997.
5. Gross L. Immunization of C3H mice against a sarcoma that originated in an animal of the same line. *Cancer Res* 1943;3:326.
6. Dunn GP, Bruce AT, Ikeda H, et al. Cancer immunoediting: from immunosurveillance to tumor escape. *Nat Immunol* 2002;3:991–998.
7. van der Bruggen P, Traversari C, Chomez P, et al. A gene encoding an antigen recognized by cytolytic T lymphocytes on a human melanoma. *Science* 1991; 254:1643–1647.
8. Koutsky LA, Ault KA, Wheeler CM, et al. A controlled trial of a human papillomavirus type 16 vaccine. *N Engl J Med* 2002;347:1645–1651.
9. Kammula US, Lee KH, Riker AI, et al. Functional analysis of antigen-specific T lymphocytes by serial measurement of gene expression in peripheral blood mononuclear cells and tumor specimens. *J Immunol* 1999;163:6867–6875.
10. Ansell SM, Stenson M, Habermann TM, et al. CD4$^+$ T-cell immune response to large B-cell non-Hodgkin's lymphoma predicts patient outcome. *J Clin Oncol* 2001;19:720–726.
11. Albert ML, Darnell JC, Bender A, et al. Tumor-specific killer cells in paraneoplastic cerebellar degeneration. *Nat Med* 1998;4:1321–1324.
12. Clynes RA, Towers TL, Presta LG, et al. Inhibitory Fc receptors modulate in vivo cytotoxicity against tumor targets. *Nat Med* 2000;6:443–446.
13. Rosenberg SA, Yang JC, White DE, et al. Durability of complete responses in patients with metastatic cancer treated with high-dose interleukin-2: identification of the antigens mediating response. *Ann Surg* 1998;228: 307–319.
14. Grosenbach DW, Barrientos JC, Schlom J, et al. Synergy of vaccine strategies to amplify antigen-specific immune responses and antitumor effects. *Cancer Res* 2001;61:4497–4505.
15. Fontaine P, Roy-Proulx G, Knafo L, et al. Adoptive transfer of minor histocompatibility antigen-specific T lymphocytes eradicates leukemia cells without causing graft-versus-host disease. *Nat Med* 2001;7:789–794.
16. Childs R, Chernoff A, Contentin N, et al. Regression of metastatic renal-cell carcinoma after nonmyeloablative allogeneic peripheral-blood stem-cell transplantation. *N Engl J Med* 2000;343:750–758.
17. Dudley ME, Wunderlich JR, Robbins PF, et al. Cancer regression and autoimmunity in patients after clonal repopulation with antitumor lymphocytes. *Science* 2002; 298:850–854.
18. Yu Z, Restifo NP. Cancer vaccines: progress reveals new complexities. *J Clin Invest* 2002;110:289–294.
19. Rosenberg SA, Yang JC, Schwartzentruber DJ, et al. Immunologic and therapeutic evaluation of a synthetic peptide vaccine for the treatment of patients with metastatic melanoma. *Nat Med* 1998;4:321–327.
20. Stoler DL, Chen N, Basik M, et al. The onset and extent of genomic instability in sporadic colorectal tumor progression. *Proc Natl Acad Sci USA* 1999;96:15121–15126.
21. Rosenberg SA. Progress in human tumour immunology and immunotherapy. *Nature* 2001;411:380–384.
22. Rosenberg SA. A new era for cancer immunotherapy based on the genes that encode cancer antigens. *Immunity* 1999;10:281–287.
23. Renkvist N, Castelli C, Robbins PF, et al. A listing of human tumor antigens recognized by T cells. *Cancer Immunol Immunother* 2001;50:3–15.
24. Hanson HL, Donermeyer DL, Ikeda H, et al. Eradication of established tumors by CD8+ T cell adoptive immunotherapy. *Immunity* 2000;13:265–276.
25. von Mehren M, Arlen P, Gulley J, et al. The influence of granulocyte macrophage colony-stimulating factor and prior chemotherapy on the immunological response to a vaccine (ALVAC-CEA B7.1) in patients with metastatic carcinoma. *Clin Cancer Res* 2001;7: 1181–1191.
26. Mackall CL, Stein D, Fleisher TA, et al. Prolonged CD4 depletion after sequential autologous peripheral blood progenitor cell infusions in children and young adults. *Blood* 2000;96:754–762.
27. Staveley-O'Carroll K, Sotomayor E, Montgomery J, et al. Induction of antigen-specific T cell anergy: an early event in the course of tumor progression. *Proc Natl Acad Sci USA* 1998;95:1178–1183.
28. Ochsenbein AF, Klenerman P, Karrer U, et al. Immune surveillance against a solid tumor fails because of immunological ignorance. *Proc Natl Acad Sci USA* 1999; 96:2233–2238.
29. Tirapu I, Mazzolini G, Rodriguez-Calvillo M, et al. Effective tumor immunotherapy: start the engine, release the brakes, step on the gas pedal, . . . and get ready to face autoimmunity. *Arch Immunol Ther Exp (Warsz)* 2002;50:13–18.

30. Keilholz U, Weber J, Finke JH, et al. Immunologic monitoring of cancer vaccine therapy: results of a workshop sponsored by the Society for Biological Therapy. *J Immunother* 2002;25:97–138.

31. Khong UT, Restifo NP. Natural selection of tumor variants in the generation of "tumor escape" phenotypes. *Nat Immun* 2002;3:999–1005.

32. Clay TM, Hobeika AC, Mosca PJ, et al. Assays for monitoring cellular immune responses to active immunotherapy of cancer. *Clin Cancer Res* 2001;7:1127–1135.

33. Disis ML, Schiffman K, Gooley TA, et al. Delayed-type hypersensitivity response is a predictor of peripheral blood T-cell immunity after HER-2/neu peptide immunization. *Clin Cancer Res* 2000;6:1347–1350.

34. McMichael AJ, O'Callaghan CA. A new look at T cells. *J Exp Med* 1998;187:1367–1371.

35. Monsurro V, Nagorsen D, Wang E, et al. Functional heterogeneity of vaccine-induced CD8(+) T cells. *J Immunol* 2002;168:5933–5942.

36. Nielsen MB, Monsurro V, Migueles SA, et al. Status of activation of circulating vaccine-elicited CD8+ T cells. *J Immunol* 2000;165:2287–2296.

37. Welsh RM. Assessing CD8 T cell number and dysfunction in the presence of antigen. *J Exp Med* 2001; 193:F19–22.

38. Hislop AD, Annels NE, Gudgeon NH, et al. Epitope-specific evolution of human CD8(+) T cell responses from primary to persistent phases of Epstein-Barr virus infection. *J Exp Med* 2002;195:893–905.

39. Miller TP, LeBlanc M, Grogan TM, et al. Major histocompatibility complex (MHC) class II antigen HLA-DR gene expression levels in diffuse large B-cell lymphoma correlate with survival. *Am Soc Hematol* 2002;100: 346a.

40. Disis ML, Gooley TA, Rinn K, et al. Generation of T-cell immunity to the HER-2/neu protein after active immunization with HER-2/neu peptide-based vaccines. *J Clin Oncol* 2002;20:2624–2632.

41. Ahlers JD, Belyakov IM, Terabe M, et al. A push-pull approach to maximize vaccine efficacy: abrogating suppression with an IL-13 inhibitor while augmenting help with granulocyte/macrophage colony-stimulating factor and CD40L. *Proc Natl Acad Sci USA* 2002;99: 13020–13025.

42. Lanzavecchia A. Immunology. License to kill. *Nature* 1998;393:413–414.

43. Gabrilovich DI, Velders MP, Sotomayor EM, et al. Mechanism of immune dysfunction in cancer mediated by immature Gr-1+ myeloid cells. *J Immunol* 2001; 166:5398–5406.

44. Hunter RL. Overview of vaccine adjuvants: present and future. *Vaccine* 2002;20[Suppl 3]:S7–S12.

45. Ahlers JD, Dunlop N, Alling DW, et al. Cytokine-in-adjuvant steering of the immune response phenotype to HIV-1 vaccine constructs: granulocyte-macrophage colony-stimulating factor and TNF-alpha synergize with IL-12 to enhance induction of cytotoxic T lymphocytes. *J Immunol* 1997;158:3947–3958.

46. Singh M, O'Hagan D. Advances in vaccine adjuvants. *Nat Biotechnol* 1999;17:1075–1081.

47. Schijns VE. Immunological concepts of vaccine adjuvant activity. *Curr Opin Immunol* 2000;12:456–463.

48. Farag SS, Fehniger TA, Ruggeri L, et al. Natural killer cell receptors: new biology and insights into the graft-versus-leukemia effect. *Blood* 2002;100:1935–1947.

49. Chen Y-T, Scanlan MJ, Obata Y, et al. Identification of human tumor antigens by serologic expression cloning. In: Rosenberg SA, ed. *Principles and practice of the biologic therapy of cancer,* 3rd ed. Philadelphia: Lippincott Williams & Wilkins 2000:557–570.

50. Offringa R, van der Burg SH, Ossendorp F, et al. Design and evaluation of antigen-specific vaccination strategies against cancer. *Curr Opin Immunol* 2000;12:576–582.

51. Pardoll DM. Spinning molecular immunology into successful immunotherapy. *Nat Rev Immunol* 2002; 2:227–238.

52. Parmiani G, Castelli C, Dalerba P, et al. Cancer immunotherapy with peptide-based vaccines: what have we achieved? Where are we going? *J Natl Cancer Inst* 2002;94:805–818.

53. Aarts WM, Schlom J, Hodge JW. Vector-based vaccine/cytokine combination therapy to enhance induction of immune responses to a self-antigen and antitumor activity. *Cancer Res* 2002;62:5770–5777.

54. Berzofsky JA, Ahlers JD, Belyakov IM. Strategies for designing and optimizing new generation vaccines. *Nat Rev Immunol* 2001;1:209–219.

55. Berzofsky JA, Ahlers JD, Derby MA, et al. Approaches to improve engineered vaccines for human immunodeficiency virus and other viruses that cause chronic infections. *Immunol Rev* 1999;170:151–172.

56. Simon RM, Steinberg SM, Hamilton M, et al. Clinical trial designs for the early clinical development of therapeutic cancer vaccines. *J Clin Oncol* 2001;19:1848–1854.

57. Korn EL, Arbuck SG, Pluda JM, et al. Clinical trial designs for cytostatic agents: are new approaches needed? *J Clin Oncol* 2001;19:265–272.

58. Schilsky RL. End points in cancer clinical trials and the drug approval process. *Clin Cancer Res* 2002;8:935–938.

59. Yang JC, Haworth L, Steinberg SM, et al. A randomized double-blind placebo-controlled trial of bevacizumab (anti-VEGF antibody) demonstrating a prolongation in time to progression in patients with metastatic renal cancer. *Proc Am Soc Clin Oncol* 2002;21:A15.

60. Hoover HC Jr, Brandhorst JS, Peters LC, et al. Adjuvant active specific immunotherapy for human colorectal cancer: 6.5-year median follow-up of a phase III prospectively randomized trial. *J Clin Oncol* 1993;11:390–399.

61. Hoover HC Jr, Surdyke MG, Dangel RB, et al. Prospectively randomized trial of adjuvant active-specific immunotherapy for human colorectal cancer. *Cancer* 1985;55:1236–1243.

62. Harris JE, Ryan L, Hoover HC Jr, et al. Adjuvant active specific immunotherapy for stage II and III colon cancer with an autologous tumor cell vaccine: Eastern Cooperative Oncology Group Study E5283. *J Clin Oncol* 2000;18:148–157.

63. Vermorken JB, Claessen AM, van Tinteren H, et al. Active specific immunotherapy for stage II and stage III human colon cancer: a randomised trial. *Lancet* 1999; 353:345–350.

64. Kirkwood JM, Ibrahim JG, Sosman JA, et al. High-dose interferon alfa-2b significantly prolongs relapse-free and overall survival compared with the GM2-KLH/QS-21 vaccine in patients with resected stage IIB-III melanoma: results of intergroup trial E1694/S9512/C509801. *J Clin Oncol* 2001;19:2370–2380.

65. Chapman PB, Morrissey DM, Panageas KS, et al. Induction of antibodies against GM2 ganglioside by im-

munizing melanoma patients using GM2-keyhole limpet hemocyanin + QS21 vaccine: a dose-response study. *Clin Cancer Res* 2000;6:874–879.

66. Mitchell MS, Kan-Mitchell J, Kempf RA, et al. Active specific immunotherapy for melanoma: phase I trial of allogeneic lysates and a novel adjuvant. *Cancer Res* 1988;48:5883–5893.

67. Elliott GT, McLeod RA, Perez J, et al. Interim results of a phase II multicenter clinical trial evaluating the activity of a therapeutic allogeneic melanoma vaccine (theraccine) in the treatment of disseminated malignant melanoma. *Semin Surg Oncol* 1993;9:264–272.

68. Mitchell MS, Harel W, Kempf RA, et al. Active-specific immunotherapy for melanoma. *J Clin Oncol* 1990;8:856–869.

69. Mitchell MS, Harel W, Groshen S. Association of HLA phenotype with response to active specific immunotherapy of melanoma. *J Clin Oncol* 1992;10:1158–1164.

70. Sosman JA, Unger JM, Liu PY, et al. Adjuvant immunotherapy of resected, intermediate-thickness, node-negative melanoma with an allogeneic tumor vaccine: impact of HLA class I antigen expression on outcome. *J Clin Oncol* 2002;20:2067–2075.

71. Zeng G, Wang X, Robbins PF, et al. CD4(+) T cell recognition of MHC class II-restricted epitopes from NY-ESO-1 presented by a prevalent HLA DP4 allele: association with NY-ESO-1 antibody production. *Proc Natl Acad Sci USA* 2001;98:3964–3969.

72. Von Hoff DD. There are no bad anticancer agents, only bad clinical trial designs—twenty-first Richard and Hinda Rosenthal Foundation Award Lecture. *Clin Cancer Res* 1998;4:1079–1086.

73. Spitler LE, Grossbard ML, Ernstoff MS, et al. Adjuvant therapy of stage III and IV malignant melanoma using granulocyte-macrophage colony-stimulating factor. *J Clin Oncol* 2000;18:1614–1621

74. Jager E, Ringhoffer M, Dienes HP, et al. Granulocyte-macrophage-colony-stimulating factor enhances immune responses to melanoma-associated peptides in vivo. *Int J Cancer* 1996;67:54–62.

75. Rosenberg SA, Yang JC, Topalian SL, et al. Treatment of 283 consecutive patients with metastatic melanoma or renal cell cancer using high-dose bolus interleukin 2. *JAMA* 1994;271:907–913.

76. Morton DL, Barth A. Vaccine therapy for malignant melanoma. *CA Cancer J Clin* 1996;46:225–244.

77. Bendandi M, Gocke CD, Kobrin CB, et al. Complete molecular remissions induced by patient-specific vaccination plus granulocyte-monocyte colony-stimulating factor against lymphoma. *Nat Med* 1999;5:1171–1177.

78. Timmerman J, Czerwinski D, van Beckhoven A, et al. A phase I/II trial to evaluate the immunogenicity of recombinant idiotype protein vaccines for the treatment of non-Hodgkin's lymphoma (NHL). *Proc Am Soc Hematol* 2000;42;A2481.

79. Small EJ, Fratesi P, Reese DM, et al. Immunotherapy of hormone-refractory prostate cancer with antigen-loaded dendritic cells. *J Clin Oncol* 2000;18:3894–3903.

80. Holmberg LA, Oparin DV, Gooley T, et al. Clinical outcome of breast and ovarian cancer patients treated with high-dose chemotherapy, autologous stem cell rescue and THERATOPE STn-KLH cancer vaccine. *Bone Marrow Transplant* 2000;25:1233–1241.

PART 8

Licensure Issues

33

Regulatory Requirements for Licensure: United States and Europe

Elaine Meaker, Bruce Feistner, and Nicole Onetto

OSI Pharmaceuticals, Inc., Boulder, Colorado 80301

OVERVIEW

Unique regulatory aspects of anticancer drug development can be attributed to the unique aspects of the disease itself, the important unmet medical needs, and, until recently, the toxicity of traditional cancer treatments (i.e., cytotoxic agents). This toxicity has precluded first use in healthy volunteers, so initial trials of cytotoxics are conducted in cancer patients who are not amenable to established forms of therapy. Further, the severity of most cancers and the limited success of available treatments lead otherwise conservative regulators to welcome new therapeutic approaches, and this situation affects the risk-to-benefit evaluation. Where the potential for benefit is great, greater risks can be tolerated; therefore, the cancer development pathway has evolved to allow higher risks than those allowed in the testing of therapies for less severe illnesses. A parallel certainly can be established with what has been observed for human immunodeficiency (HIV) drug development, but, interestingly, and maybe because of more organized activist groups, the regulatory environment has changed more rapidly for HIV than for oncology agents. Nevertheless, this supports the hope that the regulatory environment will continue to evolve for oncology agents.

A second theme of the regulatory climate is not specific to anticancer therapies but reflects the globalization of our times and of the pharmaceutical industry. Registration of today's new therapeutics typically involves a global clinical development plan and frequently aims for simultaneous submission of marketing applications in the world's larger markets (1). Drug development strategies require a global perspective on regulatory requirements; thus, the following discussion reviews regulatory aspects of anticancer development in a setting of multinational development.

REGULATORY REQUIREMENTS FOR CLINICAL TRIAL INITIATION

In considering approval of initial clinical trials, the regulatory focus is on patient safety. The regulator's evaluation of safety initially is dependent upon data developed during the nonclinical research on the selected molecular entity. *In vitro* and *in vivo* studies are undertaken to determine the target organs for toxicity in different animal species, the maximum tolerated dose (MTD), and possible schedule dependences. The main objective of the toxicology assessment is to guide the selection of a safe starting dose for the initial clinical trials and to identify potential toxicities to guide safety monitoring. The fact that phase I oncology trials start in patients with advanced cancer, who have no other options for treatment, has led to acceptance of an abbreviated toxicology package for cytotoxic cancer drugs. Chronic or reproductive toxicities are delayed until later in the development cycle. Nevertheless, cytostatic and hormonal cancer treatments, used in different settings (e.g., adjuvant use), have preclinical requirements that can be substantially different (2,3).

Interestingly, the responsibility for evaluation of patient safety has developed differently in the United States versus Europe. Both regions generally have the same elements: a national regulatory authority and medical review committees that oversee clinical trials; however, the weight of responsibility is toward the national authority in the United States and the review committee (ethics committees) in Europe. However, current trends suggest the US medical review committees [institutional review boards (IRBs)] are expected to take more responsibility in the future, whereas Europeans, with the Clinical Trial Directive (4) discussed later, are moving toward legislation strengthening the role of national authorities.

International Developments

Since 1990, regulators and industrial organizations from the United States (Food and Drug Administration [FDA] and Pharmaceutical Research and Manufacturers of America [PhRMA]), western Europe (European Union [EU] and EFPIA), and Japan (Ministry of Health, Labor and Welfare [MHLW] and Japan Pharmaceutical Manufacturers Association [JPMA]) have joined together in an effort to harmonize scientific and technical requirements for pharmaceutical development under the name of the International Committee for Harmonization (ICH). Following a five-step review process, best practices for the clinical evaluation of pharmaceuticals have been codified as ICH guidelines and provide an international standard for industry and health authorities. They are available at the ICH web site *(www.ich.org)* or at the FDA Web site *(www.fda.gov).* The ICH Guidance E8, *General Considerations for Clinical Trials,* summarizes the clinical safety and efficacy guidelines and includes a table of relevant ICH documents (Table 33.1).

The Guideline E6 *Good Clinical Practice* offers detailed information on the requirements for protocols and investigator brochures, which are key documents for clinical investigation. The M3 guideline discusses the extent and timing of nonclinical testing to support clinical trials (S6 for biotechnology products). Safety pharmacologic studies are addressed in guideline S7A (5), which notes that "for cytotoxics treating end-stage cancer patients, these studies may not be needed prior to first administration in humans."

Use of ICH guidelines is rapidly spreading to additional countries outside of the ICH regions, further facilitating the globalization the pharmaceutical industry.

United States

Within the Center for Drug Evaluation and Research (CDER) at the FDA, there are 15 review divisions, each specializing in a therapeutic area. For cancer drugs, the Division of Oncology Drug Products (DODP) reviews the applications. This division recognizes that for many cytotoxic drugs the dose difference between activity and toxicity, the therapeutic window, usually is small. As a result, they emphasize careful dosing and clinical monitoring to ensure that the side effects are less threatening than the disease.

Before initiating clinical trials, sufficient data must be provided to the FDA to convince the agency that due consideration has been given to the safety of prospective patients. For the DODP, emphasis is placed upon the safety precautions provided within the clinical protocol, which must specify both the starting dose and the escalation scheme as well as the criteria that will be used to stop the dose escalation. Toxicity studies also are necessary to identify parameters for clinical monitoring of potential adverse effects. The DODP requires that animal studies have been performed to elucidate organ effects and reversibility in both rodents and nonrodents, with histopathology in one of these species. Genotoxicity and reproductive studies are not generally needed in phase I unless healthy volunteers are enrolled in the studies. All toxicity studies must be performed under Good Laboratory Practices (GLP), and the Investigational New Drug application (IND) must contain a full tabulation of data. Final toxicology reports can be omitted from the application, but they must be submitted to the agency within 120 days from the IND submission date (6).

TABLE 33.1. *ICH E8 relevant guidelines list*

Code	Topic
E1	The Extent of Population Exposure to Assess Clinical Safety for Drug Intended for Long-term Treatment of Non–Life-Threatening Conditions
E2A	Clinical Safety Data Management: Definitions and Standards for Expedited Reporting
E2B	Clinical Safety Data Management: Data Elements for Transmission of Individual Case Safety Reports
E2C	Clinical Safety Data Management: Periodic Safety Updates Reports for Marketed Drugs
E3	Structure and Content of Clinical Study Reports
E4	Dose-Response Information to Support Drug Registration
E5	Ethnic Factors in the Acceptability of Foreign Clinical Data
E6	Good Clinical Practice: Consolidated Guidelines
E7	Clinical Trials in Special Populations—Geriatrics
E8	General Considerations for Clinical Trials
E9	Statistical Considerations in the Design of Clinical Trials
E10	Choice of Control Group in Clinical Trials
M3	Nonclinical Safety Studies for the Conduct of Human Clinical Trials
S6	Safety Studies for Biotechnology-Derived Products

Although preclinical studies in oncology often are considered of low relevance for predicting both the safety and efficacy of the drug within the clinic, they are important for establishing the starting dose. The DODP requires that toxicology studies identify the life-threatening doses within rodents and confirm that the non–life-threatening dose has been identified in a nonrodent species. The initial starting dose for phase I oncology trials traditionally is one tenth the severely toxic dose to 10% of the rodents (on a milligram per square meter basis), or, if that dose is found to be toxic in nonrodents, the starting dose is generally one sixth of the dose that does not cause severe toxicity in nonrodents (usually dogs) (7). The maximum clinical dose for cancer drugs usually is not restricted by the levels dosed in animal toxicity studies, as long as the toxicities in the clinic can be safely monitored and are reversible. Usually the dose escalation is stopped when the MTD is reached (i.e., the dose level at which one third or more of the patients experience dose-limiting toxicities). Important efforts have been made by governmental agencies [National Cancer Institute (NCI)], collaborative groups, and investigators to standardize the monitoring and evaluation of adverse events, which provide some uniformity in safety assessment of new agents among different institutions and even different territories (the NCI/CTC version 2.0 common toxicity scale now is used in most oncology protocols). Of note, the paradigm for phase I oncology studies is being challenged by the introduction of target therapies with novel mechanism of action. Phase I trials might be designed to determine an optimal biologic dose and the dose excalation might be stopped without identification of an MTD. However, the toxicology studies remain essential to determining the starting dose and guiding the clinician in monitoring drug safety in these early studies.

Prior to submission of the IND, the sponsor may request a meeting with FDA-reviewing officials to review and reach agreement on the design of animal studies, to discuss the scope and design of phase I testing, or to determine the best approach for presenting and formatting the data in the IND. The pre-IND meeting is classified as a type B meeting by the FDA and, as such, will be scheduled to occur within 60 days of the agency's receipt of the written request for the meeting. Procedures adopted by the FDA for such meetings is outlined in the FDA guidance document entitled *Formal Meetings with Sponsors and Applicants for PDUFA Products.*

The FDA provides a wealth of information on its Web site *(www.fda.gov/cder)*, including links to guidance documents, drug information, and the oncology tools database *(www.fda.gov/cder/cancer/index.htm)*. The general principles of the IND and both the content and format requirements are outlined in the Code of Federal Regulations (21 CFR 212.22 and 21 CFR 212.23). In addition, a guidance document entitled *Content and Format of Investigational New Drug Applications for Phase I Studies of Drugs, Including Well-Characterized, Therapeutic, Biotechnology-Derived Products* provides details clarifying the data and data presentation expected in the IND. It is a notification process; 30 days after the FDA receives the application, the sponsor can initiate the trial if no questions are received from the FDA. Although not required, usually sponsors are conservative and call the FDA to receive clearance. This action confirms that all review issues have been resolved and minimizes the possibility that the trial will go on clinical hold.

Western Europe

Currently, the requirements for initiating clinical trials in Europe vary among countries; however, this variability is likely to diminish when the Clinical Trials Directive is incorporated into national legislation and implemented for all member states of the EU (projected to be completed in May 2004). In the meantime, some countries require a detailed application with substantial documentation, whereas others require only ethics committee approval before clinical trial initiation. Although keeping up to date with the requirements specific for each country is onerous and even daunting, for the well-informed this heterogeneity provides an opportunity to optimize the strengths of a developmental program by selecting countries that best fit with the phase I program, thereby shortening time lines and permitting the early initiation of clinical studies.

When implemented, the Clinical Trials Directive theoretically will standardize the requirements for initiating clinical trials in member states of the EU by establishing specific provisions regarding the conduct of clinical trials by implementing Good Clinical Practice. It also provides for the following:

1. Authorization of the trial by the competent authority and ethics committees within 60 days,
2. Drug product to be manufactured in accordance with standards of Good Manufacturing Practice (GMP), and
3. Declaration from a "Qualified Person" that the manufacturing site is compliant with EU GMP.

The format and content of the request to conduct clinical trials can be found in the guidance ENTR/6418/01 at the EMEA Web site *(www.emea.eu.int)*.

The GMP requirements are provided in Annex 13, *Manufacture of Investigational Medicinal Products.* In addition, there is a specific guidance document for oncology, a *Note for Guidance on Pre-Clinical Evaluation of Anticancer Medicinal Products* (CPMP/ SWP/997/96), which defines data needed to initiate clinical trials.

REGULATORY REQUIREMENTS FOR MARKETING APPROVALS

Marketing approval requires an assessment of both safety and efficacy by the health authority. In assessing efficacy, individuals involved in drug development must remain closely attuned to the changing clinical environment, because a new therapy generally must be compared to the current standard of care for the particular indication. Although "best care" practices change as new information becomes available, these practices can vary widely by region. Drugs approved in one jurisdiction may not be used in others. In addition, there are often regional differences in reimbursement and hospitalization policies and historical differences in the practice of medicine. These differences are a constant challenge to both comprehend and take into account as clinical trials are designed and implemented.

Further complicating the design of trials is the choice of trial endpoints. Although the gold standard of endpoints is overall survival, additional endpoints such as response rate, time to progression (TTP), progression-free survival, symptom improvement, and quality of life have a valuable role in trial design. These endpoints must be prospectively defined but can be subject to cultural bias and should be discussed with prospective reviewers prior to initiation of the registrational trials. A recent review written by FDA DODP leadership clearly demonstrates that endpoints other than survival have led to full regulatory approval for oncology agents (8). Surprisingly, of 57 new drug applications (NDAs) or supplemental new drug applications (SNDAs) approved from January 1990 to November 2002, only 18 (32%) were approved on a survival endpoint. Response rate, supported or not by other endpoints such as TTP or symptom improvement, led to 26 (46%) of the approvals. However, perhaps reflecting some historical changes, among the submissions approved with a survival endpoint only three occurred before 1995, whereas the other 15 were approved between 1996 and 2002. This suggests that in recent approvals, survival was increasingly becoming the standard requirement of the FDA. According to several FDA Oncology Division written communications and oral presentations at scientific meetings, the

FDA is very interested in exploring with sponsors the possibility of a trial endpoint(s) other than survival that can clearly demonstrate patient benefit. The burden should be assumed in part by the pharmaceutical company to conduct well-controlled studies that could help regulatory agencies become more comfortable with use of an endpoint(s) other than survival to demonstrate unequivocally patient benefit.

As companies strive to develop strategies that permit the generation of uniform submission packages, lack of universal agreement in acceptable parameters for registrational trials challenge those in industry who must design and analyze trials that compare new therapies with the standards of care; however, trends are evident. The United States, with the largest share of the drug market and drug approval not contingent upon the negotiation of drug pricing, has increasingly become the market most likely to receive the first application and the first marketing approval. As a result, packages often are tailored for the United States and modified to gain acceptance elsewhere.

International Developments

An important change in the process for obtaining marketing approvals comes with implementation of an ICH program known as the common technical document (CTD). The CTD is a format for submission of technical information that will be accepted throughout the ICH regions. Unfortunately, it is not a global dossier, and differences remain in the content required for the United States, EU, and Japan, but it does provide a reusable format for summaries, reports, and data. Use of the CTD is voluntary until July 2003 (likely to be extended), a period that allows both industry and regulators an opportunity to become more familiar with its use. It consists of five modules (Fig. 33.1), with module 1 containing the unique information requested by the specific regional requirements. Guidance is available for submission of an electronic CTD, or a CTD in electronic portable document format (PDF) and extended markup language (XML). With implementation of the CTD, pharmaceutical companies can more quickly submit dossiers in the world's three major markets.

United States

The FDA has implemented a number of policies to make new therapeutics rapidly available to cancer patients in the United States. These mechanisms are briefly described here. For a more thorough discussion, see Hirschfeld and Pazdur (9) and the FDA regulations cited. Each of these mechanisms is distinct,

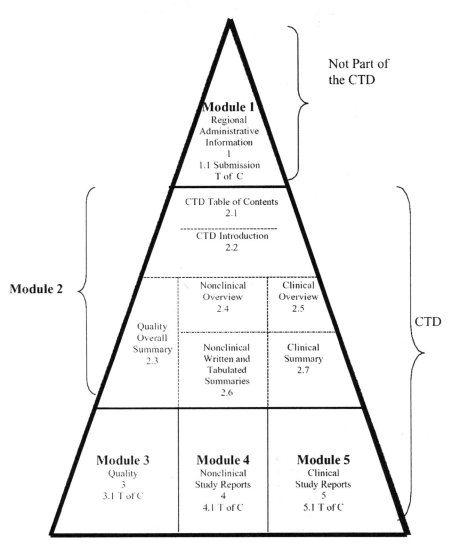

FIG. 33.1. Schematic of the common technical document.

but they can be combined when drugs qualify for more than one.

Fast Track

The FDA Modernization Act of 1997 (FDAMA) significantly changed US laws governing drug development and provided a mechanism for expediting development and review of programs for any drugs to treat a serious or life-threatening condition, which could fulfill an unmet medical need (10). Sponsors of fast track programs are eligible for consultation meetings with the FDA and for rolling submission of the appli-

cation. Usually, a fast track product's NDA or Biologics License Application (BLA) also will be eligible for priority review. The sponsor may apply for fast track status at any time during the development process by making a formal request and providing the FDA with supporting information as appropriate to the phase of development. This status will be reviewed as the development program progresses.

Accelerated Approval

The activism of HIV patients and their demand for immediate access to drugs led to the development of

TABLE 33.2. *Accelerated approvals in oncology*

Product	Year	Indication (conversion date[a])
Liposomal doxorubicin (Doxil)	1995	Second-line Kaposi's sarcoma
Dexrazoxane (Zinecard)	1995 Randomized	Reduction of doxorubicin cardiomyopathy (1998[a])
Amifostine (Ethyol)	1996	Cisplatin toxicity in NSCLC
Docetaxel (Taxotere)	1996	Second-line breast cancer (1998[a])
Irinotecan (Camptosar)	1996	Second-line colon cancer 2001[a]
Capecitabine (Xeloda)	1998	Refractory breast cancer (2001[a])
Liposomal doxorubicin (Doxil)	1999	Refractory ovarian cancer
Temozolomide (Temodar)	1999	Refractory anaplastic astroctyoma
Denileukin diftitox (Ontak)	1999	Relapsed refractory CTCL
Liposomal cytarabine (DepoCyt)	1999 Randomized	Lymphomatous meningitis
Celecoxib (Celebrex)	1999 Randomized	Reduction of adenomatous polyps
Gemtuzumab ozogamycin (Mylotarg)	2000	Second-line AML, elderly
Alemtuzumad (Campath)	2001	Third-line B-CLL
Imatinib mesylate (Gleevec)	2001	CML in BC, AC, or CP after interferon failure
Imatinib mesylate (Gleevec)	2002	Metastatic GIST
Ibritumomab tiuxetan (Zevalin)	2002 Randomized	Relapsed/refractory follicular NHL
Oxaliplatin (Eloxatin)	2002 Randomized	Second-line colorectal cancer
Anastrozole (Arimidex)	2002 Randomized	Adj. postmenopause ER+ breast cancer
Inatinib mesylate (Gleevec)	2002 Randomized	First-line CML

[a] Accelerated approval converted to full approval.

a mechanism for provisional or "accelerated" approval of drugs (11). Also known as Subpart H, accelerated approval (12) provides for approval based on a surrogate endpoint that is considered as "reasonably likely" to predict clinical benefit. The approval must be followed with definitive studies confirming clinical benefit, which for cytotoxic drugs usually means two randomized, well-controlled studies having an endpoint of survival. Response rate is the most frequently used surrogate endpoint, but FDA regulators also suggest TTP be considered (13). These are endpoints that may suffice for full approval. For example, durable complete remission has led to full approval for leukemia, and TTP has been sufficient for approval of hormonal agents for breast cancer. Pharmaceutical companies are encouraged to meet with the FDA to discuss proposed trial endpoints (14).

The FDA's experience with accelerated approval in oncology drugs was the subject of an Oncology Drug Advisory Committee (ODAC) meeting held March 2003, where industry's record of fulfilling post approval commitments was reviewed (15). At that meeting, FDA reported that of 16 drugs (and biologics) approved in 19 indications, only four approvals were converted to full approvals (Table 33.2). The FDA DODP recommended that the industry look at the HIV drug experience as a model for trials design, where an approval based on an interim analysis of surrogate laboratory marker is quickly followed with full approval based on a definitive clinical endpoint in the same trial.

Priority Review

The FDA grants "priority" review at the time of filing when a drug appears to have the potential to treat a serious or life-threatening condition, which could fulfill an unmet medical need, whether or not the sponsor has applied for fast track status. Drugs under priority review must be reviewed and acted upon in 6 months, in 90% of cases. "Standard" review times are 10 months.

FDAMA also directed the FDA to promulgate guidelines that encouraged sponsors to apply for additional indications for approved drug and promoted drug development for pediatric populations with the following mechanism.

Pediatric Exclusivity

FDAMA provided an incentive to industry for pediatric drug development in the form of an additional 6 months of exclusivity for *all* approved indications. This additional exclusivity is granted even if the study results are negative. The FDA subsequently added the Pediatric Rule (1998), which required that pediatric studies be conducted for drugs for which "meaningful therapeutic benefit and substantial" pediatric use were anticipated. These initiatives are intended to enhance access to new anticancer therapies and promote labeling for pediatric oncology indications (16). The FDA's authority to use the "stick" part of this "carrot-and-stick" approach to encourage pediatric drug development was challenged, however, and the rule was vacated in US District Court, October 2002.

The FDA's concern with the "paucity of pediatric submissions in oncology" was discussed by Hirshfeld et al. (17) in a March 2003 article in the *Journal of Clinical Oncology*. Even with these provisions, of the more than 100 FDA-approved oncology drugs, only 15 have pediatric use information in their labeling (17). FDAMA expired in December 2001, but the Best Pharmaceuticals for Children Act (BPCA) replaced and expanded the FDAMA program. It is hoped this and other FDA measures will increase the availability of pediatric oncology therapeutics.

Orphan Drug Act

The Orphan Drug Act (18) provides a mechanism for designation of drugs that are intended to treat serious or life-threatening diseases that affect fewer than 200,000 patients annually in the United States with orphan status. Orphan status provides the sponsor with special tax benefits and 7 years of marketing exclusivity (compared to 5 years for a new chemical entity without orphan designation) for development of a product with a target population of fewer than 200,000 people. It also provides incentive to develop products in areas where pharmaceutical companies would not otherwise be interested. As of November 2002, a total of 226 orphan medicines has been approved by the FDA, with 24 of these for oncologic indications.

The FDA has issued numerous guidance documents explaining procedures for the mechanisms described, as well as additional guidances of interest to those developing oncology products (Table 33.3).

It is useful to examine the ODAC transcripts for "real world" application of regulatory legislation and guidance principles and for discussions of regulatory issues that may not as yet have been addressed in the FDA guidelines. These can also be found on the FDA Web site.

TABLE 33.3. *FDA guidance documents*[a]

Title	Date
Formal Meetings with Sponsors and Applicants for PDUFA Products	February 2000
Special Protocol Assessment	December 1999
Cancer Drug and Biological Products—Clinical data in Marketing Applications	October 2001
FDA Approval of New Cancer Treatment Uses for Marketing Drug and Biological Products	March 1997 (Draft)
FDA Requirements for Approval of Drugs to Treat Non-Small Cell Lung Cancer (Report)	January 1991
Information Program on Clinical Trials for Serious or Life-Threatening Diseases: Establishment of a Data Bank (Draft)	March 2000
FDA Requirements for Drugs to Treat Superficial Bladder Cancer	June 1989 (Revised)
ODAC Discussion on FDA Requirements for Approval of New Drugs for Treatment of Ovarian Cancer	April 1988
ODAC Discussion on FDA Requirements for Approval of New Drugs for Treatment of Colon and Rectal Cancers	April 1988
Clinical Trial Sponsors on the Establishment and Operation of Clinical Trial Dada Monitoring Committees	November 2001 (Draft)
Pediatric Oncology Studies in Response to a Written Request	June 2000 (Draft)
Recommendations for Complying with the Pediatric Rule	December 2000 (Draft)
IND Exemption for Studies of Lawfully Marketed Cancer Drug or Biological Products	April 2002

[a] These documents are available at the Food and Drug Adminstration (FDA) Web site: *http://www.fda.gov/cder/guidance/index.htm*

Western Europe

In 1995, the EU created the European Medicines Evaluation Agency (EMEA) to coordinate the scientific evaluation of medicines for the community. Applications for marketing authorization in Europe may go through a centralized or a decentralized procedure.

Centralized Procedure

Under the centralized procedure, marketing applications are evaluated by the EMEA's scientific committee, the Committee for Proprietary Medicinal Products (CPMP). EMEA approval results in a single marketing authorization that is valid in all member states. This procedure, codified in the EEC Council Regulation No. 2309/93, was originally required for all biotechnology-derived products and subsequently was extended to all new chemical entities. The CPMP has addressed specific issues in cancer clinical development in *Notes for Guidance on Evaluation of Anticancer Medicinal Products in Man* (CPMP/EWP/205/95, rev 2), which provides guidance for clinical investigation, particularly with regard to cytotoxic and cytostatic drugs. It makes reference to "exceptional circumstances" where a drug could obtain approval based on noncomparative phase II data. There is precedence set for use of this mechanism in oncology. Docetaxel was the first oncology agent for which marketing authorization was granted under exceptional circumstances in 1995 for patients with breast cancer whose disease was resistant to anthracyclines. In fact, during the first 5 years (1995 to 1999) of operation of the EMEA, seven of 12 different oncology drugs submitted were approved (19), with the majority of them requiring additional clinical trials to confirm clinical benefit.

The clinical guidance document also provides guidance for pediatric drug development in the EU, which is supplemented by the *Addendum on Paediatric Oncology* (CPMP\EWP\569/02).

There is a procedure for obtaining scientific advice within the centralized system; however, it is considered to be very rigid, especially compared with the FDA's provisions allowing ongoing dialog throughout the development program (20). Drug applications are generally approved in 12 to 18 months through the centralized process.

Mutual Recognition

The decentralized process, know as *mutual recognition,* allows for approval in one country to be "recognized" by additional countries within the EU. The original directives describing these procedures have been combined into Council Directive 2001/83/EC. Application is made to the selected member state and subsequent recognition by other member states. The EMEA participates in this process when a disagreement between countries requires arbitration. An evaluation of the two procedures completed in October 2000 found that both contributed to the EU harmonization efforts, with the decentralized procedure providing flexibility that "meets the commercial needs of many companies"(20). This pathway may allow quicker access to market, particularly when there is a unique interest in the product in one of the member states. A 5-year review (20) of both procedures conducted by the European Commission in 2001 resulted in a number of proposed changes to the Regulation (21) and Directives (22) cited earlier for the sake of harmonization. If adopted, these changes likely will reduce the availability and advantages of the decentralized procedure. Proposed changes include a requirement that all new active substances utilize the centralized procedure, whereas the mutual recognition procedure would require agreement within the concerned member states before a national approval could be granted. Furthermore, member states could no longer opt out of an approval to avoid arbitration.

Orphan Medicines

In 1999, EMEA further moved to improve the development of drugs for rare diseases with legislation providing for development of Orphan Drug Regulations (EC 141/2000) and the establishment of the Committee for Orphan Medical Products (COMP). A *rare disease* was defined as one that affected not more than five in 10,000 people within the EU. A total of 58 drugs and biologic products were approved through this mechanism for 61 indications as of April 2003. Of these, 16 were approved for 18 oncology indications.

CASE STUDIES IN REGULATORY APPROVALS OF CANCER DRUGS

Capecitabine

Capecitabine (Xeloda, Roche Laboratories) is an oral fluoropyrimidine carbamate that is enzymatically converted to 5-fluorouracil (5-FU) *in vivo* and is thymidine synthesis inhibitor. The recommended dose is 2,500 mg/m^2 given orally as a divided dose (1,250 mg/m^2 administered orally twice daily), with food for 14 days on a 21-day schedule. It was first approved for use in the United States in 1998 for breast cancer after failure of paclitaxel and anthracyclines, and then for first-line metastatic colorectal cancer. Diarrhea and hand and foot syndrome are the most frequently observed adverse reactions.

The NDA for the use of capecitabine in third-line breast cancer was submitted for accelerated approval on October 31, 1997, based on a total of 163 patients in a single uncontrolled phase II trial. A response rate of 25.6% was seen in the 43 women with breast cancer resistant to both anthracyclines and paclitaxel. The submission was reviewed at ODAC March 19, 1998 and was recommended for approval. See the Summary Basis for Approval (23) for further details. This accelerated approval was later converted to full approval in second-line breast cancer.

After discussion with the CPMP in June 1996, Roche chose a different registration strategy with the EMEA, delaying submission until September 1999. The product then was submitted to the EMEA through the centralized process for first-line use in colorectal cancer. The indication claim was based on two randomized, comparative phase III studies with a total of 1,207 patients. A positive opinion was issued by the CPMP on October 19, 2000 (see European Public Assessment Report [EPAR]). This clearly illustrates a case where the CPMP was not willing to grant approval under exceptional circumstances for third-line breast cancer in a situation where the FDA had granted accelerated approval.

Oxaliplatin

Oxaliplatin for injection (Eloxatin, Sanofi-Synthelabo) is a platinum-based antineoplastic agent given in combination with 5-FU plus leucovorin (5-FU/LV) to treat advanced colorectal carcinoma.

Oxaliplatin was first approved for marketing in France for relapsed metastatic colorectal cancer in combination with 5-FU and leucovorin in September 1996. The indication was expanded to include first-line treatment in May 1998. In 1999 Sanofi-Synthelabo used the mutual recognition procedure to obtain marketing approval in Europe, with France acting as the rapporteur country.

In 1999 Sanofi Pharmaceuticals submitted an application for oxaliplatin for first-line therapy in combination with 5-FU/LV for treatment of advanced colorectal cancer in the United States. Patients in the clinical trial were dosed under the European preferred de Gramont regimen, whereas US researchers primarily utilize the Mayo regimen. The data, which demonstrated no statistical benefit in overall survival but significant improvement in response rate and TTP, were reviewed by the oncology advisory committee on March 16,

2000. The committee unanimously recommended that the drug not be approved by the FDA. The FDA followed the advice of the committee.

In 2002 Sanofi-Synthelabo submitted clinical data to the FDA from a multicenter randomized trial comparing oxaliplatin in combination with bolus 5-FU/LV versus 5-FU/LV or oxaliplatin alone in patients who relapsed within 6 months after receiving first-line therapy of bolus 5-FU/LV and irinotecan. Patients treated with a combination drug regimen of oxaliplatin and 5-FU/LV had a statistically significant increase in time to tumor progression and rate of tumor response relative to the comparators. After reviewing the application for only 7 weeks, the shortest ever for a cancer drug, the FDA approved oxaliplatin under 21 CFR 314 Subpart H for use by patients with colorectal cancer. In contrast to the capecitabine case history, this example illustrates that data that were sufficient to lead to European approval under mutual recognition did not satisfy the FDA. However, the feedback that the FDA gave to Sanofi allowed them to obtain accelerated approval very rapidly upon submission to the agency of additional data using the innovative approach of an interim analysis of TTP and response rate with survival as the definitive endpoint.

CONCLUSION

The path to marketing approval is unique for every product and must be sought through an ever-changing environment. Because clinical studies that are initiated now will not be analyzed by health authorities until many years in the future, the sponsors need to anticipate changes in standard of care, regulatory requirements, and market conditions in order to maximize chances of success. Astute regulatory intelligence and as accurate understanding of the evolution and changes in oncology medical practices are essential to designing successful regulatory strategies. In addition, a collaborative relationship among medical oncologists, cooperative groups, government agencies, patient advocate groups, and regulatory agencies is essential to continue to better advance the development of new oncology agents and ensure rapid access for patients to safe and effective new therapies. Finally, the emergence of oncology drug candidates with new mechanism of action will greatly impact design of clinical studies, patient selection for clinical trials, and possible endpoints that might be acceptable for regulatory agencies. This further underlines the need for a partnership among all parties worldwide involved in oncology drug development and drug approval to ensure that patients ultimately will benefit from the tremendous scientific progress made in recent years.

REFERENCES

1. Schwartsmann G, Ratain MJ, Cragg GM, et al. Anticancer drug discovery and development throughout the world. *J Clin Oncol* 2002;20[18 Suppl]:47S–59S.

2. Kelloff GJ, Johnson JR, Crowell JA, et al. Approaches to the development and marketing approval of drugs that prevent cancer. *Cancer Epidemiol Biomarkers Prev* 1995;4:1–10.

3. CPMP. Note for Guidance on Evaluation of Anticancer Medicinal Products in Man. In: CPMP/EWP/205/95 rev. 2, 2002.

4. EU Directive on Good Clinical Practice in Clinical Trials. 2001/20/EC, European Commission, 2001.

5. ICH. S7A: safety pharmacology studies for human pharmaceuticals. Federal Register 2001;66:36791–36792.

6. CDER/CBER. Content and format of investigational new drug applications (INDs) for phase 1 studies of drugs, including well-characterized, therapeutic, biotechnology-derived products. Food and Drug Administration, November 1995.

7. DeGeorge JJ, Ahn C-H, Andrews PA, et al. Regulatory considerations for preclinical development of anticancer drugs. *Cancer Chemother Pharmacol* 1998;41:173–185.

8. Johnson JR, Williams G, Pazdur R. End points and United States Food and Drug Administration approval of oncology drugs. *J Clin Oncol* 2003;21:1404–1411.

9. Hirschfeld S, Pazdur R. Oncology drug development: United States Food and Drug Administration perspective. *Crit Rev Oncol Hematol* 2002;42:137–143.

10. Food And Drug Administration Modernization Act of 1997. Public Law 105–115. US Public Law, 1997.

11. Podraza R. The FDA's response to AIDS: paradigm shift in new drug policy? *Food Drug Law J* 1993;48:351–375.

12. 21 Subpart H, Accelerated Approval of New Drugs for Serious or Life-threatening Illnesses. 21 CFR Parts 314 and 601. US Public Law, 1992.

13. Pazdur R. Response rates, survival, and chemotherapy trials. *J Natl Cancer Inst* 2000;92:1552–1553.

14. Beitz J. Trial endpoints for drug approval in oncology: chemoprevention. *Urology* 2001;57[4 Suppl 1]: 213–215.

15. FDA. Proceedings of the ODAC Review of Post Marketing Commitments, Bethesda, Maryland, March 12–13, 2003.

16. Hirschfeld S, Shapiro A, Dagher R, et al. Pediatric oncology: regulatory initiatives. *Oncologist* 2000;5: 441–444.

17. Hirschfeld S, Ho P, Smith M, et al. Regulatory approvals of pediatric oncology drugs: previous experience and new initiatives. *J Clin Oncol* 2003;21: 1066–1073.

18. US Orphan Drug Act. 21 CFR Part 316. US Public Law, 1983.

19. Pignatti F, Aronsson B, Vamvakas S, et al. Clinical trials for registration in the European Union: the EMEA 5-year experience in oncology. *Crit Rev Oncol Hematol* 2002;42:123–135.

20. McKenna CC, Consulting A. Evaluation of the operation of community procedures for the authorisation of medicinal products. European Commission, October 2000.

21. Proposal for a Regulation of the European Parliament and of the Council. 2001/0252. Commission of the European Communities, 2001.

22. Proposal amending Directive 2001/83/EC on the Community code relating to medicinal products for human use. 2001/0253. Commission of the European Communities, 2001.

23. CDER. Approval Package for Application Number: NDA 20-896. Food and Drug Administration, Center for Drug Evaluation and Research, April 7, 1998.

Index